Comorbidity of Mood and Anxiety Disorders

Edited by

Jack D. Maser, Ph.D.
Mood, Anxiety, and Personality Disorders Research Branch,
National Institute of Mental Health,
Rockville, Maryland

and

C. Robert Cloninger, M.D.
Department of Psychiatry,
Washington University Medical Center,
St. Louis, Missouri

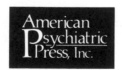

Washington, DC
London, England

Note: The authors have worked to ensure that all information in this book concerning drug dosages, schedules, and routes of administration is accurate as of the time of publication and consistent with standards set by the U.S. Food and Drug Administration and the general medical community. As medical research and practice advance, however, therapeutic standards may change. For this reason and because human and mechanical errors sometimes occur, we recommend that readers follow the advice of a physician who is directly involved in their care or the care of a member of their family.

Books published by the American Psychiatric Press, Inc., represent the views and opinions of the individual authors and do not necessarily represent the policies and opinions of the Press or the American Psychiatric Association.

The views expressed in this book are those of the authors only and do not necessarily represent the views of the National Institute of Mental Health.

American Psychiatric Press, Inc.
1400 K St., N.W., Washington, DC 20005

The paper used in this publication meets the minimum requirements of the American National Standard for Information Sciences—Permanence of Paper for Printed Library Materials ANSI Z39.48—1984.   ∞

Library of Congress Cataloging-in-Publication Data
Comorbidity of mood and anxiety disorders / edited by Jack D. Maser and
    C. Robert Cloninger.
        p.   cm.
    Includes bibliographical references.
    ISBN 0–88048–324–5 (alk. paper)
    1. Affective disorders—Complications and sequelae. 2. Anxiety.
I. Maser, Jack D.   II. Cloninger, C. Robert.
    [DNLM: 1. Affective Disorders—complications. 2. Anxiety
Disorders—complications.   WM 171 C735]
RC537.C643   1990
616.85'2—dc20
DNLM/DLC
for Library of Congress   89-17681
                                                                              CIP

British Cataloguing in Publication Data
A CIP record is available from the British Library

Contents

Section V   **Evidence for Comorbidity: Family and
               Genetic Studies**

Section VI   **Evidence for Comorbidity: Biologic Studies**

Section VII   ## Theories of and Perspectives on Anxiety and Depression

Contributors

Chul W. Ahn, Ph.D., Western Psychiatric Institute and Clinic, University of Pittsburgh, Pittsburgh, Pennsylvania

Hagop S. Akiskal, M.D., Department of Psychiatry, University of Tennessee, Memphis, Tennessee

Lauren B. Alloy, Ph.D., Department of Psychology, Temple University, Philadelphia, Pennsylvania

Jules Angst, M.D., Research Department, Psychiatric University Hospital, Zurich, Switzerland

David H. Barlow, Ph.D., Department of Psychology, State University of New York at Albany, Albany, New York

Sheri A. Berenbaum, Ph.D., Department of Psychology and Department of Psychiatry and Behavioral Sciences, University of Health Sciences/Chicago Medical School, North Chicago, Illinois

Donald W. Black, M.D., Department of Psychiatry, University of Iowa College of Medicine, Iowa City, Iowa

Roger K. Blashfield, Ph.D., Department of Psychiatry, University of Florida, Gainesville, Florida

Jack D. Burke, Jr., M.D., M.P.H., Division of Biometry and Applied Sciences, National Institute of Mental Health, Rockville, Maryland

Kimberly Christie Burke, M.S., Office of the Director, National Institute of Mental Health, Rockville, Maryland

Pamela D. Butler, Ph.D., Department of Psychiatry, Duke University Medical Center, Durham, North Carolina

Linda L. Carpenter, B.A., Western Psychiatric Institute and Clinic, University of Pittsburgh, Pittsburgh, Pennsylvania

Regina C. Casper, M.D., Department of Psychiatry, The University of Chicago and Michael Reese Hospital and Medical Center, Chicago, Illinois

Elsie Cheung, M.A., Department of Psychology, University of British Columbia, Vancouver, British Columbia, Canada

Paula J. Clayton, M.D., Department of Psychiatry, University of Minnesota Medical School, Minneapolis, Minnesota

Caroline M. Clements, M.S., Department of Psychology, Northwestern University, Evanston, Illinois

C. Robert Cloninger, M.D., Department of Psychiatry, The Jewish Hospital, Washington University Medical Center, St. Louis, Missouri

Marten W. de Vries, M.D., Social Psychiatry, University of Limburg, Maastricht, The Netherlands

Philippe A. E. G. Delespaul, Dr.S., Social Psychiatry, University of Limburg, Maastricht, The Netherlands

Chantal I. M. Dijkman-Caes, Dr.S., Social Psychiatry, University of Limburg, Maastricht, The Netherlands

Peter A. Di Nardo, Ph.D., Department of Psychology, State University of New York, College at Oneonta, Oneonta, New York

Keith S. Dobson, Ph.D., Department of Psychology, University of Calgary, Calgary, Alberta, Canada

Bruce P. Dohrenwend, Ph.D., New York State Psychiatric Institute, Columbia University, New York, New York

Jean Endicott, Ph.D., Research Assessment and Training Unit, New York State Psychiatric Institute, New York, New York

Cecile Ernst, M.D., Ph.D., Research Department, Psychiatric University Hospital, Zurich, Switzerland

Horacio Fabrega, Jr., M.D., Western Psychiatric Institute and Clinic, University of Pittsburgh, Pittsburgh, Pennsylvania

Michael B. First, M.D., Biometrics Research Department, New York State Psychiatric Institute, New York, New York

Allen Frances, M.D., Department of Psychiatry, Cornell University Medical College, New York, New York

Abby J. Fyer, M.D., New York State Psychiatric Institute, New York, New York

Minna R. Fyer, M.D., Department of Psychiatry, Cornell University Medical Center, New York, New York

Anne Gräsbeck, M.D., Department of Social and Forensic Psychiatry, University of Lund, Lund, Sweden

Samuel B. Guze, M.D., Department of Psychiatry, Washington University Medical Center, St. Louis, Missouri

Olle Hagnell, M.D., Department of Social and Forensic Psychiatry, University of Lund, Lund, Sweden

Debbie Hasin, Ph.D., College of Physicians and Surgeons of Columbia University, New York, New York

George R. Heninger, M.D., Department of Psychiatry, Yale University School of Medicine and Connecticut Mental Health Center, New Haven, Connecticut

Robert M. A. Hirschfeld, M.D., Mood, Anxiety, and Personality Disorders Research Branch, Division of Clinical Research, National Institute of Mental Health, Rockville, Maryland

Martin B. Keller, M.D., Department of Psychiatry, Brown University Medical School, Providence, Rhode Island

Robert Kellner, M.D., Ph.D., Department of Psychiatry, School of Medicine, University of New Mexico, Albuquerque, New Mexico

Kelly A. Kelly, M.S., Department of Psychology, Northwestern University, Evanston, Illinois

Kimberly Kerns, B.A., Department of Psychology, University of Health Sciences/Chicago Medical School, North Chicago, Illinois

Donald F. Klein, M.D., New York State Psychiatric Institute, New York, New York

Gerald L. Klerman, M.D., Department of Psychiatry, Cornell Medical Center, New York, New York

James H. Kocsis, M.D., Department of Psychiatry, Cornell University Medical College, New York, New York

Maria Kovacs, Ph.D., Western Psychiatric Institute and Clinic, University of Pittsburgh, Pittsburgh, Pennsylvania

Henry R. Kranzler, M.D., Alcohol Research Center, Department of Psychiatry, University of Connecticut School of Medicine, Farmington, Connecticut

David J. Kupfer, M.D., Department of Psychiatry, University of Pittsburgh School of Medicine, Western Psychiatric Institute and Clinic, Pittsburgh, Pennsylvania

Neil M. Kurtz, M.D., Central Nervous System Research, Bristol-Myers Pharmaceutical Research and Development Division, Wallingford, Connecticut

Philip W. Lavori, Ph.D., Massachusetts General Hospital, Harvard Medical School, Boston, Massachusetts

Michael R. Liebowitz, M.D., New York State Psychiatric Institute, New York, New York

John C. Markowitz, M.D., Department of Psychiatry, Cornell University Medical College, New York, New York

Ronald L. Martin, M.D., Department of Psychiatry, University of Kansas School of Medicine, Wichita, Kansas

Jack D. Maser, Ph.D., Mood, Anxiety, and Personality Disorders Research Branch, National Institute of Mental Health, Rockville, Maryland

Kathleen R. Merikangas, Ph.D., Genetic Epidemiology Research Unit, Department of Psychiatry and Epidemiology, Yale University School of Medicine, New Haven, Connecticut

Roger E. Meyer, M.D., Alcohol Research Center, Department of Psychiatry, University of Connecticut School of Medicine, Farmington, Connecticut

Juan E. Mezzich, M.D., Ph.D., Western Psychiatric Institute and Clinic, University of Pittsburgh, Pittsburgh, Pennsylvania

Susan Mineka, Ph.D., Department of Psychology, Northwestern University, Evanston, Illinois

Scott M. Monroe, Ph.D., Department of Psychology, University of Oregon, Eugene, Oregon

Jane M. Murphy, Ph.D., Department of Psychiatry, Harvard Medical School, Massachusetts General Hospital, Boston, Massachusetts

Charles B. Nemeroff, M.D., Ph.D., Departments of Psychiatry and Pharmacology, Duke University Medical Center, Durham, North Carolina

Russell Noyes, Jr., M.D., Department of Psychiatry, University of Iowa College of Medicine, Iowa City, Iowa

J. Christopher Perry, M.D., M.P.H., Department of Psychiatry, The Cambridge Hospital; Department of Psychiatry, Harvard Medical School, Cambridge, Massachusetts

Paul A. Pilkonis, Ph.D., Western Psychiatric Institute and Clinic, University of Pittsburgh, Pittsburgh, Pennsylvania

Russell E. Poland, M.D., Department of Psychiatry, Harbor-UCLA Medical Center, Torrance, California

Robert F. Prien, Ph.D., Mood, Anxiety, and Personality Disorders Research Branch, National Institute of Mental Health, Rockville, Maryland

Darrel A. Regier, M.D., M.P.H., Division of Clinical Research, National Institute of Mental Health, Rockville, Maryland

Lynn P. Rehm, Ph.D., Department of Psychology, University of Houston, Houston, Texas

Donald S. Robinson, M.D., Central Nervous System Research, Bristol-Myers Pharmaceutical Research and Development Division, Wallingford, Connecticut

Norman Sartorius, M.D., Ph.D., Division of Mental Health, World Health Organization, Geneva, Switzerland

Robert L. Spitzer, M.D., Biometrics Research Department, New York State Psychiatric Institute, New York, New York

Michael A. Taylor, M.D., Department of Psychology and Department of Psychiatry and Behavioral Sciences, University of Health Sciences/Chicago Medical School, North Chicago, Illinois

Svenn Torgersen, Ph.D., Center for Research in Clinical and Applied Psychology, Department of Psychology, University of Oslo, Oslo, Norway

Margarete Vollrath, Ph.D., Research Department, Psychiatric University Hospital, Zurich, Switzerland

Myrna M. Weissman, Ph.D., College of Physicians and Surgeons of Columbia University; Department of Clinical and Genetic Epidemiology, New York State Psychiatric Institute, New York, New York

Thomas Widiger, Ph.D., Department of Psychology, University of Kentucky, Lexington, Kentucky

Janet B. W. Williams, D.S.W., Biometrics Research Department, New York State Psychiatric Institute, New York, New York

Hans-Ulrich Wittchen, Ph.D., Dipl Psych, Max Planck Institut fur Psychiatrie Klinik, Munich, Federal Republic of Germany

Joanne Wunder, B.A., Harvard Medical School, Cambridge, Massachusetts

PREFACE

THE IDEA OF bringing together a group of clinical researchers to discuss and write on ideas related to anxiety, depression, and related disorders first arose in 1985. In that year *Anxiety and the Anxiety Disorders* (Tuma and Maser 1985) was published, and one lesson abstracted from its chapters was that the etiology and course of anxiety disorders could seldom be considered in isolation from a variety of other disorders, in particular affective or mood disorders. The present volume attempts to explore explicitly the diagnostic overlap and interaction of anxiety and mood disorders. As we quickly discovered, such an exploration could not proceed in isolation; it needed to include symptoms and at least three other types of syndromes—personality, somatoform, and substance abuse disorders.

The path to this book began—as did *Anxiety and the Anxiety Disorders*—with a conference at the Sterling Forest Conference Center in Tuxedo, New York. The timing seemed highly propitious because many of the participants in that meeting, when first contacted, said that they had been giving a lot of thought to comorbidity recently and either had just written or were thinking about writing a paper on the subject.

We made a conscious effort to select researchers from diverse backgrounds and to provide a strong emphasis on empirical findings about comorbidity and co-occurrence. Although the topic of the book focuses on anxiety and mood disorders, the viewpoint extends to other disorders. For example, the National Institute of Mental Health (NIMH) Epidemiologic Catchment Area Study revealed that schizophrenic subjects are 38 times more likely than normal subjects to have panic attacks. Does this observation raise questions about the symptoms used in the diagnosis of schizophrenia? Might it influence how the schizophrenic patient is treated? How does such information influence the nomenclature?

Although NIMH provided most of the financial support for the meeting at the Sterling Forest Conference Center, we are grateful to the Bristol-Myers Company, the Sandoz Pharmaceutical Corporation, and the Upjohn Company for contributions that allowed us to have so many distinguished clinical investigators from European countries. We thank also Dr. Darrel Regier, Director of the Division of Clinical Research, and Dr. Robert M. A. Hirschfeld, Chief of the Mood, Anxiety and Personality Disorders Research Branch, for their unwavering support of this effort. In the final stages of producing this book, Irma Maser was especially helpful in completing the Reference Section/Author Index and the Subject Index. We thank her for her effort.

Section I
Introduction

Chapter 1

Comorbidity of Anxiety and Mood Disorders: Introduction and Overview

Jack D. Maser, Ph.D.
C. Robert Cloninger, M.D.

PATIENTS WITH ANXIETY or mood disorders often have features of multiple mental disorders, but the extent and significance of this comorbidity has received surprisingly little attention in clinical practice or research in the past. However, the comorbidity of psychiatric disorders has emerged as a recent topic of major practical and theoretical significance. As more systematic attention has been devoted to psychiatric diagnosis in general, psychiatric comorbidity has commanded increasing consideration. The high frequency of multiple diagnoses has discredited the previously popular assumption that a particular patient is unlikely to have more than one disorder. Anyone interested in the assessment or treatment of psychopathology—that is, everyone in the mental health field must be concerned about psychiatric comorbidity.

This book brings together much of the recently acquired information about psychiatric comorbidity to present a systematic examination of the co-occurrence of different symptoms and syndromes in patients with disorders of anxiety or mood. The general topics of the comorbidity of syndromes and the co-occurrence of symptoms are examined at several levels: historical, descriptive, taxonomic, and etiologic. Empirical evidence is drawn from samples of the general

The opinions expressed in this chapter are those of the authors only and not necessarily those of the National Institute of Mental Health.

population and from treated cases. Theoretical implications are examined, and methodological recommendations are made for future research and clinical practice.

Comorbidity affects research and clinical practice pervasively as a result of its influence on diagnosis, prognosis, treatment, and health care delivery. Psychiatric comorbidity raises many fundamental questions about psychopathology and emerges as a test of our classification systems. Are psychiatric disorders truly discrete and independent disease entities? What does the co-occurrence of anxiety and depressive features imply about the discriminant validity of current diagnostic criteria, about course of illness, and about familial aggregation? How do genetic and environmental factors interact in the development of anxiety and mood disorders? How does comorbidity influence choice of treatment? In the final analysis, available data about psychiatric comorbidity require us to question the adequacy of many popular theoretical assumptions about psychopathology.

Unfortunately, official taxonomic systems, including both the *Diagnostic and Statistical Manual of Mental Disorders* (DSM-III-R) (American Psychiatric Association 1987) and the International Classification of Diseases (ICD) (World Health Organization 1978), do not address the many implications of comorbidity either for research or clinical practice. Clinicians soon appreciate that prototypical descriptions of patients with specific disorders are often extreme oversimplifications of the multifaceted clinical profile of patients who receive that diagnosis.

Nevertheless, the difficulties presented by psychiatric comorbidity do not imply that psychiatric diagnosis is invalid or useless. Rather, we must examine the pattern and structure of observed comorbidity to revise and improve existing methods of description and classification. Furthermore, the discriminant validity of our diagnostic criteria and the relationship of comorbidity to prognosis and treatment must undergo evaluation. In this book, the editors and contributors have tried to present available data about comorbidity to guide the efforts of clinicians working with patients who have anxiety and/or mood disorders.

Although anxiety and mood disorders are the major focus of interest here, they are considered in relation to all other forms of psychopathology. In particular, anxiety and mood disorders are considered in relation to one another and in relation to alcoholism, somatoform disorders, eating disorders, and personality disorders. For example, there are positive associations among the syndromes of anxiety, depression, and alcoholism in both the general population (Section III) and in samples of treated cases (Section IV). Accordingly, it is useful to examine the effect of comorbid anxiety and depressive disorders on longitudinal course (Sections III and IV), family history (Section V), neurobiology (Section VI), and treatment (Section VIII). Similarly, alcoholism is often comorbid with anxiety and mood disorders (Meyer and Kranzler, Chapter 17); comorbid alcoholism has a substantial effect on the clinical outcome of depressed patients (Hirschfeld, Hasin, Keller, et al., Chapter 18).

The frequent co-occurrence of symptoms of anxiety, depression, somatization, substance abuse, and eating dysfunction leads to many problems in the differential diagnosis of nonpsychotic disorders. Accordingly, chapters in this book examine clinical and longitudinal data about symptom overlap and discriminant validity of available scales and diagnostic criteria (Sections III and IV). Other chapters examine family studies (Section V), neurobiologic studies (Section VI), psychosocial studies (Section VII), and treatment studies (Section VIII) to evaluate possible causes of such comorbidity.

Finally, available data indicate that the observed pattern of psychiatric comorbidity is not random or artifactual (Section VII). Rather, certain symptoms and syndromes tend to occur together in the same individuals and families in particular patterns (Cloninger, Martin, Guze, et al., Chapter 27). For example, patients with chronic anxiety disorders tend to develop depressive syndromes after many years of disability; such secondary depressions in anxiety patients are much more frequent than are secondary anxiety disorders in patients with a history of remitted primary depression. In contrast, antisocial personality and somatization are positively associated with one another but are negatively associated with anxiety and depressive disorders.

In other words, psychopathology does not appear to be comprised of discrete, mutually exclusive disorders, as Kraepelin originally proposed. Although psychopathology involves a complex array of comorbid syndromes, this comorbidity has a stable structure. The possible etiologic basis of this stable structure is considered in this book from several perspectives, including genetic, neurobiologic, cognitive, and psychosocial theories (Section VII). We hope that such systematic examination of both empirical and theoretical information about psychiatric comorbidity will clarify our understanding of the significance of a crucial clinical phenomenon.

DEFINITIONS

Given the short history of the term *comorbidity*, there are a surprisingly large number of definitions. Feinstein (1970) coined the term *comorbidity* to mean "any distinct additional clinical entity that has existed or that may occur during the clinical course of a patient who has the index disease under study" (pp. 456–457). Strictly speaking, use of the term is restricted to diseases or disorders, not symptoms. Symptoms can associate or co-occur in a disorder, but they are not comorbid with disorders or with each other.

In psychiatric epidemiology, the term *comorbid* is used somewhat differently, the emphasis being on relative risk. When a patient has a particular index disorder, there may be a relatively greater or lesser risk of other disorders being diagnosed or other symptoms observed. For example, the likelihood (or, more strictly, the odds ratio) of a patient in a major depressive episode also having agoraphobia is more than 15 times greater than if that individual were not depressed (Boyd, Burke, Gruenberg, et al. 1984). The psychiatric epidemiologists in this book (Sections III and V) use the term *comorbidity* in this sense.

Clinical studies also use the concept of comorbidity in the sense that more than one disorder can be diagnosed in the same individual. In addition, an individual who meets the full diagnostic criteria for only one disorder may still have an increased frequency of symptoms from other categories, but to an extent that is insufficient to diagnose another disorder. Diagnostic studies may identify symptoms or relationships between syndromes that improve diagnostic precision by increasing the discriminant power of diagnostic criteria. For example, Roth and Mountjoy (1982) wrote of being able to differentiate anxious patients from depressed patients on the basis of an increased incidence of personality disorder in the anxious patients.

Kaplan and Feinstein (1974) introduced a number of distinctions about types of comorbidity that may help to clarify the concepts of comorbidity that arise in medicine in general and, possibly, in psychiatry. They distinguished between pathogenic, diagnostic, and prognostic comorbidity. *Pathogenic comorbidity* arises when a particular disease leads to certain other complications or diseases, which are therefore considered to be etiologically related. Kaplan and Feinstein gave the example of cardiovascular and renal system diseases, which are often pathogenically related to diabetes. In psychiatry, comparable examples of pathogenicity may be the development of agoraphobia secondary to recurrent panic attacks, the development of depression secondary to disability from a chronic disorder such as schizophrenia, or the development of chronic alcohol abuse as a result of repeated use of alcohol for acute relief of dysphoric mood.

For an example of two diseases that are *diagnostically comorbid*, Kaplan and Feinstein (1974) cited a patient with polyuria, which is caused by diabetes and a coexisting renal ailment. Similarly, a psychiatric patient may exhibit diminished ability to concentrate because of both depression and generalized anxiety disorder, or a patient may exhibit weight loss because of both depression and an eating disorder (see Casper, Chapter 15). Diagnostic comorbidity is likely whenever diagnostic criteria are based on patterns of symptoms that are individually nonspecific.

Disorders that predispose the patient to develop other disorders have *prognostic comorbidity*. Kaplan and Feinstein's (1974) example is the development of retinopathy in a patient with both diabetes and hypertension. The combination of diabetes and hypertension is much more likely to produce retinopathy than the effects of either disorder alone. A comparable example in psychiatry may be the possible increase in risk for alcoholism in a patient who has both panic and depressive disorders. The combination of the two disorders is more likely to precipitate alcoholism than either disorder alone.

It is often difficult to distinguish these subtypes of comorbidity, however, unless the pathogenesis of the disorders is well understood. Is a depressive disorder that occurs after many years of generalized anxiety disorder an example of pathogenic, diagnostic, or prognostic comorbidity? Accordingly, until there is a much more complete understanding of the pathogenesis of psychiatric disorders, Kaplan and Feinstein's (1974) distinctions are largely of heuristic value.

Recently clinicians and researchers have begun to use the term *comorbidity* to include the co-occurrence of symptoms as well as co-occurrence of disorders. We believe that there is value in reserving the term *comorbidity* to indicate co-occurrence of syndromes or disorders, rather than individual symptoms. Morbidity refers to a state of being diseased, and symptoms indicate that the disease is present. Therefore, one cannot have comorbidity among symptoms, but symptoms can co-occur or be associated features.

NOSOLOGY AND COMORBIDITY

Comorbidity has important implications for the classification of psychiatric disorders that are not adequately addressed by current official taxonomic systems. The DSM-III-R specifies a set of decision rules for differential diagnosis of psychiatric disorders. These decision rules include explicit inclusion and exclusion criteria about the number and type of symptoms present, as well as some criteria about age of onset and duration of the symptoms, and extent and type of disability or distress. General principles of taxonomy and the artifactual effects of classification methods for comorbidity are considered in detail in Section II of this book. Here we will emphasize some basic issues that recur frequently.

There are no individual signs or symptoms in psychiatry that are pathognomonic for a particular disease. That is, no one feature is necessary and sufficient to define a psychiatric disorder. Accordingly, diagnostic criteria are based on the natural history of a disorder, which is defined in terms of the type, number, sequence of onset, and duration of multiple nonspecific signs and symptoms. Symptoms may differ in their importance for a particular diagnosis. For example, the diagnosis of generalized anxiety disorder in DSM-III-R requires evidence of apprehensive expectation (criterion A), but any 6 of 18 other anxiety symptoms (criterion D) are also necessary. As a consequence, patients with the same diagnosis may vary widely in their clinical picture and criterion A alone seems more important than the others. Furthermore, they may differ in the extent to which they have other prominent features that are not part of the defining characteristics of the diagnosis.

Diagnostic criteria in psychiatry can be validated by means of clinical, descriptive, longitudinal, family, and laboratory studies (Feighner, Robins, Guze, et al. 1972; Robins and Guze 1970). If several symptoms tend to occur together, a syndrome is defined by the presence of that set of co-occurring symptoms. If that syndrome has a predictable clinical course, pattern of familial aggregation, and characteristic external correlates, then the diagnosis of a disorder may be considered valid. The characteristic external correlates may include any objective and reliable findings, such as neuropsychological, cognitive, or neurochemical test results. Much of the resurgence of interest in psychiatric diagnosis was stimulated when psychiatrists at Washington University in St. Louis published a set of inclusion and exclusion criteria that were reliable and validated by follow-up and family studies of psychiatric disorders (Feighner, Robins, Guze, et al. 1972). These validated criteria were able to assign a single diagnosis to about 80% of all psychiatric cases.

Unfortunately, when the Washington University criteria were expanded in DSM-III (American Psychiatric Association 1980) and DSM-III-R to provide criteria for all kinds of psychopathology, inclusion and exclusion criteria had to be added for which there was little or no evidence of validity. DSM-III-R makes "no assumption that each mental disorder is a discrete entity with sharp boundaries (discontinuity) between it and other mental disorders, or between it and no mental disorder" (p. xxii).

Accordingly, there was minimal effort to avoid multiple diagnoses, and the amount of comorbidity observed increased markedly for several reasons. First, the number of possible diagnoses ("coverage") increased substantially. Second, some of the diagnostic features were shared by multiple disorders (e.g., dysthymic disorder and major depressive disorder, or somatization disorder and generalized anxiety disorder). Third, clinicians were instructed to use each of five axes, thereby providing the possibility of comorbidity between many psychiatric syndromes on Axis I, personality disorders on Axis II, and other medical disorders on Axis III.

However, some efforts to avoid artifactual comorbidity were made following some reasonable principles in DSM-III and DSM-III-R. Whenever possible, symptoms were not included in diagnostic criteria if they were redundant with other diagnoses, even if they were commonly associated features. For example, depressive and panic symptoms are frequent in somatization disorder, but were omitted from the diagnostic criteria in DSM-III and DSM-III-R because they were not necessary and they overlapped with mood and anxiety disorders. Furthermore, there is no excess of depressive or panic disorders in the family members of patients with somatization disorder.

In DSM-III-R, certain diagnoses were excluded if a more pervasive disorder nearly always includes a more restricted syndrome. For example, conversion and hypochondriacal symptoms are consistent features of somatization disorder, so little information about a patient with somatization disorder is gained by adding symptoms of conversion disorder or hypochondriasis. Likewise, insomnia in a patient with a major depressive disorder does not justify a diagnosis of sleep disorder because insomnia is part of the more pervasive syndrome of major depression. Accordingly, reports of comorbidity that ignore exclusion rules such as these (which have been validated by follow-up and family studies), as well as their logical appeal to parsimony and efficiency of expression, would overestimate psychiatric comorbidity.

Nevertheless, even when artifactual overlap and redundancy are excluded, studies using both DSM-III and the more restricted research diagnostic criteria reveal extensive psychiatric comorbidity. If a patient is simply described as satisfying the inclusion criteria for a single diagnosis (e.g., major depressive disorder), it may be impossible to replicate results in another sample of patients who satisfy the same inclusion criteria but who differ in associated characteristics, such as personality, anxiety, or substance abuse. This condition greatly limits the growth of knowledge about psychopathology (Winokur, Zimmerman, and Cadoret 1988).

Furthermore, adequate description and classification must pay attention to the temporal sequence and course of illness. Some critics of psychiatric diagnosis have advocated abandonment of categorical diagnoses in favor of multidimensional symptom profiles. An equivalent suggestion is to eliminate all exclusion rules, regardless of their validation by follow-up and family studies or other evidence of discriminant validity. However, patients with distinct diagnoses that have been validated by follow-up, family, and treatment studies may have the same cross-sectional clinical features. For example, a patient with the first onset of panic attacks in the course of an adult-onset depression should not be classified together with a patient with a lifelong panic disorder complicated by a secondary depression. Cloninger, Martin, Guze, et al. (Chapter 27) note the importance of distinguishing among depressed patients who differ in comorbid diagnoses: the genetic epidemiology, course, and treatment of individuals with major depressive disorders depend greatly on the onset of the first (primary) disorder that affects a patient.

EPIDEMIOLOGY AND FAMILY STUDIES

Epidemiologic studies of anxiety and mood disorders have revealed several robust findings. First, the risk of depression in individuals with chronic anxiety disorders is greater than the risk of anxiety in individuals with depressive disorders (Sections III and IV). This asymmetrical comorbidity pattern arises even when no hierarchical exclusion rules are employed; the DSM-III hierarchy, in which mood disorders take precedence over anxiety disorders, actually reflect empirical patterns. Also, longitudinal studies show that depressive disorders are more likely to remain stably free of comorbid anxiety than are anxiety disorders which more often are complicated by depression after long-term follow-up (Angst, Vollrath, Merikangas, et al., Chapter 7; Cloninger, Martin, Guze, et al., Chapter 27). Furthermore, the family studies presented in Sections V and VII suggest that mixed anxiety-depressive states are genetically heterogeneous.

Together these findings suggest that mixed anxiety-depressive states are heterogeneous mixtures of primary anxiety disorders (with secondary depressions) and primary depressive disorders (with coincident anxiety symptoms). Cloninger, Martin, Guze, et al. (Chapter 27) discuss possible alternative interpretations of available data in detail in Section VII.

Most important, available epidemiologic and family study findings clearly indicate that much prior work has not adequately accounted for the temporal sequence of symptom onset and offset or for concomitant variation in personality, somatization, and substance abuse. As a result, it is often difficult to classify subjects with mixed anxiety and depression, or to accept the diagnoses advocated by earlier investigators. Simple elimination of hierarchical exclusion rules is sometimes advocated as a way of preserving more complete diagnostic information, but may actually sacrifice critical information about temporal sequence that increases discriminant validity, as exemplified by the Washington University research diagnostic criteria (Feighner, Robins, Guze, et al. 1972; Martin, Cloninger, Guze, et al. 1985). Further advances in understanding psychiatric comorbidity will require research that fully characterizes symptom onset and offset for the full range of psychopathology, as discussed in more detail in Sections VII and VIII.

Possible Causes of Comorbidity

Despite extensive efforts, there are no known biologic markers that are highly specific for a particular psychiatric disorder. This fact is not surprising in view of all the clinical and epidemiologic evidence of psychiatric comorbidity, which would be hard to reconcile with highly specific biologic or genetic findings. Rather, it appears more productive to try to characterize the complex sets of brain systems that interact in the development of a spectrum of comorbid disorders. Several neuropsychopharmacologic findings suggest the possibility of some common mechanisms in anxiety and mood disorders (Sections VI and VIII).

Likewise, several psychosocial theories have been advanced to account for observed patterns of psychiatric comorbidity (Section VII); these include psychodynamic, sociocultural, cognitive, behavioral, and neuropsychological theories. Each of these suggest fruitful areas for future research and method development. Since the facts that the theories must explain remain in some doubt because of the limitations of past research, it is premature to try to choose definitively among alternative theories. Nevertheless, it is clear that the classic Kraepelinian model in which all psychopathology is comprised of discrete and mutually exclusive diseases must be rejected or modified.

Importance of Comorbidity in Clinical Practice

Comorbidity is clearly important in patient management and treatment. Feinstein (1970) noted that researchers try to exclude patients with associated diseases from therapeutic trials for a given disease. However, findings in such presumably homogeneous samples may not apply to routine clinical practice. For example, the efficacy of antidepressant treatment of obsessive-compulsive patients depends on depressive comorbidity. Foa, Steketee, Kozak, et al. (1987) found that imipramine had little benefit for obsessive patients who were not also depressed, but was beneficial in depressed obsessive patients. In addition, psychiatric comorbidity has a major impact on the prognosis of medical and surgical patients. In a study of a large series of medical and surgical patients, those with psychiatric comorbidity had longer hospital stays than other patients (Fulop, Strain, Vita, et al. 1987). Akiskal (Chapter 33) provides practical advice for the clinician to approach the difficult problems posed by comorbidity for diagnosis and treatment planning. Robinson and Kurtz (Chapter 39) point out analogous problems faced in pharmaceutical drug development when unvalidated categorical diagnoses that neglect comorbidity become reified by government agencies.

OVERVIEW AND SUMMARY

Although interest in psychiatric comorbidity is only recent, available data have accumulated to indicate that anxiety and depressive disorders often occur together with one another or with other psychiatric disorders (including personality, somatoform, and substance abuse disorders) and with other medical disorders. Furthermore, this comorbidity has a stable structure in that particular sets of disorders are positively associated with one another (e.g., anxiety and depressive disorders) and negatively associated with other disorders (e.g., antisocial personality and anxiety disorders).

Future assessment must focus attention on lifetime chronology of symptom onset and offset. Also future assessment methods would be improved by more comprehensive attention to the full range of psychopathology, including inclusion and exclusion criteria that take into account disorders that are frequently comorbid with anxiety and depression (e.g., somatization, substance abuse, and eating disorders).

It is clear that the classic Kraepelinian model in which all psychopathology is comprised of discrete and mutually exclusive diseases must be rejected or modified. However, as discussed in more detail in Section VII, this does not mean that diagnostic exclusion rules should be indiscriminately ignored. Neither does it mean that the many unvalidated exclusion rules of DSM-III or DSM-III-R should be reified. Despite their limitations, DSM-III and DSM-III-R have greatly stimulated the advance of interest and knowledge about psychiatric comorbidity, which ultimately should lead to a sounder understanding of the nature of psychopathology and improved clinical management.

Chapter 2

Approaches to the Phenomena of Comorbidity

Gerald L. Klerman, M.D.

THIS BOOK REFLECTS a growing interest in the phenomenon of comorbidity. The term refers to the joint occurrence of two or more mental disorders occurring with each other and/or with medical conditions. The concept originated in general medicine and is increasingly being applied in psychiatry. Comorbidity can occur within an episode of illness for an individual and/or within the lifetime of an individual, and among patients, the general population, and families. Interest in comorbidity is relatively new. The term itself did not enter psychiatric discourse until less than a decade ago, although it has a longer history of use in medical epidemiology and biomedical research.

This chapter will examine the topic of comorbidity within the larger context of recent trends in psychopathology and mental health research. My thesis is that interest in comorbidity is a consequence of the recent paradigm shift in psychopathology. A "neo-Kraepelinian" paradigm has become dominant in research centers concerned with psychopathology, diagnosis, and nosology. The major features of the neo-Kraepelinian paradigm are shown in Table 1. The neo-Kraepelinian model includes the concept of multiple, discrete mental disorders and the use of operational criteria. Structured interviews and diagnostic algorithms derive from these premises, allowing for reliable assessment of psychopathology. This paradigm shift has had a significant impact on research in psychopathology as well as in epidemiol-

Supported in part by grants U-01-MH-43077 and R-01-MH-43044 from the National Institute of Mental Health; Alcohol, Drug Abuse, and Mental Health Administration; Public Health Service, Department of Health and Human Services, Washington, DC.

Table 1.   The Neo-Kraepelinian Paradigm

Multiple, discrete mental disorders
Operational criteria
Structured interviews (PSE, SADS, DIS)
Diagnostic algorithms (RDC, DSM-III)
Reliability (kappa statistics)
Validity (internal/external)

Note.   PSE = Present State Examination; SADS = Schedule for Affective Disorders and Schizophrenia; DIS = Diagnostic Interview Schedule; RDC = Research Diagnostic Criteria.

ogy, therapeutics, nosology, and clinical investigations.

The new paradigm arose in the United Kingdom and in North America during the period after World War II. It was a reaffirmation, as well as a modification, of the 19th century continental European approach to psychiatry, often called the "medical model." The culmination of the paradigm shift occurred with the publication in 1980 of the third edition of the *Diagnostic and Statistical Manual of Mental Disorders* (DSM-III) (American Psychiatric Association 1980). Subsequently, there was a wide application of DSM-III criteria in clinical practice and research activities.

I will review the historical changes leading to this paradigm shift and discuss a number of current approaches to the comorbidity phenomenon, including those approaches that accept the neo-Kraepelinian paradigm and some that do not.

THE HISTORICAL CONTEXT

To understand the recent scientific changes that have led to the current interest in the phenomenon of comorbidity, I have made use of the terms *paradigm* and *paradigm shift*. These concepts derive from the views of Thomas Kuhn (1970) and his theory of scientific progress. At this point, it is worthwhile to summarize briefly Kuhn's theory and its application to research in psychopathology.

Kuhn's Theory of Scientific Progress

The views of Thomas Kuhn (1962) on the nature of change and progress in science appear particularly appropriate to the current American mental health research scene. Kuhn proposed that the history of a scientific field is punctuated by "revolutions," the essence of a scientific revolution being the emergence of a new paradigm that produces a significant restructuring of the ways in which the scientific field defines its problems. Kuhn (1970) described a paradigm as having two components: cognitive and communal. The *cognitive* component refers to the theories, hypotheses, and ideas by which a scientific field is delineated, and the rules employed to conduct research and evaluate evidence. The *communal* component refers to the collectivity of scientists who share the ideas and values and acknowledge the validity of a particular form of scientific "truth."

Kuhn's theory has been the subject of much controversy. It has been criticized for using the physical sciences as the standard for evaluating other sciences, for too closely identifying subject matters with scientific communities, and for overstating the allegiances of individual scientists to specific paradigms. Nonetheless, Kuhn's ideas provide a broad framework for understanding change within a scientific field—particularly one as diverse as psychiatry and mental health, where no unifying paradigm is, as yet, accepted by the whole field.

Origin of Scientific Interest in Psychopathology

Anthropologists, historians, and investigators of cross-cultural psychopathology have observed that every society has its own view of health and illness and its own classification of diseases. Some of these views are consistent with those that have emerged in Western scientific medicine; others are culturally unique (Good and Kleinman 1985).

Although descriptions of many symptoms and illnesses appear in ancient Egyptian, Greek, and Roman texts (particularly those codified by Hippocrates), modern concepts of medical disease and nosology emerged in Western Europe in the late 18th century, influenced by the period of Enlightenment. The development of general scientific thinking and experimental investigation contributed to the concept of multiple illnesses, each with its own signs, symptoms, and natural course outcome and prognosis. This concept was most clearly enunciated in England by Thomas Sydenham, who had been called the father of modern medical nosology.

In the 19th century, these general views of illness were afforded scientific support and intellectual and societal acceptance by discoveries in the biologic sciences. Four discoveries were particularly noteworthy. First was the correlation of clinical syndromes with morphological changes noted at autopsy, by either morbid anatomy or histopathology. Pathology emerged as a basic medical science in France, Germany, and Austria in the mid-19th century, and its rationale was codified in the writings of Virchow.

Second, the discoveries of Pasteur, Koch, and others resulted in delineation of many clinical disorders associated with specific bacteria or other microorganisms. The spectacular success in control of many infectious diseases by treatment with antibiotics or their prevention by sanitary measures or immunization offered the most powerful validation of the concept of discrete disorders.

Third, toward the end of the 19th century, advances in diagnostic radiology followed the discovery of X-rays and contributed to improved clinical assessment.

Fourth, biochemical tests, such as the determination of serum glucose, provided independent assessment of pathologic processes in the living organism that could be correlated with clinical signs and symptoms and surgical or autopsy findings.

The Medical Model Paradigm: Hierarchical Classification of Psychopathologic Conditions

These advances in biology gave medicine a scientific basis and were applied to understanding lunacy, insanity, folie, and other mental conditions. Attempts were made to correlate mental syndromes with autopsy and bacteriologic findings, particularly in France, Germany, and Austria, in the second half of the 19th century.

There were many notable successes from these searches for biologic causes of specific mental conditions, three of which are worthy of attention.

Syphilis. By 1895, clinical and epidemiologic studies had shown that infection with syphilis was associated with the syndrome of general paresis. This association was confirmed by the development of the Wasserman Test in 1905, and the isolation of the spirochete in the brain by Noguchi in 1911. Soon afterward, therapeutic efforts involved the use of mercurial compounds, fever therapy, and ultimately, treatment with penicillin in the 1940s.

Pellagra. After World War I, Goldberger and his associates in the U.S Public Health Service discovered the relationship between pellagra and vitamin B deficiency. In addition to elucidating the biologic basis of this disorder, the discovery paved the way for effective treatment and, ultimately, the prevention of pellagra.

Senile dementia. The anatomic basis of one form of senile dementia was demonstrated by the studies of Alzheimer in Munich, who identified the characteristic tangle and plaques in brains at autopsy. Recently, the techniques of molecular biology have been applied to this disorder, and chromosomal location of a putative gene has been identified.

From the 1920s through the early 1950s, there were relatively few discoveries of biologic correlates of the functional psychoses, particularly schizophrenia and manic-depressive illness. At the same time, however, psychiatry and psychology extended their activities into other disorders of psychopathology, including neuroses and personality disorder, where biologic approaches appeared less relevant. Biologic approaches fell into disrepute, contributing to an erosion of confidence in the medical model in general and the concept of multiple discrete mental disorders in particular.

This situation was not true for the field of mental retardation. The discovery of forms of chromosomal anomalies led to the understanding of Down's syndrome and other retarded states. Advances in biochemistry resulted in the discovery of multiple forms of aminoacidurias and other "inborn errors of metabolism," further contributing to the elucidation of multiple causes of mental retardation.

The medical model paradigm, which was widely accepted between World War I and World War II, is depicted in Table 2. Individual mental disorders were grouped into larger classes—organic, psychotic, neurotic—and these classes were ordered in a hierarchy. This hierarchy was seldom stated explicitly, but was evident in the organization of almost all textbooks in psychiatry and the official diagnostic systems, particularly the International Classification of Diseases (ICD), ninth revision (World Health Organization 1977); the DSM-I

Table 2. Medical Model Hierarchical Classification

Organic mental disorders
  Trauma
  Infection (AIDS)
  Degenerative diseases (Alzheimer's)

Psychoses
  Schizophrenia (dementia praecox)
  Manic-depressive insanity

Neuroses
  Anxiety neuroses
  Obsessive-compulsive
  Phobia
  Hysteria

Personality disorders
  Psychopathic personality
  Cyclothymic personality

Transient/reactive states
  War neuroses
  Traumatic states

and DSM-II (American Psychiatric Association 1952, 1968); and the Veterans Administration.

The order in which the various classes of disorders are presented represents hierarchies reflective of value judgments and principles of classification. First, Spitzer, and Williams (Chapter 5) discuss hierarchies in some detail. Next is the principle of causation—causation being the highest standard of classification in modern medicine. By this criteria, the organic mental disorders come first in any classification of mental conditions. Organic disorders are due to diseases of the central nervous system, diseases where brain pathology has been demonstrated by methods of autopsy, histopathology, or experimental induction. Some examples are mental disorders due to hereditary causes (Huntington's disease); infectious disorders, trauma, and degenerative diseases of the brain (parkinsonism, Alzheimer's disease); and alcohol and drugs.

Organic conditions are usually, but not always, manifested clinically by the syndromes of delirium or dementia. Where evidence for one of these organic disorders exists, it takes precedence over all other diagnoses, according to this hierarchical principle.

The Nonorganic (or Functional) Disorders

Having defined a group of organic conditions, the remaining conditions were often called nonorganic or functional. There was, and continues to be, much ambiguity in the use of the term *functional*. Originally, it referred to biologic changes in the central nervous system that were not apparent by the usual histopathologic means. Hence the impairment was in the functioning, rather than in the structure of the nervous system. Later, the term became synonymous with environmental, or nonbiologic, causes.

As a further classification principle, the functional disorders have usually been subdivided according to the psychotic-neurotic distinction. The criteria for the distinction between psychotic and neurotic states were crystalized at the turn of the century in the writings of Freud and Kraepelin. Freud, in particular, wrote a series of influential papers correlating differences between neurotic and psychotic states according to type of symptoms, degree of social impairment, and, from the psychodynamic point of view, level of regression and extent of the loss of secondary process and manifestation of primary process thinking.

The psychotic-neurotic distinction had considerable appeal because it seemed to combine five aspects of psychopathology simultaneously: (1) descriptive symptoms, (2) presumed causation, (3) psychodynamics, (4) justification for hospitalization, and (5) treatment recommendation (Table 3).

The psychotic disorders had in common: impairment of higher mental faculties, as manifested by delusions, hallucinations, disorientation, and impairments of perception, memory, and thought. It was presumed they were due to constitutional (i.e., biologic) causes—hereditary, biochemical, or physiologic—and provided justification for hospitalization. Where treatments were available, these would usually be somatic (biologic) treatments, such as lobotomy, insulin coma treatment, electroconvulsive therapy (ECT), and the psychopharmacologic agents, which became available in the 1950s.

In contrast, the neurotic conditions were characterized descriptively by the absence of impairment of higher mental faculties and by the patient's subjective experience of distress, which often provided the impetus to seek medical care. It was generally agreed that the neurotic conditions were due to learning experiences—the two dominant etiologic theories being learning theory and psychodynamics. Moreover, treatment seldom required hospitalization, but rather some form of psychotherapy (i.e., individual, group, family) based on behavioral, psychodynamic, or interpersonal principles.

The Nosologic Status of Other Disorders: Personality Disorders and Reactive States

As psychiatry expanded, the field became increasingly concerned with other disorders, such as personality disorders and various types of stress response and adjustment reactions. These forms of pathologic behavior were usually considered low on the hierarchy and

Table 3. The Psychotic-Neurotic Distinction in Classification of Functional Disorders

	Psychoses	Neuroses
Description	Impaired higher mental faculties	Reality-testing intact
Causation	Organic	Environmental
Psychodynamic	Severe regression to one process	Ego functions intact
Hospitalization	Often	Seldom
Treatment	Somatic therapy (ECT, lobotomy)	Psychotherapy

Note. ECT = electroconvulsive therapy.

considerable debate was often generated as to the legitimacy of their status as psychopathology. Often they were considered on the boundary between normal adjustment problems and psychopathology. In this controversy, there was a mixture of scientific and social policy issues. Scientifically, there was disagreement over the descriptive features of personality disorders and reactive states and over the criteria to be employed in their diagnoses. Socially, there was disagreement over the legitimacy of these conditions as falling within the province of medicine and psychiatry. Many critics argued that these were essentially "problems of living" and of social adjustment and should not be considered pathology and medical concepts. Consequently, they appeared last in classifications and at the end of textbooks, reflecting their lower status in the classification hierarchy.

Challenges to the Medical Model Paradigm

The medical model came under considerable criticism both in and out of the psychiatric profession. Six lines of criticism were debated during the 1960s and 1970s.

The most fundamental criticism was the challenge to the legitimacy of mental illness as a concept and to psychiatry as part of medicine. Led by Szasz (1961), the antipsychiatrists and the antilabeling theorists in sociology and psychology denied the basic premise that mental disorders such as psychoses, neuroses, and personality disorders are true "illnesses." In the absence of anatomic or physiologic evidence of some biologic abnormality, the application of the concept of illness to behavioral, emotional, and cognitive states served society's need for control of deviance rather than the needs of individual patients.

The second line of criticism pointed to the adverse social and psychological consequences of psychiatric diagnosis. This view was expressed forcefully by Karl Menninger (1963) in his influential book *The Vital Balance* in which he drew attention to the dehumanizing and depersonalizing manner in which psychiatric diagnoses were often employed. This unfortunate consequence of diagnostic practice was expanded on by a group of sociologists who came to be referred to as "labeling theorists"—in particular Scheff and Lemere—who saw diagnosis labeling as part of the social control function of psychiatry. Many labeling theorists went even further, denying the existence of any intrinsic differences between those people who later came to be "labeled" mentally ill and those people with other forms of deviance. The most dramatic effort to document this view was reported by Rosenhan (1973) in his widely cited article: "On Being Sane in Insane Places."

The third line of criticism came from mental health professionals in developing countries and from cultural anthropologists who criticized the medical model's diagnostic system as being rooted in Western European culture and not relevant to, or valid in, other cultures. Anthropological investigations described cultures that had different concepts of medical illness and presented criteria for abnormality that varied both from culture to culture and with historical change. Cultural relativism served to undermine the universality of any diagnostic system.

The fourth line of criticism came from social critics such as Illich (1976) who cited the growing scope of mental illness to include adjustment reactions, stress reactions, and transient states related to life events. It was argued that this extension of the medical model into problems of living and social adjustment was promoting dependency and extending the expertise of medical and mental health professionals beyond their proper role. Rather than these conditions being seen as issues of psychopathology, Illich felt they should be seen as social and personal problems.

The fifth line of criticism focused on the low reliability of psychiatric diagnosis made by clinicians and researchers. The absence of agreement on diagnoses among clinicians, especially in dramatic court cases, undermined the credibility of the mental health profession.

The sixth line of criticism came from within the research community, mainly from psychologists and statisticians experienced in multivariate statistical techniques. These critics did not challenge the existence of mental illness or the legitimacy of research in psychopathology, but they did question the categorical or typological nature of the medically dominated diagnostic systems. They pointed out there are indistinct boundaries between the normal and the abnormal, and that many of the phenomena seen in clinical states are quantitative extensions of normal phenomena, such as anxiety and depression. This group advocated the use of dimensional approaches to classify mental disorders.

This older paradigm was often called the *medical model*, a term that was widely used through the 1950s and 1960s. Discussion of the scientific issues of this model is difficult because of the confounding of scientific problems with professional tensions and ideological controversies. In the period after World War II, the medical model came into dispute. The medical model paradigm, which postulated multiple disorders and the search for predominantly biologic causes, had arisen within 19th-century medicine. The social sciences became increasingly involved in psychiatric research during and after World War II. Moreover, with the rapid growth of other mental health professions (clinical psychologists, psychiatric social workers, psychiatric nurses), interprofessional rivalries occurred, and issues of diagnosis and psychopathology came to be associated with the struggles of the newer professional groups for autonomy, prestige, funds, and client referrals.

The medical model and hierarchical approaches to classification began to break down during World War II. Many psychiatrists came to question the concept of separate mental disorders. The strong psychotherapeutic orientation led to attempts to treat even the psychoses, such as schizophrenia, with intensive individual and family psychotherapy. Moreover, research on life events and stress, initiated during World War II, and epidemiologic research on social class questioned the constitutional basis of the psychoses.

Dimensional approaches to personality assessment were the most popular. Psychiatric epidemiology and community surveys (e.g., the Midtown Manhattan study [Srole and Fisher 1980]) did not attempt to estimate the rates of specific disorders, such as depression or schizophrenia, but instead judged degrees of mental impairment. Sociological forces, particularly the stress of living, were emphasized as the major causative factors. In clinical practice, attention to psychopathology and diagnosis was considered irrelevant for decision making and treatment planning, particularly if the mode of treatment was dynamic psychotherapy.

Revival of Interest in Diagnosis and Classification

Confronted by these challenges, groups within the research community responded vigorously. By the late 1960s there was a growing awareness among clinicians and researchers that one reason for the limited progress in the description of psychopathology and diagnosis was the absence of an objective and reliable system. In 1965 the National Institute of Mental Health (NIMH) Psychopharmacology Research Branch sponsored a conference on classification in psychiatry, noting the problems created by inadequate knowledge of diagnosis and classification (Katz, Cole, and Barton 1968).

In the 1970s, commenting on the long period of neglect of diagnosis, nosology, and classification in North American psychiatry, Lehmann (1970), predicted a renaissance of interest. His words were prophetic: within a few years the Washington University criteria for operational diagnosis were published. The Schedule for Affective Disorders and Schizophrenia (SADS) (Endicott and Spitzer 1978) and Research Diagnostic Criteria (RDC) (Spitzer, Endicott, and Robins 1978a) were then developed by the NIMH Collaborative Program on Psychobiology of Depression.

Biologic treatments, notably psychopharmacologic drugs, were shown to be useful, not only in psychotic states such as mania, paranoia, and schizophrenia, but also for obsessive-compulsive states, phobias, and anxiety disorders. Findings from these therapeutic studies, in addition to family aggregation studies and pathophysiology research, suggest biologic bases for many of the neurotic conditions and for some of the personality disorders.

A number of other factors contributed to the interest in diagnosis and classification: (1) the advance of new psychosocial therapeutic modalities, especially new behavioral and brief psychotherapeutic methods; (2) the availability of high-speed electronic computers allowing the management of large-scale data sets and the application of multivariate statistics; and (3) the use of rating scales and other psychometric techniques for quantitative assessment of symptoms, behavior, and personality.

The Neo-Kraepelinian Paradigm

By themselves, however, these factors could not have constituted a paradigm shift. They created the climate for change, but did not define the nature of the change. That was to be the role of the neo-Kraepelinians.

At this point it is useful to return to Kuhn's (1962, 1970) theory of scientific progress. To recapitulate: Kuhn proposed that scientific progress occurs when a new paradigm emerges to resolve an impasse or to solve a crisis. A crisis had occurred in psychopathology after World War II. The new paradigm that emerged in the early 1970s involved the reaffirmation of the concept of multiple discrete disorders and the use of operational criteria for making diagnostic judgments of a categorical (i.e., typological) nature.

A large number of reliable and valid scales were developed in the late 1950s and 1960s, first, for psychotic patients and then for depressed and anxious patients. Beck (1967), Hamilton (1960), Lorr, McNair, Klett, et al. (1962), and Zung (1965) were leaders in these developments. In this effort there was active interchange among psychiatrists, clinical psychologists, psychopathologists, and psychopharmacologists. They were able to draw on the extensive knowledge in psychometrics, initially developed in the assessment of intelligence and other areas of educational and social performance.

By the late 1960s, considerable difficulty in clinical research was encountered because of the lack of reliable, valid, and standardized techniques for individual patient diagnosis required for the selection of samples for research and treatment studies. Psychiatrists and other clinicians had been relying heavily on categorical (typological), nosologic approaches in contrast to the dimensional methods employed in rating scales and personality inventories. There was considerable dissatisfaction with the unreliability of existing diagnostic practices, both in clinic and research settings. In addition to the scientific issues, considerable social and political criticism was expressed in the many lawsuits brought by civil rights advocates, by the continuing criticisms of Szasz and other antipsychiatrists, and by the antilabeling positions taken in sociology and social psychology.

The development of a new paradigm helped to resolve the "crisis" in Kuhn's sense. The operational criteria formulated by the Washington University group, codified by Feighner, Robins, Guze, et al. (1972), led the way for improved reliability and empirical tests of validity. The new development of operational criteria constituted the main technical innovation of the new paradigm; operational criteria reduced the problems of reliability that paralyzed research on psychopathology and diagnosis and classification through the 1950s and 1960s. Another innovation came out of statistics. Fleiss, Spitzer, Endicott, et al. (1972) developed the kappa technique for quantifying diagnostic reliability and categorical judgments, and this technique was applied by Spitzer, Endicott, and Robins (1978a) to a wide range of data on psychopathology.

The neo-Kraepelinian point of view was first articulated in the first edition of the influential textbook by Meyer-Gross, Slater, and Roth (1954). Strongly critical of psychoanalysis, psychotherapy, and social psychiatry, this textbook was an aggressive reaffirmation of the Kraepelinian approach. In the United States, neo-Kraepelinian activity originated at Washington University in St. Louis. Its main psychiatric spokespersons were Lee Robins and his colleagues George Winokur and Samuel Guze. Lee Robins has been instrumental in developing new psychiatric epidemiologic methods (1978). Winokur has been active in familial-genetic studies of affective disorder (Winokur, Behar, and Van Valkenburg 1978). Guze is best known for his research on Briquet's syndrome and the reformulation of the categoria "hysteria" (Guze and Roth 1986).

Although the neo-Kraepelinians tend to be most interested in biologic especially genetic, explanations for mental illnesses, a focus on a categorical approach is not, in my opinion, necessarily unique to the biologic school of psychiatry. For example, Freud and many of his early followers, such as Abraham (1927) and Glover (1956), proposed a classification of mental illness based on psychosexual stages of development (Freud 1917). In current research and clinical practice, however, most neo-Kraepelinians emphasize the biologic bases of mental disorders. As a group, they are neutral, ambivalent—at times even hostile—toward psychodynamic, interpersonal, or social approaches.

The Significance of DSM-III

The DSM-III may be regarded as the culmination of the process of change and the profession's acknowledgment of the paradigm shift that had taken place during the 1970s. Robert Spitzer, the chair of the American Psychiatric Association Task Force that generated the DSM-III, has denied any personal inclination to be considered a neo-Kraepelinian. However, the approach to the DSM-III, particularly the emphasis on operational criteria, the elimination of a separate category of neurosis, and the development of the multiaxial system, all represent ideas and methods from the neo-Kraepelinian paradigm.

The DSM-III was criticized from many sources. The psychoanalysts were critical of the elimination of neurosis as a diagnostic category and critical of the principle of psychodynamic conflict as causative of anxiety neuroses and other states. Psychologists, social workers, and other mental health professionals were skeptical and suggested that the DSM-III represented an attempt by psychiatrists to assert dominance in the field of diagnosis. One of the controversial issues was whether the conditions in the DSM-III should be regarded as "medical" disorders, as distinct from "mental" disorders. Many European psychiatrists have been critical of the American Psychiatric Association for not accepting the World Health Organization's ICD-9. The DSM-III has proven to be a major challenge to the ICD-9. The DSM-III has been translated into many languages and many of the features novel to the DSM-III are to be incorporated in the proposed draft of the ICD-10.

Progress in Psychopathology Since the DSM-III

After the promulgation of the DSM-III, the new paradigm became the standard, and a period followed that Kuhn (1970) would call "normal science." There was expansion of structured interviews and application to epidemiology and family/genetics follow-up studies and a marked increase in research on personality disorders as conceptualized in Axis II.

It soon became apparent that patients had multiple disorders. The conventions used in the DSM-III—including the limited use of certain hierarchies within Axis I, the encouragement of multiple diagnoses, and multiaxial assessment—proved only partially successful in dealing with the problems. In 1987, the American Psychiatric Association promulgated the DSM-III-R (American Psychiatric Association 1987). In a number of diagnoses, notably depressive and anxiety disorders, hierarchical diagnostic rules were modified to allow multiple diagnoses of comorbid states, i.e., panic disorder and major depression.

In this context, the concept of comorbidity entered psychiatric research from medical research and epidemiology. The writings of Feinstein (1984) were influential, and the discipline of clinical epidemiology grew.

A number of investigators modified the RDC and DSM-III criteria to eliminate various hierarchies and to encourage multiple diagnoses, both as a lifetime and current episode. Having done so, the frequency with which various disorders coexisted became increasingly apparent and a matter of concern in the design of nearly all aspects of clinical investigation.

APPROACHES TO COMORBIDITY WITHIN THE NEO-KRAEPELINIAN PARADIGM

There are a number of approaches to problems of comorbidity that accept the basic neo-Kraepelinian paradigm (Table 4).

The Multiaxial System

The history of multiaxial systems in the classification of psychiatric disorder has been reviewed by Spitzer and Williams (1980), and by Mezzich (1980). The DSM-III and DSM-III-R attempted to deal with this system with five axes (Table 5).

Most difficulties with comorbidity occur with respect to conditions within Axis I. The introductions in DSM-III and DSM-III-R

Table 4. Approaches to Comorbidity Within the Framework of the Neo-Kraepelinian Paradigm

Multiaxial system
Primary-secondary distinction
Spectrum disorders
Empirical approach:
Suspend all hierarchies

Table 5. DSM-III-R Multiaxial System

Axis I	Clinical Syndromes and V Codes[a]
Axis II	Developmental Disorders and Personality Disorders
Axis III	Physical Disorders and Conditions
Axis IV	Severity of Psychosocial Stressors
Axis V	Global Assessment of Functioning

[a]V Codes = conditions not attributable to a mental disorder that are a focus of attention or treatment.

explicitly encourage multiple diagnoses to be made. Assignment of personality disorders in Axis II and associated medical conditions in Axis III acknowledge the comorbidity phenomena and encourage the clinician to use all of the axes. However, there is no implication as to causation; in this sense, the multiaxial system is "agnostic" with respect to any implications of a causative relationship for specific conditions listed in Axis I and Axis II.

The split of Axis II from Axis I conditions is, in part, a mode of dealing with the long-standing controversy over the etiologic relationship of personality and symptoms. The psychodynamic school has proposed that symptom states fluctuate and co-vary, but that the "underlying" condition is a disordered personality or character pathology. Others, more biologically oriented, have felt that many of the personality conditions classified in Axis II represent subclinical, attenuated forms of Axis I psychopathology. DSM-III partially responded to this issue by moving two personality disorders—dysthymic disorder (depressive personality in earlier editions; dysthymia in DSM-III-R) and cyclothymic disorder (cyclothymia in DSM-III-R)—into Axis I and grouping them together with the affective disorders (mood disorders in DSM-III-R).

In addition, the multiaxial system has helped alleviate a major discomfort that many practitioners have felt using previous diagnostic systems. It is the long-standing dilemma that exists for all medicine: Whereas the unit of scientific interest is pathology (the disorder or disease), the unit of clinical practice is the individual patient. Put another way, medicine studies diseases but treats patients.

This dilemma has contributed to a continuing controversy about the relevance of diagnostic systems for humane clinical practice. Practitioners have complained that medical model approaches to psychopathology had hindered patient care in at least two ways. First, they alleged that diagnostic categories were inadequate for understanding the complexity of individual patients and for clinical decision making. For example, it is argued that in evaluating the need to hospitalize suicidal patients, in addition to knowing whether the patient is depressed or psychotic, it is also necessary to assess personality dynamics, such as the patient's impulsivity or degree of self-control, and to have an adequate understanding of that patient's life circumstances, particularly current stresses, family, income, and social supports. Second, some clinicians have asserted that assigning patients to categories contributes both to depersonalization and deindividualization of the doctor-patient relationship and to social stigmatization.

DSM-III incorporated a multiaxial framework to deal with these objections and to expand the realm of diagnostic assessments. This system consists of clinical psychiatric syndromes, entailing chronicity and periodic aspects as well as symptoms (Axis I); personality disorders that include those of children and adolescents (Axis II); physical illness (Axis III); psychosocial stressors (Axis IV); and level of adaptive functioning (Axis V). The first three axes are typological; the last two are dimensional.

DSM-III has gone a long way toward meeting some of the hesitations and criticisms of clinicians with regard to previous diagnostic systems. It is likely that further axes will be proposed, particularly axes dealing with psychoanalytic defenses, ego functions, and family pathology.

In some ways, the multiaxial system has contributed to the problems of comorbidity: at least it made the problems evident. If there is encouragement to make diagnoses on Axes I, II, and III, the question arises as to what relationship, if any, these axes have? What relationship do these multiple diagnoses have to each other? Is there any implication of causation or relative importance? Problems arise within axes, since many patients will have comorbidity within each axis as well as across axes. Moreover, there is no coding system for the conditions to be listed in Axis III. There are no criteria to indicate whether the comorbidity of mental disorders with medical disorders is coincidental, or whether it is believed relevant in causation, prognosis, outcome, or modifying treatment decisions.

The Primary-Secondary Distinction

Another approach to the phenomenon of comorbidity has been the use of the primary-secondary distinction. This distinction was initially articulated by the Washington University group, which explicitly restricted *primary* and *secondary* terms to chronology. There are three uses of the primary-secondary distinction (Table 6).

First, the chronological criteria, as embodied in the Washington University-St. Louis criteria, has the facilitation of research as its main purpose. Here the primary-secondary use is to generate homogeneous groups that would reduce variability in subject selection and contribute to the knowledge of etiology. In this use, the primary condition is the one that came first chronologically. No inference as to

Table 6. Uses of the Primary-Secondary Distinction

Chronological sequence	Washington University criteria
Causal inference ("due to")	DSM-III-R organic mood disorders
Symptomatic predominance	Clinical judgment (past and current episode)

causation is implied, nor is any inference as to which condition requires the major clinical attention.

Second, in general medical classification systems, the primary-secondary distinction carries with it causal implications. Secondary conditions are usually regarded as having a "due to" causation. Thus with "anemia secondary to infection" or "hypoglycemia secondary to tumor," the implication is clear that the condition of major etiologic importance should take precedence in diagnosis and treatment planning. Probably the medical condition in which this is most widely embodied is the distinction between essential hypertension and symptomatic hypertension; the term *symptomatic hypertension* being analogous to the concept of secondary. Thus, in the classification of hypertension, symptomatic hypertension includes those conditions resembling renal disease, tumors (e.g., pheochromocytoma), or other conditions. The DSM-III-R incorporates this version of the primary-secondary distinction in criteria for a number of conditions (e.g., where the clinical syndrome is clearly the consequence of organic mental disorder). Thus DSM-III-R has categories of organic mood disorder, organic anxiety disorder, and organic personality disorder in which the implication of causation is explicit. Again, the hierarchical principle is retained, with the organic condition being considered causal or etiologic and thus overriding in the hierarchy. Furthermore, in the new criteria for dysthymia, distinction is made between primary and secondary dysthymia, with an implication of "due to."

A third use places emphasis on the predominance of the clinical feature. This requires the clinician's judgment as to which condition is of major importance, particularly for treatment decisions. This use has been less accepted in research, but there are no studies of the reliability of this judgment either for research or in clinical practice.

The Concept of Spectrum Disorders

This approach to the problem of comorbidity makes use of concepts from genetics. In the Danish adoption studies, Kety, Rosenthal, Wender, et al. (1968) proposed the concept of schizophrenic spectrum disorders linking chronic schizophrenia with borderline personality disorder. This concept was subsequently modified to include DSM-III schizotypal personality disorder and schizoid personality. The evidence for grouping these disorders together lies in their increased rates among the adopted offspring whose biological parents were schizophrenic.

The spectrum concept extends the classic genetic distinction between genotype and phenotype. The genotype is the presumed genetic predisposition to schizophrenia, which, according to the concept of spectrum disorder, manifests itself in a number of different clinical states: chronic schizophrenia, schizotypal personality, and schizoid personality. It was originally formulated from studies of adoption and cross-rearing, but subsequently was extended in twin studies by Kendler and Hays (1981) and in family aggregation studies by the NIMH-Danish group (Wender, Kety, Rosenthal, et al. 1986).

There is also some confusion in the use of the term *spectrum*. Sometimes it refers to "dimension," sometimes "variation." However, the unique feature of the spectrum concept in diagnosis is similar to its use in optics and vision. In the visual spectrum, there are separate colors (i.e., red, blue, green), which are the perceptual reflection of an underlying optical variable—the light spectrum measured in Angstrom units. Extending the parallel to mental disorders, schizophrenia, schizotypal personality, and schizoid personality represent different clinical presentations, which have in common a shared, "underlying" genetic predisposition.

Although DSM-III has not fully adopted this concept of schizophrenic spectrum disorder, it partly accepted the spectrum concept in the decision to group cyclothymic disorder (previously called cyclothymic personality and hypomanic personality; cyclothymia in DSM-III-R) with bipolar disorder on Axis I, and to include dysthymic disorder (previously called depressive personality; dysthymia in DSM-III-R) on Axis I.

If this concept is extended in the future to DSM-IV, it is likely that schizotypal personality and schizoid personality would be moved to Axis I as part of the schizophrenia category. Similar proposals have also been made for a relationship between avoidant personality and agoraphobia. Avoidant personality has many phenomenological features in common with earlier descriptions of "phobic character" in the psychoanalytic literature. There is growing evidence that avoidant personality represents a subclinical and/or chronic variation of phobic states; in the creation of DSM-III-R, there was active discussion about the proposal to move avoidant personality from Axis II to Axis I anxiety disorders.

The Radical Empirical Approach: Complete Suspension of Hierarchies

A number of researchers feel uncomfortable even with the modification of hierarchies in DSM-III-R. They feel that the existing evidence does not allow *any* prior judgment as to causative relationships among syndromes. Furthermore, in the application of diagnostic hierarchies in field studies of clinical populations, epidemiologic community surveys, or family studies, hierarchies often obscure important information and preclude testing of the causal hypotheses implicit in the hierarchies. These researchers advocate suspension of all hierarchies and encourage the assessment of all aspects of comorbidity. They would await the results of future research to indicate the extent to which the hierarchies are supported by further empirical evidence.

One instance where elimination of hierarchies is controversial is the relationship of anxiety disorders to mood disorders. In DSM-III-R the hierarchy for major depression precludes an independent diagnosis of generalized anxiety disorder or of panic disorder if these symptom syndromes occur co-terminus with the depressive condition. Others, adopting a strict nonhierarchical approach, advocated that a patient, client, or subject be coded as having major depression with generalized anxiety disorder and/or a panic disorder if these symptom complexes were present during the index episode or in the past.

APPROACHES TO COMORBIDITY THAT DO NOT ACCEPT THE NEO-KRAEPELINIAN PARADIGM

The high occurrence of comorbidity within episodes, throughout the lives of individual patients, and within population samples and their families has prompted many researchers and theorists to question the assumption of multiple discrete episodes, the basic assumption of the medical model and its modification in the neo-Kraepelinian paradigm.

These theorists and investigators are searching for "underlying," "fundamental," or "basic" processes that are, in some sense, causal or etiologic to the clinical symptom complexes. Kraepelin (1974), himself, expressed this point of view toward the end of his career:

> On the other hand, we must seriously consider how far the phenomena on which we normally base our diagnosis really do afford insight into the basic pathological process. While it may be admitted that this procedure is generally valuable, there is a fairly extensive area in which such distinguishing criteria are lacking: either they are insufficiently well-marked or they are unreliable. This is understandable if we assume that the affective and schizophrenic forms of mental disorder do not represent the expression of particular pathological processes, but rather indicate the areas of our personality in which these processes unfold. (p. 107)

I have identified five approaches (Table 7) that seek to delineate the "basic pathologic process" (to use Kraepelinian terms). All five reflect a dissatisfaction with the current diagnostic system, which they feel relies heavily on symptoms and behavioral manifestations. In support of their dissatisfaction, they point out the high degree of comorbidity.

Table 7.   Approaches to Comorbidity Outside the Neo-Kraepelinian
Paradigm

Mental health–mental illness continuum
Stress
Psychodynamic character structure
Genetic (genotype-phenotype)
Psychobiologic

The Mental Health–Mental Illness Continuum

As stated previously, a number of psychiatrists who participated in
World War II came away from that experience considerably dissatis-
fied with the medical model and the Kraepelinian diagnostic system.
This dissatisfaction was most evident in the United States and the
United Kingdom.

In the United States there was an alliance between psychodynamic theorists, particularly those holding to the Menninger view,
and social psychiatrists. The strongest statement of this point of view
was Karl Menninger's (1963) book, *The Vital Balance*, which was extremely critical of classification systems through the centuries. Menninger proposed a unitary continuum between states of mental health
and mental illness. This proposal was embodied empirically in the
Menninger health-illness scale, which was the forerunner of the
Global Assessment Scale (GAS) developed by Endicott, Spitzer,
Fleiss, et al. (1976) and the new code for Axis V in DSM-III.

Dissatisfaction with the medical model was widespread among
psychodynamic, social psychiatric, and epidemiologic researchers
after World War II. Their awareness of diagnostic unreliability made
them decide against using existing psychiatric nosology and substitute measures of overall mental impairment for traditional diagnostic
categories. The use of general impairment scales rather than diagnostic judgments made it easier and more economical to execute epidemiologic surveys. Furthermore, highly trained psychiatrists were no
longer required to make diagnostic judgments, and unreliability of
diagnosis and nosologic disputes could be avoided. The general impairment scales usually included a list of 20 or more symptoms that
were scored additively, providing an index of mental status, independent of specific diagnosis.

Mental health and mental illness were said to fall along a gradient. This view became widely accepted in the period during and
after World War II. The most dramatic public acceptance of this view
was the decision by the Congress in 1947 to create a National Institute

of Mental *Health*. They did not create a National Institute of Mental *Illness*. In this respect, NIMH was different from the other National Institutes of Health, which were named after specific diseases or illnesses. The NIMH had a more visionary scope—the encouragement of mental health—and not just the investigation and treatment of mental illness. A succinct expression of this viewpoint was offered in 1955 by the National Advisory Mental Health Council: "The concept of etiology as embraced by modern psychiatry differs from the simple cause and effect system of traditional medicine. It subscribes to a 'field theory' hypothesis in which the interactions and transactions of multiple factors eventuate in degrees of health and sickness."

Having rejected the use of discrete psychiatric disorders and psychiatric diagnostic procedures, many American investigators adopted inventories that had been developed during World War II. These inventories measured nondifferentiated severity of psychiatric impairment. Rejection of categories of psychiatric diagnosis and the use of measures of impairment was consistent, in part, with thinking expressed during the influential series of conferences on psychiatric epidemiology sponsored by the Milbank Memorial Fund and the World Health Organization as early as 1956. For example, in a report published by the World Health Organization, Lin and Standley (1962) noted the reliability problem in psychiatric diagnosis and suggested that:

> Instead of attaching a firm diagnosis to each patient, the physical, psychological and psychiatric findings can be used to isolate symptoms or personality traits that go together and a label can be applied to such aggregates. This approach has been advocated by some workers who think little of psychiatry and may be better suited to psychological rather than to psychiatric investigation; but it may be worth trying to see how much psychiatry can gain from it, even though it implies some reversion to pre-Kraepelinian ideas. The quantitative aspect of morbid psychiatric states—the degree of impairment—also requires attention, an aspect rather neglected in the past. (p. 65)

The unitary concept of mental illness in the United States was usually combined with theories of social causation of mental illness. This approach emphasized the importance of life experience for understanding the psychopathology of individuals and the role of economics, social class, and social stress in the etiology of mental disorders. The American approach was heavily influenced by the teachings of Adolph Meyer at Johns Hopkins University. Diagnostic groups were considered merely quantitatively different manifestations of the same causes of mental functioning, since common etiologic factors (e.g., social stress) underlay psychiatric disorders.

Stress

In the "golden era" of social epidemiologic research of the 1950s and 1960s, the mental health–mental illness continuum dimension was often related to environmental stress and its impact on the individual and on society. The hypothesis stated that a correlation between the degree of stress and a person's position on the mental health–mental illness continuum existed. This hypothesis has been accepted as proven by many segments of the general public; the concept of stress is often invoked as an explanation, not only of the occurrence of mental illness, but of physical illnesses such as hypertension, coronary artery disease, and peptic ulcer.

The concept of "stress" originated in the endocrinologic research of Selye (1956), who induced unexposed various laboratory animals to external stressors and documented the response of the pituitary and adrenal organs to the "general adaptation syndrome." Selye's endocrinologic concept was rapidly expanded to a general view of the relationship between the individual and the environment and proved particularly useful during World War II.

The U.S. Army organized a group of talented scientists who used the best available sampling methods and survey techniques to conduct a wide range of studies. One aspect of their work was to develop neuropsychiatric screening questionnaires relating neurotic symptoms to combat stress and morale problems. These scales became the basis of the impairment scales used in community surveys after the war.

The observation that rates of psychiatric reactions varied in relation to combat stress was of practical as well as theoretical importance. These combat reactions occurred in psychiatrically screened young men for whom manifest preexisting disability factors would seem to have been eliminated. These methods for screening were far from ideal by today's standards; however, for post-World War II, they were highly important. The planners of mental health research and service programs in the post-World War II period concluded that predisposing vulnerability and concurrent mental and physical illness had been adequately screened. Therefore, it seemed reasonable at that time to conclude that precipitant stress, rather than predisposition or vulnerability, was a major factor in mental illness.

The role of stress as a precipitant of mental illness was supported powerfully by wartime observations, and stress was to become a major unifying concept in the post-World War II studies in civilian settings. Poverty, urban anomie, rapid social change, and social class were to become the civilian stress equivalents of combat and threat of death in the military.

Today the concept of stress has more credence and acceptability in the general public than among mental health researchers. Attempts to explain all mental illness in terms of the general concept of stress have proven too all-encompassing. Research on life events and chronic social stressors continues, but it has become methodologically more rigorous, and the nature of the hypotheses more limited and better specified.

Psychoanalytic Approaches to Underlying Personality Organization and Character Structure

In current psychoanalytic thinking, disturbances of character structure and personality organization are the basic psychopathologic process. Character pathology determined symptom formation. Early psychoanalytic writers through World War I accepted the Kraepelinian approach. However, the attempt was made to relate the psychopathologic conditions and diagnoses to the developmental stage postulated by psychoanalysis. There was a hypothesis that the severity of illness correlated with the degree of regression to infantile psychosexual stages, and that the propensity to illness in adulthood was the consequence of childhood experiences reflected in the concept of fixation. Elaborate charts can be found in the writings of Abraham (1927) and Glover (1956) that relate adult predispositions to fixations at childhood stages of psychosexual development.

Since World War II, the focus on psychosexual stages has given way to a psychosocial developmental approach. Nevertheless, the concept of an underlying hierarchy of personality organization persists, explicitly articulated in the writings of Kernberg (1975). He proposed a general theory in which there are three levels of personality organization (from highest to lowest): neurotic to borderline to psychotic.

It is to be noted that Kernberg's (1975) concept of borderline personality organization has only a limited approximation to DSM-III and DSM-III-R categories of borderline personality disorder. Kernberg hypothesized a structural organization of personality functioning and character pathology that underlies variations in symptom formation and clinical manifestations. Within this view, the phenomenon of comorbidity is seen as evidence for and supportive of the search for underlying psychopathologic and psychopathogenic processes located in the personality organization of the individual.

Genetic Approaches: The Genotype-Phenotype Distinction

Psychiatric genetic research, particularly with the successes of molec-

Section II
Classification Issues

Chapter 3

The Influence of Classification Methods on Comorbidity

Allen Frances, M.D.
Thomas Widiger, Ph.D.
Minna R. Fyer, M.D.

T HE PURPOSE OF this chapter is to explore the ways in which methods used in classifying psychiatric disorders influence the reported rates and directions of comorbidity occurring among them. Our conclusion will be that the levels and types of comorbidity vary greatly, depending on the decisions that are made in classifying and defining the various psychiatric disorders. Many of the innovations introduced by the third edition of the *Diagnostic and Statistical Manual of Mental Disorders* (DSM-III) (American Psychiatric Association 1980) and its revision (DSM-III-R) (American Psychiatric Association 1987) have the (usually unintended) result of increasing the likelihood of comorbidity. The weight given in interpreting comorbidity data determined under our current system should be tempered by an awareness that results might differ considerably were we to use different, but equally plausible, classification methods, assumptions, and definitions. Our chapter is divided into 10 separate sections, each of which presents a different methodological issue that impacts on the determination of comorbidity. We will then discuss how these issues interact with one another and their implications for future classification, research, and clinical practice.

COVERAGE

The extent of coverage of a given diagnostic system is likely to affect dramatically the comorbidity reported within it. Systems differ greatly in their coverage, and there is a trend for the DSMs to broaden their coverage with each new edition, both with respect to subsuming new domains of psychopathology (e.g., tobacco use and sleep disorders) and to increasing the number of differentiations within existing domains (e.g., panic disorders). In general, the more categories a system includes, the wider will be its "coverage." DSM-III has many more categories than the Research Diagnostic Criteria (RDC) (Spitzer, Endicott, and Robins 1978a) in large part because, as an official system of classification, it has the responsibility for providing diagnostic information on the wide variety of patients seen in differing kinds of clinical practice. For this reason, conditions with low prevalence are included even if their usefulness is restricted to a relatively narrow segment of clinical practice (Spitzer and Williams 1985a; Williams and Spitzer 1982). RDC had the much narrower goal of providing homogeneous subjects for research protocols. It could therefore focus its attention on a much less extensive list of categories. The DSM-III and DSM-III-R have also included a number of newly defined disorders that were not present in previous nomenclatures. It is thus not surprising that a recent study (Van der Brink, Koster, Ormel, et al. unpublished manuscript) found DSM-III to have 87% coverage compared to only 69% for the eighth revision of the International Classification of Diseases (ICD-8) in an outpatient sample (World Health Organization 1969).

It should be recognized that the degree of coverage in any given psychiatric classification will have a direct and possible profound influence on the level of comorbidity (Blashfield 1984). As the variety of disorders that are included within a diagnostic system increases, the more likely is it that a patient will meet criteria for any one diagnosis and therefore become a "case." Also, patients will meet criteria for multiple diagnoses and therefore demonstrate comorbidity. This coverage issue is likely to become even more important in future systems because the level of coverage provided psychiatric classifications seems to be increasing over time. This trend toward increased coverage is, in part, a consequence of the recent increased interest in psychiatric diagnosis to describe new entities. It is also, in part, the result of the recent clinical attention that has been focused on individuals who might previously not have been considered psychiatric patients (i.e., smokers, "paraphilic rapists," self-defeating personalities, and those with premenstrual disorders). The bigger the total diagnostic pie, the greater will be the reported comorbidity.

SPLITTING VERSUS LUMPING

This issue might have been included under the coverage issue above but is perhaps more conveniently presented in a separate discussion. Two systems of classification may attain equally wide coverage but include a very different number of individual disorders if one system has fewer, but broader, categories than the other. DSM-III-R has the most categories of any of the current alternatives both because it has the widest coverage but also because it is a splitter's dream and a lumper's nightmare. DSM-III-R describes 8 kinds of anxiety disorder (with subspecifications), 19 kinds of substance abuse disorder, and 13 kinds of personality disorder. Any system that would be content with making fewer fine distinctions within broadly defined general categories would generate less comorbidity, both within major categories and also across major categories. Under most conditions, the more slices there are in the diagnostic pie, the higher will be the rates of comorbidity.

The choice of a splitter's strategy in DSM-III reflects its distrust of the organizing principles that have been used previously to group disorders. This choice has the advantage of keeping open for empirical study questions of possible relationships among disorders. It has the possible disadvantage of creating what may be artificially narrow categories whose association with one another reflects the excessive splitting to which they have been subjected.

A possible example of the splitting issue is the distinction among the DSM-III anxiety disorders of panic disorder, agoraphobia, and generalized anxiety disorder (GAD). Panic disorder was included in DSM-III in large part because of Klein's research demonstrating that imipramine blocks recurrent panic attacks but has no apparent effect on associated anxiety or nonassociated phobic anxiety (Klein 1981; Klein, Zitrin, Woerner, et al. 1983; Spitzer and Williams 1985b). GAD was created to cover the domain of DSM-II (American Psychiatric Association 1968) anxiety neurosis not covered by panic. There is now considerable interest in assessing the comorbidity of panic disorder with a variety of syndromes, including GAD. Data supporting the validity of the panic disorder diagnosis are extensive, and the diagnosis provides valid and useful information. However, much of the research on the comorbidity of panic and agoraphobia may be due to their mapping a common, overlapping domain of psychopathology (Thyer, Himle, Curtis, et al. 1985). Barlow, Blanchard, Vermilyea, et al. (1986) suggested that panic attacks may not be spontaneous or unpredictable but may be associated with subtle cues of which the patient is unaware, such as mild exercise, sexual relations, sudden temperature changes, or stress. Tyrer (1986a) suggested that agoraphobia with panic is more common than agoraphobia alone because the situational cues necessary to exclude a panic disorder are too restrictive. If unexpected panic means not occurring "immediately before" or "on exposure" to a situation that "almost always" causes anxiety (American Psychiatric Association 1987, p. 238), then most agoraphobia (by European thinking) is panic disorder (by American thinking). Comorbidity is not due to agoraphobia resulting from panic disorder (Klein 1981), but to covering a common and overlapping domain.

MULTIPLE DIAGNOSES

Comorbidity is greatly and progressively enhanced in recent DSM systems because of new ground rules that encourage, rather than discourage, multiple diagnoses. Previous systems tended to establish an a priori diagnostic hierarchy, with the more severe and/or pervasive conditions taking diagnostic priority over the less severe and pervasive when both are present. DSM-III removed some of the exclusion criteria to the diagnoses of the lower hierarchy condition, but retained a number of them that substantially affected comorbidity. DSM-III-R has gone even further in permitting (in fact, insisting) that the different conditions each be assessed on its own merits and that each be diagnosed independently when present together. This strategy has been chosen because it saves possibly important information (Spitzer and Williams 1985b), but some critics believe that it results in reduced attention to differential diagnosis and artificially high rates of comorbidity.

As part of this same tendency, the DSMs have established a multiaxial system so that separate consideration is given to the possible presence of the Axis I clinical syndromes and to the Axis II personality disorders. This separation has given great impetus to personality research and to studies of comorbidity between Axis I and Axis II syndromes. It must be recognized, however, that the distinction between Axis I and Axis II is often artificial and difficult to make on both practical and theoretical grounds (Widiger and Frances 1987a). Conceiving of the independence between Axis I and Axis II diagnosis in a naive fashion results in an artificial comorbidity with distinctions that lose clinical meaning; for example, avoidant personality and early onset generalized social phobia are often impossible to distinguish and really are more identical than they are comorbid.

This problem is clearly evident in some of the comorbidity reported within the anxiety disorders both among themselves and with the depressive disorders (Barlow, Di Nardo, Vermilyea, et al. 1986; Boyd, Burke, Gruenberg, et al. 1984; Leckman, Merikangas, Pauls, et al. 1983, Leckman, Weissman, Merikangas, et al. 1983; Spitzer and Williams 1985c; Tyrer 1986a). DSM-III included a number of exclusion criteria in the criteria sets for various anxiety disorders that disallowed comorbidity. The principle guiding these hierarchical exclusions was that it would be redundant, uninformative, and even misleading to provide two diagnoses if the symptoms of one are the result of the other (see First, Spitzer, and Williams, Chapter 5). A hierarchical structure was therefore imposed: a diagnosis was not given if its inclusion symptoms were felt to be the symptoms of a more pervasive, severe, or dominant disorder (Spitzer and Williams 1985c). Agoraphobia, for example, could not be diagnosed if it were "due to" a major depressive, obsessive-compulsive, paranoid personality, or schizophrenic disorder. Major depression, in fact, took priority and therefore excluded most of the anxiety disorders.

Difficulties with these hierarchies quickly become apparent, both logically (Spitzer and Williams 1985c) and empirically (Boyd, Burke, Gruenberg, et al. 1984). Leckman and colleagues (Leckman, Merikangas, Pauls, et al. 1983; Leckman, Weissman, Merikangas, et al. 1983) indicated how a hierarchical scheme might obscure a familial relationship between anxiety disorders and depression through the exclusion of subjects with overlapping diagnoses (e.g., eliminating atypical cases that were not homogeneous with respect to their disorders and the reduction of multiple diagnoses to a single diagnosis through the use of hierarchical conventions). They found that relatives of probands with major depression and panic disorder showed markedly increased rates of major depression, anxiety disorders (phobia, panic disorder, and generalized anxiety disorder), and alcoholism compared with the first-degree relatives of depressed probands without an anxiety disorder. This finding did not emerge if only the probands with depression without an anxiety disorder were studied. The thrust of the findings was replicated in a subsequent study on parent and offspring associations (Weissman, Leckman, Merikangas, et al. 1984).

Hierarchical conventions obscure comorbidity rates (Barlow, Di Nardo, Vermilyea, et al. 1986; Boyd, Burke, Gruenberg, et al. 1984). One cannot demonstrate that an anxiety disorder is comorbid with major depression if the former cannot be diagnosed in the presence of the latter (Buller, Maier, and Benkert 1986; Finlay-Jones and Brown 1981). Boyd, Burke, Gruenberg, et al. demonstrated that there is a general tendency for the presence of any one disorder to increase the odds of having almost any other disorder. Although DSM-III was presumably atheoretical and without assumptions regarding etiology, the hierarchical system assumes that co-occurrence is etiologic and that the causality is in one direction. DSM-III required clinicians to make unreliable and debatable judgments regarding whether an obsessive-compulsive disorder, GAD, or panic disorder were due to major depression.

Because of the above problems, many of the exclusionary criteria were eliminated in DSM-III-R. Spitzer and Williams (1985b) suggested that some hierarchical structure remains necessary lest the classification of mental disorders be reduced "to a list of symptom complexes or syndromes" (p. 764). They provided three principles that guided the exclusionary criteria in DSM-III-R: (1) "When a syndrome has a known organic etiology, the diagnosis of an organic mental disorder takes precedence" (p. 764); (2) "a symptomatically more pervasive disorder preempts the diagnosis of a less pervasive disorder that is based on a symptom that is part of the essential features of the more pervasive disorder" (p. 765); and (3) "a diagnosis is not given if its essential features are typically associated features of another disorder whose essential features are also present" (p. 765). Spitzer and Williams acknowledged that "this is the most problematic principle because it requires knowledge about the relative frequency of associated features" (p. 765).

GAD provides an example of the impact of hierarchical rules. It contains more exclusionary criteria than any other anxiety disorder because it is commonly present as an associated feature of other disorders (Barlow 1985). Because the anxiety of GAD is relatively nonspecific (neither circumscribed in time as in panic disorder nor in situations as in phobia or agoraphobia), it is considered by some to represent a residual, leftover category. In fact, Barlow, Blanchard, Vermilyea, et al. (1986) suggested that GAD not be diagnosed in patients with other anxiety disorders when the generalized anxiety is due to an "anticipatory anxiety" with respect to the panic or phobia of the "primary" diagnosis (a policy that was incorporated into DSM-III-R). They indicated that many of their patients with anxiety disorder (except simple phobia) would not meet the criteria for GAD when this exclusion rule is in place.

PROVISION OF DIAGNOSTIC CRITERIA

The provision of diagnostic criteria in DSM-III and DSM-III-R also increases reported rates of comorbidity, especially since the availability of these criteria has stimulated the use of semistructured interviews. Clinicians' diagnoses, based on general impression and unstructured interviewing, are likely to highlight the most prominent presenting syndrome at the expense of all other possibly diagnosable conditions. To the degree that diagnostic criteria are clearly specified and detailed interviews are used to tap systematically each of the items, comorbidity will be increased because the more subsidiary conditions receive equivalent attention and are more likely to be diagnosed. For example, rates of comorbidity were enhanced in the National Institute of Mental Health (NIMH) Epidemiologic Catchment Area study because of its use of a semistructured interview tapping simple phobia with explicit criteria and questions. Under most clinical conditions the presence of simple phobia is overlooked, and rates of anxiety disorders and of comorbidity are lower.

ITEM OVERLAP

The degree of comorbidity among diagnoses is directly influenced by the degree to which they share similar or identical items within their definitional criteria sets. To some extent item overlap may be a technical or artifactual issue. Overlapping items may appear in different sets because these were created by different groups with insufficient attention to the possibilities of confusion and overlap. More often, however, the question of definitional overlap touches on one of the most fundamental questions underlying classification strategy: Should criteria sets be devised with the primary purpose of providing discriminant validity? Discriminant validity is achieved by emphasizing those items that provide distinction among disorders, even if this means sacrificing some of the essential features of the given disorders when these features are present across a variety of different categories. Choosing this strategy could increase the specificity of the various criteria sets, heighten the value placed on differential diagnosis, and, in the process, reduce the reported rates of comorbidity.

Or, should each category be defined by those features that are felt to be most essential to it, whether or not these are present in other diagnoses? This strategy will increase the sensitivity and clinical utility of the diagnostic system, but in the process will reduce the meaningfulness of differential diagnosis and will increase the comorbidity that may be based on nothing more than a definitional overlap. Furthermore, it is rarely clear, when a given symptom serves as a defining feature for two different categories, whether the resulting overlap between them reflects the true state of their relationship or is an unnecessary artifact based on the choice of the identical definitional items in both sets. For example, the criteria set for borderline personality disorder includes items that tap affective symptomatology. It is unclear whether the frequently reported comorbidity between borderline personality disorder and affective disorder is the result of some underlying true affinity between the two syndromes or reflects a superficial descriptive similarity creating a definitional overlap (Akiskal, Yerevanian, Davis, et al. 1985; Widiger and Frances

1987a). Does it make sense to alter the criteria for GAD because many individual definitional items are seen in most other anxiety disorders and in major depression? We will be stuck with these questions until our diagnostic system goes beyond the descriptive level.

The comorbidity of anxiety and depression may be inflated by overlapping features (Foa and Foa 1982; Tellegen 1985). Is the comorbidity artifactual, or does the overlap in criteria sets reflect the actual commonalities of the disorders? If to compensate for this problem comorbidity is reassessed with overlapping items excluded, one may then artifactually diminish comorbidity by failing to assess the constructs in a valid fashion.

A variety of multivariate analyses have attempted to identify the items that are most effective in differentiating between anxiety and depression. Items that have been identified as being particularly efficient have included panic, situational phobias, depressed mood, pessimistic outlook, suicidal tendencies, fatigue, and sexual disinterest (Breslau and Davis 1985; Mountjoy and Roth 1982b; Roth and Mountjoy 1982). However, the discriminability of items will likely vary across settings and differential diagnoses, and items that are most useful in differentially diagnosing a disorder may not be the most useful in defining a disorder (Widiger and Frances 1987b; Widiger, Hurt, Frances, et al. 1984). If the constructs of anxiety and depression overlap, then perhaps the criteria sets should as well. Until the criteria sets assess the underlying pathology of the disorder directly, or an infallible means of independently identifying the presence of the disorder is available, then disentangling actual from artifactual comorbidity with descriptive data will be difficult or often impossible.

THRESHOLDS

The degree of comorbidity among syndromes within a classification will be greatly influenced by the thresholds used to determine the presence or absence of any given criterion and the thresholds for the cutoffs specifying the proportional number of criteria necessary to establish the presence or absence of the disorder. If it is relatively easy to fulfill the requirements of the individual criteria and if only a relatively small proportion of the criteria are necessary to make the diagnosis, then patients will more likely meet criteria for several diagnoses and the chances for comorbidity are increased. Thresholds are generally set to establish the expected severity, frequency, impairment, and duration of the pertinent symptoms or behaviors. DSM-III has provided definitions for a number of diagnoses with relatively low thresholds that may be relatively easy to meet (e.g., major depression, simple phobia, substance abuse, personality disorder). Setting low thresholds may be useful from a number of standpoints, but it has the risk of artificially raising comorbidity. Some critics have argued that the DSM-III criteria for these and many other conditions should require longer durations, greater severity, or increased frequency of symptoms to raise the thresholds for these diagnoses and thus reduce artificial comorbidity.

The absence of a nonarbitrary cutoff point to identify clinical anxiety and clinical depression from normal mood complicates comorbidity research. Lay interviewers, for example, may employ a lower threshold than professional clinicians, resulting in higher comorbidity when they do the assessments. Depression, as a symptom or as a subjectively unpleasant state, is common to almost all mental disorders, but the point at which it is considered to be a syndrome is debatable and variable across nosologies (Blashfield 1984). This judgment can be particularly difficult when many of the indicators that suggest a mental disorder (e.g., social or occupational dysfunction) may be due, in part, to the comorbid syndrome.

Depressive symptomatology below an apparent clinical threshold for dysthymia (or major depression) is seen in many patients with anxiety disorder (e.g., Barlow, Di Nardo, Vermilyea, et al. 1986), and comorbidity would be increased if the full range of depression were included. Similarly, the threshold for panic disorder is difficult to demarcate, with perhaps many false negatives below the DSM-III cutoff point (Katon, Vitallano, Russo, et al. 1987). Given that the threshold is to a large extent arbitrary, it may be preferable to measure anxiety and affective disorders on a continuum to allow the full range to be included in analyses. Much information is lost in a nominal distinction of simply the presence versus the absence of dysthymia. It is apparent that patients vary in the extent to which they display dysthymia, panic disorder, and other anxiety and affective disorders. Why not use this information? If more homogeneous samples are desirable for particular research purposes, then analyses can focus on patients who are above a particular cutoff point on the primary diagnosis of interest, and below cutoff points on particular comorbid disorders or other diagnoses often confused with the disorder of interest.

HALO EFFECTS

Semistructured interviews are helpful in curtailing clinical biases against multiple diagnoses and in allowing more valid assessment of comorbidity (Roth and Mountjoy 1982), but they are not without their problems. One example is halo effects. Conditions may artifactually

Dimensional Versus Categorical Classification

We have discussed the possibility that at least some of the comorbidity reported using our currently categorical psychiatric classification may result from the inherently overlapping "fuzzy set" nature of psychiatric diagnosis (Cantor and Genero 1986; Frances 1982). An alternative methodological approach would be to determine and rate the underlying dimensions that may best account for the surface correlation among clinical categories. This approach most applies to the diagnosis of personality disorders (Frances 1980; Frances and Widiger 1986a). Most available studies suggest that patients meeting criteria for any given personality disorder are quite likely to meet criteria for two or more, and that there are substantial and relatively systematic correlations across specific disorders. The high degree of comorbidity within Axis II reflects the high level of both actual and artifactual overlap across the personality disorders and is exacerbated by the fact that so many different individual disorders are available for rating. A dimensional system that provided ratings of only three or four more "basic" dimensions that are found to cut across all of the correlated categories would be an alternative way to address, and reduce, the comorbidity question. Similarly, one might consider rating all patients on both dimensions of anxiety and depression rather than having multiple subcategories of anxiety and depression, with varying degrees of overlap, comorbidity, and heterogeneity of membership.

The DSM-III-R classification of the anxiety and affective disorders follows the medical tradition of categorical distinctions. One either has a panic disorder or one does not. This categorical form of classification is useful in simplifying case discussions and in defining homogeneous groups for research purposes (Andreasen 1982). For example, the biogenetic covariates and contributions to the construct of depression may be most apparent in the pure cases—those without anxiety, schizophrenia, or other pathology (Robins and Guze 1970). But gleaning these homogeneous groups (e.g., panic disorder) from the broader domain (e.g., anxiety disorders) results in problematic borderline, residual, and wastebasket categories (e.g., GAD and anxiety disorder not otherwise specified).

There has been a recent increase in discussions of dimensional, spectrum models of Axis I pathology (e.g., Dobson 1985c; Dobson and Cheung, Chapter 34; Fabrega, Mezzich, Mezzich, et al. 1986; Mirsky and Duncan 1986). Even the distinction between bipolar and unipolar affective disorders is being questioned and reinterpreted as a continuum (Khouri and Akiskal 1986). Difficulties with a number of the problematic diagnoses, such as GAD, may be due in part to an imposition of an unnecessary categorical model on a dimensional variable. A useful analogy is intelligence. One could diagnose mental retardation by the various specific etiologies and homogeneous syndromes that are associated with mental retardation (e.g., Down's syndrome). But this would lose sight of the fact that intelligence is itself a dimensional variable with no clear, absolute boundary between levels of retardation and normality. One would also be left with a variety of boundary, overlapping, and residual categories to account for the mental retardation cases that have a nonspecific and multifactorial etiology and are not easily placed within a homogeneous category with distinct boundaries. Identification of the specific etiologies and homogeneous syndromes is clearly useful and important, but retaining the dimensional classification is useful as well.

It may similarly be the case that the DSM-III-R categories of panic disorder with agoraphobia, panic disorder without agoraphobia, and agoraphobia with panic are also better expressed within a dimensional rather than categorical system. It has been suggested in a number of studies (e.g., Garvey and Tuason 1984; Sheehan and Sheehan 1983; Thyer, Himle, Curtis, et al. 1985) that panic disorder and agoraphobia with panic are only different manifestations or expressions of a common, underlying pathology. Turner, Williams, Beidel, et al. (1986) found that there is not a sharp boundary between groups of patients with these two disorders with respect to the intensity of panic and agoraphobic symptoms: "It appears that these two groups vary along the dimensions of panic and agoraphobia . . . suggesting that a categorical classification . . . may be incorrect" (p. 386). The DSM-III-R classification retains the categorical format, but now provides the beginning of dimensional scoring by including a rating of severity of agoraphobic and panic symptoms.

A problem with imposing a categorical model on a dimensional variable is that leftover categories begin to become reified and elevated to the status of a new disorder, distinct from the rest. To some, borderline personality disorder is a distinct pattern of personality disorder pathology (Gunderson 1984), while to others it represents literally borderline cases that lie across the boundary of existing categories (Widiger 1982). Similarly, there are a number of alternative labels for those patients who display symptoms of both anxiety and depression, such as atypical depression, masked depression, and anxiety depression. These literally borderline cases may be interpreted eventually as distinct disorders (e.g., Van Valkenburg, Akiskal, Puzantian, et al. 1984), and their comorbidity with anxiety and depression will be assessed, even though they may, in fact, be simply the heterogeneous leftovers after removal of the more distinct members along the underlying dimensions.

Comorbidity is difficult to study and interpret under these circumstances. Is it meaningful to discuss the comorbidity of borderline with affective and histrionic personality disorder if borderline selects patients who overlap with the histrionic and affective disorders? Is it meaningful to discuss the comorbidity of GAD and panic if GAD is the collection of residual anxiety neuroses after panic disorder is removed? Is it informative to say that panic patients exhibit a greater comorbidity with major depression than GAD (Brier, Charney, and Heninger 1985a), if panic disorder is an extreme variant of GAD? The comorbidity of some anxiety and affective disorders may be due in large part to where along the affective and anxiety multidimensional pie they are sliced.

A variety of multivariate (e.g., discriminant function and factor analytic) studies have differentiated affective and anxiety dimensions (e.g., Derogatis, Lipman, Covi, et al. 1972; Mendels, Weinstein, and Cochrane 1972; Mountjoy and Roth 1982b; Mullaney 1984; Prusoff and Klerman 1974; Roth, Gurney, Garside, et al. 1972; Roth and Mountjoy 1982), but these findings do not necessarily suggest that the disorders are qualitatively distinct. In fact, each study has typically obtained a considerable degree of correlation and overlap (Dobson 1985c).

A variety of multidimensional models of anxiety and depression have been proposed (Barlow 1985; Izard and Blumberg 1985; Lang 1985; Russell 1980; Tellegen 1985). Space limitations prevent a comprehensive review of each of them. We will briefly describe the models of Russell and Tellegen and discuss how they relate to comorbidity.

Russell (1980) proposed a circular (circumplex) array that is defined by the dimensions of pleasure-displeasure and degree of arousal. Depression, sadness, tension, distress, and fear are all displeasurable emotions (versus excitement, joy, happiness, and delight) and hence are often correlated and co-occurring. The anxiety emotions of tension, distress, and fear, however, are additionally characterized by relatively higher levels of arousal, whereas the depressed emotions of sadness, depression, and sluggishness are characterized by low levels of arousal, and hence are often distinguished in factor analytic studies and in patient populations. Some patients will be characterized by high arousal and displeasure (panic disorder), some by low arousal and displeasure (major depression), some by high arousal and pleasure (mania), and some by low arousal and pleasure (normality, or at least no anxiety or affective disorder). Some may alternate (cyclothymia) and some will present mixtures (e.g., anxious, agitated depression). One can attempt to carve sections within and around the circumplex to form 10 to 15 categories to characterize various sections, pieces, and mixtures, but this would lose sight of the simplicity of the underlying structure and the arbitrariness of the categories, distinctions, and comorbidity.

In an independent investigation, Tellegen presented a remarkably similar two-dimensional model (Tellegen 1985; Watson, Clark, Tellegen 1984; Zevon and Tellegen 1982). Tellegen proposed the two dimensions of positive affect and negative affect. High positive affect is characterized by being active, elated, and enthusiastic (pleasurable engagement); low positive affect is characterized by being drowsy, dull, and sleepy (nonpleasurable disengagement). High negative affect is characterized by being distressed, fearful, hostile, and jittery (unpleasurable engagement); low negative affect is characterized by being calm, placid, and relaxed (pleasurable disengagement). If one rotates the dimensions by 45 degrees, one essentially has the same dimensions as Russell (1980).

Tellegen (1985) suggested that the correlation and overlap of anxiety and depression scales and criteria sets may be due in large part to anxiety and depression being characterized by the rotated dimensions that share in subjective discomfort and demoralization. This emphasis is understandable; it is subjective discomfort and demoralization that is of most concern and focus clinically. However, Tellegen suggested that this emphasis contributes to the confusion and covariation of anxiety and depression (and perhaps to their comorbidity), and may be optimally replaced by measures of negative and positive affect. Anxious mood would be characterized as heightened negative affect (or unpleasurable engagement) with a particularly salient fear component, and depressed mood as lowered positive affect (or nonpleasurable disengagement) with salient features of sadness and fatigue.

It may be that different latent class taxons (e.g. genotypes) underlie the constructs of anxiety and depression and that discontinuity would be obscured by a dimensional model (Andreasen 1982; Barlow, Di Nardo, Vermilyea, et al. 1986). We are not arguing here for the dimensional model. We are suggesting that comorbidity research has been dominated by categorical assumptions and that the dimensional alternative should receive further consideration. One suggestion is to include dimensional ratings and analyses along with the categorical in comorbidity studies—for example, measures of the octants or quadrants of Tellegen (1985) or Russell (1980)—and to analyze and interpret the results with respect to both models. Direct comparisons of the categorical and dimensional models may be particularly informative.

INTERPRETATION OF COMORBIDITY

When two disorders (A and B) appear to be associated on descriptive grounds, it is impossible, without outside validators, to determine which of the following interpretations is most relevant: (1) A predisposes to or somehow causes B; (2) B predisposes to or somehow causes A; (3) A and B are both influenced by another underlying predisposing or causal factor C; (4) the apparent association of A and B is the chance result of their relatively frequent presentation in the sample or the result of other chance factors; (5) A and B are associated because they share overlapping definitional criteria items, with sharing of descriptive features that may or may not reveal real underlying relationships on other grounds; or (6) A and B should not be considered "comorbid" so much as they are best included within one larger underlying syndrome that has been artificially split into parts by the classificatory system. The considerable interest in the comorbidity of anxiety and depressive disorders is largely an attempt to determine which of the above explanations accounts for the comorbidity. We will not try, nor could we hope, to offer an explanation. The intent of our chapter is only to indicate how classificatory problems and decisions impinge on efforts to choose among the various possible explanations. It is usually impossible, on the basis of descriptive classification alone, to determine which of these interpretations is most pertinent.

Comorbidity determined by descriptive studies can never be understood until information on course, pathogenesis, family loading, and treatment response provides an independent means of determining the causal relationships underlying surface associations. Until such data are available, we must allow that the determination of descriptive comorbidity may reflect little more than difficulty in defining disorders at the descriptive level of abstraction.

DISCUSSION

Although there was certainly no deliberate intention during the creation of DSM-III and DSM-III-R to increase the frequency of comorbidity of psychiatric disorders, the innovations introduced by these systems have progressively had this result. Influenced as we are by the results generated by the first wave of clinical and epidemiologic studies using the DSM-III categorical diagnoses, it is therefore no great surprise that the question of comorbidity has commanded such a great recent interest. Let us begin by summarizing the ways in which DSM-III and DSM-III-R have established conditions that enhance the likelihood of comorbidity, and then discuss the implications for future classifications, research, and clinical practice.

DSM-III (and DSM-III-R even more) greatly expanded the coverage of psychiatric disorders, and therefore the number of people assessed who become cases and who have multiple diagnoses. DSM-III (and DSM-III-R even more) exhibited a splitters predilection to divide major categories into many separate disorders, thus increasing and perhaps artifactually creating comorbidity within and across major disorders. Moreover, the provision of a separate assessment for personality disorders greatly enhanced Axis II comorbidity. DSM-III-R especially encourages multiple diagnoses as a general principle and specifically eliminates many of the diagnostic hierarchies that restricted multiple diagnoses in the past. Explicit diagnostic criteria, and the semistructured interviews spawned by them, increased comorbidity by encouraging systematic evaluation and equal treatment for accessory symptoms in the patient's presentation, and perhaps by providing halo effects across domains of assessment. The item overlap frequently present across criteria sets ensures a correlation among disorders that is reflected in increased comorbidity. Finally, DSM-III and DSM-III-R have relatively low severity and duration thresholds for a number of conditions, resulting in their frequent diagnosis and, consequently, frequent comorbidity.

Is the comorbidity encouraged by our current methods of description good or bad? Like most things, it is both and neither, and the relative merits depend on the particular goals one has in mind in a given situation. DSM-III and DSM-III-R diagnoses are almost exclusively based only on descriptive criteria. To say that conditions are comorbid in a given patient means no more than that the defining descriptive features tend to associate with one another. We must not reify the DSM syndromes into distinct disease entities and assume that comorbidity means the presence of two different even if presumptively related diseases. Our high rates of comorbidity are just as likely to emerge from simply the descriptive overlap included in DSM-III and DSM-III-R. The encouragement to make multiple diagnoses inherent in DSM-III and DSM-III-R is useful in saving information if it is understood that such information is only at the descriptive level and that causal inference requires data that must come from outside of our classification system.

The danger in the current state of affairs is that some observers may reify the descriptive conventions. They may naively believe, for instance, that anxiety and depressive disorders are necessarily separate, distinct, and comorbid rather than holding open the possibility that these are the related surface manifestations of underlying unitary syndromes. It is also important to recognize that reports of comorbidity are greatly influenced by the classification system with which we work and by the samples tested. Moreover, such reports may not be very robust across classificatory schemes and differences in sampling.

What are the implications for future psychiatric classifications? There are no established grounds on which to base decisions about the degree to which a given classification system should encourage or discourage high rates of comorbidity. We do, however, have some sense of how nosologic decisions, made largely for other reasons, will impact on this question. Their impact on the comorbidity question should become part of future discussions concerning coverage, lumping versus splitting, hierarchies and multiple diagnoses, and the use of diagnostic criteria. Perhaps the most obvious immediate need is for systematic review of the performance characteristics of the various diagnostic criteria sets to determine their internal consistency and discriminant validity. Such data would provide a basis for future decisions regarding definitional overlap and the collapsing and reorganization of categories. DSM-III and DSM-III-R are clearly informed by a splitter spirit and by the lack of data on which to define empirically more general syndromes. As we know more, both descriptively and about underlying pathogenesis, it seems likely that we will have a simpler system, lumping together categories now considered separate and comorbid. Dimensional systems may be useful to reduce artificial comorbidity, particularly in classifying personality disorders.

What are the implications for research? Most clearly, the finding of comorbidity among disorders is a call to determine the degree to which this comorbidity reflects a true underlying relationship and to determine the nature of that relationship. Such efforts will help separate the comorbidity due to fundamental relationships from that which results from definitional artifact, and will suggest new and higher-order methods of organizing the classification of psychiatric disorders. Descriptive research helps to determine the internal consistency and correlation of criteria sets, but must be supplemented by other approaches that determine the meaning of these relationships.

What are the implications for clinical practice and education? One of the problems created by the DSM-III penchant for splitting has been the the tendency for the newly created categories quickly to take on a life of their own and become "distinct entities." At times, this tendency to reification leads to a fragmentation of the view of the patient who may appear to present with six or seven different disorders. The target symptom approach to treatment can be very valuable in many situations, but at times results in a reductionistic and/or unintegrated approach to treatment planning. Clinicians and trainees must become aware of the meaning and the limitations in their interpretations of the high levels of descriptive comorbidity generated by the use of DSM-III system.

It is important for all of us to remember that our classification system provides no more than a set of very useful conventions for defining disorders that has improved our reliability, clinical communication, and ability to generalize from research studies. By and large, our system is not based on pathogenesis and does not define distinct diseases. Small changes in classification decisions result in large changes in reported rates and types of comorbidity. The underlying meaning of this comorbidity and the determination of better methods of classification await advances in our understanding of pathogenesis.

Chapter 4

Comorbidity and Classification

Roger K. Blashfield, Ph.D.

Comorbidity IS A TERM from medicine that refers to the co-occurrence of different diseases in the same individual. Comorbidity has been recognized as an important clinical phenomenon in medicine, both because of its negative implications for prognosis in individual cases and because empirical studies on comorbidity can help elucidate the causal mechanisms that lead to the development of different diseases.

In psychiatry, comorbidity has been a topic of recent interest. During the 1970s and 1980s, there was a major revolution in psychiatry, which Klerman (1978b) associated with a group of research-oriented psychiatrists he described as the neo-Kraepelinians. These psychiatrists have stimulated increased research of psychiatric classification and were instrumental in the formation of the DSM-III (American Psychiatric Association 1980) and DSM-III-R (American Psychiatric Association 1987). Moreover, because of their concern with diagnosis and description, these researchers have supported the development of a number of structured interviews that will permit the systematic assessment of clinical pictures of patients. One of the results of the use of these structured interviews and the application of diagnostic criteria in the DSM-III is that high degrees of diagnostic overlap have been noted in a number of empirical studies. For instance, Boyd, Burke, Gruenberg, et al. (1984) analyzed data using the Diagnostic Interview Schedule, which had been administered to 11,519 subjects in four communities. They found that if an individual

This chapter was completed while the author was being supported by NIMH grant #R01-MH-41081 entitled "Prototype Research on Personality Disorders."

was assigned one DSM-III diagnosis, in many cases the person met the diagnostic criteria for at least one other DSM-III diagnosis. Widiger, Hurt, Frances, et al. (1984) conducted a study of personality disorder diagnoses in a state hospital population and found that these patients met the diagnostic criteria for an average of 3.75 Axis II disorders.

Because of the descriptive studies that have found high levels of diagnostic overlap, the concept of comorbidity has been attracting attention in the psychiatric literature. In this chapter, the phenomenon of comorbidity will be briefly reviewed by discussing one particular journal article on this topic. Then the relevance of comorbidity for issues in psychiatric classification and for possible future research on psychopathology will be discussed.

THE PHENOMENON OF COMORBIDITY

The phenomenon of comorbidity and its relevance for psychiatric classification are exemplified in a recent journal article by Barlow, Di Nardo, Vermilyea, et al. (1986) entitled "Co-morbidity and depression among the anxiety disorders: issues in diagnosis and classification." In this article, the authors reported on 126 patients who were referred to the Center for Stress and Anxiety Disorders in Albany, New York. These patients were administered systematic interviews—the Anxiety Disorders Interview Schedule (ADIS)—on two separate occasions by different interviewers. A subsequent staff meeting was held to assign a primary diagnosis and any additional diagnoses using the DSM-III. The only exception to the DSM-III diagnostic rules was that the authors modified the exclusion criteria because this was a study of comorbidity, and strict use of the exclusion rules would limit the potential diagnostic overlap.

Of the 126 patients interviewed, 108 patients were assigned one of seven diagnoses that fit within the anxiety-affective disorder spectrum. Of these 108 patients, 65% were given at least one additional diagnosis. More specifically, 39% of the patients with agoraphobia also met the criteria for major affective disorder or dysthymic disorder.

In discussing their results, Barlow, Di Nardo, Vermilyea, et al. (1986) made a number of comments about the relevance of comorbidity for psychiatric classification. Their first comment was directed at the concept of *hierarchy*. They noted that since a goal in psychiatric classification is to isolate discrete categories of mental disorders, hierarchical rules had been introduced into the decision rules for the DSM-III. These hierarchical rules are based on the long-standing clinical tradition that there is a "pecking order" among general categories of mental disorders and that the diagnosis of certain, more pervasive disorders should have precedence over other disorders. For instance, the diagnosis of an organic brain syndrome is considered to be higher in this clinical pecking order than the diagnosis of depression. Moreover, since a patient with an organic brain syndrome such as Alzheimer's disease might present with a significant depressive picture, this hierarchical arrangement of disorders would imply that only the Alzheimer's disease should be diagnosed because the depressive syndrome could be due to this organic disorder. Thus the hierarchical arrangement of mental disorders as recognized within the DSM-III led to the specification of exclusionary rules in which certain diagnoses would not be made if the syndromes represented by these diagnoses could be due to disorders that were higher in the hierarchical system.

After the 1980 publication of the DSM-III, the exclusionary rules in this classification became a focus of major criticism. Critics argued that the exclusionary rules often were arbitrary, and their blanket use could hide important descriptive relationships that might be noted among different mental disorders. In particular, Boyd, Burke, Gruenberg, et al. (1984) showed that, when the exclusionary rules were dropped, then patients who were assigned one DSM-III diagnosis are likely to meet the criteria for at least one additional DSM-III diagnosis. These authors noted that the use of the arbitrary exclusionary rules of the DSM-III would hide any important patterns that might be noted by studying diagnostic overlap.

Contrary to Boyd, Burke, Gruenberg, et al. (1984), Barlow, Di Nardo, Vermilyea, et al. (1986) commented that the reasonable solution is not simply to drop all exclusion rules. In the area of the anxiety disorders, patients with an obsessive-compulsive disorder might have a fear of contamination (a common fear of obsessives) sufficiently strong that they would develop a phobic response to dirt. In such an instance, the additional diagnosis of a simple phobia would not be relevant, and the treatment program for such patients would focus on the obsessive-compulsive syndrome. In contrast, they mentioned an example of a patient who has a generalized anxiety disorder with associated features of anxiety, tension, and worry. This individual happened to witness a gruesome suicide and developed a phobic response to blood. An additional diagnosis of simple phobia was made for this patient. The difference between the two cases is important. In the first instance, an additional diagnosis was not made because the dirt phobia was *functionally related* to the primary diagnosis. In the second instance, this functional relationship was not observed—that is, the fear of blood was not precipitated by the generalized anxiety disorder but by the witnessing of a suicide—and

From a set theory perspective, each of the categories of dogs mentioned above is a class whose members are individual organisms. For instance, the species of domestic dogs (*Canis familiaris*) contains my niece's dog named Penny as a member. An important feature of a hierarchy from a set theory perspective is that categories at higher levels in the classification include categories at lower levels. For instance, since the genus *Canis* (true dogs) includes the species *Canis familiaris*, then every organism that is a member of *Canis familiaris* is also a member of *Canis*. What this means is that the further up a category is in the hierarchy, the larger (in terms of membership) is that category. For example, *Canis* has more organisms as members than does *Canis familiaris*. However, the sheer number of categories is larger at lower levels of the hierarchies. For example, there are only 10 genera under *Canidae* while there are 33 species in this same family.

Another important feature in biologic classifications is that the categories at the same level in these systems are mutually exclusive and exhaustive. The property of being mutually exclusive means that an organism can be a member of one and only one species. My niece's dog, Penny, cannot be both a member of *Canis familiaris* and a member of *Canis lupus* (despite how often Penny tries to scare me into thinking she is a wolf when I visit). Moreover, the property of being exhaustive means that all organisms can be classified into a species. All organisms that fit under the dog family (*Canidae*) must be assigned to one of the 33 species under this family.

The final important distinction that is made in biologic classification that will have relevance to the discussion of comorbidity concerns types of definitions. Biologic taxonomists discuss two types of definitions of categories: intensional definitions and extensional definitions. Extensional definitions are definitions in terms of the membership of the categories. For instance, an extensional definition of *Canis familiaris* would list all the organisms that are and have been members of this species. However, since there are millions of domestic dogs, extensional definitions are impractical and are not used in biologic classification. The other type of definition is intensional. Using this type of definition, a category is defined by the features that are associated with membership in the category. Thus the intensional definition of *Canis familiaris* would list the morphological features that are used to decide whether a particular dog was a member of this species as opposed to some other species.

In biologic classification, the intensional definition of a category contains the features that are used to differentiate that category from all other categories that are included in the same branch of the hierarchical system. The features that are important for defining *Canis familiaris* are those morphological features that discriminate between

Canis familiaris and other species under the genus *Canis*. These morphological features include overall body size, the relative size of the brain, and the size and shape of the eyes. In the same way, the defining features for *Canis* contain those features that discriminate between *Canis* and *Vulpes*. Of course, since my niece's dog is both a member of *Canis familiaris* and a member of *Canis*, Penny must demonstrate the defining features for both categories.

COMORBIDITY AND THE STRUCTURAL MODEL APPLIED TO PSYCHIATRIC CLASSIFICATION

Now that a structural model of biologic classification has been briefly presented, this model will be applied to psychiatric classification and to the concepts used by Barlow, Di Nardo, Vermilyea, et al. (1986) when discussing comorbidity.

Figure 2 presents a partial representation of the categories in the anxiety-affective disorder spectrum of mental disorders as contained in DSM-III. Notice that these categories have a hierarchical organization that follows a rather similar outline to the hierarchical organization of categories under the dog family. Any patient, for instance, who would be diagnosed as having a simple phobia would also be considered as having a phobic disorder (the next level higher in the hierarchy) as well as having an anxiety disorder (the second level up). The nesting of mental disorders is parallel to the nesting of categories as represented by the hierarchical structure of biologic classification. However, the meaning of the concept of *hierarchy* as represented in Figure 2 can easily be shown to be different from the meaning of *hierarchy* as discussed by Barlow, Di Nardo, Vermilyea, et al. (1986).

As presented in the beginning of this chapter, *hierarchy*, as it has been used in the comorbidity literature, refers to a pecking-order relationship among categories. However, as extrapolated from biologic classification and as shown in Figures 1 and 2, the concept of *hierarchy* refers to a nesting relationship among categories. Consider a patient who meets the diagnostic criteria for agoraphobia and major depressive disorder. According to the Barlow, Di Nardo, Vermilyea, et al. (1986) data, patients with these clinical features are relatively common. Using the pecking-order approach to hierarchy, this patient might be diagnosed as having major depressive disorder, since it has precedence over agoraphobia. However, from the perspective of the hierarchical arrangement analogous to biologic classification, the presence of such a patient is problematic. Agoraphobia is not nested under major depressive disorder. In fact, agoraphobia and major depressive disorder are disorders that occur in separate branches of the classification. To find a patient who appears to be a member of

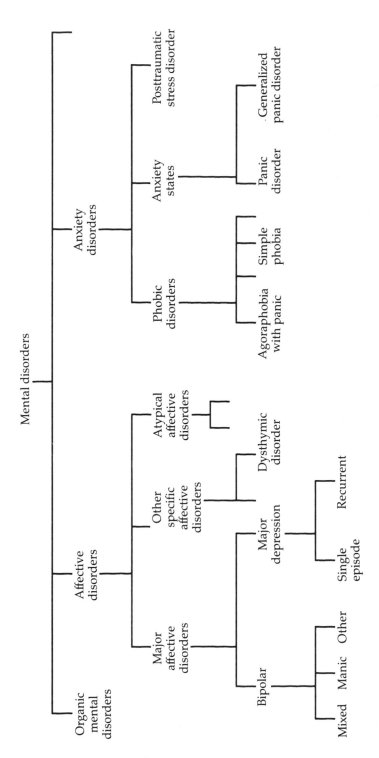

Figure 2. A partial representation of the categories in the anxiety-affective disorder spectrum of mental disorders as contained in DSM-III.

both categories is analogous to finding an animal that is both a pet dog (*Canis familiaris*) and a red fox (*Vulpes vulpes*). Moreover, in biologic classification, no branches of a hierarchical tree have precedence over others; for example, *Canis* is not higher in some pecking order over *Vulpes*.

What this analysis suggests is that the concept of *hierarchy* as used in discussions of psychiatric classification has two meanings. The first meaning, which is best understood in terms of the analogy to biologic classification, is what will be described in this chapter as the nesting or inclusion interpretation. Under this use of the term *hierarchy*, any entity (i.e., a patient) who is a member of a lower level category is by definition also a member of a higher level category, which includes the lower level category. In other words, if a patient has a dysthymic disorder, that patient can be said to have an affective disorder.

The second meaning of *hierarchy*, the meaning used by Barlow, Di Nardo, Vermilyea, et al. (1986), is described as a pecking-order interpretation. The pecking-order meaning can be best understood by making analogy to the hierarchical organization of rank among military officers. A colonel is higher in rank than is a major, who in turn is higher in rank than a lieutenant. In this pecking-order structure, a colonel can give orders to a lieutenant but a lieutenant cannot issue orders to a colonel. Thus the pecking-order nature of the hierarchical arrangement in military rank concerns lines of authority. A colonel has authority over a lieutenant. Notice, however, that there is no membership nesting in these categories. If a particular individual is a lieutenant, then that individual is not a colonel even though a colonel is higher in the hierarchy than a lieutenant. However, in terms of responsibility, there is a nesting relationship. Suppose Colonel Alpha is in charge of a regiment and Lieutenant Bravo is one of the officers in that regiment. Under this circumstance, Colonel Alpha is responsible for the behavior of Lieutenant Bravo. If Lieutenant Bravo fails to achieve a particular objective during a military encounter, not only is Lieutenant Bravo held responsible for that failure but so is Colonel Alpha.

To understand how this analogy to the hierarchical arrangement of military rank can be applied to psychiatric classification, consider the following order of general mental disorders:

Organic mental disorders
Schizophrenic disorders
Affective disorders
Anxiety disorders

In terms of pecking order, this means that disorders that are higher in this order should be diagnosed over disorders lower in the hierarchy.

Thus, in terms of standard diagnostic practice, the presence of organic mental disorders should be ruled out first, then the schizophrenic disorders, and then affective disorders. This principle of diagnostic precedence is analogous to the authority relationship among different levels of rank in the military.

Notice that the pecking-order relationship among the four general mental disorders also carries another implication. If a patient has an organic mental disorder, the patient can (and often does) have the symptoms associated with disorders that are lower in the hierarchy. A patient with Alzheimer's disease can develop hallucinations, become severely depressed, and perhaps develop agoraphobia. On the other hand, a patient with agoraphobia will not show the disturbed memory patterns and disorientation of a patient with an organic mental disorder. In short, there is a nesting relationship to the pecking-order hierarchy of mental disorders, but the nesting occurs among symptoms (features, characteristics, signs, abnormal behaviors) and not among patients (entities). This nesting relationship is analogous to the lines of responsibility with the hierarchical structuring of military rank.

The distinction between nesting of features and nesting of entities is important and can be stated somewhat differently. The inclusion interpretation of hierarchy (analogous to biologic classification) concerns the extensional definition of categories. The nesting that occurs involves the entities (organisms, patients) who are members of the various categories. In the pecking-order interpretation of *hierarchy* (analogous to military rank), the nesting involves the intensional definitions of the categories. Nesting occurs among the defining features (symptoms).

Having made this distinction between nesting of features and nesting of entities, it is useful to reconsider the data that Barlow, Di Nardo, Vermilyea, et al. (1986) presented on comorbidity of the anxiety and affective disorders. What their data demonstrated was that there was a high degree of overlap among a number of diagnostic categories in the anxiety-affective disorder spectrum. In the terms of the structural model introduced earlier, the Barlow, Di Nardo, Vermilyea, et al. data showed *the memberships of the categories* in terms of entities (patients) were not mutually exclusive. What their data did not demonstrate is that the *nesting of features* (symptoms) among these different categories either confirmed or disconfirmed the nesting implied by the exclusionary rules used in the DSM-III. In general, this methodological pattern is true in other studies. Empirical studies that have led to criticisms of the exclusionary rules in the DSM-III have been studies about the overlap of category memberships rather than studies about the nesting of features (Sturt 1981).

DIMENSIONS VERSUS CATEGORIES

The preceding distinction between a hierarchical system referring to the nesting of features as compared to a hierarchical system referring to the nesting of entities leads to a more general issue that was raised near the end of the Barlow, Di Nardo, Vermilyea et al. (1986) article. The issue concerns a dimensional approach to psychiatric classification versus a categorical approach. A dimensional approach is often favored by those researchers who focus on the measurement of symptoms (i.e., on features). Moreover, the dimensional approach is often associated with factor analysis, which is a multivariate statistical procedure that groups similar features (behaviors, self-report answers, symptoms) together to form general dimensions (relatively abstract features). In contrast, the categorical approach is generally favored by researchers who are concerned with understanding etiology and predicting treatment response. Their focus is on patients (on entities). The multivariate method associated with the categorical approach is a cluster analysis that attempts to form relatively homogeneous groups by putting similar patients together.

Interestingly, the issue of dimensional versus categorical approaches has been an extremely heated issue that has appeared over and over again in the literature on psychopathology (Eysenck 1970; Garside and Roth 1978; Skinner 1979). The consistent and recurrent debate between these two approaches is particularly interesting, since most theoreticians who have attempted to compare these approaches have found them to be complementary rather than oppositional (Cattell 1966; Skinner 1986). Because of the complexity of the debate surrounding these two approaches and because of the possible relevance of this debate for comorbidity, a brief review will be provided of both approaches.

A dimensional model is concerned with finding a small set of dimensions (abstract variables) that will account for the observed co-variation among features and that can be used to visualize the relationships among patients. These dimensions or abstract variables are usually estimated through linear equations combining the data about the features. A specific example may help explain the dimensional approach.

Suppose that a researcher systematically assessed a number of symptoms occurring within a sample of psychotic patients. In particular, this researcher examines the following 10 features: alcoholism in parents, euphoria, excitement, irritability, mutism, negativism, refusal of food, stereotypism, suicidal tendency, and tantrums. When this researcher correlates the symptoms, he notes that some symptoms form collections of highly correlated symptoms. For instance, mutism, negativism, refusal of food, and stereotypism are all highly correlated. These four symptoms, visually represented by the two-dimensional system seen in Figure 3, all form a cluster of features and appear along the horizontal dimension of this figure. We might call this dimension "negative schizophrenic symptoms." On the other hand, the vertical dimension might be named "manic symptoms" (Moore 1933).

Now that the two dimensions have been formed from these 10 symptoms, it would also be possible to plot patient data. This relationship is shown in Figure 4. Notice that the patient data tend to clump into groups in this figure. One relatively small cluster of patients appear near the top of the figure and might be thought of as the manic patients. In the lower right quadrant are another group of patients that might be described as the depressed patients. Finally in the middle right portion of the figure is a more diffuse collection of patients that might be thought of as the disorganized schizophrenic cluster. In addition, there are other patients whose symptoms do not clearly fit into any of these three groups.

The data shown in Figure 4 are consistent with a categorical model. These data suggest that patients can be assigned to relatively homogeneous groups (categories) and that there are relatively clear boundaries (zones of rarity) that appear between the categories. The presence of these relatively discrete groups identified by descriptive data would imply that these groups represent different disorders that require different causal mechanisms to explain their symptomatology.

On the other hand, suppose that when the patient data are plotted into the two-dimensional space as defined by these 10 psychotic symptoms, Figure 5 is obtained instead of Figure 4. Notice that in Figure 5 there are no clear clusters in the data. Instead, the data appear amorphous with no obvious boundaries or zones of rarity occurring. In Figure 5, to draw boundaries separating the patients into categories would seem arbitrary and to have no descriptive justification (at least with these data). In this figure, a dimensional model would seem more plausible since the dimensional model would not force the assignment of patients into some procrustean categorical solution (Frances and Widiger 1986b). (Procrustes was a giant, according to Greek myth, who would force travelers to fit in his bed by stretching them if they were too short or cutting off parts of their legs if they were too tall.)

The above example suggests why a number of theoreticians have suggested that a dimensional approach and a categorical approach are complementary. As can be seen in Figures 4 and 5, the dimensional approach can be used to help visualize the categorical structure of the data (or the lack of a categorical structure). Together, these two figures

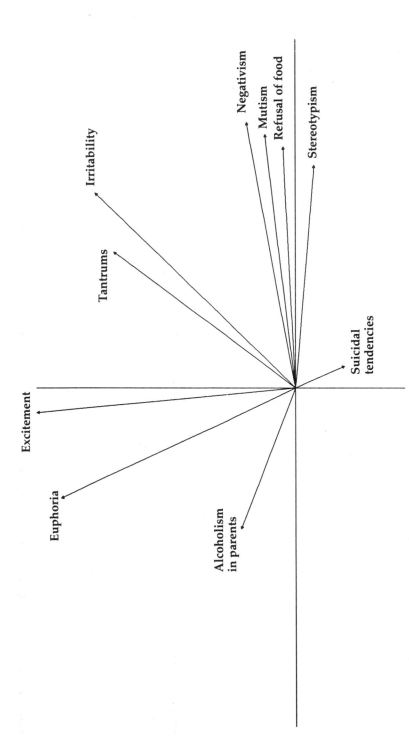

Figure 3.　Relationship between symptoms occurring within a sample of psychotic patients (i.e., mutism, negativism, refusal of food, and stereotypism), visually represented by a two-dimensional system.

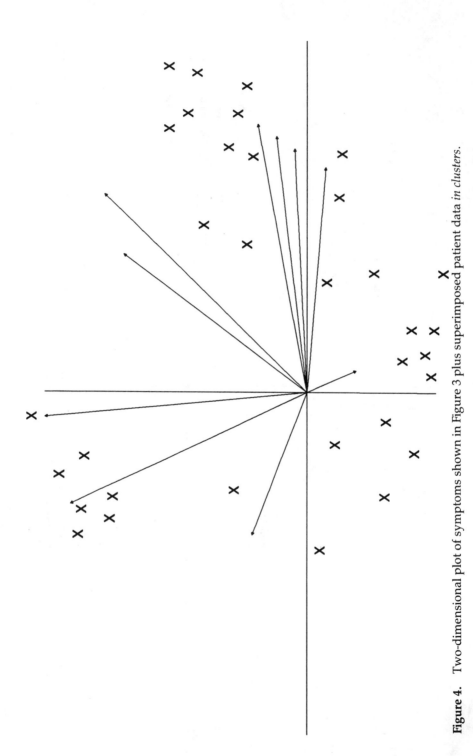

Figure 4. Two-dimensional plot of symptoms shown in Figure 3 plus superimposed patient data *in clusters*.

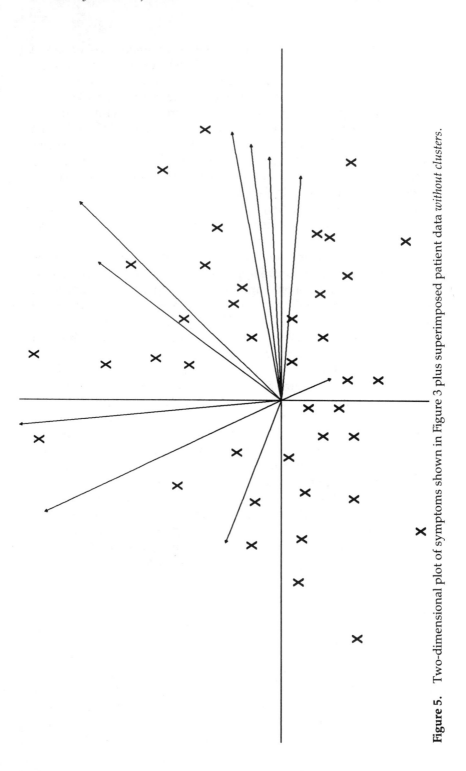

Figure 5. Two-dimensional plot of symptoms shown in Figure 3 plus superimposed patient data *without clusters.*

suggest why the dimensional model has maintained a collection of advocates. In both figures, the use of a dimensional model is appropriate and does not sacrifice or misrepresent data about the patients. It is the categorical model that appears to be the more restrictive of the two. The categorical model assumes that there exist relatively homogeneous groups with zones of rarity among them (Kendell 1975). The categorical model is useful only when the patient data match this assumption. However, regardless of whether there are homogeneous groups or not, the dimensional model is appropriate. Restated, the dimensional model generally is the more agnostic (i.e., it makes fewer assumptions), the more parsimonious (i.e., is a simpler model), and the more descriptive (i.e., it does not impose the structure of discrete categories onto the data).

What does the phenomenon of comorbidity have to do with the dimensional versus categorical approach to psychiatric classification? As noted earlier, the major empirical finding that is stimulating the discussions of comorbidity in the literature is the high degree of diagnostic overlap (among DSM-III categories). In the Barlow, Di Nardo, Vermilyea, et al. (1986) data, for instance, almost two-thirds of the patients were assigned more than one diagnosis in the anxiety-affective disorder spectrum. Graphically, this would seem similar to a situation depicted in Figure 6. This figure contains the same dimensions and the same data as Figure 5. In addition, outlines depicting the diagnostic boundaries of the three psychotic disorders are shown. Notice the significant amount of overlap among these three disorders. Of all patients who fit under the boundaries of one of these diagnoses, only one-third fall into portions of the dimensional space associated with only one diagnosis. This is similar to the Barlow, Di Nardo, Vermilyea, et al. situation in which two-thirds of the patients fit more than one diagnosis. High amounts of diagnostic overlap can be interpreted as suggesting that a dimensional approach to classification would be more parsimonious than would a categorical model.

If the dimensional model is generally the more descriptive, parsimonious, and agnostic, why has not this model gained ascendancy in psychiatric classification, especially given the high degree of diagnostic overlap that is being found in current research? There are a number of reasons for the continued resilience of the categorical model. First, the categorical model is more consistent with the language of classification. When dealing with stimuli in the real world, our linguistic tendency is to use nouns to talk about these stimuli, as if all stimuli can be subdivided into different classes of objects. For instance, color is clearly a dimensional concept that is associated with the wavelength of visible light. When we talk of color, we talk of red, blue, magenta, and so on as if these nouns referred to different classes of hues. In

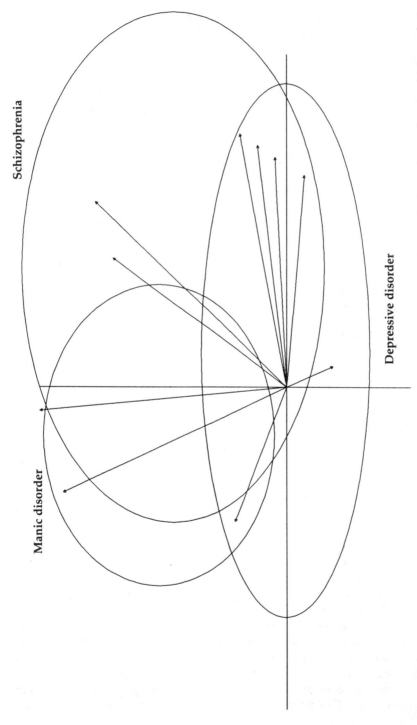

Figure 6. Two-dimensional plot of symptoms shown in Figure 3 plus superimposed disorder boundaries showing high overlap.

psychiatric classification, there have been concepts introduced into the language of psychopathology that were clearly dimensional (at least, at first). For instance, introversion-extroversion was a dimensional concept originally introduced by Jung in the early 1900s (Hempel 1965). Over time this dimension has been altered in our language to become categorical; that is, we now talk about introverts and extroverts as if these nouns referred to categories of people.

A second reason for the resiliency of the categorical model is its association with the medical model. An implicit assumption, sometimes explicit, is that the categories in a psychiatric classification refer to different diseases. The etiologic bases of the different disorders, as well as the treatment approaches, will differ across disorders. The DSM-III and the DSM-III-R were formed primarily by a group of psychiatrists whom Klerman (Chapter 2) described as neo-Kraepelinians. These psychiatrists believe that mental disorders are discrete and are associated with different disease processes. Since the adoption of a dimensional model would be a repudiation of the neo-Kraepelinian approach, this model has attracted little acceptance within current psychiatric classification.

IMPLICATIONS FOR CLASSIFICATORY RESEARCH

The phenomenon of comorbidity has a number of implications for future research concerning psychiatric classification. Two of these implications will be discussed in some detail below. These two implications concern (1) research strategies that can be used to investigate the hierarchical (pecking-order) structure of psychiatric classification, and (2) the issue of the severity dimension in descriptive research on psychopathology.

Relatively little research has been conducted on the pecking-order interpretation of hierarchy within psychiatric classification, despite the fact that the history of this view of a hierarchical organization can be traced back to the writings of Jaspers (Morey 1987). The major research that has been conducted on the pecking-order model has focused on a particular classificatory scheme suggested by a British author named Foulds (1964, 1965). Foulds advocated a psychiatric classification system in which there are four broad categories: (1) delusions of disintegration, (2) integrated delusions, (3) neurotic symptoms, and (4) dysthymic states. In addition, there is a fifth category that Foulds named non-personally ill. Within each of these broad categories are specific categories of mental disorders. For example, the category of integrated delusions contains the specific categories of delusions of grandeur, delusions of persecution, and delusions of contrition. Foulds postulated a strongly hierarchical (pecking-order) relationship among the four general categories. According to Foulds, any patient who would fit in a higher-level category would necessarily have the symptoms associated with categories lower in the system. Thus a patient who met the definition for delusions of contrition would also meet the definition for inclusion into a neurotic states category as well as a dysthymic states category.

Research on Foulds' (1964, 1965) hierarchical model has been generally positive. Most of this research has used the Delusions-Symtoms-States Inventory (DSSI), a self-report instrument developed by Bedford and Foulds (1977) to test this model. Foulds and Bedford (1975), McPherson, Antram, Bagshaw, et al. (1977), and Morey (1985) have all reported positive results using the DSSI. For instance, Morey (1985) studied 52 inpatients at the Yale Psychiatric Institute and found that 47 fit the pecking-order pattern explicitly predicted by Foulds (i.e., that a patient belonging in a higher-level category would have symptoms fitting categories lower in the hierarchical order).

Sturt (1981) published an interesting empirical study of the relationship among psychiatric symptoms that contained a useful methodological analysis of Foulds' (1964, 1965) classificatory system. She noted that the use of the DSSI was problematic since a response bias (yea-saying) could account for any positive results. Surtees and Kendell (1979) published a study of the Foulds system using a structured interview, the Present State Examination (PSE) (Wing, Cooper, Sartorius 1974a). Almost 80% of their patient sample fit the Foulds' hierarchical model, although half of the schizophrenic patients within the sample did not.

In comparison to Foulds' hierarchical model, the pecking-order model in DSM-III is largely implicit. DSM-III does not stipulate that patients who are diagnosed with a higher-order disorder (such as schizophrenia) are likely to meet the diagnostic criteria for a lower-order disorder (such as dysthymic disorder). Nor does DSM-III clearly state which disorders are higher or lower in the pecking order. As noted earlier, DSM-III-R contains fewer exclusion rules than did DSM-III. By postulating a classification in which there are fewer exclusion rules, the authors of DSM-III-R apparently were moving away from a pecking-order structure among mental disorders. Yet some exclusion rules still exist in this most recent system. Again, this state of affairs suggests that the authors of DSM-III-R need to be more explicit in the specification of the hierarchical model(s) used in this system.

To conclude the first point to be made about comorbidity and research on psychiatric classification, the pecking-order interpretation of hierarchical structures among psychiatric diagnoses suggests that future research should focus on the relationships among different *symptoms* and *symptom patterns* rather than emphasizing studies of diagnostic overlap. Moreover, if future research is to help clarify the DSM-III-R classifications of psychopathology, then the hierarchical models need to be made explicit so that the appropriateness of the various exclusionary rules can be empirically tested.

If future research does not support a pecking-order model among mental disorders, then an important phenomenon will need to become the focus of future classificatory research. This phenomenon is the *severity dimension*. Commonly, descriptive studies of psychopathology that have used factor analysis have found a ubiquitous first dimension that can be described as a severity dimension. On this dimension there are some patients who score high and who have many, if not most, of the symptoms being studied. On the low end of this dimension are other patients who have relatively few of the symptoms being studied. In most descriptive studies of psychopathology, a severity dimension will account for 25% to 40% of the variance in the symptom data. A severity dimension is evident in factor analytic studies of the Minnesota Multiphasic Personality Inventory (MMPI) (Jackson and Messick 1962), in early factoring studies of psychotic symptoms (Moore 1933), and in descriptive studies of alcoholics (Morey, Skinner, Blashfield 1984).

To understand the relevance of the severity dimension for the phenomenon of comorbidity, a return to Sturt's (1981) study is instructive. Sturt administered the PSE to four samples: a community sample from southeast London, a series of patients seen in an emergency room for self-poisoning, an outpatient psychiatric sample, and an inpatient psychiatric sample. Sturt found that every symptom in the PSE had a positive correlation with the total PSE score. Moreover, relatively rare symptoms (e.g., "guilty ideas of reference") were associated with higher total PSE scores than were relatively frequent symptoms. What these results mean is that the combined patient sample in Sturt's study were distributed along a severity dimension ranging from a relatively small number of patients with a large number of symptoms to a relatively large number of patients with few symptoms.

From the perspective of a pecking-order hierarchical model of psychopathology, the existence of this severity dimension is not surprising. Since the pecking-order model specifies that symptoms are nested within categories according to their hierarchical arrangement, the model would predict a strong severity dimension in any descriptive study of psychopathology. If future research does not support some version of a pecking-order model, then the explanation of a consistent severity dimension in descriptive research will need to be handled through an alternative classificatory model. Eysenck's

(1987) three-dimensional, threshold model of psychopathology, for instance, could be used to explain a severity dimension.

In addition to the two major implications for psychiatric classification noted above, the phenomenon of comorbidity does lead to other implications. For instance, recent data demonstrating high levels of diagnostic overlap suggest that continued emphasis needs to be placed on improving the assessment of psychopathologic symptoms and the diagnostic criteria that are used to define mental disorders. As Frances, Widiger, and Fyer note (Chapter 3), a major reason for the current interest in comorbidity has been the appearance of structured interviews and the use of diagnostic criteria. The continued refinement and use of these assessment instruments will provide more data on diagnostic overlap. As more data become available, perhaps it will be possible to search for patterns in overlap so that any necessary revisions can be made in DSM-IV.

As a corollary of the continued emphasis on improved assessment devices for psychopathology, future descriptive research should also emphasize the identification of symptoms that are optimally discriminating in diagnostic decisions. These symptoms can then be incorporated in future diagnostic criteria. DSM-III emphasized identification of core features of different mental disorders and using these core features in the diagnostic criteria. The core features are those symptoms that almost always occur in the disorder (i.e., symptoms that have high sensitivity). However, as can be shown in a brief analogy to biologic classification, the use of core features is not always optimal for diagnosis. Suppose that a researcher who wanted to develop "diagnostic criteria" for *Canis familiaris* decided to rely on core features. One feature that is common to all domestic dogs is that they are warm blooded. This feature will not serve a useful exclusionary purpose for this category since all other species within the genus *Canis* contain warm-blooded animals. As noted in the discussion of intensional definitions, biologists use features in these definitions that serve to differentiate categories occurring at the same hierarchical (inclusion) level.

Another implication of comorbidity for research on classification concerns the type of data that will be used in this volume. Frances, Widiger, and Fyer (Chapter 3) note that comorbidity of two disorders, A and B, could suggest any of the following interpretations:

A predisposes to or somehow causes B;
B predisposes to or somehow causes A;
A and B are both influenced by another underlying predisposing or causal factor C;
the apparent association of A and B is the chance result of their relatively frequent presentation in the sample or other chance factors;

A and B are associated because they share overlapping definitional items;

A and B should not be considered "comorbid" so much as they are best included within one larger underlying syndrome that has been artificially split into parts by the classificatory system.

The differentiation of these interpretations is a difficult process, and Frances, Widiger, and Fyer discuss a series of methodological issues associated with classificatory research that can affect this differentiation. One important addition to their comments is the importance of using longitudinal data. The diagnostic approach implicit in DSM-III and DSM-III-R could be described as a "snapshot" perspective. Most mental disorders in these two classifications are defined using symptoms that can be ascertained in one interview. Thus diagnoses in these symptoms can be said to result from a clinical "snapshot" taken of the patient at one point in time. It is well recognized that clinical pictures can and usually do change over time. Moreover, Kraepelin made clinical course an important classificatory principle when deciding what clinical presentations were associated with separate disorders and what clinical presentations were simply variations on a common theme. Longitudinal, descriptive research is expensive. Nonetheless, the potential of this type of research to examine clinical course and explain the phenomenon of comorbidity would seem to justify the cost.

Chapter 5

Exclusionary Principles and the Comorbidity of Psychiatric Diagnoses: A Historical Review and Implications for the Future

Michael B. First, M.D.
Robert L. Spitzer, M.D.
Janet B. W. Williams, D.S.W.

IN THE CONTEXT OF diagnostic classification, comorbidity refers to the assignment of more than one diagnosis to an individual to account for symptoms of illness occurring during a given period of time. As discussed elsewhere in this book (Frances, Widiger, and Fyer, Chapter 3), different classification methods can have a profound effect on apparent rates of comorbidity. The use of exclusion rules is the method with perhaps the most significant impact on comorbidity (i.e., diagnosis A not given in the event of condition X). In general, the fewer and more limited the exclusion rules in a classification system, the greater the number of multiple diagnoses that must be assigned to account for a given set of symptoms. A move toward such an increase in comorbid diagnoses has been advocated by those who claim that exclusion rules artificially obscure the independence of certain syndromes, resulting in a loss of potentially valuable information. For example, in the third edition of the *Diagnostic and Statistical Manual of Mental Disorders* (DSM-III) (American Psychiatric Association 1980), panic disorder was excluded from being diagnosed in the presence of schizophrenia, even though there was no empirical evidence that these two disorders cannot co-occur. Therefore, an individual with symptoms meeting criteria for both schizophrenia and panic disorder was given only the single diagnosis of schizophrenia, with the implication being that the presence of multiple panic attacks did not warrant any different diagnostic consideration of this individual from those without this symptom. Making such a diagnosis might result in such an individual not receiving treatment specific for the panic attacks (e.g., the addition of tricyclic antidepressants to a regimen of neuroleptic medication).

Exclusion rules cannot be completely removed without the elimination of many of the fundamental diagnostic concepts underlying modern psychiatry. For example, the fundamental distinction between bipolar disorder and major depression is operationalized by an exclusion rule in the criteria for major depression requiring that the diagnosis not be given if the criteria for bipolar disorder are met. If this rule were to be eliminated, then an individual with one or more major depressive episodes and one or more manic episodes would be given two separate diagnoses—major depression and manic disorder—implying the co-occurrence of two different disorders. The basic nosologic distinction between unipolar and bipolar mood disorders, with its well-established prognostic, biologic, and genetic correlates, would be ignored.

The fundamental nosologic concept of schizophrenia would similarly be compromised in a classification system without exclusion rules. Schizophrenia is conceptualized as a pervasive disorder that interferes with many aspects of an individual's functioning, causing disturbances in affect, mood, perception, reality testing, interpersonal relations, motivation, and thought processes. Even though the basic pathophysiologic mechanisms underlying this disorder have yet to be established, its nosologic validity has been amply supported empirically (Cloninger, Martin, Guze, et al. 1985; Kendler 1987; Spitzer, Andreasen, and Endicott 1978). With the elimination of exclusion rules, the concept of a single unifying disorder that can affect multiple areas of functioning is also eliminated, with such an individual being diagnosed as having multiple disorders. For example, an individual with schizophrenia who has nonbizarre delusions, social isolation, peculiar behavior, chronic depressed mood, and chronic anxiety might be diagnosed in an exclusion-rule-free system as having schizophrenia, delusional disorder, schizotypal personality disorder, dysthymia, and generalized anxiety disorder.

A balance must be reached between these two approaches. In this chapter, we examine how classifications of mental disorders have dealt with this problem historically, and, with the benefit of hindsight, we propose a taxonomy of exclusion rules that may be useful to the developers of DSM-IV.

DEFINITIONS OF TERMS

Before proceeding with a historical review of how exclusion rules have been used in psychiatric classification systems, some definitions of terms are in order. In discussions about the use of exclusion rules, these rules are usually referred to as operationalizations of "diagnostic hierarchies." According to *Webster's Dictionary*, a *hierarchy* is defined as a "ruling body organized into orders or ranks each subordinate to the one above it," or in its most general sense as: "a group of persons or things arranged in order of rank, grade, class, etc." The key concept is that a hierarchical relationship implies an ordering among items.

In the field of nosology, diagnostic hierarchies are based on the principle of set inclusion; that is, nosologic entities are arranged so that, for any two nosologic entities A and B, entity A is considered to be higher than entity B in the hierarchy when entity B is a subset of entity A. In most classifications of mental disorders, however, there are actually two coexisting types of diagnostic hierarchies, each based on a different sense of the word *subset* (see also Blashfield, Chapter 4).

In the first type of hierarchy, a class membership hierarchy, *subset* refers to the concept of class membership; that is, if set B is a subset of set A, then all members of set B are members of set A. This is best illustrated outside the field of nosology in Linnaeus' familiar classification of species, in which general concepts (e.g., kingdom, phylum) are at the top of the hierarchy and more specific concepts (e.g., genus, species), which are subsets of the general concepts are at the bottom. Class membership hierarchies have traditionally been employed to provide the fundamental organizational structure of classifications of medical disorders, for example, the World Health Organization's International Classification of Diseases (ICDs) and the American Psychiatric Association's DSMs.

The DSM-III-R (American Psychiatric Association 1987) classification contains general categories at the top of its hierarchy (e.g., mood disorders), each of which are subdivided into more specific categories (e.g., mood disorders subdivides into bipolar disorders and depressive disorders) until the most specific categories (i.e., particular disorders) are reached on the bottom level (e.g., depressive disorders finally divides into major depression, dysthymia, and depressive disorder not otherwise specified). Therefore, under the DSM-III-R class membership hierarchy, cases meeting the criteria for major depression have the disorder major depression, which is a depressive disorder, which in turn is a mood disorder.

The second type of diagnostic hierarchy is based on a conceptualization of subset that focuses on the sets of features that are characteristic of the disorders. These feature hierarchies rank disorders based on the subset relationships between their respective sets of characteristic features. Disorder A is placed higher in the feature hierarchy than disorder B when the set of features that defines disorder B is a subset of the set of features characteristically associated with disorder A. For example, bipolar disorder is higher in the hierarchy than major depression since the set of features defining major depression is a subset of the set of features that define bipolar disorder. In contrast with the more traditional class membership hierarchy, in which both major depression and bipolar disorders are subsets of (i.e., members of) the class mood disorders, the disorder major depression is not a subset of the class, bipolar disorder. Also note that in a feature hierarchy, hierarchical relationships are defined exclusively among entities at the same level of specificity (i.e., disorders), whereas in a class membership hierarchy, the relationships are always between entities at different levels of specificity (e.g., mood disorders and major depression).

Feature hierarchies form the basis for many of the exclusionary relationships in a psychiatric classification system. An *exclusionary relationship* between disorder A and disorder B is defined as a relationship between the two disorders such that in some set of circumstances, disorder A precludes the diagnosis of disorder B, or disorder B precludes the diagnosis of disorder A. Each relationship in the feature hierarchy corresponds to a hierarchical exclusionary relationship in the classification in the following way: if disorder A is higher than disorder B in the feature hierarchy (i.e., the set of defining features of disorder B is a subset of the set of defining features of disorder A), then the diagnosis of disorder B is excluded by the presence of disorder A. Put another way, the diagnosis of disorder B necessarily implies the absence of the defining features of disorder A.

For example, the set of characteristic features of schizophrenia contains nonbizarre delusions, among other psychotic symptoms. Since the set of defining features of delusional disorder (i.e., nonbizarre delusions) is a subset of the set of features characteristic of schizophrenia, schizophrenia is higher than delusional disorder in the feature hierarchy. Therefore, a hierarchical exclusional relationship exists between schizophrenia and delusional disorder, in that schizophrenia excludes the diagnosis of delusional disorder, and the diagnosis of delusional disorder implies the absence of any other defining features of schizophrenia.

Note that the traditional organic exclusion rule in which the presence of an established organic factor precludes the diagnosis of the corresponding functional disorder is, in fact, an example of a hierarchical exclusionary relationship as described above. For example, delusions developing after the use of amphetamine are diagnosed as amphetamine-induced delusional disorder, precluding the diagnosis of delusional disorder, and conversely, the diagnosis of delusional disorder implies the absence of any established etiologic organic factors. By considering the etiologic organic factor to be a "feature" of the disorder, then the set of features of the functional delusional disorder (e.g., delusions) is a subset of the set of features of the organic delusional disorder (e.g., delusions plus the etiologic organic factor).

Hierarchical exclusionary relationships are a fundamentally important construct in classification systems. Without them, it would be impossible to formulate a definition of a disorder that includes the set of defining features of another disorder. Different disorders have different ranges of symptomatic expression. For example, disorders that have a wide range of symptomatic expression, like schizophrenia, can be considered more pervasive than disorders with a narrower range of symptomatic expression, like dysthymia. Exclusionary relationships allow for the suspension of the diagnosis of the more narrowly defined disorder in favor of the more pervasive disorder. Therefore, the narrowly defined disorder dysthymia is not diagnosed if it occurs only in the presence of the more pervasive schizophrenia, since the defining feature of dysthymia (i.e., chronic mild depression) is an extremely common associated feature of schizophrenia. This ability to construct distinct disorders out of syndromes that are themselves disorders is more than just a nosologic convenience. As described earlier, the very existence of the concepts of bipolar disorder (which includes features that define major depression) and schizophrenia (which includes features that define delusional disorder, dysthymia, etc.) requires it.

The term *diagnostic hierarchy* is often used as if it encompasses all relationships among disorders in which one diagnosis precludes another diagnosis. Hierarchical relationships are only a special case of the more general concept of exclusionary relationships; that is, if two disorders have an exclusionary relationship, then under some set of circumstances, one disorder precludes the diagnosis of another. There are other instances, however, in which the exclusionary relationship is not a strictly hierarchical relationship but a mutual exclusionary relationship, in which two disorders share all of the same features with the exception of one feature that acts as a cut point between the two disorders. For example, the feature that distinguishes between conduct disorder and antisocial personality disorder in DSM-III and DSM-III-R is the age of the individual. If the individual's age is less than 18, antisocial personality disorder is excluded in favor of conduct disorder; if the age is greater than 18 and criteria are met for antisocial personality, conduct disorder is excluded.

In summary, to avoid the confusion caused by the different uses of the phrase "diagnostic hierarchy," we propose that the term *hierarchical exclusionary relationship* be used when referring to the rank ordering among disorders that precludes the diagnosis of a disorder lower in the hierarchy when the defining criteria are met for a disorder higher in the hierarchy, and the term *mutual exclusionary relationship* to describe the mutually exclusive relationship between disorders that exists when there is a single feature that determines which of two disorders (with an otherwise common set of features) should be diagnosed.

HISTORICAL REVIEW

According to Foulds (1976), allusions to a hierarchical ranking can be found as early as 1845, when Ernst Von Feuchtersleben wrote: "Every psychosis is, at the same time, a neurosis . . . but every neurosis is not a psychosis." Even though his use of the terms *psychosis* and *neurosis* differed from current use, it is clear that a hierarchical relationship was being described. Implicit in Kraepelin's classifications (beginning in 1883, with the final edition in 1919) are hierarchical exclusionary relationships among the classes of disorders, based on the range of symptomatic expression. Highest in the exclusionary hierarchy are the organic psychoses; if there is evidence of an organic etiology in addition to the psychotic and neurotic symptoms, organicity takes precedence over all disorders lower in the hierarchy, and all psychotic and neurotic symptoms are considered features of the organic disturbance. Next in the exclusionary hierarchy is schizophrenia. The position of schizophrenia in the hierarchy is the basis for the concept of the pathognomonic nature of the Schneiderian first-rank symptoms (Schneider 1959); that is, the presence of any of these symptoms excludes a diagnosis of a manic-depressive illness by virtue of the fact that schizophrenia takes precedence over manic-depressive illness, even if the full picture of manic-depressive illness is present.

An examination of DSM-I (American Psychiatric Association 1952) provides examples of the different ways in which the hierarchical relationships among disorders were depicted. Like its Kraepelinian precursors, most of the hierarchical structure is implicit in the order in which the disorders are listed in the classification. Disorders caused by or associated with impairment of brain tissue function (i.e., acute brain disorders and chronic brain disorders) are listed first and, therefore, at the top of the hierarchy. The remaining classes of disorders are ranked in order of the severity of the "reaction of the personality, in its struggle for adjustment to internal and external stresses." Psychoses, which include schizophrenic, affective, and paranoid reactions, are the highest ranked of the nonorganic disorders. This is followed by psychoneuroses, the personality disturbances (which include drug and alcohol addiction), and the transient situational reactions.

This implicit hierarchy was not always strictly followed. In some situations, DSM-I allowed the assignment of multiple diagnoses that violated the basic hierarchy; for example, drug intoxication and depressive reaction were allowed to be diagnosed together. In other situations, some exclusionary relationships, the precursors to exclusion rules in diagnostic criteria, were explicitly specified. Some of these were mentioned in the descriptions of disorders (for example, alcohol addiction is given only in those cases "without recognizable underlying disorder"), whereas some were described in the section giving guidelines to the recording of psychiatric conditions (for example, psychoneurotic and psychotic reactions cannot occur together).

In addition, disorders within certain classes were considered to be mutually exclusive. For example, "only one type of psychoneurotic reaction can be used as a diagnosis, even in the presence of symptoms of another type . . . the diagnosis being based on the predominant type, followed by a statement of its manifestations, including symptoms of the other types of reactions." Therefore, a patient with predominantly depressive symptoms and some anxiety symptoms would be diagnosed as having "depressive reaction with anxiety symptoms." Overall, while it is clear that DSM-I was designed with many hierarchical and mutual exclusionary relationships in mind, these relationships were not always consistently applied or made explicit.

Jaspers (1962) was the first to identify formally the concept of a hierarchical exclusionary relationship among diagnoses and to use the term *diagnostic hierarchy* with his proposal for a synthesis of disease entities. His system included a hierarchical exclusionary ordering between three groups of disorders, which roughly correspond to organic, psychotic, and neurotic-personality disorders. Jaspers believed that a basic principle of medical diagnosis is that all of the disease phenomena should be characterized by a single diagnosis and viewed the convention of hierarchical exclusion as a means to that end. He wrote:

> Where a number of different phenomena co-exist, the question arises which of these should be preferred for diagnostic purposes so that the remaining phenomena can be considered secondary or accidental. . . . The phenomena which occur in their own right in the subsequent

groups of our schema also occur in the previous groups and are then devalued either to symptoms of the . . . basic [psychotic] process or to unimportant phenomena. . . . Thus in diagnosis, the previous group always has preference over the latter. We diagnose neurosis and personality disorder [only] when we have no evidence of a [psychotic] process and no physical symptoms of any organic illness which could explain the whole. (pp. 611–612)

The use of a completely hierarchically structured classification was taken to its logical extreme by the work of two British clinicians, Foulds and Bedford (Foulds 1965, 1976; Foulds and Bedford 1975). They proposed a classification that differs radically from the Kraepelinian-influenced classifications such as the ICDs and DSMs, called the "personal illness model." Rather than being a classification of psychiatric disorders, this sytem consists of four "classes of personal illness" that have an explicit hierarchical exclusionary order. Unlike Jaspers (1962), Kendell (1975), Wing (Wing, Cooper, and Sartorius 1974a), and others who considered these exclusionary hierarchies to be a utilitarian convention adopted by nosologists to handle issues of comorbidity, Foulds and Bedford considered these hierarchical exclusionary relationships to be phenomena of nature with important implications in the prognosis, treatment, and course of the patient's illness. These classes of personal illness, which are based on certain characteristic symptoms, are: class 4—delusions of disintegration (highest in the hierarchy); class 3—integrated delusions; class 2—neurotic symptoms; and class 1—dysthymic states, which include anxiety, depression, and elation. It was their contention that not only does a patient with a disorder not have symptoms characteristic of disorders higher in the hierarchy, but that such a patient would necessarily have symptoms characteristic of all disorders lower in the hierarchy.

Foulds and Bedford (1975) empirically demonstrated some validity to this model by showing that, using a self-report inventory, psychiatric patients who reached a threshold score for a particular class also achieved a threshold score for all of the classes lower in the hierarchy. Their study was subsequently replicated by some investigators (Bagshaw and McPherson 1978; Bedford and Presly 1978; McPherson, Antram, Bagshaw, et al. 1977; Morey 1985), but not by others (Sturt 1981; Surtees and Kendell 1979). Sturt proposed that Foulds and Bedford's findings could be explained on the basis of an association between prevalence rates of symptoms and the total symptom score, without needing to invoke a hierarchical exclusionary ordering between classes of illness. Morey (1985, 1987) confirmed Sturt's conclusions by finding that reordering the Foulds classes according to prevalence resulted in 94% of cases fitting the assumptions of the Foulds model (as compared to 90% when using the Foulds hierarchy). However, in a cross-method validation assessment study using the Brief Psychiatric Rating Scale, Morey found that the Foulds taxonomy significantly outperformed the prevalence model, suggesting that the power of the Foulds model goes beyond the artifactual interpretation offered by Sturt and that the model be investigated further.

The developers of DSM-II (American Psychiatric Association 1968) made a decision to move toward limiting exclusionary hierarchical relationships among diagnoses and increasing comorbid diagnosis, specifically encouraging clinicians to make multiple diagnoses, "even if one is the symptomatic expression of another disorder." The need for some hierarchical exclusionary relationships was not ignored, and clinicians were admonished "not to lose sight of the rule of parsimony and diagnose more conditions than are necessary to account for the clinical picture." Unfortunately, virtually no explicit guidelines were given to help the clinician with this difficult judgment. The fundamental hierarchical exclusionary principle of Kraepelin was retained (albeit implicitly), with the nonorganic conditions being excluded by their organically induced counterparts. Most of the other hierarchical exclusionary relationships were eliminated, so that it became possible to diagnose alcoholism along with any other disorder. Even though DSM-II made no mention of the traditional hierarchical exclusionary relationship between psychoses and neuroses, in clinical practice this exclusion continued.

The development of explicit exclusion rules began with the development of specified diagnostic criteria. Diagnostic criteria for psychiatric research were first proposed in 1972 by a group at Washington University School of Medicine in St. Louis (Feighner, Robins, Guze, et al. 1972). It is important to keep in mind that these criteria were not intended to constitute a classification system for mental disorders, but rather to act as guidelines for researchers attempting to create homogeneous groups of patients. Exclusion rules were provided for 6 of the 15 disorders, the purpose being to provide boundaries between disorders so that "patients with other illnesses are not included in the group to be studied," and to permit the exclusion of "borderline and doubtful cases" (Feighner, Robins, Guze, et al. 1972). The exclusion criteria were hierarchical or mutually exclusionary. The hierarchical exclusion rules operationalized certain assumed hierarchical relationships; for example, "patients with primary or probable primary affective disorder, or with schizophrenia or probable schizophrenia, who manifest obsessive-compulsive features do not receive the additional diagnosis of obsessive compulsive neurosis." Other exclusion rules defined mutually exclusive relationships between disorders to ensure diagnostic homogeneity. For example, schizophrenia and primary affective disorders were mutually exclusive, so that primary affective disorder had an exclusion rule requiring "no preexisting schizophrenia" and schizophrenia had an exclusion rule requiring the "absence of a period of depressive or manic symptoms."

The Research Diagnostic Criteria (RDC) (Spitzer, Endicott, and Robins 1978a, 1985) modified and expanded the work of the Washington University group, establishing diagnostic criteria for 25 major diagnostic categories, with the emphasis on diagnoses of importance in the differential diagnosis of affective disorders and schizophrenia. As the criteria became increasingly more elaborate and complex, so did the exclusion criteria. While most of the exclusion criteria (as in the "Feighner criteria") served to operationalize certain hierarchical exclusionary relationships among disorders, there was no consistent terminology used to indicate these relationships; in fact, 10 different phrases (listed in Table 1) were used to express such exclusionary

Table 1. Examples of Phrases Used in the Research Diagnostic Criteria to Indicate Exclusion Rules

---

"at no time did the subject meet the full criteria for . . ."
(schizophrenia)

"none of the following criteria which suggest condition X is present"
(manic disorder, major depressive disorder)

"does not meet the criteria for . . ."
(hypomanic disorder, major depressive disorder, minor depressive disorder, unspecified functional psychosis)

"cannot be completely accounted for by any other psychiatric condition such as . . ."
(intermittent depressive disorder)

"not limited to an episode of . . ."
(panic disorder, phobic disorder)

"not limited to the two months prior to or after . . ."
(generalized anxiety disorder)

" . . . cannot be attributed to any other psychiatric condition . . ."
(labile personality)

"this diagnosis should not be made when a diagnosis of disorder X is made"
(antisocial personality)

"episode may be superimposed only if it can be distinguished from the subject's usual condition"
(minor depressive disorder)

"does not coincide with an episode of . . ."
(obsessive-compulsive disorder)

Note. Disorders in parentheses indicate in which diagnostic criteria the exclusion rule appears.

relationships. It is interesting to note that the historically fundamental hierarchical exclusionary relationship of organic mental syndromes over functional mental disorders was not included with the diagnostic criteria for each disorder. Instead, the introduction to the RDC noted:

> All of the conditions in the RDC (with the exception of Alcoholism, Drug Use Disorder, and Other Psychiatric Disorder) are to be diagnosed only when there is no likely known organic etiology for the symptoms; therefore . . . subjects should be screened to exclude those in whom known organic factors . . . may play a significant role in the development of the psychiatric disturbance.

In 1980, DSM-III was published. Following the lead of the "Feighner criteria" and the RDC, diagnostic criteria were presented for each disorder. Exclusion criteria were included in the diagnostic criteria of 60% of the DSM-III disorders (Boyd, Burke, Gruenberg, et al. 1987), with the vast majority of them indicating hierarchical exclusionary relationships. According to Spitzer and Williams (1987), these exclusion criteria reflected DSM-III hierarchical exclusionary relationships that were organized on the assumption that disorders higher in the hierarchy are more pervasive than disorders lower in the hierarchy. These relationships have been operationalized by the DSM-III exclusion criteria, so that a diagnosis ("the excluded diagnosis") is not given if its inclusion symptoms are considered to be a symptom of a more pervasive disorder. For example, social phobia has an exclusion criterion specifying that the disorder is "not due to another mental disorder, such as Major Depression," since the inclusion criterion of a "persistent irrational fear of . . . a situation in which the individual is exposed to possible scrutiny of others" was assumed to be a frequently associated feature of the more pervasive disorder, major depression.

The use of structured diagnostic interviews—for example, the Schedule for Affective Disorders and Schizophrenia (SADS) (Spitzer and Endicott 1978) and the National Institute of Mental Health (NIMH) Diagnostic Interview Schedule (DIS) (Robins, Helzer, Croughan, et al. 1981)—has facilitated research investigating the empirical validity of the DSM-III exclusion criteria by encouraging comprehensive and systematic collection of diagnostic data, while allowing for the suspension of the exclusion rules if the investigator so chooses. Boyd, Burke, Gruenberg, et al. (1987) used data from the Epidemiologic Catchment Area (ECA) program to investigate the validity of the exclusion rules by empirically testing whether the dominant disorder in a hierarchical exclusionary relationship is a "risk factor" for the excluded disorder. For example, panic disorder (the excluded disorder) cannot be diagnosed in the presence of major depression (the dominant disorder), since the panic attacks are as-sumed to be an associated feature of the major depression. So it would be expected that individuals with major depression are more likely to have panic attacks than individuals without major depression (i.e., major depression would be a risk factor for panic disorder). The study found that while the presence of a dominant disorder (e.g., major depression) greatly increased the likelihood of the presence of an excluded disorder (e.g., panic disorder), the presence of *any* DSM-III disorder increased the odds of having almost any other disorder, although to a lesser degree. They argued that, given this general tendency, the justification for a hierarchical exclusionary relationship between two disorders would be empirical studies showing that the "two disorders have the same prognosis, that they wax and wane together, and that the excluded disorder has different risk factors and responds to different treatment than it would if it occurred in the absence of the dominant disorder" (pp. 422–423).

The validity of the particular DSM-III hierarchical exclusionary relationship that gives major depression precedence over the anxiety disorders has been questioned in several studies. Breier, Charney, and Heninger (1984) conducted a retrospective study of 60 patients with panic disorder, agoraphobia, or mixed phobia and found that one-third of them had depression considerably before the onset of panic attacks. Secondary depression did not always coincide with the times of the most severe anxiety symptoms and often resolved while anxiety symptoms persisted. They concluded that the findings are consistent with a dual etiology for anxiety and depressive disorders, with an interaction effect, or with a common shared diathesis, a situation not reflected by the DSM-III hierarchical exclusionary rela-tionship.

A case-control family study by Leckman, Merikangas, Pauls, et al. (1983) examined the lifetime psychiatric diagnoses of relatives of individuals with major depression. Relatives of probands with major depression plus clear symptoms of anxiety (sufficient to meet the criteria for an anxiety disorder) were found to be at greater risk for both depression and anxiety disorders than the relatives of probands with major depression alone. The rates were equally high whether the anxiety symptoms were separate from the depressive episodes or always associated with depressive episodes, a fact that is at variance from what would be predicted from the DSM-III hierarchical relation-ship. This finding would appear to invalidate the DSM-III exclusion criterion in the anxiety disorders, which prevents the diagnosis of the anxiety disorder being made if "due to" major depression. Although this study indicates that major depression with an associated anxiety disorder appears to be a different disorder than major depression without an associated anxiety disorder, both would be diagnosed as major depression under the DSM-III exclusion rules.

The DSM-III exclusion criteria were also criticized for their lack of precision and the inconsistent way in which they are applied (Boyd, Burke, Gruenberg, et al. 1987; Spitzer and Williams 1987). These hierarchical exclusion criteria are in the form of "not due to disorder A or disorder B," meaning that when considering whether to make a diagnosis of a particular disorder, it should not be diagnosed (i.e., it should be excluded) if it is "due to" disorder A or disorder B. While this single construct is more uniform than the nine different constructs used in the RDC, it is less precise; the phrase "not due to" is not explained in DSM-III, so its meaning is left to idiosyncratic interpretation. Boyd, Burke, Gruenberg, et al. (1987) described the discussion among members of the ECA project who needed to operationalize these exclusion criteria as follows:

> Discussions . . . have attempted to operationalize the phrase ["not due to"] as meaning "not always occurring during an episode of." However, some ECA investigators take exception to the operationalization, because they interpret . . . DSM-III to mean that a disorder at one period of time might "cause" a disorder at another period of time, even if there is a symptom-free interval of many years in between. These investigators point to the possibility that a disorder such as major depression might recur, and present with panic symptoms when it recurs. In this way, an earlier episode of major depression can "cause" a subsequent episode of panic disorder. (p. 404)

Spitzer and Williams (1987) noted that some of the DSM-III exclusion principles were not applied consistently. For example, a psychotic disorder in DSM-III, such as schizophrenia, takes precedence over all of the anxiety disorders except social phobia and posttraumatic stress disorder. They also noted that, in some instances, the goal of operationalizing hierarchical exclusionary relationships was being confused with the goal of clarifying the interpretation of symptoms for the purposes of differential diagnosis. For example, the DSM-III exclusion criterion for agoraphobia lists obsessive-compulsive disorder and paranoid personality disorder as disorders that exclude a diagnosis of agoraphobia, because people with these disorders are sometimes afraid of going out of the house alone. In fact, the fear of going out of the house alone in agoraphobia is rooted in a fear of sudden incapacitation, which is quite different from a fear of contamination (as in obsessive-compulsive disorder) or a fear of being taken advantage of (as in paranoid personality disorder).

In response to these findings, it was decided that research and clinical practice would be improved by eliminating many of the DSM-III hierarchical exclusionary relationships that have prevented giving multiple diagnoses when different syndromes occur in one episode of illness. In revising DSM-III, two principles governing the appropriate use of exclusion rules were formulated (Spitzer 1987):

1. When an organic mental disorder can account for the symptoms, it preempts the diagnosis of any other disorder that could produce the same symptoms (e.g., Organic Anxiety Disorder preempts Panic Disorder).

2. When a more pervasive disorder [i.e., with a wide range of symptomatic expression,] such as Schizophrenia, commonly has [essential or] associated symptoms that are the defining symptoms of a less pervasive disorder, such as Dysthymia, only the more pervasive disorder is diagnosed if both its defining symptoms *and* associated symptoms are present. For example, only Schizophrenia (not Schizophrenia and Dysthymia) should be diagnosed when defining the symptoms of Schizophrenia are present along with chronic mild depression (which is a common associated symptom of Schizophrenia). (p. 8)

The systematic application of these principles to DSM-III-R has resulted in far fewer excluded diagnoses in DSM-III-R as compared to DSM-III. Table 2 compares the number of excluded diagnoses in the two classification systems. Note that while the number of disorders excluded by organic factors has actually increased from 22 to 24 because of a more systematic attempt to consider organic factors, there is a significant decrease in the number of disorders excluded by

Table 2. Numbers of Excluded Disorders in DSM-III-R as Compared to DSM-III for Selected Dominant Disorders

Dominant disorder	Number of excluded disorders in DSM-III	Number of excluded disorders in DSM-III-R
Schizophrenia	29	17
Organic factors	22	24
Major depression	11	5
Pervasive developmental disorder	9	11
Delirium	8	4
Bipolar disorder	8	7
Cyclothymia	8	5
Mental retardation	7	2
Dementia	7	2
Dysthymia	7	3
Antisocial personality disorder	7	3
Conduct disorder	6	3
Agoraphobia	5	1
Somatization disorder	4	2

schizophrenia (decreased from 29 to 17) and major depression (decreased from 11 to 5). Given the relationship between exclusion rules and the appearance of comorbidity (i.e., the fewer the exclusion rules, the more comorbidity), it is expected that studies determining diagnoses using DSM-III-R criteria should report higher rates of comorbidity. Researchers investigating comorbidity must therefore take care when comparing comorbidity rates between studies using different diagnostic criteria.

The criticisms concerning the validity of excluding anxiety disorders in the presence of major depression have been addressed by the elimination of most of the exclusion rules giving major depression precedence over the anxiety disorders. Table 3 indicates the differences in the exclusion rules for the anxiety disorders in DSM-III and DSM-III-R. A notable exception is generalized anxiety disorder, in which the diagnosis is not made if the anxiety symptoms occur only during the course of a mood disorder or a psychotic disorder.

A TAXONOMY OF EXCLUSIONARY RELATIONSHIPS

As discussed in the previous section, the exclusionary relationships that appear in DSM-III-R have evolved from the hierarchical exclusionary relationships implicit in the order in which Kraepelin listed the categories in his classification, to the exclusion criteria in DSM-III-R, reflecting hierarchical relationships based on the range of symptomatic expression. These exclusion criteria are of significant importance in that they are one of the primary determinants of the degree of comorbidity produced by a classification system. However, most of the exclusionary relationships in DSM-III-R are based on clinical wisdom rather than empirical findings, leading to a call for more attention to be paid to the examination of the validity of these exclusion rules (Barrett 1987; Boyd, Burke, Gruenberg, et al. 1987; Regier 1987).

A prerequisite to any research on the validity of the exclusion criteria is the establishment of precise rules that can be used in a consistent and unambiguous way. Close inspection of the exclusionary relationships contained in DSM-III-R, however, shows that the current exclusion criteria are not always consistently worded. In the revision of DSM-III, the imprecise nature of the phrase "not due to" was recognized and in most instances was replaced by a number of different phrases, including "does not meet the criteria for," "has never met the criteria for," "does not occur exclusively during the course of," "not sufficiently pervasive and persistent to warrant a diagnosis of," "not superimposed on," "not a symptom of," "it cannot be established that an organic factor initiated or maintained the disturbance," as well as some instances of the holdout "not due to." The

Table 3. Comparison of Exclusion Criteria for the Anxiety Disorders in DSM-III and DSM-III-R

Disorder	DSM-III	DSM-III-R
Panic disorder	Not due to a physical disorder or another mental disorder, such as major depression, somatization disorder, or schizophrenia.	It cannot be established that an organic factor initiated and maintained the disturbance, e.g., amphetamine or caffeine intoxication, hyperthyroidism.
Agoraphobia	Not due to a major depressive episode, obsessive-compulsive disorder, paranoid personality disorder, or schizophrenia.	No exclusions
Social phobia	Not due to another mental disorder, such as major depression or avoidant personality disorder.	If the person is under 18, the disturbance does not meet the criteria for avoidant disorder of childhood or adolescence.
Simple phobia	Not due to another mental disorder, such as schizophrenia or obsessive-compulsive disorder.	No exclusions
Obsessive-compulsive disorder	Not due to another mental disorder, such as Tourette's disorder, schizophrenia, major depression, or organic mental disorder.	No exclusions
Posttraumatic stress disorder	No exclusions	No exclusions
Generalized anxiety disorder	Not due to another mental disorder, such as depressive disorder or schizophrenia.	The disturbance does not occur only during the course of a mood disorder or a psychotic disorder. It cannot be established that an organic factor initiated and maintained the disturbance, e.g., hyperthyroidism, caffeine intoxication.

definitions of most of these phrases (exceptions being "it cannot be established" and "not exclusively during the course of," which are discussed in "Use of This Manual" in DSM-III-R), as well as the distinctions among them, are not specified, potentially leading to incorrect speculation and confusion. We propose a taxonomy of exclusionary relationships, which, as shown in Figure 1, can be arranged hierarchically (in a class membership sense). For each class of exclusionary relationship, we recommend standard phraseology that can serve to facilitate research on the validity of these criteria and that we hope will be considered for use in DSM-IV.

As defined earlier, a hierarchical exclusionary relationship between disorder A and disorder B implies that if certain features of both disorder A and disorder B are present during an episode of illness, only disorder A is diagnosed. These relationships are operationalized in exclusion criteria that appear *only* in the set of criteria for the excluded diagnosis (i.e., disorder B); there is no mention of this exclusionary relationship in the criteria of the dominant disorder (i.e., disorder A). For example, there is a hierarchical exclusionary relationship between schizophrenia and delusional disorder, such that delusional disorder is excluded by schizophrenia, the dominant disorder. This relationship is operationalized by the exclusion criterion in the criteria set for delusional disorder: "has never met criterion A for Schizophrenia"; there is no reference to delusional disorder in the criteria for schizophrenia.

Hierarchical exclusionary relationships can be further subgrouped based on the presence or absence of an established organic

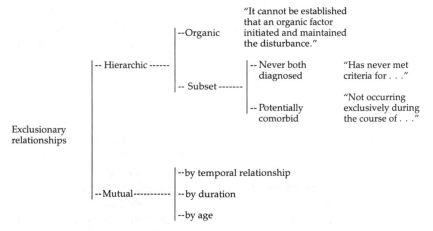

Figure 1. The proposed taxonomy for exclusionary relationships with suggested phraseology.

etiology. Even though an organic hierarchical exclusionary relationship can be considered to be an example of a disorder with a more broad symptom set (i.e., psychological symptoms plus organic factor) taking precedence over a less broad symptom set (i.e., psychological symptoms without an organic factor), the clinical importance of ruling out organic factors warrants special consideration of organic exclusion rules. As has been discussed, the principle of organic exclusion has its origins in the original Kraepelinian classification schemes. In DSM-III-R, three different wordings are used to indicate this relationship: "not due to a physical disorder" (e.g., chronic urinary tract infection causing functional enuresis); "not occurring exclusively during known central nervous system disease" (e.g., Huntington's chorea causing a syndrome resembling Tourette's disorder); and "it cannot be established that an organic factor initiated and maintained the disturbance." This latter phrase is preferred because it serves to operationalize the process of determining whether there are any known organic factors. We therefore propose that "it cannot be established . . ." be used uniformly to indicate the concept of causality by a physical condition or psychoactive substance.

While this phrase has operationalized some aspects of the process of determining the presence of a known organic factor, there remain many problems with the existing organic-nonorganic distinction in DSM-III-R, most importantly the erroneous implication that the etiology of a "nonorganic" disorder is necessarily psychological. We have proposed a radical new reorganization of the classification to address this problem (Spitzer, Williams, First, et al. 1989).

Nonorganic hierarchical exclusionary relationships can be further subgrouped, based on the potential for the dominant and excluded disorders to both be diagnosed in the same individual. For a few of these exclusionary relationships, by definition the two disorders cannot ever *both* be diagnosed even if the two disorders occur at distinctly different points in the individual's lifetime, so that if the criteria have *ever* been met for the dominant disorder, the criteria can *never* be met for the excluded disorder. For example, bipolar disorder excludes major depression, and schizophrenia excludes delusional disorder by this principle; if the criteria are ever met for bipolar disorder (i.e., if a manic syndrome has ever been present), then the diagnosis of major depression is forever preempted. For this type of relationship, we propose the phrase "[the disturbance] has never met criteria for. . . ."

For the majority of the hierarchical exclusionary relationships, there is the potential for both the dominant and excluded disorders to be diagnosed in the same individual. In these cases, the exclusionary relationship is relevant only in situations in which the excluded disorder occurs exclusively during the course of the dominant disorder. Put another way, both the dominant and excluded disorders can be diagnosed in the same individual only if, at some point, the excluded disorder occurs in the *absence* of the dominant disorder. For example, dementia is preempted by delirium for the same episode of illness because the essential features of dementia (memory loss and other forms of cognitive impairment) are included as either essential or associated features of delirium. However, since the exclusion criterion states that dementia is diagnosed only if it is "not occurring exclusively during the course of delirium," if there is a distinct period of time when dementia is present without the delirium, then dementia can be diagnosed in addition to the delirium. We recommend the phrase that is most often used in DSM-III-R, namely, "not occurring exclusively during the course of."

Note that a criterion of the form "if another Axis I disorder is present, symptom X is not related to it," while similar in form to the exclusion rules, does not define an exclusionary relationship but rather restricts the intended meaning of the defining criteria. For example, one of the DSM-III-R criteria for obsessive-compulsive disorder states that "if another Axis I disorder is present, the content of the obsession is unrelated to it; e.g., the ideas, thoughts, impulses, or images are not about food in the presence of an Eating Disorder . . . ." This does not define an exclusionary relationship between the two disorders because an eating disorder and obsessive-compulsive disorder can co-occur in the same individual if the criteria for each are met. In a number of cases, DSM-III-R uses an exclusion criterion when a nonexclusionary restricting definition would be more appropriate. For example, one of the criteria for body dysmorphic disorder states "occurrence not exclusively during the course of Anorexia Nervosa or Transsexualism." It is, however, possible, albeit unlikely, to have body dysmorphic disorder exclusively during the course of either anorexia nervosa or transsexualism, as long as the focus of preoccupation is with a part of the body not related to either anorexia nervosa or transsexualism. All of the exclusionary relationships in DSM-III-R that should be restricting definitions are indicated in Table 4 (which lists all of the DSM-III-R exclusionary relationships).

A mutual exclusionary relationship between disorder A and disorder B implies that if the features for both disorder A and disorder B are present, disorder A is diagnosed under certain conditions and disorder B is diagnosed under other conditions. This type of relationship is employed to delimit disorders that share essential features from one another, and form the basis for the decision trees in DSM-III-R (First, Williams, and Spitzer 1987). For example, although schizophrenia and schizophreniform disorder do not include explicit criteria to exclude one another, the duration criterion in each disorder func-

Table 4.   Hierarchical Exclusionary Relationships in DSM-III-R

Mental Retardation

--possbl-co-->	Developmental Articulation Disorder
--nevr-both-->	Reactive Attachment Disorder

Pervasive Developmental Disorder (Autistic Disorder and Pervasive Developmental Disorder Not Otherwise Specified)

--nevr-both-->	Developmental Articulation Disorder
--nevr-both-->	Developmental Expressive Language Disorder
--nevr-both-->	Developmental Receptive Language Disorder
--nevr-both-->	Attention-Deficit Hyperactivity Disorder
--nevr-both-->	Separation Anxiety Disorder
--nevr-both-->	Overanxious Disorder
--nevr-both-->	Pica
--nevr-both-->	Reactive Attachment Disorder
--nevr-both-->	Stereotypy/Habit Disorder
--nevr-both-->	Schizophrenia [only if no prominent delusions or hallucinations]
--nevr-both-->	Schizotypal Personality Disorder

Conduct Disorder

--possbl-co-->	Oppositional Defiant Disorder
--possbl-co-->	Intermittent Explosive Disorder
--possbl-co-->	Kleptomania

Anorexia

Body Dysmorphic Disorder
(incorrectly listed as excluded in DSM-III-R)

Transsexualism

--nevr-both-->	Gender Identity Disorder of Adolescence or Adulthood, Nontranssexual Type
	Body Dysmorphic Disorder
	(incorrectly listed as excluded in DSM-III-R)
--nevr-both-->	Transvestic Fetishism

Gender Identity Disorder of Adolescence or Adulthood, Nontranssexual Type

--possbl-co-->	Transvestic Fetishism

Tic Disorders

--possbl-co-->	Stereotypy/Habit Disorder

Table 4. (continued)

Organic Mental Disorders/Physical Disorders

--organic---->	Specific Developmental Disorders
--organic---->	Encopresis
--organic---->	Enuresis
--organic---->	Tic Disorders
--organic---->	Schizophrenia
--organic---->	Delusional Disorder
--organic---->	Brief Reactive Psychosis
--organic---->	Schizophreniform Disorder
--organic---->	Schizoaffective Disorder
--organic---->	Bipolar Disorder
--organic---->	Cyclothymia
--organic---->	Major Depression
--organic---->	Dysthymia
--organic---->	Panic Disorder
--organic---->	Generalized Anxiety Disorder
--organic---->	Psychogenic Amnesia
--organic---->	Depersonalization Disorder
--organic---->	Vaginismus
--organic---->	Dream Anxiety Disorder
--organic---->	Sleep Terror Disorder
--organic---->	Sleepwalking Disorder
--organic---->	Intermittent Explosive Disorder

Delirium

--possbl-co-->	Dementia
--possbl-co-->	Organic Delusional Disorder
--possbl-co-->	Organic Hallucinosis
--possbl-co-->	Organic Anxiety Syndrome

Dementia

--possbl-co-->	Amnestic Syndrome
--possbl-co-->	Organic Personality Syndrome

Amnestic Syndrome

--possbl-co-->	Intoxication
--possbl-co-->	Withdrawal

Organic Delusional Disorder

--possbl-co-->	Intoxication
--possbl-co-->	Withdrawal

Organic Hallucinosis

--possbl-co-->	Intoxication
--possbl-co-->	Withdrawal

Table 4.   (continued)

Major Depression

--possbl-co-->   Oppositional Defiant Disorder
--possbl-co-->   Brief Reactive Psychosis
--possbl-co-->   Generalized Anxiety Disorder
--possbl-co-->   Undifferentiated Somatoform Disorder
--possbl-co-->   Sexual Dysfunctions

Dysthymia

--possbl-co-->   Oppositional Defiant Disorder
--possbl-co-->   Generalized Anxiety Disorder
--possbl-co-->   Undifferentiated Somatoform Disorder

Panic Disorder

--nevr-both-->   Agoraphobia Without History of Panic Disorder
                   Undifferentiated Somatoform Disorder
                   (incorrectly listed as excluded in DSM-III-R)
--possbl-co-->   Depersonalization Disorder

Agoraphobia Without History of Panic Disorder (with limited symptom attacks)

--possbl-co-->   Depersonalization Disorder

Body Dysmorphic Disorder

                   Undifferentiated Somatoform Disorder
                   (incorrectly listed as excluded in DSM-III-R)
--possbl-co-->   Psychological Factors Affecting Physical Condition

Conversion Disorder

                   Undifferentiated Somatoform Disorder
                   (incorrectly listed as excluded in DSM-III-R)
--possbl-co-->   Psychological Factors Affecting Physical Condition

Hypochondriasis

--possbl-co-->   Undifferentiated Somatoform Disorder
--possbl-co-->   Psychological Factors Affecting Physical Condition

Somatization Disorder

--possbl-co-->   Undifferentiated Somatoform Disorder
--possbl-co-->   Psychological Factors Affecting Physical Condition

Somatoform Pain Disorder

--possbl-co-->   Conversion Disorder
                   Undifferentiated Somatoform Disorder
                   (incorrectly listed as excluded in DSM-III-R)
--possbl-co-->   Psychological Factors Affecting Physical Condition

Table 4. (continued)

Undifferentiated Somatoform Disorder

--possbl-co-->   Psychological Factors Affecting Physical Condition

Multiple Personality Disorder

--nevr-both-->   Psychogenic Fugue
--nevr-both-->   Psychogenic Amnesia

Vaginismus

         Undifferentiated Somatoform Disorder
         (incorrectly listed as excluded in DSM-III-R)
--possbl-co-->   Dyspareunia

Insomnia

         Undifferentiated Somatoform Disorder
         (incorrectly listed as excluded in DSM-III-R)

Hypersomnia

         Undifferentiated Somatoform Disorder
         (incorrectly listed as excluded in DSM-III-R)

Sleep-Wake Schedule Disorder

         Undifferentiated Somatoform Disorder
         (incorrectly listed as excluded in DSM-III-R)
--possbl-co-->   Insomnia
--possbl-co-->   Hypersomnia

Dream Anxiety Disorder

         Undifferentiated Somatoform Disorder
         (incorrectly listed as excluded in DSM-III-R)
--possbl-co-->   Insomnia

Sleep Terror Disorder

         Undifferentiated Somatoform Disorder
         (incorrectly listed as excluded in DSM-III-R)
--possbl-co-->   Insomnia

Sleepwalking Disorder

         Undifferentiated Somatoform Disorder
         (incorrectly listed as excluded in DSM-III-R)
--possbl-co-->   Insomnia

Any Specific Axis I Disorder

--possbl-co-->   Adjustment Disorder

Evidence for Comorbidity: Population-Based Studies

Chapter 6

Comorbidity of Affective and Anxiety Disorders in the NIMH Epidemiologic Catchment Area Program

Darrel A. Regier, M.D., M.P.H.
Jack D. Burke, Jr., M.D., M.P.H.
Kimberly Christie Burke, M.S.

THE CO-OCCURRENCE OF multiple symptoms in the same person has been an issue of long-standing importance to physicians. The challenge of differential diagnosis has been to recognize symptoms in several different physiologic systems that may be part of a common underlying illness. Hence the presence of a fever, skin rash, joint pain, headache, and irritability in many viral illnesses does not require multiple dermatologic, rheumatological, neurologic, and psychiatric diagnoses but one etiologically based infectious disease diagnosis. However, even before viruses were discovered, careful observations of symptoms and clinical course permitted definition of syndromes and diagnoses.

A parsimonious diagnosis that will encompass multiple symptoms is a more efficient way of describing clinical phenomena. Careful observations of the co-occurrence of symptoms, and the formulation of hypotheses that such symptoms will tend to occur together as syndromes in future cases, are an important use of the scientific method in medicine. The validity of these syndrome and diagnostic hypotheses is determined in part by their usefulness in predicting clinical course and response to treatment. Robins and Guze (1970)

113

described several approaches to establishing the validity of psychiatric diagnoses. These include the following steps: (1) a careful clinical description, (2) laboratory studies, (3) development of exclusion criteria to delimit the index disorder from other disorders, (4) study of longitudinal clinical course, and (5) an assessment of the degree to which these illnesses are shown to run in families.

Despite the preference for single, parsimonious diagnostic categories, effective treatments for many acute illnesses and longer life expectancy increase the probability of multiple diagnoses being found in the same person. In statistical terms, longer exposure periods increase the probability of additional illnesses—some of which may appear at the same time. In lay terms, if a man is itching, he may have lice or he may have fleas, but it is also possible that he could have both. Bringing the analogy closer to home, where clear etiologic agents are harder to find, if a patient has a symptom of psychomotor agitation, the patient may have a major depressive disorder or a generalized anxiety disorder but it is also possible that the patient could have both.

Epidemiologic research in community populations has the potential for complementing the observations and descriptions carried out in clinical settings, if certain conditions are met. Of particular importance is coverage of the same symptoms and use of the same diagnostic criteria in both community and clinical settings. If this central condition can be met, then the possibility exists for clinically relevant epidemiology research. The clinical relevance of epidemiologic research has been cogently summarized by Morris (1964) in his classic book *The Uses of Epidemiology*. Of particular significance for this chapter are the following: (1) the use of community diagnoses to determine base rates, (2) the determination of individual risk for developing a disorder, (3) the identification of syndromes, and (4) the completion of the clinical picture by identifying mild and subclinical cases in the community. The other three potential uses—the study of historical change in rates over time, the identification of causes, and the determination of the working of health services—will be given less attention in this chapter.

The possibility of using the same diagnostic criteria in community epidemiologic studies and clinical studies was given a major boost by the publication of the St. Louis or Feighner criteria (Feighner, Robins, Guze, et al. 1972), followed in rapid succession by the Research Diagnostic Criteria (RDC) of Spitzer, Endicott, and Robins (1978a) as well as the criteria of the 1980 edition of the *Diagnostic and Statistical Manual of Mental Disorders* (DSM-III) (American Psychiatric Association 1980). Diagnostic criteria based more on observable symptoms, rather than relying on etiologic inference, greatly increased the possibility of reliable application in multiple settings. The subsequent step of incorporating such criteria in semistructured clinical interviews—such as the Schedule for Affective Disorders and Schizophrenia (SADS) (Endicott and Spitzer 1978) for clinicians and the highly structured National Institute of Mental Health (NIMH) Diagnostic Interview Schedule (DIS) (National Institute of Mental Health 1981) for lay interviewers—was an essential part of "operationalizing" the criteria for use in clinical and epidemiologic research studies. Application of the DSM-III criteria via the DIS was an essential component of the Epidemiologic Catchment Area (ECA) study, which will serve as the data base for the remaining discussion.

METHODS

Because the objectives, design, and methods of the NIMH ECA program have been described previously in considerable detail (Eaton and Kessler 1985; Eaton, Holzer, VonKorff, et al. 1984; Regier, Myers, Kramer, et al. 1984), only the essential facts relevant to this chapter will be discussed.

The NIMH ECA has now completed interviews with more than 20,000 community and institutionalized adult subjects (age 18 and over) in five sites including part or all of New Haven, Connecticut; Baltimore, Maryland; St. Louis, Missouri; Durham, North Carolina; and Los Angeles, California. At least two interviews using the DIS were conducted at 1-year intervals to elicit the presence of symptoms of sufficient severity, duration, and combination to meet selected DSM-III criteria. The presence of these criteria were determined by subject recall for periods extending from 2 weeks prior to interview to the person's entire lifetime. In addition, information was collected on the use of specialty mental health, general medical, and other human services over comparable time intervals.

Data from all five sites have recently been merged and standardized to the 1980 U.S. population to provide a single best estimate of national 1-month prevalence rates for specific mental disorders (Regier, Boyd, Burke, et al. 1988). To study the rates of individual disorders, DSM-III diagnostic exclusion rules were not used in collecting the symptom information from subjects who potentially could have multiple diagnoses. Such hierarchical rules could be applied in the analysis if certain assumptions were made about what the criteria "due to another disorder" can mean in operational terms. For example, the diagnosis of panic disorder could be suppressed if schizophrenia were also diagnosed. However, in this chapter we will use the combined five-site data, without diagnostic hierarchies, standardized to the U.S population. The estimates presented in this chapter represent data for all household respondents from all five sites in the ECA. These summary rates have been determined using a set of weights that standardize the five-site sample to the 1980 U.S. adult population on the basis of age, sex, and race/ethnicity (Regier, Boyd, Burke, et al. 1988).

RESULTS

Prevalence of Disorders

Any study of comorbidity should begin by understanding the base rates of disorders in the community. Since disorders with high prevalence rates are more likely to be found in a given community subject, it follows that two disorders with high prevalence rates are more likely to be found in the same person than two disorders with lower prevalence rates. Hence, it is first necessary to identify the random probability of two disorders occurring together in the population before one can begin to assess any increased probability of a second disorder occurring if a first is already present.

It is not sufficient to look at the co-occurrence of disorders in patients who come to clinical settings to determine base-rate comorbidity. A strong bias exists for individuals with multiple disorders to present themselves to clinical settings (Berkson 1946). As can be seen from the ECA study, individuals with specific clinical disorders do not automatically request treatment. In the ECA study, about 30% of those with a 6-month diagnosis of any affective disorder and about 20% of those with any anxiety disorder sought mental health services over the same prior 6-month period (Regier and Burke 1987). Other analyses have shown that increases in the total burden of symptoms and disability levels are associated with higher service use rates (Shapiro, Skinner, Kessler, et al. 1984). As a result of this bias, the co-occurrence of such disorders as panic disorder and agoraphobia have been shown to be much greater in clinical settings than in the ECA community study (Boyd, Regier, and Burke 1985).

The 6-month and lifetime prevalence rates for the affective disorders are reported in Table 1. Major depressive episode is found in 3.0% of the population over 6 months and in 5.8% on a lifetime basis. Bipolar illness, based on the presence of a manic episode only, was found in 0.5% of the population at 6 months and in 0.8% of the population on a lifetime basis. This table also demonstrates that virtually all of the respondents with a 6-month diagnosis of bipolar illness also had major depression, whereas one-quarter of those respondents with bipolar illness on a lifetime basis (0.2/0.8) had a manic episode only.

Dysthymic disorder, which in DSM-III requires a 2-year duration of symptoms compared to 2 weeks for major depressive episode and 1 week for manic episode, was diagnosed on a lifetime basis only. However, because of the greater likelihood of recalling recent dysthymic symptoms and to avoid a serious undercount of this affective disorder, many of the ECA analyses have included dysthymia in the 1-month and the 6-month overall categories of any affective disorder. About one-quarter (24%) of those respondents with a diagnosis of dysthymia have a 6-month diagnosis of major depression. Almost one-half (48%) of those respondents with dysthymia have a lifetime diagnosis of major depression; this comorbidity has been referred to as double depression (Keller and Shapiro 1982). In the ECA, overall rates of any affective disorder are 5.8% for the 6-month period and 8.3% lifetime.

Table 1 also reports the 6-month and lifetime prevalence rates for the anxiety disorders. As a group, these disorders have the highest overall prevalence rate of any in the study, with a 6-month rate of 8.9% and a lifetime rate of 14.6%. The major component of these relatively high rates are the phobic disorders, which contribute 7.7% to the 6-month rate and 12.5% to the lifetime rate. These rates are obviously subject to the threshold of the A criteria (a persistent

Table 1. Prevalence of Affective and Anxiety Disorders DIS/DSM-III Diagnoses, Rates per 100

	Six-month	Lifetime
Major depressive episode	3.0 (0.2)	5.8 (0.3)
Unipolar illness only	2.5 (0.2)	5.2 (0.2)
Bipolar illness	0.5 (0.1)	0.8 (0.1)
Dysthymic disorder	3.3 (0.2)	3.3 (0.2)
Without major depression	2.5 (0.2)	1.7 (0.1)
With major depression	0.8 (0.1)	1.6 (0.1)
Any affective disorder	5.8 (0.3)	8.3 (0.3)
Panic disorder	0.8 (0.1)	1.6 (0.1)
Phobic disorder	7.7 (0.3)	12.5 (0.3)
Obsessive-compulsive disorder	1.5 (0.1)	2.5 (0.2)
Any anxiety disorder	8.9 (0.3)	14.6 (0.4)
Any anxiety and any affective disorder	1.9 (0.1)	3.6 (0.2)
Any anxiety or any affective disorder	12.8 (0.4)	19.2 (0.4)

Note. These estimates are for all household respondents in the National Institute of Mental Health Epidemiologic Catchment Area Program and are standardized to the 1980 U.S. Census on the basis of age, sex, and race/ethnicity. Standard errors are in parentheses. DIS = Diagnostic Interview Schedule.

irrational fear of, and compelling desire to avoid. . .) and the B criteria (significant distress and recognition that the fear is excessive or unreasonable) of DSM-III and to their operational interpretation in the DIS. In addition, there were significantly higher rates at two of the five sites, which may involve systematic threshold differences in the training of interviewers—a methodological issue that remains unclear at this time. In the ECA, panic disorder is found at a rate of 0.8% for a 6-month diagnosis and 1.6% for a lifetime diagnosis. Obsessive-compulsive disorder rates are somewhat higher in the community study than were expected from clinical experience; in the ECA, the 6-month prevalence rate was found to be 1.5% and the lifetime rate was 2.5%.

Table 2 reports the prevalence of the affective and anxiety disorders for males and females separately. In the ECA, the higher rate for any affective disorder for females (10.7%), approximately twice the 5.4% rate found in males, is consistent with the well-known belief that women report higher rates of the affective disorders compared to men.

Prevalence of Multiple Disorders

In an article by Boyd, Burke, Gruenberg, et al. (1984), it was shown that the odds of having a 1-month anxiety disorder if one had a

Table 2. Prevalence of Affective and Anxiety Disorders, by Sex, DIS/DSM-III Lifetime Diagnoses, Rates per 100

	Male	Female
Major depressive episode	3.5 (0.3)	7.9 (0.4)
Unipolar illness only	3.0 (0.2)	7.2 (0.4)
Bipolar illness	0.7 (0.1)	0.9 (0.1)
Dysthymic disorder	2.2 (0.2)	4.2 (0.2)
Without major depression	1.4 (0.2)	2.0 (0.2)
With major depression	0.8 (0.1)	2.2 (0.1)
Any affective disorder	5.4 (0.3)	10.7 (0.4)
Panic disorder	0.9 (0.2)	2.1 (0.2)
Phobic disorder	8.4 (0.4)	15.8 (0.5)
Obsessive-compulsive disorder	1.9 (0.2)	3.0 (0.2)
Any anxiety disorder	10.2 (0.4)	18.6 (0.5)
Any anxiety and any affective disorder	2.2 (0.2)	4.8 (0.3)

Note. These estimates are for all household respondents in the National Institute of Mental Health Epidemiologic Catchment Area Program and are standardized to the 1980 U.S. Census on the basis of age, sex, and race/ethnicity. Standard errors are in parentheses. DIS = Diagnostic Interview Schedule.

1-month major depressive episode ranged from 9.0 for simple phobia, to 10.8 for obsessive-compulsive disorder, to 15.3 for agoraphobia, and up to 18.8 for panic disorder. That is, someone with a major depressive episode has from 9 to 19 times the odds of having an anxiety disorder compared with someone who does not have a major depressive episode. From these data it is relatively clear that anxiety and depressive disorders are not randomly distributed in the population but have a higher probability of occurring in the same individuals.

Table 1 reports that 1.9% of the population have both an anxiety disorder and an affective disorder in a 6-month period, and that 3.6% of the population report the presence of both disorders in their lifetime. Because of the lower base rate of affective disorders, this comorbid group represents 33% of those with affective disorders and 21% of those with anxiety disorders over a 6-month period. Over the course of the lifetime, the comorbid group represents 43% of those with affective disorders and 25% of those with anxiety disorders. These prevalence rates for these disorders are also reported by sex in Table 2.

In Table 3, the lifetime prevalence rates for the co-occurrence of major depressive episode and the anxiety disorders with substance use disorders are reported. The highest lifetime prevalence rate occurs for those ECA respondents with both alcohol abuse/dependence and

Table 3. Co-Occurrence of Selected DIS/DSM-III Mental Disorders, Rates per 100

Disorder	Lifetime Prevalence		
	Total	Male	Female
Major depressive episode with alcohol abuse/ dependence	1.2 (0.1)	1.5 (0.2)	0.9 (0.1)
Major depressive episode with drug abuse/dependence	1.2 (0.1)	1.0 (0.1)	1.3 (0.1)
Anxiety disorders with alcohol abuse/dependence	2.5 (0.2)	3.6 (0.3)	1.6 (0.1)
Anxiety disorders with drug abuse/dependence	1.7 (0.2)	1.7 (0.2)	1.6 (0.2)
Alcohol abuse/dependence with drug abuse/dependence	2.7 (0.2)	4.2 (0.3)	1.4 (0.2)

Note. These estimates are for all household respondents in the National Institute of Mental Health Epidemiologic Catchment Area Program and are standardized to the 1980 U.S. Census on the basis of age, sex, and race/ethnicity. Standard errors are in parentheses. DIS = Diagnostic Interview Schedule.

drug abuse/dependence at 2.7%. The prevalence rate for those respondents with an anxiety disorder and alcohol abuse/dependence is almost as high at 2.5%.

DISCUSSION

There has been a major benefit of having epidemiologic data on symptoms and diagnoses that did not follow a theoretically designed diagnostic hierarchy incorporated in DSM-III. There is now an empirical data base to look at the co-occurrence of disorders before deciding whether one disorder is due to another. The value of this approach was immediately apparent after the Boyd, Burke, Gruenberg, et al. (1984) article, and a change in approach is reflected in the criteria without hierarchies in DSM-III-R (American Psychiatric Association 1987). At this time in the history of psychopathology research, there is no benefit in suppressing information on the co-occurrence of multiple disorders. Such complex diagnoses may represent multiple separate diagnoses, or they may represent different syndromes, or, at the very least, different subtypes of a disorder that may have different treatment responses.

A careful review of several international studies examining the prevalence of affective and anxiety disorders indicates that the prevalence rates found in the ECA are similar. Table 4 reports the 1-month prevalence rates for the affective and anxiety disorders found in five different international studies using the Present State Examination— London (Bebbington, Hurry, Tennant, et al. 1981); Australia (Henderson, Duncan-Jones, Byrne, et al. 1979); Athens (Mavreas, Beis, Mouyias, et al. 1986); Edinburgh (Dean, Surtees, and Sashidharian 1983); and Uganda (Orley and Wing 1979).

There are many issues raised by the comorbidity of mental disorders. It has been suggested by Kendler and Eaves (1986) that there may be a common genetic etiology or predisposition for both affective and anxiety disorders in which different environmental exposures are responsible for expression of one or both of the disorders. It is also possible that one disorder could cause another disorder (e.g., individuals with anxiety disorders becoming depressed over their agoraphobic condition). Another consideration is whether or not there could be a subtype of major depression with onset before age 30 associated with an anxiety disorder, such as panic disorder. In this chapter, we began to investigate the prevalence of the affective and anxiety disorders both as single occurring disorders and as co-occurring disorders. Clearly, the prevalence of having more than one mental disorder is not uncommon in the community, and there are obviously many unanswered questions regarding the comorbidity of mental

Table 4. International Epidemiologic Studies: One-Month Prevalence Rates for Selected Mental Disorders, in Percentages

Disorder	Place of study						
	US/ECA	London	Australia	Athens	Edinburgh	Uganda
Any DIS/DSM-III disorder	15.4	—	—	—	—	—
Total mental disorders[a]	11.2	10.9	9.0	16.0	8.7	25.0
Affective disorders	5.1	7.0	4.8	7.4	5.9	18.9
Anxiety disorders	7.3	2.9	3.5	8.2	2.8	3.4

Note. ECA = Epidemiologic Catchment Area; DIS = Diagnostic Interview Schedule.
[a] Except substance use, cognitive impairment, or antisocial personality.

disorders that may be addressed with further analyses of the ECA data and by follow-up studies of cohorts identified in this study. Future epidemiologic studies on the comorbidity of disorders in the community should include investigations that would complement the studies being done with clinical populations.

Chapter 7

Comorbidity of Anxiety and Depression in the Zurich Cohort Study of Young Adults

Jules Angst, M.D.
Margarete Vollrath, Ph.D.
Kathleen R. Merikangas, Ph.D.
Cecile Ernst, M.D., Ph.D.

W ITH THE INTRODUCTION of the third edition of the *Diagnostic and Statistical Manual of Mental Disorders* (DSM-III) (American Psychiatric Association 1980) classification of mood and anxiety disorders, the relationship between anxiety and depression has received renewed attention in psychiatric research. Although the overlap in symptoms of anxiety and depression is well known (Hamilton 1986), the existence and prevalence of pure forms of depression and anxiety and their overlap remain controversial. Reviews of the evidence regarding the association between anxiety and depression provide no clear evidence favoring either the unitary or dichotomous classification of these two disorders. However, the lack of consistent findings across studies could be partially attributed to semantic inconsistencies and methodological differences concerning sampling and procedures

This project was supported by grant 3.948.0.85 from the Swiss National Science Foundation; and also supported by a Research Scientist Development Award (MH-00499) from the United States Public Health Service, National Institute of Mental Health (Dr. Merikangas).

123

(Angst and Dobler-Mikola 1985; Stavrakaki and Vargo 1986).

Data from the longitudinal epidemiologic cohort study of young adults in Zurich, Switzerland (Angst, Dobler-Mikola, and Binder 1984) provide information on (1) the external validity of concepts derived from clinical samples to that of the general population; and (2) the validity of the association of anxiety and depression through the longitudinal assessment of diagnostic stability. Previous cross-sectional analyses of the data from the 1981 interview of this sample showed a strong overlap between anxiety disorders and major or recurrent brief depression (Angst and Dobler-Mikola 1985). This chapter will examine the association between anxiety and depression with cross-sectional interview data from the same subjects in 1986 and longitudinal data over a 7-year follow-up from 1979 to 1986.

OVERVIEW OF METHODOLOGY

The subjects for the study, which began in 1978, consist of a cohort of 292 males and 299 females aged 19 to 20 from the Canton of Zurich in Switzerland (Figure 1). The sample was selected according to scores on the 90-item Hopkins Symptom Checklist (SCL-90) (Derogatis 1977) in 1978. Subjects with high scores (i.e., greater than the 85th percentile) comprised two-thirds of the sample. The remainder of subjects were randomly selected from those who scored below the 85th percentile on the SCL-90. The two groups comprised the high- and low-risk groups, respectively. The subjects were interviewed at three

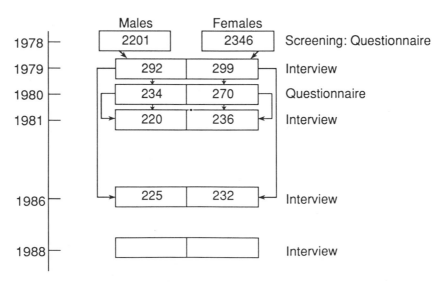

Figure 1.   Breakdown of cohort for Zurich longitudinal study.

times with a semistructured interview, the Structured Psychopathological Interview and Rating of the Social Consequences for Epidemiology (SPIKE), in 1979, 1981, and 1986. This instrument, which was developed for epidemiologic studies, collects information on 21 psychic and somatic syndromes and on consumption of various substances. Symptoms, length and frequency, subjective suffering, treatment, and social consequences are assessed for each syndrome. Different diagnostic algorithms can then be applied to the data on each syndrome (for further details on the methodology, see Angst, Dobler-Mikola, and Binder 1984).

The 1986 interview was conducted by trained psychiatric residents and clinical psychologists. As of this writing, 457 subjects of the 1979 sample have been reinterviewed. The dropout rate after the third interview wave and 7 years after the first interview is 23%. The subsample for the present analysis consists of the 395 subjects (189 males, 206 females) who were interviewed at all three times (in 1979, 1981, and 1986) over 7 years. The proportion of ratios of high versus low scores on the SCL-90 and the sex composition of the sample were comparable at all three interviews.

Diagnostic Assessment

The operational criteria for assignment of diagnoses are shown in Table 1. DSM-III definitions were applied when sufficient information was available. Major depression was defined according to DSM-III criteria in both 1981 and 1986. The category of recurrent brief depression as introduced and defined by Angst and Dobler-Mikola (1985) was also examined (Angst 1988, in press; Angst, Vollrath, and Koch 1987). This diagnosis requires a monthly recurrence of depression over 1 year, subjective impairment at work, and the presence of four of the eight possible depression symptoms in 1981 and 1986 and three of the six possible symptoms of depression in 1979. Thus, although the symptomatic criteria are the same for recurrent brief depression and DSM-III major depression, recurrent brief depression requires less duration, increased frequency, and functional impairment. These two categories of depression are mutually exclusive.

The group of anxiety disorders consists of panic disorder, mild panic disorder, generalized anxiety disorder (GAD), agoraphobia, social phobia, and simple phobia. In the third interview, the DSM-III criteria were applied. A weekly occurrence of panic attacks was required for the diagnosis of panic disorder at the first two interviews. Mild panic disorder was based on spontaneous panic attacks that occurred at least four times over the past 12 months. GAD was diagnosed if anxiety states with somatic symptoms of anxiety states

Table 1. Diagnostic Criteria Over the Three Interviews

	1979	1981	1986	
Major depression				
Number of symptoms	3/6	4/8	4/8	
Length $\geq$ 2 weeks	+	+	+	
		DSM-III	DSM-III	
Recurrent brief depression				
Number of symptoms	3/6	4/8	4/8	
Length < 2 weeks	+	+	+	
Frequency: monthly	+	+	+	
Work impairment	+	+	+	
Generalized anxiety disorder				
Anxiety	+	+	+	
Somatic anxiety	+	+	+	
Length: 1 month	o	o	+	
Frequency: monthly	+	+	o	
			DSM-III	
Panic				
Panic attacks	+	+	4/12	symptoms
Somatic symptoms	+	+	4/12	symptoms
Frequency: weekly	+	+	3/3	weeks
			DSM-III	
Mild panic				
Panic attacks	+	+	4/12	symptoms
Somatic symptoms	+	+	4/12	symptoms
Frequency: < weekly				
> 4–8 × per year	+	+	+	
Agoraphobia/social phobia				
Situational phobia	+	+	+	
Phobic symptoms[a]	+	+	+	
Avoidance behavior	+	+	+	
Major impairment in daily life	o	o	+	
			DSM-III	
Simple phobia				
Animal phobia	+	+	+	
Other phobic symptoms	o	o	+	
Avoidance behavior	+	+	+	
Recognition that fear is				
unreasonable	o	o	+	
			DSM-III	

[a] Hopkins Symptom Checklist (SCL-90).

occurred at least monthly. Agoraphobia and social phobia were combined in a single category. Both DSM disorders were defined by the presence of a situational phobia specified by items 13, 25, 47, and 70 of the SCL-90 plus avoidance behavior.

Family history of each syndrome was also routinely obtained separately for fathers, mothers, and siblings, irrespective of the subjects' response to the initial probes to each section. However, diagnostic criteria could not be assessed because information regarding specific symptoms and duration was not obtained for family members other than the probands. It is likely that this method of collection of family history resulted in an underestimate of psychopathology among relatives, particularly when the index subjects did not report the presence of a syndrome themselves.

Cross-Sectional Analysis Results

The raw frequencies of the diagnostic categories stratified by sex at each of the three interviews in 1979, 1981, and 1986 are given in Table 2. Except for major depression and recurrent brief depression, these categories are not mutually exclusive; that is, subjects with more than a single diagnosis can be counted multiple times.

There was a two- to threefold greater prevalence of major depression and anxiety disorders among females. However, the sex difference was less prominent for brief depression. The weighted 1-year prevalence rates for the population are given in Table 3. The weighting factor was derived from the original sampling procedure based on the proportion of high and low scores on the SCL-90 at intake. Three of 44 major and one of 52 recurrent brief depressive patients are bipolar. The rates of each of the diagnostic categories were quite stable across time. As one would expect, there is a slight increase in the 1-year rates of depression with the increase in the age of the sample. The decrease in panic disorders is likely to be attributable to the application of stricter diagnostic criteria in the latter interviews.

Table 2. Frequencies of Diagnosis at Interviews in 1979, 1981, and 1986 by Sex

	1979		1981		1986	
Diagnosis	Male ($N = 189$)	Female ($N = 206$)	Male ($N = 189$)	Female ($N = 206$)	Male ($N = 189$)	Female ($N = 206$)
Major depression	7	20	8	29	12	32
Recurrent brief depression	28	33	18	27	19	33
Generalized anxiety disorder	7	18	4	9	5	8
Panic disorder	9	28	7	11	3	15
Phobias	7	24	8	24	9	32

Table 3. Weighted 1-Year Prevalence Rates of Diagnoses at Interviews in 1979, 1981, and 1986, in Percentages

Diagnosis	1979	1981	1986
Major depression	4.0	6.8[a]	7.8[a]
Recurrent brief depression	7.0	6.1	10.7
Generalized anxiety disorder	2.0	1.3	1.9[a]
Panic disorder	5.7	1.6	2.2
Phobias	5.3	7.1	8.3[a]

[a] DSM-III.

Cross-Sectional Overlap Within the Anxiety Disorders

There was very little overlap within the specific categories of anxiety disorders irrespective of the diagnostic criteria applied for panic disorder (DSM-III panic or mild panic) as depicted in Figure 2. This figure presents the association between the DSM-III categories of panic, GAD, and all phobias that were assessed at the 1986 interview.

The distinction among the specific categories of the phobias could not be analyzed because of limitations of information in the interview itself and because of the small number of persons ($N = 3$) who met criteria for agoraphobia at the 1986 interview. However, at all three interviews, a trend for an association between agoraphobia and/or social phobia, and GAD and panic disorder was observed. In contrast, simple phobias did not appear to be associated with either GAD or panic disorder.

Cross-Sectional Overlap Between the Anxiety Disorders and Depression

In the following section, the overlap between anxiety and depression is examined at each of the three interviews. For this analysis, the categories of major and recurrent brief depression and the categories of anxiety disorders are combined. Because of the rather low association between GAD, panic, and phobias, their overlap with depression is presented in two ways: (1) combining the three categories of anxiety disorders to increase the group sizes and (2) restricting the analysis to panic alone.

Associations between the anxiety disorders and depression at each of the three interviews are presented in Table 4. There was a strong association between depression and the anxiety states, with a threefold increase in the prevalence of the simultaneous manifestation of both disorders beyond that expected by chance. Indeed, the

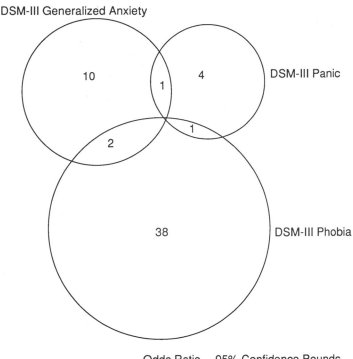

DSM-III Generalized Anxiety

DSM-III Panic

DSM-III Phobia

10

1

4

1

2

38

	Odds Ratio	95% Confidence Bounds
Generalized anxiety and phobia	1.6	0.3 – 7.4
Panic and phobia	1.7	0.2 – 14.9
Generalized anxiety and panic	6.3	0.7 – 58.0

Figure 2. The association between the DSM-III anxiety disorders assessed at the 1986 interview.

combination of anxiety and depression was nearly as common as anxiety alone at each of the three interviews.

When the overlap between depression and panic disorder was examined, an even stronger association emerged (Table 5). At each of the three interviews, rates of the combination of panic and depression exceeded the rate expected by chance by at least a factor of five.

Logistic regression analysis was applied to examine the effects of the three subgroups of anxiety disorders on depression as the dependent variable (Table 6). Logistic regression, a type of log-linear analysis, yields a logit or log-odds by logistic transformation of the dependent variable. The multiplicative factor by which the odds increase or decrease with changes in the predictor variable is then determined. The contribution of each predictor can be assessed independently of the possible effects of other predictors (Bishop, Fienberg, and Holland 1975; Cox 1970).

Table 4. Cross-Sectional Association of Anxiety and Depression

Diagnosis	1979		1981		1986	
	n	%	n	%	n	%
Anxiety and depression	30	7.6	20	5.1	31	7.8
Anxiety only	39	9.9	31	7.8	36	9.1
Depression only	58	14.7	62	15.7	65	16.5
Neither	268	67.8	282	71.4	263	66.6
Odds ratio	3.6		2.9		3.5	
95% confidence bounds	2.1–6.1		1.6–5.4		2.0–6.0	

Table 5. Cross-Sectional Association of Panic and Depression

Diagnosis	1979		1981		1986	
	n	%	n	%	n	%
Panic and depression	20	5.1	10	2.5	13	3.3
Panic only	17	4.3	8	2.0	5	1.3
Depression only	68	17.2	72	18.2	83	21.0
Neither	290	73.4	305	77.2	294	74.4
Odds ratio	5.0		5.3		9.2	
95% confidence bounds	2.6–9.6		2.2–12.7		3.8–22.6	

Table 6. Logistic Regression for the Effects of Anxiety Subgroups, Risk, and Sex on Depression in 1986

Variable	β	SE	χ^2	p
Panic and mild panic	1.96	0.55	12.60	0.000
Generalized anxiety	0.49	0.63	0.62	0.431
Phobias	0.71	0.36	3.95	0.047
Risk[a]	0.53	0.28	3.52	0.061
Sex	0.66	0.26	6.52	0.011
Intercept	−2.78	0.48	32.96	0.000

[a] Hopkins Symptom Checklist (SCL-90).

After controlling for the effects of sex and of risk group at the time of the original interview, it was found that the association between anxiety and depression could be attributed mainly to panic disorder. Indeed, generalized anxiety was not significantly associated with depression after controlling for panic disorder, sex, and risk group in all three interviews.

A significant association was also observed between major or recurrent brief depression and phobias at the 1986 interview (i.e., odds ratio = 2.5 [1.3–4.7] (Figure 3). Despite some difficulty distinguishing clearly between subtypes of phobia, the data suggest that the association between depression and phobias can be attributed to the overlap between depression and agoraphobia or social phobia rather than between depression and simple phobia alone.

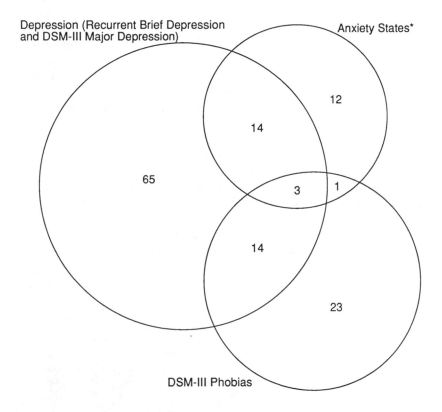

*GAD, Panic, Mild Panic

Figure 3. The association between depression, phobias, and anxiety states (generalized anxiety disorder, panic, and mild panic) assessed at the 1986 interview.

LONGITUDINAL ANALYSIS

Longitudinal Association Between Depression and Anxiety Disorders

A major methodological feature of the Zurich study is the prospective design in which the stability of the comorbidity of anxiety and depression can be examined over time. Three different approaches were applied to examine the stability of subjects with either pure anxiety or pure depression in 1979. First, the subjects were classified by the following diagnostic outcomes in 1981 or 1986: (1) the same "pure" disorder; (2) a diagnostic switch to the other "pure disorder"; (3) development of the other disorder in conjunction with the original disorder; or (4) no diagnostic episode at follow-up. The results of this analysis are shown in Table 7.

In 1979 there were 39 subjects with a diagnosis of an anxiety disorder alone, and 58 subjects with a diagnosis of depression alone. The results in Table 7 show that there were similar proportions of subjects with pure depression or pure anxiety who manifested the pure form of the other diagnosis at one of the follow-up interviews. Subjects with pure anxiety tended more often to develop depression in conjunction with anxiety (36%) at follow-up than did subjects with pure depression (19%). Nearly one-half of the cases with pure anxiety suffered from major depression or recurrent brief depression over the 7-year follow-up period. Moreover, subjects with pure depression manifested pure depression at follow-up more frequently (28%) than subjects with pure anxiety (13%). However, these differences are statistically nonsignificant.

A second approach to the assessment of the longitudinal data was classification of subjects with comorbid diagnosis according to the

Table 7. Stability of Diagnoses of Anxiety and Depression Among Subjects With "Pure" Diagnoses in 1979

Diagnosis in 1979	Diagnosis at follow-up	%
Anxiety only (N = 39)	Depression only	13
	Anxiety + depression	36
	Anxiety only	10
	None	41
Depression only (N = 58)	Depression only	28
	Anxiety + depression	19
	Anxiety only	14
	None	40

order of occurrence of the two disorders. The finding that persons with anxiety disorders were more likely to develop depression over time than the converse situation was suggested by taking into account the ages at onset of the respective disorders. Among subjects who manifested both disorders longitudinally, the onset of anxiety disorders was more likely to precede that of depression than the converse situation. That is, 62% of those with pure anxiety as a first diagnosis later developed depression, as compared to 18% of those with pure depression who later developed anxiety.

In a third approach to the assessment of longitudinal comorbidity, longitudinal diagnoses were made for each subject over the three interviews in the following ways: Probands who suffered from depression only (major or recurrent brief), but who never met the criteria for an anxiety disorder, were assigned to the category of depression only. The same procedure was applied to subjects with anxiety disorders who never met criteria for depression. A further group consisted of subjects with both diagnoses of anxiety and depression. The diagnoses could be present either cross-sectionally or at subsequent follow-up. In the latter cases, for instance, the subject was diagnosed as suffering from an anxiety disorder at the interview in 1981 and from depression at the interview in 1986. A final category consisted of subjects without either of these diagnoses.

In Table 8, these four categories were broken down into mutually exclusive classes of subtypes of depression. The overlap between anxiety and depression was quite similar for subjects with either major depression or recurrent brief depression, with odds ratios of 2.5 (1.5–4.0) for major depression and 2.3 (1.5–3.7) for recurrent brief depression. The overlap with anxiety disorders was stronger when both groups of depressive patients were considered (i.e., odds ratio = 3.9 [2.5–5.9]). Similar results emerged when the anxiety disorders were restricted to panic disorder alone (Table 9).

Family History of Depression and Anxiety

The information from the subjects regarding a history of depression and anxiety in their parents was also analyzed to determine whether there was specificity of transmission of the two disorders and their combination. These results are shown in Table 10, in which the diagnoses of anxiety and depression among the subjects and either or both parents are broken down into mutually exclusive categories. These data suggest that there does not appear to be specificity of transmission of these diagnoses between the subjects and their parents. Neither the rates of pure depression nor those of pure anxiety are greater among parents of subjects with these disorders. Further-

Table 8.   Longitudinal Diagnostic Overlap Between Anxiety Disorders and Depression Broken Down by Type of Depression, in Percentages

	Type of depression		
Longitudinal diagnosis	I + II	I	II
Anxiety and depression	23.0	11.4	11.9
Anxiety only	11.0	23.0	22.5
Depression only	23.0	10.9	12.1
Neither	42.5	54.7	53.4
Odds ratio	3.9	2.5	2.3
95% confidence bounds	2.5–5.9	1.5–4.0	1.5–3.7

Note.   Type of depression: I = depression defined as DSM-III major depression; II = depression defined as recurrent brief depression; I + II = DSM-III major depression or recurrent brief depression.

Table 9.   Longitudinal Diagnostic Overlap Between Panic and Depression, in Percentages

	Type of depression		
Longitudinal diagnosis	Major or recurrent brief	Major	Recurrent brief
Panic and depression	11.9	5.1	6.8
Panic only	4.1	10.9	9.1
Depression only	34.4	17.2	17.2
Neither	49.6	66.8	66.8
Odds ratio	4.2	1.8	2.9
95% confidence bounds	2.3–7.8	1.0–3.3	1.7–5.1

Table 10.   History of Anxiety Disorders and Depression Among Parents of 395 Subjects With and Without Anxiety and Depression at 1986 Interview

Subject's diagnosis	N	Parents' diagnoses (%)			
		Anxiety + depression	Anxiety only	Depression only	Neither
Anxiety + depression	92	29	12	28	30
Anxiety only	44	18	14	25	43
Depression only	91	29	10	22	40
Neither	168	6	13	20	61

more, rates of anxiety alone or depression alone are not elevated among the parents of subjects with either of these conditions, as compared to those of subjects without depression and anxiety. In contrast, there is a fivefold greater risk of anxiety and depression among the parents of subjects with these two conditions and those with depression only, and a threefold increase among parents of subjects with anxiety alone, as compared to those of subjects with neither disorder. These findings were confirmed when diagnoses were limited to parents who had received psychiatric treatment for anxiety and depression (Table 11).

IMPLICATIONS OF THESE DATA

The data from this epidemiologic cohort of young men and women from the Canton of Zurich, Switzerland, provide cross-sectional and longitudinal information about presence or absence of diagnostic overlap within the anxiety disorders and between the anxiety disorders and depression. The three categories of anxiety disorders that were found to be distinct at three separate interviews consisted of panic, GAD, and phobia. The phobias, which were comprised of simple phobias in the majority of the subjects, exhibited very little overlap with either panic disorders or GAD.

In contrast, cross-sectional comorbidity for depression and anxiety consistently exceeded chance expectations at all three interviews. There was even a stronger association between panic and depression. The overlap was the same for recurrent brief depression as it was for major depression. To our surprise, the association of depression with GAD was not significant in the multivariate analysis after controlling for the effects of panic and phobia.

The prospective design of the study permitted assessment of the

Table 11. History of Treatment for Anxiety Disorders and Depression Among Parents of 395 Subjects With and Without Anxiety and Depression at 1986 Interview

Subject's diagnosis	N	Parents' treatment history (%)			
		Anxiety + depression	Anxiety only	Depression only	Neither
Anxiety + depression	92	9	2	6	83
Anxiety only	44	5	0	5	91
Depression only	91	4	1	13	81
Neither	168	1	1	6	92

stability of the diagnostic categories across a 7-year interval. There are three major findings that emerged from the longitudinal data. First, there was a significant association between depression and anxiety—especially panic—within the total sample of subjects for whom diagnostic assessments were made at all three interviews. Second, there was a tendency for stability of pure depression across the 7 years of follow-up. Nearly one-third of the subjects who manifested the disorder in 1979 were diagnosed as having pure depression at follow-up again. Subjects starting with pure anxiety tended to develop additional depressive disorders at follow-up. However, these differences of course in subjects with pure anxiety and subjects with pure depression are statistically nonsignificant and should be interpreted with caution. Third, subjects who started with "pure" anxiety disorders exhibited a substantially lower degree of stability across time than did those with pure depression, with nearly half of those persons with pure anxiety states in 1979 developing either major or recurrent brief depression during the follow-up interval.

These findings have methodological and clinical implications. Methodologically, they suggest that the DSM-III distinctions between the anxiety disorders are relevant in an epidemiologic population in which the overlap of categories is small between the individual diagnostic categories themselves. Our data do not negate that there may be an association between agoraphobia and panic. However, agoraphobia is so rare that the association does not appear in this epidemiologic sample.

Furthermore, as this population proceeds through the peak risk period of onset of the affective disorders, the stability of the pure anxiety disorders decreases, with half of the subjects already having developed depression over a 7-year follow-up. In contrast, for persons with the diagnosis of depression, the data provide evidence of longitudinal stability.

These findings, when taken together with those from other epidemiologic studies, may yield clinical applications. Estimates of the degree to which diagnostic categories are switched, or the risk of developing a second disorder in a basically untreated population, are crucial in interpreting the effects of clinical intervention. In addition, treatment strategies may differ for subjects with comorbid coexisting disorders as compared to those with either disorder alone.

There are several limitations to the study to be considered when evaluating the findings. First, the diagnostic criteria for the earlier interview (1979) did not strictly adhere to the DSM-III categories published in 1980. Furthermore, some of the sections of the 1986 interview did not permit the strict assessment of these categories. Second, attrition of subjects from the original sample, a liability in nearly all longitudinal studies of this type, may lead to unknown biases in the remaining sample. Third, although the design of the study was truly prospective, the longitudinal assessments yielded three separate 12-month prevalence rates rather than incidence rates. Fourth, the family history data should be interpreted with caution because the information was not blindly obtained, nor were systematic diagnostic criteria assessed for the relatives.

Nevertheless, these findings are consistent with those of other epidemiologic surveys that have been conducted throughout the world. The results of the National Institute of Mental Health Epidemiologic Catchment Area study (Boyd, Burke, Gruenberg, et al. 1984) and the longitudinal follow-up of the Stirling County Study in Nova Scotia (Murphy, Sobol, Neff, et al. 1984) have also demonstrated a substantial degree of overlap between both symptoms and diagnoses of anxiety and depression, but they did not control for age and sex.

The longitudinal data of the present study provide evidence for the validity of a common subtype of affective disorder that is comprised of prominent symptoms of both anxiety and depression. Subjects who manifest this subtype are likely to meet the criteria for a pure anxiety disorder initially and then to develop depression either in conjunction with or distinct from the anxiety later. However, these findings do not demonstrate a lack of validity for the pure forms of either anxiety or depression. Rather, these results are consistent with the interpretation that a substantial proportion of cases on the anxiety-depression spectrum manifest mixed clinical features both cross-sectionally and longitudinally. Data from the next follow-up interview will continue to provide valuable information on these young adults as they progress through the risk period for these disorders.

Chapter 8

Comorbidity of Anxiety and Depression in the Lundby 25-Year Prospective Study: The Pattern of Subsequent Episodes

Olle Hagnell, M.D.
Anne Gräsbeck, M.D.

THE MAJORITY OF people ill with anxiety or depression pass their lives undiagnosed and untreated because of poor understanding by treating facilities and by society in general. They live a life filled with limitations because of this lack of treatment. People who have never experienced panic attacks or phobias find it difficult both to realize the feelings evoked by these syndromes and to comprehend the social consequences involved. By means of various epidemiologic, psychiatric studies—such as the Epidemiologic Catchment Area (ECA) study in the United States (Regier, Burke, and Burke, Chapter 6), the Stirling County study in Canada (Murphy, Chapter 9), and the Lundby study in Sweden (considered here)—convincing support has accrued for the large extent to which people in a general population, treated or untreated, contract anxiety or depression. New classifica-

This study has been supported by the following grants: The Bank of Sweden Tercentenary Foundation Nos. 71/2, 89/71; The Swedish Medical Research Council Nos. 3474, 6881, 4803, 9116; and The Swedish Ministry of Health and Social Affairs, Delegation of Social Research No. 83/64.

tion systems like the International Classification of Diseases (ICD-9) (World Health Organization 1987) and the revised third edition of the *Diagnostic and Statistical Manual of Mental Disorders* (DSM-III-R) (American Psychiatric Association 1987) have directed attention to the role these illnesses are playing in society today.

In Scandinavia the concept of comorbidity has been considered mainly within clinical or recently hospitalized populations, but little is known from general psychiatric population studies. One way to understand better the syndromes of anxiety, depression, and their comorbidity is by performing longitudinal population studies. Since 1957 Hagnell has been conducting an epidemiologic, longitudinal study of mental disorders, personality traits, and social conditions in a total general population. The Lundby study, as it has come to be called, was initiated 40 years ago by Essen-Möller. Within the framework of this study, it is possible to study subsequent episodes of morbidity across a quarter of a century.

In 1947 Essen-Möller and three other psychiatrists made a prevalence study of all 2,550 inhabitants registered in a geographically delimited area in southern Sweden (Essen-Möller, Larsson, Uddenberg, et al. 1956). In 1957 Hagnell began a follow-up study (Hagnell 1966) of the original population, irrespective of domicile (700 were now living elsewhere), and in addition investigated 1,013 newcomers to the Lundby area. In 1972 Hagnell and Öjesjö performed a second follow-up (Hagnell 1986a, 1986b; Hagnell, Essen-Möller, Lanke, et al. in press). Again, the study was accomplished irrespective of the subject's domicile, but then only of those examined in 1947 and/or 1957. Since in Sweden everyone must appear in a local community register, and not more than one, this method of defining the sample precludes missing some individuals as well as including too many.

A preliminary report on the syndromes of anxiety and depression and their symptom comorbidity will be presented here, covering that part of the Lundby study that deals with those 2,550 persons who were followed during the 25 years from 1947 to 1972. At the second follow-up in 1972, half of the 1947 cohort had moved from Lundby and were now living elsewhere, 20% of them in cities with more than 100,000 inhabitants. We also collected information on 673 subjects who had died. In 1972, as in 1947 and 1957, attrition from the study was negligible, a few percent (Table 1).

When the Lundby study started 40 years ago, few psychiatric diagnostic systems existed. Some examples from that time are the U.S Army classification and Essen-Möller's three-dimensional system (Essen-Möller and Wohlfahrt 1949). In the course of any longitudinal study, classification systems are likely to develop and change. In the Lundby study we found it suitable to make our own diagnostic

Table 1. Proportion of Participants in the Lundby Field Studies

1947 cohort	Number of living persons	Personally examined	
		N	%
In 1947	2,550	2,520	98.8
In 1957	2,297	2,274	99.0
In 1972	1,877	1,839	98.0

system (Hagnell 1966). This desire resulted in 18 diagnostic groups, which we have kept to over the years because they have proved useful for purposes of psychiatric research. However, since our data bank is extremely comprehensive, it is possible to reevaluate the material according to other classification systems, such as ICD and DSM.

By means of this three-wave study with field examinations in 1947, 1957, and 1972, we have been able to study first episodes as well as relapses of mental disease during a quarter of a century. We can, therefore, answer topical questions such as: what happened to those with a first episode of anxiety or depression: did they recover or did they fall ill again? The information that formed the basis for our diagnostic evaluations at the three field examinations was collected from the population living in the two adjoining parishes that we call "Lundby." It is located in one of the most developed parts of southern Sweden, not far from a big city (Malmö) and the university town of Lund.

All field examinations were performed by psychiatrists from the Department of Psychiatry at the University of Lund. The psychiatric evaluation was based on the joint information gathered from two main sources: (1) a field examination by a psychiatrist, consisting of a semistructured, focused interview together with a written description of the proband and environment; and (2) information collected from supplementary sources. A list of the sources from which further information was gathered follows:

Parish and central population registration
The Swedish central bureau of statistics
Social insurance office
National tax board
Criminal register
County temperance boards
Hospital case notes, psychiatric
Hospital case notes, nonpsychiatric
Key informants

Official death certificates
Autopsy reports
Regional archives
Postal investigation in 1962

As already mentioned, 18 diagnostic groups were established:

Anxiety proper
Anxiety plus other psychiatric symptoms
Tiredness proper
Tiredness plus other psychiatric symptoms
Tiredness plus gastrointestinal discomfort
Depression proper
Depression plus other psychiatric symptoms
Mixed neurosis
Mixed neurosis, more serious plus other psychiatric symptoms
Mental disorder plus somatic illness
Child neurosis
Schizophrenia
"Other psychosis" (confusion, paranoia, etc.)
Organic syndrome
Psychiatric symptoms and epilepsy
Multi-infarct dementia
Senile dementia
Age neurosis

In addition to these 18 categories, we also evaluated another set of mental disorders:

Psychopathy
Mental retardation
Character neurosis
Psychosomatic diseases
Alcoholism

It is impossible to define a disease clearly by means of one or two words. What one can do is to describe, as carefully as possible, the condition in question to enable those with about the same training as yourself to understand your meaning. Since anxiety and depression are central themes of this presentation, we will here quote our description of these conditions (Hagnell 1966).

ANXIETY

"The main symptom in the Anxiety group is anxiety, a feeling of danger, disaster, dissolution, and the feeling of 'being blown to bits.' The cause of this anxiety is unknown to the patient, and he feels helpless against it.

"In addition to a more or less constant anxious nervousness, expressing itself as mental or psychosomatic signs, the patient has anxiety attacks. They are often delimited, and may be seen as a type of panic reaction, in which the patient clings to a member of his family. The anxiety attacks are often accompanied by tachycardia, nervous sensations around the heart, feelings of suffocation, sensations or pain in the chest, dizziness, feelings of fainting, anxiety often described by the patient as 'death anxiety,' and fear of dying from heart trouble" (Hagnell 1966). The patient also suffers from anxiety feelings in the epigastrium; diarrhea, and frequent urination.The symptoms usually come from organs in which there is normally a certain degree of sensation—not from 'mute' organs—and often give rise to fear of having a serious illness. The patient may suffer from restlessness and sleep difficulties: may often wake up at night with anxiety, although the anxiety may come at any time.

Subgroups of Anxiety

Anxiety proper. "Anxiety is a prominent symptom in the case history. More acute anxiety is episodically demarcated without any prominent psychiatric symptomatology. Often attacks of cardiac anxiety, 'death anxiety,' and feelings of suffocation (Hagnell 1966)."

Anxiety plus other psychiatric symptoms (cosyndrome). "Anxiety is a prominent symptom, and occurs in addition to other psychiatric symptoms, such as depression (Hagnell 1966)."

DEPRESSION

"Lowered mood, depressive feelings, tendency to guilt feelings, gloomy outlook, reduced activity, reduced self-esteem, lowered enjoyment of life and feeling of low vitality, anxiety, fear, terror, lack of initiative; has more difficulty than usual, and is unable to carry out his daily responsibilities. Many patients continue their usual work; however, the symptoms become an increasing strain and the work suffers. Sometimes motor or mental retardation is present. Pertaining to daily rhythm the patient is worse in the morning and better towards the evening. Often he has sleep disturbances and wakes up early in the morning. Loss of appetite and weight (Hagnell 1966)."

Subgroups of Depression

Depression proper. "This depressive syndrome is well demarcated without other more prominent psychiatric symptoms (Hagnell 1966)."

Depression plus other psychiatric symptoms (cosyndrome).
"Depression occurs with other psychiatric symptoms."

Impairment, duration, onset age, and certainty (that a case was a psychiatric case) were evaluated in addition to diagnosing the syndromes. For a more extensive description of our classification and for examples of what is meant by various kinds of syndromes in the Lundby study, we refer the reader to Hagnell (1966).

We are quite aware of the possible drawbacks connected with this kind of study. There are many assets, however. Psychiatrists with similar training have examined all persons in a general population, whether or not they had sought help. Moreover, the psychiatrist completed an interview and a description of the proband's behavior in the proband's own environment. In addition, a large amount of information from different sources have supported the diagnostic accuracy.

Using the above Lundby classification, this chapter is a report of what happened to those of our probands who had their first psychiatric episode diagnosed as anxiety or depression. We emphasize that this longitudinal investigation is only one approach to studying comorbidity and should be seen as an additional perspective to studies performed with other techniques.

INCIDENCE AND LIFETIME RISK OF CONTRACTING ANXIETY OR DEPRESSION

From our figures, a lifetime risk (probability) of contracting a mental disorder during the 25-year period of 1947 to 1972 can be calculated. Note that the risk is conditional, the condition being that of a newborn living to the age of 90. All other figures of cumulative risks in our presentation are handled according to the same principle.

The probability of falling ill with anxiety proper during any time of life up to age 90 is 2.6% for men and 6.1% for women. For anxiety plus other psychiatric symptoms, the lifetime risk is 8.6% for men and 16.8% for women. Thus the probability of contracting an anxiety disorder is about double for women (Hagnell, Lanke, Rorsman, et al., in press; Merikangas and Weissman 1986; Rorsman, Hagnell, Lanke, et al. 1987).

The calculated lifetime risk of developing depression proper is 6.8% for men and 15.5% for women. For depression plus other psychiatric symptoms, the lifetime risk for men is 17.3% and 32.1% for women. As with anxiety disorders, there is a doubled risk for women of falling ill with depression (Hagnell, Lanke, Rorsman, et al. 1982, in press).

RELAPSE PATTERN OF ANXIETY AND DEPRESSION

Using our own classification, a summary of the findings on relapse rate is given here by looking at the course of disease. The analysis includes probands with a first-time episode of any of these illnesses. We have also looked into the interactive role played by other diagnoses, such as alcoholism, psychosomatic illnesses, and our tiredness diagnoses.

Anxiety Proper

Forty-two individuals, 13 men and 29 women, had a first-time episode of anxiety proper (Table 2); 14 persons had only one episode. Of the remaining 28, 19 persons relapsed into anxiety and the rest into different mental disorders. Only 1 of 9 men and 1 of 19 women relapsed with depression. Two of 3 men and 5 of 8 women with more than one relapse into mental illness had some kind of psychosomatic disease. These figures may seem rather dramatic and will be further

Table 2. The Lundby Longitudinal 1947–1972 Episode Study: Anxiety Proper ($N = 42$)

	n	Syndromes	n
Men	13		
Single episode	4		
Subsequent episodes	9		
One relapse	6	Anxiety proper or with cosymptoms	3
		Depression proper or with cosymptoms	1
		Other psychiatric diagnosis	2
More than one relapse	3	Anxiety proper or with cosymptoms	3
Women	29		
Single episode	10		
Subsequent episodes	19		
One relapse	10	Anxiety proper or with cosymptoms	7
		Other psychiatric diagnosis	3
More than one relapse	9	Anxiety proper or with cosymptoms	6
		Anxiety/depression[a]	1
		Other psychiatric diagnosis	2

[a]Changes between episodes of anxiety proper or with cosymptoms and episodes of depression proper or with cosymptoms.

explored. Until this analysis is done, we want to underline the fact that anxiety often accompanies various kinds of bodily sensations. This association certainly has some connection with our high rate of psychosomatic diseases.

None was diagnosed as an alcoholic. This finding goes against most other findings. An explanation might be that the majority of probands with anxiety proper are women who have a very low rate of alcoholism in this study. However, further investigation seems warranted.

Anxiety Plus Other Psychiatric Symptoms

The anxiety plus other psychiatric symptoms group contains 125 individuals, 45 men and 80 women (Table 3); 64 had only one episode.

Table 3.   The Lundby Longitudinal 1947–1972 Episode Study: Anxiety + Other Symptoms (Cosyndrome) (N = 125)

	n	Syndromes	n
Men	45		
Single episode	21		
Subsequent episodes	24		
		Anxiety proper or with cosymptoms	4
One relapse	10	Depression proper or with cosymptoms	1
		Other psychiatric diagnosis	5
More than one relapse	14	Anxiety proper or with cosymptoms	11
		Anxiety/depression[a]	3
Women	80		
Single episode	43		
Subsequent episodes	37		
One relapse	10	Anxiety proper or with cosymptoms	4
		Other psychiatric diagnosis	6
More than one relapse	27	Anxiety proper or with cosymptoms	11
		Anxiety/depression[a]	11
		Other psychiatric diagnosis	5

[a]Changes between episodes of anxiety proper or with cosymptoms and episodes of depression proper or with cosymptoms.

Among those 61 who had one or more relapses, anxiety was a very common diagnosis. However, altogether 25%, 4 of 24 men and 11 of 37 women, developed depression. The figures for men are small, but a tendency toward relapses into depression may be traced. In the subgroup of women with more than one relapse, more than 40% had episodes with depression. The relapses into depression occur mostly in the group with depression plus other psychiatric symptoms.

About 30% of both men and women had a psychosomatic disease. No woman was classified as alcoholic, but 1 of the 14 men was. This is about the same proportion as among all men in the Lundby population (Hagnell and Tunving 1972; Öjesjö, Hagnell, and Lanke 1982).

Depression Proper

The depression proper group contains 60 individuals, 21 men and 39 women (Table 4). After an initial episode of depression proper, almost

Table 4. The Lundby Longitudinal 1947–1972 Episode Study: Depression Proper (N = 60)

	n	Syndromes	n
Men	21		
Single episode	13		
Subsequent episodes	8		
One relapse	2	Depression proper or with cosymptoms	1
		Other psychiatric diagnosis	1
More than one relapse	6	Depression proper or with cosymptoms	6
Women	39		
Single episode	28		
Subsequent episodes	11		
One relapse	4	Depression proper or with cosymptoms	3
		Other psychiatric diagnosis	1
More than one relapse	7	Depression proper or with cosymptoms	6
		Other psychiatric diagnosis	1

all relapses are with the same diagnosis. None of those with an initial episode of depression proper developed anxiety.

Half of the men and 2 of 7 women with more than one relapse into mental illness had some kind of psychosomatic disease. The rate of alcoholism seems rather low in this group. Only one case of depression proper was diagnosed an alcoholic. This was a man with many episodes of depression proper (endogenous depression, unipolar) who eventually committed suicide.

Depression Plus Other Psychiatric Symptoms

There are 202 individuals, 73 men and 129 women, in the depression plus other psychiatric symptoms group (Table 5). A majority of the

Table 5. The Lundby Longitudinal 1947–1972 Episode Study: Depression + Other Symptoms (Cosyndrome) ($N = 202$)

	n	Syndromes	n
Men	73		
Single episode	37		
Subsequent episodes	36		
One relapse	17	Depression proper or with cosymptoms	12
		Other psychiatric diagnosis	5
More than one relapse	19	Depression proper or with cosymptoms	16
		Depression/anxiety[a]	2
		Other psychiatric diagnosis	1
Women	129		
Single episode	63		
Subsequent episodes	66		
One relapse	35	Anxiety proper or with cosymptoms	2
		Depression proper or with cosymptoms	18
		Other psychiatric diagnosis	15
More than one relapse	31	Depression proper or with cosymptoms	21
		Depression/anxiety[a]	4
		Other psychiatric diagnosis	6

[a]Changes between episodes of depression proper or with cosymptoms and episodes of anxiety proper or with cosymptoms.

probands with subsequent episodes of mental disease (36 men and 66 women) relapsed into the same disease as earlier (i.e., depression plus other psychiatric symptoms). Two men and six women developed anxiety episodes in the course of their illness.

About one-fifth of the men and one-third of the women had some kind of psychosomatic disease. Only one woman and slightly more than one-fourth of the men were diagnosed as alcoholics.

An example of each proband's individual pattern of relapses, where depression plus other psychiatric symptoms was the first diagnosis and there were at least two relapses of mental illness, can be seen in Table 6. The psychosomatic and alcoholic diseases have been placed last in the rows because of uncertainty of onset of these diseases. It seems as if the depressions come prior to alcoholism and psychosomatic diseases, but this is still under investigation.

TIREDNESS AS COMORBIDITY TO DEPRESSION

Depressions often appear as atypical or masked. One of our tiredness diagnoses, that of tiredness with cosymptoms, seems to be a group from which many obvious depressions originate (Hagnell 1989). A description of our tiredness diagnoses after Hagnell (1966) is given below.

Tiredness

"Nervous fatigue, low threshold for fatigue, wearies quickly, feels weak and worn out. Tendency for headaches, 'like a pressure or band around the head and pain in the neck.' Subjective memory difficulties owing to reduced ability to concentrate, but without such objective signs as found in organic syndromes. Hypochondriac sensations and imaginings. Insomnia is often prominent. Irritability and a certain degree of tearfulness, feelings of displeasure, vagueness, general feelings of disinclination, feelings of being stressed, of being overworked, lack of energy, feeling of tension, inadequate ability to relax, trembling and shaking. The last mentioned symptoms, of course, merge into those labelled 'Anxiety,' but there are no attacks, and tiredness is the dominant symptom. There is often a multitude of different symptoms, but many men complain about epigastric pain (Hagnell 1966)."

Subgroups of Tiredness

Tiredness proper. "Nervous fatigue is by far the dominant symptom (Hagnell 1966)."

Table 6. The Lundby Longitudinal 1947–1972 Episode Study: Depression + Other Psychiatric Symptoms as First Diagnosis in Life

MEN No. of cases	Relapse 1	2	3	4	5	6	7	8	9	10	11
1	A+	Oth Psych									
1	T+Gast	A+									
1	D+	D+	(Alc)								
1	D+	D+									
1	D+	MDS									
1	D+	MID									
1	Org Syndr	Oth Psych	(Psychosom)[a]								
1	D	D	D								
1	D+	A+	D+	(Alc)							
3	D+	D+	D+								
1	D+	D+	D+	(Psychosom)[a]							
1	Oth Psych	D+	MN	(Alc)							
1	D+	D+	D+	D+	(Alc)						
1	MN	MN	MN	D+	(Alc)						
1	D+	D+	D+	D+	D+						
1	MN+	MN+	MN+	MN+	MN+	(Psychosom)[a]	D+	MN+			
1	T+	D+	T+	T+	D	(Psychosom)[a]	D	D	D	D	D
19											

Note. Only cases with more than one relapse were included. A = anxiety; Alc = alcoholism; D = depression; Gast = nervous gastrointestinal complaints; MDS = mental disorder plus somatic illness; MID = multi-infarct dementia; MN = mixed neurosis; Oth Psych = other psychosis; Org Syndr = organic syndrome; Psychosom = psychosomatic diseases; T = tiredness.
[a] Gast.

Tiredness plus other psychiatric symptoms. "Nervous fatigue together with other psychiatric symptoms, such as Anxiety (Hagnell 1966)."

Tiredness plus gastrointestinal discomfort. "Nervous fatigue is present with psychosomatic symptoms expressed as epigastric pain (Hagnell 1966)."

In our terminology, tiredness does not include any similar syndrome appearing as a part of any other physical or mental disease.

Our diagnosis of tiredness has much in common with the concept of neurasthenia, which was especially discussed at the end of the 19th century, (e.g., Kraepelin 1899). Although used in various settings since that time, there has been a renewed interest in this diagnosis during recent years, often referring to it as chronic fatigue syndrome (Byrne 1988; Holmes, Kaplan, Gantz, et al. 1988; Kennedy 1988; Portwood 1988).

Ten out of 16 men and 13 of 34 women with two or more episodes subsequent to tiredness with cosymptoms of different kinds were diagnosed with depression in the subsequent course of illness. This calls for further analysis of our material.

CONCLUSION

Judging from these analyses of the Lundby data, it seems as if some syndromes have a tendency to change into another during the course of life. Diagnoses that have this tendency are those that include an obvious amount of "other psychiatric symptoms" and signs (cosyndromes). Stable within the original category are those with a more distinct syndrome.

For probands who started with the diagnosis of anxiety plus other psychiatric symptoms, there is a 25% chance of depression emerging in the course of illness. This tendency is stronger among women (30%) and still stronger among women with more than one relapse (40%). Such a shift into other diagnoses is not found in the diagnostic group of anxiety proper.

Depression shows another pattern: Depression proper maintains a diagnostic stability over time; no proband had any episode of relapse into anxiety. Among those with depression plus other psychiatric symptoms, only 7% switched to anxiety. Angst, Vollrath, Merikangas, et al. (Chapter 7) reported a similar stability over time for those with "pure depression" and a lower degree of stability over time among those who started with anxiety.

The cosyndromes of anxiety seem important for developing a depression and need to be further analyzed. Do they contain a depressive equivalent? Can this syndrome as a whole be prodromal to a depression? Has this category a more severe and debilitating course than anxiety proper? This last question could be investigated with regard to impairment, duration, and frequency of episodes within our population. Psychosomatic diseases and alcoholism appear with anxiety and with depression to a fairly equal degree. Other findings like ours suggest a possible relationship between certain anxiety and depressive disorders (Angst, Vollrath, Merikangas, et al., Chapter 7; Merikangas and Weissman 1986).

Prospective, longitudinal, psychiatric population studies should be given the highest priority and the security of long-range support. Experience has shown that longitudinal studies are very hard to carry through without this type of commitment. The Lundby study is unique in surviving for four decades. This is our first attempt to analyze anxiety and depression and their subsequent episodes of diseases. Even if the results are drawn from a period 25 years in duration, further studies of syndrome and symptom relationships will be needed to improve our knowledge of the complex patterns of cosyndromes.

Chapter 9

Diagnostic Comorbidity and Symptom Co-Occurrence: The Stirling County Study

Jane M. Murphy, Ph.D.

T HERE ARE SEVERAL issues about relationships among psychiatric symptoms and diagnostic categories that can be explored in a long-term epidemiologic study of a general population. Insofar as large numbers of subjects are asked about the psychiatric symptoms they may have experienced, evidence can be gathered about the degree to which symptoms that figure in the clinically defined syndromes do, in fact, occur naturally together. Research can be carried out to investigate the value of different kinds of classification principles. Questions can be asked about the possibility, for example, that combinations of syndromes are more important than single syndromal entities.

The purpose of this chapter is to discuss some of these issues on the basis of information from the Stirling County Study. The focus will be on symptom co-occurrence as it relates to the syndromes of depression and anxiety and on diagnostic comorbidity between these two syndromes and, to some extent, other types of diagnoses as well. The materials include structured interviews with subjects and reports

The analysis on which this chapter is based has been supported by grant MH-39576 from the National Institute of Mental Health, Rockville, MD. Earlier funds were provided by National Health Research and Development project 6603-1154-44, Department of Health and Welfare of Canada, and by the Sandoz Foundation and the Milbank Memorial Fund. Grateful acknowledgment is made to Richard R. Monson, Donald C. Olivier, Arthur M. Sobol, Lisa A. Pratt, and Alexander H. Leighton for assistance in the preparation of this report.

from general physicians. The kinds of assessments on which the discussion draws include statistical measures, computer algorithms, and longitudinal follow-up of community samples. One of the main findings is that while both co-occurrence and comorbidity are prominent in this general population study, depression irrespective of whether or not it is accompanied by anxiety appears to be a more serious disorder than anxiety alone.

Background Information on the Stirling County Study

The site of the study is a town-and-country area of Atlantic Canada for which "Stirling County" is a fictitious name. The historical period covered is a major portion of the third quarter of this century, with 1952 being its opening date and 1970 being the year of our most recent prevalence estimates (Beiser 1971; Hughes, Tremblay, Rapoport, et al. 1960; Leighton 1959; Leighton, Harding, Macklin, et al. 1963a; Murphy 1980).

The study consists of both repeated cross-sectional surveys of samples of the the adult residents of the county and cohort follow-up investigations of persons selected in earlier samples. At the present time, the study involves 2,848 subjects about whom we have gathered various types of information. For example, the subjects have been interviewed by trained personnel using a structured questionnaire that contains an inventory of questions about the symptoms of neurotic depression and anxiety. The county's general physicians have been interviewed by psychiatrists about the medical and psychiatric histories of these sample members. A case register of specialized psychiatric care has been prepared from records kept for a local community mental health center, and death certificates have been assembled for those who died.

For comparative purposes, we have used similar methods for cross-sectional investigations in other sites. One is an urban area in New York, which we named "Queensbrook," and the others are non-Western areas (Beiser, Benfari, Collomb, et al. 1976; Benfari, Beiser, Leighton, et al. 1972, 1974; Leighton, Lambo, Hughes, et al. 1963; Murphy 1976; Zahner 1983).

In the early 1950s, when information about our first sample from Stirling County was available, analytic decisions that bear on the topics of comorbidity and co-occurrence were made. In preparation for reading and evaluating materials from the interviews with subjects as well as reports from general physicians, a group of psychiatrists worked out an assessment plan so that consistent criteria could be applied for determining which subjects should be enumerated in a prevalence rate of psychiatric disorders (Leighton, Harding, Macklin, et al. 1963a). Some of the key points of this procedure were:

1. "Causal inferences should be eliminated as a basis for classifying the behaviors noted in the protocols. . . . This decision constituted our most radical revision of the psychiatrists' customary way of thinking and proceeding" (p. 48).
2. "The aim became that of detecting and classifying *symptom patterns* [italics added] of psychiatric interest" (p. 48).
3. "If a person exhibited *more than one* [italics added] [category of symptom pattern] this should be shown rather than masked by the system of evaluation" (p. 48). This approach was different from the "prevailing clinical view," which suggested "that a person has as a rule only one psychiatric disorder at a time and that an important responsibility of the psychiatrist is differential diagnosis—an attempt to determine which disorder is the essential one in each particular case" (p. 160).
4. "Illness stands for more than the presence of symptoms; it means a certain intensity of them and usually also a certain amount of interference with ordinary functioning" (p. 73).

Thus, for research purposes, a scheme was designed that departed in some ways from clinical practice in the 1950s even though it made use of the language of the *Diagnostic and Statistical Manual of Mental Disorders*, first edition (DSM-I) (American Psychiatric Association 1952) for describing symptom patterns. I have suggested that this plan resembles several features of contemporary approaches to classification, such as in the third edition of the *Diagnostic and Statistical Manual of Mental Disorders* (DSM-III) (American Psychiatric Association 1980; Murphy 1980, 1986a, 1986b). Its orientation was nonetiologic; and it focused on syndromal configurations or patterns of co-occurring symptoms, on their duration and intensity, on the impairment in functioning that they engendered, and on the use of multiple categories for revealing diagnostic comorbidity.

SYMPTOM CO-OCCURRENCE

Recognizing symptom patterns was one of the main tasks carried out by the psychiatrists for our original analysis of the data from Stirling County, and the symptom patterns were, in turn, the building blocks on which the remainder of the evaluation procedure stood. By *symptom pattern* we mean a model or mental image of a cluster of symptoms that psychiatrists have learned to use as an aid in identifying a specific syndrome. An illustration we used is the collection of symptoms that make up the symptom pattern called an anxiety attack as, for example, palpitations, dyspnea, sensations of choking, marked fear of dying, and concern about the heart. Such models are based on clinical experience and figure in a psychiatrist's training through the words of mentors and descriptions provided in textbooks.

Since syndromes embody what can be termed the conventional wisdom of clinical psychiatry, questions have been raised about whether symptoms such as palpitations, choking sensations, and fear of dying actually co-occur in nature or whether they partly reflect the clinical expectation that they should co-occur. Because psychiatry lacks biologic markers for most diagnoses, the data leading to clinical diagnoses tend to be the *observations* made by a psychiatrist or the patient's family members and the *verbal answers* that the patient and/or family members give in response to a psychiatric interview. Since World War II, there has been an impressive growth of schedules and questionnaires developed to systematize the way patients and research subjects are asked about psychiatric symptoms (Murphy 1981, 1988). The availability of responses from large numbers of subjects who have been asked standard questions has encouraged investigation of the empirical basis for clinical syndromes.

One of the early methods used to assess the degree to which symptoms co-occur was the Guttman test employed by U.S. Army researchers in the development of the Neuropsychiatric Screening Adjunct, which was one of the first instruments used in this country for large-scale studies (Star 1950a, b). The Guttman technique is a form of deterministic ordinal or hierarchical assessment that has rarely again been used in psychiatric studies, perhaps because its requirements are extremely stringent (Guttman 1947, 1950). If a scale of symptoms passes this test, a positive response to a question about the most severe symptom in a domain predicts positive responses to all other questions relevant to the domain.

The Army's approach was to construct a long inventory of questions drawn from the extant clinical literature. The questions were organized and then tested in terms of their approximations to Guttman scales. The inventory consisted of about 100 questions with separate scales for worrying, oversensitivity, personal adjustment, psychosomatic complaints, and various childhood experiences. The scale that achieved the best discrimination between soldiers in hospitals with diagnoses in the psychoneurotic categories and active-duty soldiers was the psychosomatic complaints scale. In fact, this scale of 15 questions, which constitutes the core of the Neuropsychiatric Screening Adjunct, discriminated about as well as the entire combination of scales. Its internal consistency ranged from .82 to .87, and its test-retest reliability ranged from .90 to .93.

The name *psychosomatic complaints* appears to have been an unfortunate choice, and it has obscured the fact that the symptoms queried are indicators of autonomic anxiety that parallel, to a remarkable degree, the symptoms shown in DSM-III under panic disorder and generalized anxiety. They include, for example, nervousness, dizziness, cold sweats, nightmares, hands trembling, hands sweating, heart beating fast, and shortness of breath.

In constructing this scale, the Army researchers reasoned that if a soldier reported incontinence in a panic-provoking situation, he would probably also report trembling, sweating, and so on, possibly in a hierarchical fashion with a milder symptom such as palpitations being endorsed by almost all subjects in such situations. While the Army's scale did not display full Guttman properties and did not, in fact, include a question about incontinence, the evidence that the symptoms tended to co-occur was ample. Evidence also existed that the scale had good psychometric properties and, at the same time, allowed patients to report about themselves in ways that distinguished them from "normals."

The inventory of neurotic symptoms that constitutes the psychiatric portion of the questionnaire interview used in the Stirling study was constructed in a fashion similar to the Neuropsychiatric Screening Adjunct. The goal was to design and standardize an instrument that would be appropriate for women as well as men and for persons of a broader age range than pertained in the Army study. Our instrument was prepared by Macmillan (1957) and is named the Health Opinion Survey. Its items were selected from a longer inventory that contained the Army's questions as well as questions from other inventories available at that time (Eysenck 1947; Rimoldi 1950). The selection procedure involved comparisons between responses from psychiatric patients diagnosed as psychoneurotic, mainly as having generalized anxiety states, and responses from a healthy community sample. Twenty questions were identified by this means. Among them, items from the Neuropsychiatric Screening Adjunct were 16 times more likely to appear in the new selection than were questions from the other inventories.

Several factor-analytic studies of the Health Opinion Survey were subsequently carried out by members of the Stirling group as well as others (Beiser, Benfari, Collomb, et al. 1976; Benfari, Beiser, Leighton, et al. 1972; Butler and Jones 1979; Murphy 1977; Spiro, Siassi, and Crocetti 1972). A factor reflecting autonomic anxiety has almost always appeared and has been composed of at least some of the Army's items. These studies have not, however, focused solely on the 20 questions of the original Health Opinion Survey. In fact, even the questions that have consistently been asked in the longitudinal study in Stirling County are not exactly identical to those published by Macmillan (1957). This was partly due to the fact that Macmillan's study was not entirely completed when our first survey was carried out. It was also due to the fact that while the questions seemed adequate for anxiety, and most of the concomitants of depression were represented, a question about dysphoric mood was absent. Such a question was therefore added to the version used in our first study in Stirling County and thereafter.

As the study has progressed through time, we have added still other questions about symptoms we thought were affiliated with depression and anxiety. Some of the factor-analytic work has been based on these expanded versions. In an analysis of information from 2,527 subjects studied in the United States and Canada, as well as in Nigeria, Senegal, and South Vietnam, we found that positive responses to questions about "being in poor spirits," "feeling that life was no longer worthwhile," "feeling that people are trying to pick quarrels with you," and "feeling weak all over" formed a factor that could be interpreted as depression in these diverse cultural areas (Murphy 1977).

The work of the Stirling study has not, however, been primarily concerned with developing an improved instrument, since for a longitudinal study it has been important to use consistent data-gathering procedures. In this regard, our work has differed from that of a group of researchers at Johns Hopkins University who have carried out a programmatic sequence of factor-analytic studies leading to an inventory of 90 questions—the Hopkins Symptom Checklist (Derogatis and Cleary 1977; Derogatis, Lipman, Rickels, et al. 1974; Parloff, Kelman, and Frank 1954). The Hopkins Symptom Checklist has benefitted from a long history of building on the results of successive factor-analytic studies and of adding questions as needed (Derogatis, Covi, Lipman, et al. 1970; Derogatis, Lipman, Covi, et al. 1972; Lipman, Rickels, Covi, et al. 1969; Mattsson, Williams, Rickels, et al. 1969; Williams, Lipman, Rickels, et al. 1968).

A 25-item version of the Hopkins Symptom Checklist incorporates factors for depression and anxiety (Hesbacher, Rickels, Morris, et al. 1980). As can be seen in Table 1, the anxiety factor is very similar to the Army's Neuropsychiatric Screening Adjunct, and the depression factor overlaps to a large extent with the symptoms described in DSM-III under major depression and dysthymia. While it would overreach the conclusions of most investigators to say that factor-analytic studies have confirmed clinical syndromes, studies such as those at Hopkins have identified factors that bear a reasonable degree of correspondence to the symptom profiles now available in DSM-III.

Table 1. Depression and Anxiety Factors From the 25-Item Version of the Hopkins Symptom Checklist

Depression	Anxiety
Low energy	Suddenly scared
Blaming self	Feeling fearful
Cry easily	Dizziness
Loss of sexual pleasure	Nervous
Poor appetite	Heart pounding
Trouble sleeping	Trembling
Feeling hopeless	Feeling tense
Feeling blue	Headaches
Feeling lonely	Panic spells
Suicidal thoughts	Feeling restless
Feeling trapped	
Worrying too much	
Feeling no interest	
Feeling everything is an effort	
Feeling worthless	

Note: The questions shown here are paraphrased versions of items that appear in the Patient Symptom Checklist as described by Hesbacher, Rickels, Morris, et al. (1980).

In addition to factor analysis, other multivariate statistical techniques, such as cluster analysis, have been used to explore the relationships between self-reported symptoms and nosologic categories (Benfari, Beiser, Leighton, et al. 1974). A new method, called grade-of-membership (GOM) analysis, has recently been employed to investigate somatization disorder as part of the National Institute of Mental Health (NIMH) Epidemiologic Catchment Area (ECA) program in which information has been gathered by means of the Diagnostic Interview Schedule (Regier, Myers, Kramer, et al. 1984; Robins, Helzer, Croughan, et al. 1981; Swartz, Blazer, Woodbury, et al. 1986; Woodbury and Manton 1982). A characteristic of GOM analysis is that individuals are grouped in terms of "fuzzy" (in contrast to "crisp") categorical definitions. This allows a certain degree of heterogeneity in symptom expression while at the same time providing an examination of the clustering of symptoms free of assumptions about these relationships. The ECA researchers indicate that the emergence of a "pure" type that "is nearly identical to DSM-III somatization disorder represents a strong validation of the natural occurrence of an entity resembling somatization disorder" (Swartz, Blazer, Woodbury, et al. 1986, p. 608).

Diagnostic Algorithm for Syndrome Recognition

Factor analysis and GOM analysis deal with intercorrelations of responses to questions, and the results indicate the degree to which the symptoms form coherent dimensions of psychopathology. The concept of a *syndrome* is different from a *dimension* in that some symptoms in the syndrome are considered to be essential and others to be associated. Sad or disinterested mood is essential to depression just as fearful or apprehensive mood is essential to anxiety. When scales, dimensions, and factors are used to identify cases, a cutting point on a symptom enumeration score is almost always employed, and in such procedures each symptom is given the same weight. Recognition of a clinical syndrome involves an algorithm whereby it is determined *if* the essential features are present, and *then if* sufficient associated symptomatology is exhibited. The use of an operationalized algorithm can help overcome the well-known problems related to differentiating between depression and anxiety (Klerman 1978a).

For the longitudinal study in Stirling County, we decided to try to build a computer algorithm that would simulate the analysis carried out earlier by psychiatrists and that would, at the same time, be sufficiently explicit so that our diagnostic categories could be compared to those in DSM-III. Because discriminant function analysis gives results that to some extent reflect which symptoms should be given the greatest weight to effect the replication of an a priori category, we used this form of multivariate analysis for parts of the program construction (Murphy, Neff, Sobol, et al. 1985).

We named the program DPAX; the DP standing for depression and the AX standing for anxiety. It was designed to analyze the responses given by subjects themselves. In this latter regard, the program addressed the corollary goal of providing a means of analyzing the subject information separately from the general physician information. In the early publications of our study, this separation was not made.

The DPAX program has two basic aspects, the first of which deals with *case-identification* and the second with *diagnosis*. In regard to case identification, the first step involves the application of linear coefficients from discriminant function analysis. The a priori categorization involved a division provided earlier by psychiatrists for separating those subjects who were shown in our earliest data sets for the Stirling study as having a psychoneurotic symptom pattern at the definite level of confidence from those in which there was no evidence of this symptom pattern. We tested the results of discrimination using a split-half approach as well as by repeating the procedures using data from our Queensbrook sample.

The Queensbrook sample was selected in 1964, and we interviewed its members with a questionnaire that is similar to that of the Stirling study. The responses were also analyzed by procedures fashioned on those of our first study in Canada except, in this instance, by a different team of psychiatrists. These psychiatrists had been trained to focus on syndromes and to record their judgments by the same method of documentation used in our other studies. Our plan in using this information was to make the DPAX program as generalizable as possible over time and place.

Four categories are used in the DPAX program's routines for case identification: well, conceivable, borderline, and cases (Murphy, Sobol, Olivier, et al. 1989). The program can be thought of as casting a net, the mesh of which is made successively smaller and tighter so that in the final step only the cases remain. The first step leaves behind those who are well (i.e., those so classified by both the Stirling and Queensbrook coefficients); the second leaves behind those in the conceivable category who mainly have physiologic concomitants in the absence of mood disturbance; the third leaves behind those in the borderline category who have not experienced the preestablished standards for impairment, duration, and symptom intensity. The fourth step identifies the cases.

Using the original evaluations as the standard, the first step of the program has a sensitivity (i.e., proportion of true cases detected as such) of 99% and a specificity (i.e., proportion of non-cases properly excluded) of 64%. At the second step, sensitivity is 97% and specificity is 82%. At the third step, sensitivity is still 97% and specificity is 93%. When all four steps have been carried out, the cases reflect a sensitivity of 92% and a specificity of 98%. These values indicate that the case-identification portion of the program consists mainly in improvements in specificity without undue loss of the initially high sensitivity.

Employing a method of test evaluation derived from medical decision analysis and called receiver operating curve analysis, we found that the DPAX program was a significantly better approximation ($p < .001$) of the decisions of clinical psychiatrists than was the use of a cutting point on scores for the questions about symptoms (Murphy, Berwick, Weinstein, et al. 1987). The difference can be conveyed by reference to a measure called area under the curve (AUC). For the DPAX program the AUC value is .97; for the other scoring systems it is approximately .91. We interpret this information as suggesting that, while co-occurring constellations of symptoms are fundamental to psychiatric judgments, more is involved than simply counting them and applying a cutting point to the scores.

Following the case-identification procedures, the diagnostic aspects of the DPAX program are implemented through an algorithm by means of which depression and anxiety are diagnosed. In Table 2, the components of the algorithm are presented along with the symptoms used in the two syndromes. For depression the first requirement is that the subject report being in poor spirits at least sometimes. The second requirement has two parts and concerns associated symptoms. The first part is a requirement that three characteristic types of associated symptoms be present (i.e., disturbances of sleep, energy, and appetite) following which a threshold on a frequency-weighted score for these symptoms is applied. The third requirement concerns impairment and establishes that the subject has indicated reduced functioning in his or her ordinary work role. The fourth requirement

Table 2. Analytic Components and Syndromes Used in DPAX

Analytic components	Depression	Anxiety
Orienting features	Nervous trouble Nervous breakdown	Nervous trouble Nervous breakdown
Essential features	Poor spirits	Frightening dreams Palpitations Trembling
Associated symptoms	Sleep difficulty Loss of appetite Food tasteless Fatigue Many ailments	Sweating Paresthesias Cold sweats Sick headaches Upset stomach Bad taste in mouth
Impairment	Going easy on work	Going easy on work
Duration	At least one month	At least one month

Note: The criteria for severe depression are given here to illustrate the procedures of DPAX. Step 1 for essential features requires that the subject report that he or she was almost never in good spirits (assigned a value of 3) or that he or she was only sometimes in good spirits (assigned a value of 2). Step 2 for associated symptoms has two components. Step 2a requires that a positive response (value 2 for "sometimes" or value 3 for "often") be given to at least one question in each of the three clusters concerned with sleep, appetite, and energy. Step 2b requires a sum of 11 if Step 1 equals 3 and a sum of 13 if Step 1 equals 2. Step 3 for impairment requires a positive response. Step 4 for duration requires a response of "at least one month."

Source. Reprinted from Murphy, Sobol, Neff, et al. 1984, with permission from the American Medical Association. Copyright 1984, and Murphy, Sobol, Neff, et al. 1985, with permission from the Cambridge University Press.

deals with duration and uses a threshold to determine that the impairment has lasted at least a month. The algorithm for anxiety is similar but the symptoms deal with autonomic hyperactivity and motor tension.

Eight of 10 subjects identified as cases by the program, whether as depressed or as anxious, either say that they are troubled by their "nerves" or respond positively to a question about fearing they may have a nervous breakdown. While such information is neither sufficient nor essential for a diagnosis to be made, its commonness among the cases made us believe that it deserved to be named as an orienting feature. The information about "nerves" is also the basis for a residual diagnostic category, which we call ill-defined affective disorder. This diagnosis is for subjects who are bothered by "nerves" but whose other symptomatology is scattered across both the depressive and anxious syndromes but does not fulfill the complete criteria for either.

Using as a standard the diagnostic decisions of the psychiatrists who made the initial evaluations, the DPAX definition of depression has a sensitivity of 89% and that for anxiety is 96%. The values for specificity are lower (79% and 48%, respectively) due to the fact that we compared the depressed cases, for example, to other cases and not to "well" subjects. The relatively low specificity values also point to the fact that there is a substantial degree of comorbidity among these cases of depression and anxiety, as will be explained more fully below.

The fact that we were able to construct a computer program that performs adequately in terms of sensitivity, specificity, and receiver operating curve analysis stems, to a large extent, from the fact that the evaluating psychiatrists were quite reliable in applying the principles of syndromal recognition, intensity, impairment, and duration from case to case. Also the fact that the symptoms used by the program to identify syndromes tend to be those that factor-analytic studies have shown to cluster together empirically offers an element of validity to the procedures. For example, there is a fair degree of congruence between our symptom profiles and the factors for depression and anxiety in the Hopkins Symptom Checklist. As Robins and Guze (1970) have indicated, however, diagnostic validity needs demonstration from multiple vantage points. These diverse vantage points involve etiology, pathophysiology, course, and outcome. In the next section, some information about outcome is described as it relates to our follow-up of persons diagnosed as depressed and/or anxious.

DIAGNOSTIC COMORBIDITY

In reporting and analyzing findings that involve comorbidity, there are three main strategies of classification: (1) hierarchical, in which categories presumed to be the most informative subsume other categories; (2) comprehensive, in which each diagnosis is shown, irrespective of the presence of other categories; and (3) mutually exclusive, in which unique categories are used for solo and comorbid diagnoses.

It is traditional in clinical psychiatry to apply *hierarchical* rules whereby the presumed most essential syndrome is used irrespective of the other syndromes that may be subsumed (Foulds 1976; Jaspers 1962; Kendall 1975; Sturt 1981). In using the word *essential* to describe a hierarchical principle pertinent to the relationship among syndromes, it is important to link the discussion to what was said earlier about the role of essential features as a diagnostic principle pertinent to the relationship among symptoms. In each case, a category or a symptom takes precedence over another because of its presumed greater importance. Where syndrome recognition is concerned, there are also requirements for the presence of a certain number of associated symptoms. Where a diagnostic hierarchy is concerned, this second level is absent. The hierarchy does not require, for example, that schizophrenia be accompanied by anxiety. Rather the hierarchy states that if schizophrenia *is* accompanied by anxiety, the appropriate diagnosis remains schizophrenia.

In the large sense, the meaning of *essential* as a basis for selecting one diagnosis in preference to another refers to those various attributes that may ultimately lead to the determination that a particular syndrome or a particular combination of syndromes constitutes a valid diagnostic category. To simplify the discussion and relate it to the type of information available in our study, we will focus on seriousness as the essential attribute of interest here. By *seriousness* we refer to poor prognosis in terms of continuing illness or death.

The use of a strict hierarchy in an epidemiologic study means that each case is counted in one and only one category, and the summation of prevalence rates for these specific categories equals overall prevalence. A hierarchical classification is a tidy way of presenting findings. Questions have been raised, however, about whether the exclusion rules needed to implement a hierarchy are valid. For example, DSM-III hierarchies gave precedence to depression over anxiety on the assumption that depression, irrespective of whether it is accompanied by anxiety, is a more serious disorder than anxiety alone. This assumption, however, may be false; and one of the reasons for interest in comorbidity is to formulate the assumption in terms of a testable hypothesis. An alternate hypothesis, for example, is that coexisting depression and anxiety constitute a categorical entity that in and of itself is more serious than either syndrome separately.

Comprehensive classifications are becoming customary for reporting research findings, especially for general population epidemiology (Myers, Weissman, Tischler, et al. 1984; Robins, Helzer, Weissman, et al. 1984). Because of interest in the multiplicity of syndromes, a comprehensive classification was also used in our original publications (Leighton, Harding, Macklin, et al. 1963a). In a comprehensive system, *each* case is shown in *each* category where the information on *that* case satisfies the criteria of *that* category. Since one case can be counted in several categories, summation of the prevalence rates for specific categories usually exceeds overall prevalence.

This approach does not involve assumptions about one category being more important than another. When information is presented in this fashion, visual inspection of the results does not, however, reveal which particular categories are most frequently in coexistence with another category. Nevertheless, computerized statistical approaches, such as those involved in log-linear analysis, can assess the interactive effect of two categories on a dependent variable while also assessing the main effect of a given category (Bishop, Fienberg, and Holland 1975; Olivier and Neff 1976).

A *mutually exclusive* set of diagnostic categories, in which solo syndromes and combining syndromes are shown, is rarely feasible for psychiatric epidemiology studies. This lack of feasibility is due to the fact that when all possible types of psychiatric disorders are involved, the large number of unique categories thwarts both visual and statistical assessment. Nevertheless, an exercise of this type is useful in that it gives empirical evidence about which categories are frequently combined and which are not. Furthermore, if the number of diagnostic categories is limited to a few that are of special interest, statistical interactions can be readily observed in the results.

We designed the DPAX program in a flexible manner so that each of these systems of classification could be used to show findings. Even mutually exclusive categories are feasible since DPAX involves only four categories: (1) comorbid depression/anxiety; (2) solo-depression; (3) solo-anxiety; and (4) residual ill-defined affective.

COMORBIDITY AND PREVALENCE

Our first use of the DPAX program concerned an assessment of the prevalence of depression and anxiety disorders at two points in time, based on two separate samples of Stirling County (Murphy, Sobol, Neff, et al. 1984). The first sample, drawn in 1952, consisted of 1,003 adults who had given complete interview information; the more recent sample, drawn in 1970, involved 1,094 subjects. For the presentation of point prevalence rates, we used a hierarchical arrangement of categories, as shown in Table 3. These rates make use of the DPAX program's diagnostic distinctions as well as its criteria for severe and moderate levels of symptomatology.

We found that current overall prevalence was remarkably similar in the two samples (12.5% for 1952 and 12.7% for 1970) as were also the prevalence rates for the specific diagnoses. Based on the hierarchy, the prevalence of depression (plus or minus anxiety) was approximately 5% in each sample, that of solo-anxiety was about 5% in each, and that for residual ill-defined affective was about 2%.

Not only did year of study lack a main effect according to our use of log-linear analysis, there were also no significant interactive effects between year of study, age of subject, and subject's gender. The degree to which depression and anxiety were comorbid in the sense of being temporally coexisting also did not change markedly, and we

Table 3. Prevalence Rates per 100 Subjects: Depression and Anxiety Disorders by Year of Study

	1952	1970
Diagnostic categories		
Severe depression	1.4	1.5
Moderate depression	3.9	4.1
Severe anxiety	1.3	1.7
Moderate anxiety	3.7	2.9
Ill-defined affective disorder	2.2	2.5
Aggregated categories	12.5	12.7
95% Confidence intervals		
Severe depression	1–2	1–2
Moderate depression	3–6	3–6
Severe anxiety	1–2	1–3
Moderate anxiety	3–5	2–4
Ill-defined affective disorder	1–4	2–4
Aggregated categories	10–15	11–15

Note. There were no sampling zeros in the full contingency table based on age, sex, and nine sampling districts for 1970. For 1952, the following three cells lacked a respondent: women ≥ 70 years of age, men < 30 years of age, and men 60 to 69 years of age. The 1952 standardization was carried out in the following two ways: a lower bound was calculated by filling the empty cell with a fictitious healthy subject and an upper bound by a fictitious ill subject. Because the probability of being healthy is greater than the probability of being ill, the lower-bound rates are shown. To illustrate the difference between the two bounds, the upper-bound rate for the aggregated categories in 1952 is 12.8 and the lower-bound rate is 12.5.

Source. Reprinted from Murphy, Sobol, Neff, et al. 1984, with permission from the American Medical Association. Copyright 1984.

commented that "it is of interest to note that in both years of study, most of the episodes diagnosed as depression also involved anxiety (72% in 1952 and 75% in 1970)" (Murphy, Sobol, Neff, et al. 1984, p. 994). Thus in both of these community samples where prevalence was the focus, it was rare to find a person who reported solo-depression while it was quite common to find a person reporting solo-anxiety. The same relative frequency of solo-anxiety also pertained in our study of incidence (Murphy, Olivier, Monson, et al. 1988).

COMORBIDITY AND CLINICAL OUTCOME

Shortly before selecting the separate sample for 1970, we also began a follow-up of the 1952 sample. The 12.5% standardized overall prevalence of DPAX disorders for 1952 involved 121 cases among the 1,003 adults. Of those who were alive in 1968 when the follow-up began, we were able to re-interview 81%, a proportion that was the same for the cases and non-cases. From the original 121 cases, 79 were living at the time of follow-up and 64 were re-interviewed.

The analysis of clinical outcome among those 64 cases was based on the application of the DPAX program to the responses given in the interviews of 1968 (Murphy, Olivier, Sobol, et al. 1986). Not only does the DPAX program record who has met the criteria of a disorder at the time of inteview, but also it records whether or not the criteria had been met earlier even though the subject had recovered by the time of interview. For a definition of poor outcome involving subsequent morbidity, we used evidence of a DPAX disorder having occurred at some time during the follow-up interval. The durations of these disorders were variable, but about one-fourth of the disorders were chronic in that their sufferers were rarely free of symptoms and impairment. In all, 56% had a poor outcome when those persons with at least one subsequent episode were added to the chronic cases.

Our presentation of the results about the relationships between the 1952 diagnoses and outcome by 1968 involved mutually exclusive categories, as shown in Table 4. Nearly 80% of those who suffered from comorbid depression-anxiety in 1952 had a poor outcome while nearly 85% of those with residual ill-defined affective disorder had a good outcome. It will be recalled that ill-defined affective is different from comorbid depression-anxiety because the symptomatology in the residual category does not fulfill the complete criteria of either depression or anxiety. A log-linear analysis indicated that while diagnosis had a significant effect on outcome ($p < .005$), age and sex lacked both main and interactive effects.

The diagnostic findings raise the issue that comorbid depression-anxiety may carry a poorer prognosis than either diagnosis singly.

Table 4. Effects of Initial Diagnosis on Outcome

Categories	Subjects	Poor outcome (%)
Depression and anxiety	24	79.2
Depression only	8	75.0
Anxiety only	26	38.5
Mixed affective	6	16.6

Source. Reprinted from Murphy, Olivier, Sobol, et al. 1986, with permission from Cambridge University Press. Copyright 1986.

When the effect of depression was controlled for anxiety, however, the significance of depression in regard to poor outcome was prominent ($p = .00025$). On the other hand, anxiety controlled for depression was not significant ($p = .37$). It is possible that this result was influenced by the rarity of solo-depression in the naturalistic environment of a general population study. Nevertheless, the difference between depression and anxiety is brought to light by noting that "depression-plus-or-minus-anxiety" was associated with a rate of 78% poor outcome whereas "anxiety-plus-or-minus depression" was associated with a rate of 58% poor outcome. These latter figures (involving "one category plus-or-minus the other") show the use of a comprehensive system of classification.

COMORBIDITY AND MORTALITY

In describing prevalence at two points in time, I noted above that depression did not interact with sex; that is, the relationship between depression and gender did not change in the two samples. Furthermore, depression was almost equally common in the two sexes at both time periods. In addition, sex did not interact with poor outcome as seen in the perspective of the follow-up study; that is, depressed men and depressed women were about equally likely to have a poor outcome. It should be noted that our prevalence findings are dissimilar to numbers of epidemiologic investigations where the prevalence of depression has been found to be more common among women than men (Boyd and Weissman 1981; Myers, Weissman, Tischler, et al. 1984; Robins, Helzer, Weissman, et al. 1984; Weissman and Klerman 1977b). There is some evidence that this sex difference may relate to methodological conventions or may be changing over time (Hagnell, Lanke, Rorsman, et al. 1982; Kessler and McRae 1981; Murphy 1986c; Srole and Fisher 1980). Nevertheless, the similarity between men and women in regard to depression at the beginning of our study is shown in Table 5. The higher overall prevalence among women of

Table 5. Standardized Point-Prevalence Rates (1952) per 100 Subjects
Depression and Anxiety Disorders

Disorders	Men (n = 456)	Women (n = 547)
Depression and anxiety	3.7	4.8
Depression only	1.0	1.2
Anxiety only	2.3	7.6
Residual mixed-affective	1.2	3.1
Aggregated disorders	8.2	16.7

Note. These rates have been standardized for age and for sampling districts.
Source. Reprinted from Murphy, Monson, Olivier, et al. 1987, with permission from the American Medical Association. Copyright 1987.

the disorders identified by the DPAX program is due to solo-anxiety and residual ill-defined affective disorder.

A relationship between sex and depression *did* appear in the Stirling study, however, when we turned to the topic of mortality. In this regard we found that depressed men were more likely to have an increased risk of death than were depressed women (Murphy, Monson, Olivier, et al. 1987). When all DPAX disorders were grouped together, we found that those diagnosed in 1952 experienced 1.5 times the number of expected deaths, which is a significant elevation of risk (p = .01). When all depression disorders were assessed together (i.e., using the comprehensive classification approach), they bore a significant association with mortality (p = .03). All anxiety disorders grouped together did not have a significant relationship to mortality (p = .21), and the interaction between depression and anxiety also lacked significance (p = .89). The effect of residual ill-defined affective disorder was not significant (p = .07).

With one exception, sex and age did not interact with the diagnoses or with their aggregation. The exception is that the interaction of sex and depression was significant (p = .05), indicating that the risk for men was higher than for women. In presenting these results, we continued to use mutually exclusive categories, as shown in Table 6. This table gives the mortality findings in two ways. One is in terms of standardized mortality ratios based on comparing the Stirling findings with death rates for the province using a life-table computer program prepared by Monson (1974). The other is in terms of the effects estimates from survival regressions based on comparisons within the sample itself using an adaptation of log-linear analysis described by Laird and Olivier (1981).

The findings in Table 6 are suggestive that comorbid depression-

Table 6. Observed and Expected Deaths From All Causes: Depression and Anxiety

Disorders	Men					Women				
	n	OBS	EXP	SMR	EE	n	OBS	EXP	SMR	EE
Depression and anxiety	16	11	4.8	2.3	2.9	27	5	5.3	0.9	0.9
Depression only	8	4	2.4	1.6	2.0	9	4	2.2	1.8	1.6
Anxiety only	12	1	2.4	0.4	0.5	31	9	7.2	1.3	1.2
Residual mixed-affective	4	1	0.9	1.1	1.3	14	7	2.3	3.1	2.5
No affective disorder	416	109	137.2	0.8	1	466	91	95.7	0.9	1

Note. OBS = observed number of deaths; EXP = expected number of deaths based on age, sex, and time of death using provincial standards; SMR = standardized mortality ratio; EE = effects estimate from survival regression.

Source. Reprinted from Murphy, Monson, Olivier, et al. 1987, with permission from the American Medical Association. Copyright 1987.

anxiety may be especially associated with death for men, and solo-depression for women. The meaning of the significance of the findings is revealed, however, in the fact that depressed men irrespective of whether they were also anxious had a standardized mortality ratio of 2.1 (15 observed deaths divided by 7.2 expected deaths equals a standardized mortality ratio of 2.1). The ratio for women who were similarly depressed (i.e., irrespective of anxiety) was only slightly above the expected (standardized mortality ratio of 1.2).

In our study of mortality, we investigated still another type of comorbidity, the coexistence of a DPAX disorder with a physical disorder. The information on physical disorders was derived from the health section of the interviews. We counted as prevalent physical disorders those that met the same criteria for impairment and duration as used for the DPAX disorders; that is, that the physical disorder was associated with "going easy on work" for at least one month.

There was a substantial degree of comorbidity in these terms: 5% of the men and 10% of the women reported that they were impaired in 1952 by both a psychiatric and a physical disorder. The prevalence of physical disorders was associated with increased age. When age was taken into account, however, physical disorders did not bear a significant association with death 16 years later ($p = .60$), nor did they interact with the effect of the DPAX disorders. While the vast majority of the death certificates showed an organic disease as the immediate cause of death, the results about self-reported disorders suggested that "what community residents describe about their physical problems does not seem to have as much long-range meaning for mortality as what they reveal about their psychiatric health problems in regard to the moods and feelings of depression and anxiety" (Murphy, Monson, Olivier, et al. 1987, p. 479).

The association between death and depression among men raised another question about comorbidity. We speculated that some of these men might suffer from both depression and alcohol abuse, and that the risk we found associated with depression might actually reflect the greater lethality of comorbid alcoholism. While our interviews with subjects have been limited in coverage to depression and anxiety, the interviews with general physicians covered all types of psychiatric disorders. The physician information confronted us with several other issues about comorbidity, which we will now describe even though it ultimately led to the discovery that, in our data, depression and alcohol abuse were rarely coexisting disorders.

COMORBIDITY IN PSYCHIATRIC REPORTS PROVIDED BY GENERAL PHYSICIANS WITH A FOCUS ON MORTALITY

In our first publications on the Stirling study, we indicated that when all information was taken into account, 20% of the adults suffered from some kind or kinds of psychiatric disorders (Leighton, Harding, Macklin, et al. 1963b). This is quite similar to the 23% prevalence reported for the Midtown Manhattan study (Srole, Langner, Michael, et al. 1962) and is generally in line with the range from 15% to 19% reported as 6-month prevalence for three sites of the ECA studies (Myers, Weissman, Tischler, et al. 1984).

Originally our rate of 20% was not broken down in terms of which cases came from the subject interviews and which from the physician interviews. Aided by the DPAX program and a computer-assisted procedure for analyzing the physician interviews, we have now been able to present findings for each source of information separately.

As shown in Table 7, the physicians gave a current prevalence rate of 13% pertinent to the 1,029 subjects known to at least one physician (Murphy, Monson, Olivier, et al. 1989). This rate comprised diverse types of disorders, some of which had very low prevalence. While each psychiatric syndrome described by a physician is carried in the data sets for this analysis, we found it impossible to construct a meaningful set of mutually exclusive categories. If we had shown the physician information in absolutely unique categories for solo and multiple diagnoses, the number of categories would have been about half the number of cases. At the same time we believed it unwise to use a hierarchical classification. Thus the diagnoses shown here involve comprehensive classification, and summation of the specific

Table 7. Standardized Prevalence Rates (1952) per 100 Subjects: Types of Psychiatric Disorders Described by General Physicians

Categories	Disorders	Men (n = 469)	Women (n = 560)	Total (n = 1,029)
One	Organic psychosis	0.2	0.0	0.1
	Organic brain syndrome	0.5	0.1	0.3
	Schizophrenia	0.3	0.6	0.5
	Other functional psychosis	0.1	0.7	0.4
	Anorexia nervosa	0.0	0.2	0.1
Two	Alcohol abuse	9.4	0.5	4.9
	Drug abuse	0.1	0.2	0.2
Three	Personality disorder	1.3	2.1	1.7
	Mental retardation	1.8	1.4	1.6
Four	Depression disorder	0.5	2.8	1.7
Five	Anxiety disorder	1.3	4.7	3.0
Six	Somatization disorder	1.8	6.0	4.0
	Other neurotic disorder	0.1	0.5	0.3
Any psychiatric disorder		14.5	12.1	13.3

Note. These rates have been standardized by methods described elsewhere for districts in which different sampling rates were used and for age as well as sex (Murphy, Sobol, Neff, et al. 1984). The rates refer to all subjects described as belonging in that category whether or not they also suffered from a disorder of another type. In the original publications of the Stirling study, information was given about 1,010 subjects who gave at least part of an interview. Subjects who were not interviewed but were known to a physician were not included among the 1,010 but are included here.

Source. Reprinted from Murphy, Monson, Olivier, et al. 1989, with permission from Social Psychiatry and Psychiatric Epidemiology. Copyright 1989.

rates exceeds the overall prevalence since each case is counted in its appropriate category irrespective of whether it is also counted in another category.

The effort to construct mutually exclusive categories was useful in that it disclosed that none of the physicians had reported comorbid depression and alcohol abuse, even though their information indicated that alcohol abuse was sometimes combined with a personality disorder or mental retardation. Furthermore, none of the men who described themselves as depressed were reported to be alcohol abusers by the physicians.

The category that the physicians most frequently gave in combination with another was personality disorder. This seems to fit well with the fact that personality disorders constitute a separate axis in

DSM-III to accommodate their frequent alliance with Axis I disorders. Over and above this, the combinations of specific diagnoses that were most commonly given by the physicians came from the neurotic domain and involved depression, anxiety, and somatization disorder. Somatization disorder in our data means that the physician reported the subject to have multiple physical complaints for which he or she was unable to find an organic basis and which he or she interpreted to be due to accompanying depression or anxiety or simply to the subject's emotional state.

While mutually exclusive categories seemed clearly unrealistic for the physician information, even the comprehensive categories shown in Table 7 seemed too large in number and too uneven in frequencies to allow an interpretable analysis using a dependent variable such as mortality. For this reason, we grouped the specific diagnoses into six categories. The first category is the most heterogeneous, but it has the logic that patient studies have shown that the organic and functional psychoses as well as anorexia nervosa carry an increased risk for death (Innes and Millar 1970; Schwartz and Thompson 1981; Tsuang and Woolson 1977). The second category contains the affiliated disorders of alcohol and drug abuse. The third is for the lifetime patterns of mental retardation and personality disorders. Theoretically a person could have both a psychosis and anorexia, or both mental retardation and personality disorders. Moreover, at the present time, it is not unlikely for a case to involve both drug abuse and alcoholism. For our 1952 sample, however, there was no duplication of cases "within" the six categories, and all the duplication that represents comorbidity occurred "between" the six categories.

In Table 8 we show the mortality risks associated with these six categories as standardized mortality ratios and effects estimates. The highest risk was associated with depression, followed by the organic and functional psychoses. The risk associated with alcohol and drug abuse was quite similar to that for mental retardation and personality disorders. The risks associated with these four categories are significant. While somatization disorder has a modest elevation of risk, it is not significant. Anxiety does not appear to increase the risk of death at all in this sample.

When all those persons with a physician-identified psychiatric disorder were grouped together, we found that they experienced 1.6 times the number of expected deaths, which is a standardized mortality ratio approximately the same as that which pertained to the DPAX cases. Because the physicians had frequently given anxiety as an accompaniment to depression, we carried out further analyses regarding depression, anxiety, and somatization, controlling each for the others and testing their interactions. Depression retained its sig-

Table 8. Observed and Expected Deaths From All Causes: Types of
Psychiatric Disorders Identified by General Physicians

Disorder categories	n	OBS	EXP	SMR	EE	p
Organic brain disorders, psychoses, anorexia	14	9	3.8	2.4	2.4	.025
Alcohol and drug abuse	47	20	12.4	1.6	2.1	.005
Personality disorder, mental retardation	40	14	6.4	2.2	2.4	.006
Depression	17	6	1.8	3.3	3.6	.012
Anxiety	27	6	7.1	0.8	1.0	.920
Somatization, other neurotic	41	12	9.0	1.3	1.4	.300
No disorder	887	206	234.5	0.9	1	

Note. OBS = observed number of deaths; EXP = expected number of deaths based on
age, sex, and time of death using provincial standards; SMR = standardized mortality
ratio; EE = effects estimates from survival regression. A summation of the numbers
under "n" exceeds 1,029 because all subjects described as belonging in a given category
are enumerated whether or not they suffered a disorder of another type. The levels of
statistical significance are derived from survival regressions in which persons in a given
category are compared to well persons. The levels refer to the main effect of that
category when the effects of sex and age were controlled. These main effects did not
interact significantly with sex or age in any category.

Source. Reprinted from Murphy, Monson, Olivier, et al. 1989, with permission
from Social Psychiatry and Psychiatric Epidemiology. Copyright 1989.

nificance as associated with mortality despite these controls, and there
were no significant interactions. In this latter regard, the physician
results also resembled DPAX results. In interpreting the findings from
both studies, we suggested that the cautiousness and avoidance of
risk taking that often characterize anxiety, especially generalized anxiety, might contribute to the absence of risk for death. We also suggested that self-neglect and disinterest in life might be factors that
help explain the association between depression and death.

Summary and Conclusions

Considerable evidence exists that the symptom clusters traditionally employed to define the syndromes of depression and anxiety have roots in empirical correlations based on self-report information. Clinical tradition also, however, gives greater weight to some of the symptoms than others and uses an algorithmic form of decision analysis for diagnosis. For the Stirling study, we constructed a computer program that replicates the procedures by which psychiatrists applied such criteria to identify cases and make diagnoses.

Using this program to assess information gathered longitudinally from subjects in personal interviews and drawing also on reports from general physicians, our findings suggest that depression is a more serious disorder than anxiety. Irrespective of whether it was accompanied by anxiety, depression was more predictive of both subsequent psychiatric morbidity and of subsequent mortality than was anxiety alone. This information supports the traditional hierarchy where depression takes precedence over anxiety. Our findings indicate that it is the depressive component of these often affiliated syndromes that makes for poor prognosis rather than their coexistence. Furthermore, it also appeared that when depression co-occurred with a physical disorder, it was again the depressive component that carried the main risk for death. Lastly, it appeared that depression and alcohol abuse were rarely coexistent, and that depression carried a risk at least as great if not greater than alcohol abuse in this community study.

These points not only summarize our findings about comorbidity focused on depression, they also indicate lines of further research that could profitably be pursued. Of special importance is the need to assess the generalizability of these findings. In a cohort study of young adults in Zurich, for example, it has been reported that a substantial degree of overlap between depression and anxiety was observed in each cross-sectional assessment (Angst, Vollrath, Merikangas, et al., Chapter 7). In this regard, there is similarity to what we have described about Stirling County, but there are also differences between the two studies. For example, the prevalence of depression was about 5% in each of our samples, and about three-fourths of the depressed subjects reported accompanying anxiety. The prevalence of depression in the Zurich study was about 11% at the first assessment, and only about one-third of these depressed subjects reported a coexisting anxiety disorder. It is possible that differences such as these accurately reflect the epidemiology of depression in an urban population of young Swiss adults investigated mainly in the 1980s in contrast to a rural population of young, middle-aged, and older Canadian adults investigated somewhat earlier in historical time. It is more probable, however, that the differences in findings are at least partly influenced by differences in data-gathering techniques and in the criteria used for diagnosis. Although comparability in definitions of disorders is much greater in psychiatric epidemiology studies at the present time than earlier, more research is needed to assess the validity of criteria for diagnosis and to determine whether findings differ because of methods or as a reflection of the empirical situation.

A number of other specific research needs are discernible. Although the results of factor analysis and other correlational assessments support the validity of symptom clusters insofar as they correspond to clinical concepts, the validity of weighting procedures and algorithms as used in our study and in other epidemiologic investigations is still in need of testing. It would also be useful to conduct research on outcome in a study where solo-depression, solo-anxiety, and comorbid depression-anxiety were more equally represented among the cases than has been true of our investigation. Where comorbidity with a physical disorder is concerned, there is need to go beyond subjective assessment and draw on information from physicians or laboratory results. Where depression and alcoholism are concerned, the independence of the two disorders needs further investigation in urban areas and in more recently drawn samples of the population.

While we hope to conduct some aspects of such further research, the work we have carried out to date impresses us with the overall seriousness of a psychiatric condition in which dysphoric mood is central, and characteristic disturbances of sleep, appetite, and energy are its accompaniments.

Chapter 10

Notes on Some Epidemiologic Studies of Comorbidity

Bruce P. Dohrenwend, Ph.D.

T HIS DISCUSSION IS in three parts. The first is concerned with my work on the development of screening scales for epidemiologic research; the second focuses on three of the epidemiologic presentations in this volume; and the third has to do with some preliminary findings from an ongoing epidemiologic study my colleagues and I are conducting in Israel. Unfortunately, each part is more analogous to a one-act play than a three-act drama. I will, however, suggest a scenario by which the separate parts might be converted into a coherent whole.

SCREENING SCALES AND THE PROBLEM OF THE INTERCORRELATION OF SYMPTOMS OF ANXIETY AND DEPRESSION

Over 20 years ago, I had occasion to work with data obtained from a 22-item screening scale developed in the course of the Midtown Manhattan study (Langner 1962). This scale, like the Health Opinion Survey (HOS) constructed during the Stirling County study (Macmillan 1957), consisted of items tapping anxiety, depressed mood, and psychophysiologic symptoms. Like the 15-item Psychosomatic Scale developed for psychiatric screening during World War II (Star 1950)

Work on this chapter was supported by Grants MH-30710, K05–MH 14663, and MH-30906 from the National Institute of Mental Health.

from which these screening scales were descended, the items in them were selected because they discriminated between known psychiatric cases and noncase controls more strongly than the larger pools of test items in which they were originally included.

There now exists a large family of such scales. All have high internal consistency reliabilities, and each tends to be highly correlated with every other (Link and Dohrenwend 1980b). One of the first things that I tried to do when working with one such scale was to construct separate subscales of anxiety, depressed mood, and psychophysiologic disturbance. It was not possible to do so. Each of the resulting subscales was correlated as highly as its reliability would permit with every other subscale. In further research, my colleagues and I constructed 25 scales for use in epidemiologic research with general population samples (Dohrenwend, Shrout, Egri, et al. 1980). Again, we found it impossible to develop empirically distinct scales of anxiety and depressed mood. Rather, these scales correlated as highly as their reliabilities permitted not only with each other, but with six other scales that included low self-esteem, helplessness/hopelessness, dread, confused thinking, psychophysiologic disturbance, and perceived poor physical health.

We were puzzled as to why these particular scales were so highly intercorrelated that none of them was distinct from the others. What, indeed, were they measuring? I was discussing these matters one day with Donald Klein, and he asked if I had ever heard of Jerome Frank's (1973) concept of "demoralization." I had not, but made it my business to do so without delay. On the basis of what I found, I have concluded that all of these highly intercorrelated scales were measuring an underlying dimension of nonspecific psychological distress that is probably best described by Frank's concept.

The Three Epidemiologic Chapters

Since the turn of the century, there have been close to 100 epidemiologic studies in which investigators have attempted to count cases of psychiatric disorders in the general population regardless of whether individuals have ever been in psychiatric treatment (Dohrenwend 1983). Less than 10 of these have been longitudinal.

The reason there are so few is that longitudinal studies are extremely difficult to do. They require generous and stable funding for long periods of time and long-term commitments by research staff. They often face serious problems of sample attrition. Longitudinal studies are, however, extremely valuable for investigating comorbidity. Given the serious problems with trying to use recall to obtain information about past disorders (e.g., Bromet, Dunn, Connell, et al.

1986; Pulver and Carpenter 1983), longitudinal investigations are the best way to obtain knowledge of comorbidity of disorders over time. It is our good fortune to have read in this volume about two of these longitudinal studies (Angst, Vollrath, Merikangas, et al., Chapter 7; Hagnell and Gräsbeck, Chapter 8) together with information from the cross-sectional stage of a third important investigation (Regier, Burke, and Burke, Chapter 6).

Ideally, of course, all three studies would have covered similar and substantial periods of time, all would have used the same state-of-the-art case identification and classification procedures (would that we could agree on what these are), and all would have assessed the same types of anxiety and depressive disorders according to the same diagnostic system. Given the state and stage of this field, that would be too much to ask.

Rather, we read about data from two longitudinal studies covering 7 years (Zurich, Chapter 7) and 25 years (Lundby, Chapter 8) and a third study (five Epidemiologic Catchment Area [ECA] sites in the United States, Chapter 6) with retrospective lifetime coverage. The methodology differs among them, with first-stage screening scales followed by a clinical examination by clinicians in one study (Zurich), diagnostic examinations by clinicians in another (Lundby), and a lay interview designed to yield diagnoses in the third (ECA). In the Lundby study, the diagnostic conventions are those developed by the investigators for research that began before there was general concern with objectively defined research diagnostic criteria. The Zurich study used the *Diagnostic and Statistical Manual of Mental Disorders*, third edition (DSM-III) (American Psychiatric Association 1980) criteria, but had to apply these criteria retrospectively to data collected at the beginnings of the study without benefit of DSM-III. The ECA uses DSM-III criteria. There are differences as well in the types of disorder reported. For example, in the Lundby study, anxiety disorder in general and depression are reported; the ECA chapter reports data on phobia and panic disorder, but not generalized anxiety disorder; the Zurich study includes generalized anxiety disorder as well as phobia and panic disorder. What they all appear to have in common is diagnoses that would probably meet criteria for major depression.

Given this diversity of time period, diagnostic approach, and coverage, it is unproductive to focus on inconsistencies in the results as they bear on correlations between anxiety and depressive disorders. Rather, one hopes that, despite the methodological diversity, there will be consistencies worth our attention. There do appear to be important *inter*-episode relationships that hold up in the longitudinal data from the Zurich and Lundby studies: (1) depression seems to go to depression more often than depression goes to anxiety or anxiety to depression, and (2) anxiety is more likely to evolve into depression than depression into anxiety.

The data on *intra*-episode consistencies are less clear, due partly to differences in the diagnostic subtypes of depression and anxiety counted in the three studies and partly to DSM-III hierarchical conventions with respect to the intra-episode co-occurrence of anxiety and depression. While there appears to be considerable evidence of intra-episode comorbidity of depression and anxiety in the Zurich results, this comorbidity is based largely on phobia and panic disorders rather than generalized anxiety. The ECA findings on phobia and panic disorder seem consistent with the Zurich findings. Unfortunately, these two types of anxiety disorder were not reported separately in the Lundby chapter.

THE ISRAEL STUDY

For the past 7 years, my colleagues and I have been engaged in a large-scale project involving epidemiologic, case-control, and family studies in Israel (Dohrenwend, Levav, Shrout, et al. 1987). A 2-year pilot study to test and calibrate a variety of screening and diagnostic procedures and life stress measures developed in the United States laid the groundwork for the present project (Dohrenwend, Levav, and Shrout 1986; Levav, Krasnoff, and Dohrenwend 1981; Shrout, Dohrenwend, and Levav 1986). The project got underway in 1982 when fieldwork began. Data collection is now nearing completion on the epidemiologic and case-control investigations, and initial analyses have been conducted. I want to discuss some results of one of these analyses of the epidemiologic study. First, however, let me tell you a little about the overall project.

One of the reasons for our choice of Israel as the setting for this research was that we needed a site with a population register. A register would make it possible to draw samples of birth cohorts on the basis of information that was recorded prior to the age of risk for developing the disorders in which we are interested. Such a resource allows unbiased estimates of rates of schizophrenia and antisocial personality, and even some neurotic types of disorders that tend to disappear from contemporary samples because of migration, institutionalization, and early death (e.g., Kendler 1986; Martin, Cloninger, Guze, et al. 1985).

Our focus is on a birth cohort of Jews of European background born in Israel between 1949, just after it became a state, and 1958. They are to be contrasted with Jews of North African background born in Israel during the same period. This gives us a cohort of respondents ranging in age at the time we began the study in 1982 from 24 (following 3 years of obligatory military service and usual completion of formal education) through 33 (maximum age possible). Our main procedures for studying this cohort have involved:

1. Using full probability sampling procedures to select about 5,500 individuals representing the birth cohort of about 177,000 persons from the population register.
2. Using a specially developed set of scales taken from the Psychiatric Epidemiology Research Interview (PERI) to screen this sample for the disorders in which we are interested (Shrout, Dohrenwend, and Levav 1986).
3. Following all screened positives and a sample of screened negatives with a second-stage diagnostic interview by psychiatrists, an adaptation of the Schedule for Affective Disorders and Schizophrenia (SADS) (Endicott and Spitzer 1978) that yields information required for diagnoses according to the Research Diagnostic Criteria (RDC) (Spitzer, Endicott, and Robins 1978a).
4. Selecting subsamples of 100 cases from persons with each of five types of psychopathology and 200 well controls for intensive investigation of social and psychological risk factors.
5. Screening and diagnosing the adult siblings of the above cases and controls to get a measure of the various types of psychopathology in first-degree relatives.

Our procedures have been described in more detail elsewhere (Dohrenwend, Levav, Shrout, et al. 1987). Suffice it to say that more than 40 psychiatrists, trained by Itzhak Levav, have been involved in the diagnostic work. Preliminary evidence from blind reviews of tapes of 64 of their interviews indicates quite satisfactory interrater reliability (Dohrenwend, Levav, Shrout, et al. 1987). Although the fieldwork in the epidemiologic study for respondents living in Israel is not quite complete, we are confident in projecting final completion rates. It is expected that 97% for demographic prescreening of eligible sample members selected from the population register, 93% for the first-stage psychiatric screening interviews, and 95% for the SADS clinical examination will be obtained by the end of the fieldwork, for an overall completion rate of about 86% for respondents alive and residing in Israel. We have only barely begun the diagnostic work with migrants and the deceased via records and informants. In the aggregate, these make up about 10% of the cohort sample.

Although all data collection operations are still underway, preliminary analyses of data from the Tel Aviv metropolitan area, which contains about 40% of the entire population of Israel, are available. Fieldwork and data processing are further along in Tel Aviv than in some of the other areas, and we have checked and cleaned data files for slightly more than 90% of the Tel Aviv sample on PERI screening scores and a little more than 80% on SADS diagnostic examinations.

Of the 1,829 respondents from the Tel Aviv sample who were available for the present analysis, our focus is on the subgroup of 894 (all screened positives and 15% of the screened negatives) who received SADS clinical examinations by the research psychiatrists. Forty-one of this subgroup met RDC criteria for probable or definite current major depression, and 44 met RDC criteria for probable or definite generalized anxiety disorder. Unfortunately, only 5 respondents met criteria for panic disorder and 3 for social phobia, too few to include in the analysis.

Table 1 compares the 41 respondents diagnosed as suffering from major depression and the 44 respondents diagnosed as showing generalized anxiety disorder; 506 respondents were rated as definitely having no current disorder. (An additional 13 were rated as probably no current disorder and are not included.) Both unadjusted means and tests of differences in means adjusted for differences in demographic variables are shown for scaled variables. The statistical method used to adjust for demographic differences is the general statistical model with least-squares estimation. For the two categorical variables of frequent drinking and any use of unprescribed drugs, an analogous procedure, maximum likelihood logistic regression, is used.

The contrasts between major depression and generalized anxiety disorder in Table 1 are striking. Except for frequent drinking, where proportions are extremely small in all three groups (alcohol use is low in Israel), the respondents with depression show more symptomatology on the PERI screening measures than those with anxiety disorder. The respondents with anxiety disorder tend to be about midway between the respondents with no disorder and those with depression on symptom measures. If number and variety of symptoms are the criteria, it would seem that major depression is more severe than generalized anxiety disorder. This is consistent with Murphy's conclusion (Chapter 9).

The question must be raised, however, of whether these results are an artifact of the diagnostic conventions involved in distinguishing major depression from generalized anxiety disorder. In the RDC, anxiety disorder can be a diagnosis only when the full set of criteria for unipolar depression is not met. DSM-III follows a similar convention.

I have no great faith in the accuracy of diagnoses of past disorder based on data involving long-term recall by respondents, at least in general population studies where most cases have never been in psychiatric treatment (Link and Dohrenwend 1980a), which helps

Table 1. Scores on PERI Symptom Measures for Tel Aviv Sample Respondents With Current RDC Diagnoses of Major Depression (Definite or Probable) Versus Generalized Anxiety Disorder (Definite or Probable) Versus No Disorder (Definite)

PERI screening measure	Unadjusted means ± SD			Significance of overall F	Adjusted differences between groups		
	A No disorder (n = 506)	B Generalized anxiety disorder (n = 44)	C Major depression (n = 41)		A versus B	A versus C	B versus C
Demoralization	.98 ± .48	1.45 ± .54	1.83 ± .77	.000	−.39***	−.75***	.36***
Enervation	1.01 ± .62	1.41 ± .76	1.87 ± .82	.001	−.35***	−.78***	.42***
Suicidal ideation and behavior	.19 ± .68	.34 ± 1.01	1.05 ± 1.52	.001	−.12	−.82***	−.70***
False beliefs and perceptions	.29 ± .32	.48 ± .44	.73 ± .57	.000	−.16**	−.42***	−.26***
Schizoid tendencies	.94 ± .57	1.15 ± .76	1.33 ± .77	.000	−.27**	−.42**	−.15
Antisocial history	.46 ± .61	.46 ± .58	.78 ± .83	.000	−.03	−.34***	−.30*
Problems due to drinking	.02 ± .10	.02 ± .07	.10 ± .26	.000	−.01	−.07***	−.07**
	Unadjusted porportions				Adjusted difference in log odds		
"Frequent" drinking	.01 ± .11	.02 ± .15	.02 ± .15	NS	−.70	−.87	−.17
Any unpresceibed use of drugs	.04 ± .20	.05 ± .21	.12 ± .33	NS	−.09	−1.17*	−1.08

Note. PERI = Psychiatric Epidemiology Research Interview; RDC = Research Diagnostic Criteria. *p<.05, **p<.01, ***p<.001. NS = not significant.

Table 2.   Past Major Depression and Generalized Anxiety Disorder in Tel Aviv Sample Respondents With Current RDC Diagnoses of Major Depression (Definite or Probable) Versus Generalized Anxiety Disorder (Definite or Probable) Versus No Disorder (Definite), in Percentages

	Current RDC diagnosis		
Past RDC diagnoses	Major depression ($n = 41$)	Generalized anxiety disorder ($n = 44$)	No disorder ($n = 506$)
Major depression	63.4	22.7	16.6
Generalized anxiety disorder	0	15.9	11.9
Both	2.4	6.8	1.8
Other disorder(s)	19.5	29.5	25.9
No past disorder	14.6	25.0	43.9

Note.   RDC = Research Diagnostic Criteria.

them define the disorder. However, there is no reason why the problem of recall should be more severe for respondents suffering current generalized anxiety than for those suffering from current major depression. Comparing the past disorders diagnosed for respondents in these groups may be instructive. Table 2 shows that 65.8% of those with current major depression have diagnoses of past major depression (63.4% past depression only plus 2.4% with both past depression and anxiety) by contrast with only 29.5% of those with current generalized anxiety disorder (22.7% past depression only plus 6.8% both). Moreover, the rate of past depression for the anxiety group (29.5%) is nearer that of those with no current disorder (18.4%) than that of the depressives (65.8%). Nevertheless, 29.5% is a sizable number, suggesting that it may be useful to look further for etiological and subgroup implications.

Only 22.7% of those with current generalized anxiety have diagnoses of past generalized anxiety. While this is substantially more than the 2.4% figure for those with current unipolar depression, it differs only marginally from the 13.7% in the no disorder group who were diagnosed as having past generalized anxiety.

CONCLUSION

It is tempting to see a common theme in the three parts of this discussion that would make them more like a three-act drama than three one-act plays. The scenario might go like this:

Act I.	There is strong evidence of intra-episode co-occurrence or correlation of symptoms of anxiety and symptoms of depression. There is evidence from research on relations among symptom scales that some of this correlation is due to the presence of underlying nonspecific distress or demoralization.
Act II.	There is evidence, from longitudinal epidemiologic studies especially, of inter-episode comorbidity or correlation of syndromes of anxiety and syndromes of depression. The direction of this relationship over time is more likely to be of anxiety going to depression than depression to anxiety. While depression tends to go to depression, anxiety tends to evolve into either anxiety or depression.
Act III.	Generalized anxiety disorder (and probably other types of anxiety) may be much more analogous to nonspecific distress or demoralization than major depression. It may, in fact, be a risk factor for major depression.

Before a convincing case can be made for this last possibility, however, it will be necessary to have some much-needed missing information. While we have considerable information about the intra-episode correlation of symptoms and syndromes, we know almost nothing about the day-to-day, week-to-week, or month-to-month temporal relations among these symptoms of anxiety and symptoms of depression. Perhaps the methodology developed by de Vries, Dijkman-Caes, and Delespaul (Chapter 40) will be valuable in this effort. If anxiety is, indeed, a nonspecific risk factor for depression and other disorders, there should be an indication of this fact in the temporal sequence of anxiety symptoms and symptoms of depressions within episodes for persons diagnosed as being comorbid for anxiety disorder and depression.

Evidence for Comorbidity: Treated Samples and Longitudinal Studies

Chapter 11

Patterns of Psychiatric Comorbidity in a Large Population Presenting for Care

Juan E. Mezzich, M.D., Ph.D.
Chul W. Ahn, Ph.D.
Horacio Fabrega, Jr., M.D.
Paul A. Pilkonis, Ph.D.

CLINICAL EXPERIENCE REVEALS that individuals showing more than one recognizable psychiatric disorder are not an infrequent occurrence. Such patterns challenge the neatness of our nosologic notions, in regard to both the cross-sectional picture and longitudinal unfolding. Furthermore, they are often perceived as requiring more complex treatment strategies (e.g., Kofoed, Kania, Walsh, et al. 1986).

Documentation of comorbidity has been obtained through both community surveys and clinical studies, as well as by the contents of this volume. For example, Weissman and Merikangas (1986), on reviewing epidemiologic data on adult populations, reported considerable co-occurrence of anxiety and affective disorders. However, it has been in patient care settings where the thrust and diversity of comorbid conditions have been most evident. Particularly prominent has been the documentation of comorbidity indexed to substance use disorders, including alcohol-related conditions (e.g., Schuckit 1983b) and dependence to other substances (e.g., Khantzian and Treece 1985; Weiss, Mirin, Michael, et al. 1986). Also conspicuous have been reports on the comorbidity of emotional conditions of both affective (e.g., Feinberg and Goodman 1984) and anxiety (e.g., Barlow, Di Nardo, Vermilyea, et al. 1986) types, among themselves as well as with other psychiatric disorders. In children, the coexistence of mental retardation and other developmental disabilities, on one hand, and various other mental disorders such as conduct and attention deficit disorders, on the other, has received significant attention (e.g., Sigman 1985). Finally, a major form of psychiatric comorbidity is that reported between personality disorders and several classes of nondevelopmental psychiatric syndromes (e.g., Dahl 1986; Koenigsberg, Kaplan, Gilmore, et al. 1985).

Interest in psychiatric comorbidity seems to have been catalyzed by the development of the third edition of the *Diagnostic and Statistical Manual of Mental Disorders* (DSM-III) (American Psychiatric Association 1980) and its wide implementation and use (Mezzich 1987). Features of DSM-III that facilitate the identification of comorbidity cases are the formulation of mental disorders into separate axes, which has pointedly enhanced the elucidation of personality disorders (Frances 1980), and the organization of most diagnostic categories into phenomenologically based syndromes (Spitzer, Williams, and Skodol 1980). The latter has been influential in the elucidation of comorbidity despite the restrictions on multiple diagnoses imposed by the use of exclusionary diagnostic criteria (Boyd, Burke, Gruenberg, et al. 1984).

Although documentary information on cases of comorbidity is relatively abundant, as noted above, it is also quite fragmented. Understandably, most of the pertinent reports have focused on the identification and description of a specific form of comorbidity (e.g., panic disorder and alcoholism). This situation limits the possibilities of comparing the magnitude, scope, and implications of co-occurring diagnoses. Furthermore, the scarcity of systematic explorations of syndromic co-occurrence across the broad range of psychopathologic conditions points out the possibility of our missing some interesting and potentially useful comorbid patterns. The critical requirement for such systematic explorations is the availability of large populations of psychiatric patients experiencing a wide diversity of pathology and evaluated in a systematic way.

In response to this need, the purpose of this chapter is to display and discuss patterns of comorbidity noted in a large population of patients presenting for care at a comprehensive psychiatric institution during an 18-month period. These patients were diagnostically assessed with a semistructured procedure that allowed the use of all pertinent sources of information and the formulation of judgments covering all diagnostic categories and axes in DSM-III.

EVALUATION SETTING AND PROCESS

The immediate setting for this study was the Diagnostic Evaluation Center, a 24-hour-a-day, 7-day-a-week, walk-in clinic, and the assessment components of the Clinical Modules of the Western Psychiatric Institute and Clinic (WPIC). This houses the Department of Psychiatry of the University of Pittsburgh, located in Allegheny County of the Commonwealth of Pennsylvania. The above-mentioned units conduct the initial comprehensive evaluations of all patients presenting for care prior to clinical dispositions (inpatient or outpatient treatment or no care needed). WPIC is a large, comprehensive, urban-based university psychiatric facility that also serves as a community mental health center. It admits approximately 2,000 inpatients a year and has more than 100,000 outpatient visits a year. This clinical population belongs to all age groups and experiences a wide diversity of forms and levels of psychopathology. It is served through specialized child, adolescent, adult, and geriatric treatment programs.

Patient evaluations are typically conducted by a primary clinician (a resident, medical student, mental health professional trainee, or nurse clinician especially trained in psychiatric assessment) and a supervising psychiatrist. The primary clinician reviews available past records and any documents arriving at that time, interviews the patient and accompanying people, and, if pertinent, makes telephone contact with relatives and health professionals. This clinician then presents the case to the supervising psychiatrist who conducts a brief complementary interview of the patient and accompanying people to clarify diagnostic formulation and dispositional issues. Finally, clinical and legal disposition are jointly made.

The whole assessment process is conducted according to the guidelines of the Initial Evaluation Form (IEF) (Mezzich, Dow, Rich, et al. 1981). This is a standardized instrument that specifies and defines the items to be covered and allows flexibility for the clinician to adjust the order of the interview and probe the patient as needed. As noted above, all live and documentary sources of information available are used. The recording format includes narrative and structured components complementing one another. The IEF was designed to cover all psychiatric disorders and is keyed to DSM-III criterion markers. In an ongoing reliability study, a kappa coefficient of 0.61 was obtained for Axis I and for Axis II across diagnostic categories. The diagnostic format provides space and guidelines for statements along all axes of the DSM-III system. For Axis I, slots are provided for up to four main formulation diagnoses ranked according to importance for evaluation and care. For Axis II, two such slots are provided. There is also space for four and two rule-out diagnoses in each axis, respectively. Completed IEFs are checked regularly by a senior clinician, and their structured components are computerized as part of WPIC's clinical information system (Mezzich, Dow, and Coffman 1981; Mezzich, Dow, Ganguli, et al. 1986).

PATIENT POPULATION

The subjects of this study consisted of the 4,141 new patients presenting for care at WPIC from January 1985 through June 1986. On completion of the IEF, 38% were admitted to inpatient care at WPIC, 26% were referred to WPIC outpatient clinics, and 36% were referred to other health facilities or social agencies.

Table 1 presents a demographic profile for the study population. All ages were represented, adults accounting for 72% of the cases, and the children and adolescents and the geriatric patients about equally complementing the sample. Females at 58% outnumbered males. The largest marital status groups were never married (43%) and married (32%). Ethnically, 80% of the patients were white. The most frequent religious denominations were Catholic (36%) and Protestant (32%). In

Table 1. Demographic Profile of the Study Population of 4,141 Patients

Demographic variables	n	%
Age		
Less than 19 years	547	13.2
19–59 years	2,977	71.9
Older than 59 years	617	14.9
Gender		
Female	2,411	58.2
Male	1,730	41.8
Marital status		
Never married	1,791	43.3
Married	1,309	31.6
Separated	247	6.0
Divorced	408	9.9
Widowed	305	7.4
Unknown	81	2.0
Ethnic grouping		
White	3,314	80.0
Non-white	827	20.0
Religion		
Roman Catholic	1,496	36.1
Protestant	1,324	32.0
Other/none	1,321	31.9

general, the social grouping of the patient population exhibited most aspects of the social spectrum in the metropolitan area where the institute is located.

RESULTS

First, the complexity of the main formulation in Axis I of DSM-III was examined. Here, 23% of the patients received more than one diagnosis. Table 2 shows a list of Axis I categories and their distribution as single versus multiple diagnoses. The categories with highest rates as single diagnoses were senile and presenile dementias (88%), psychotic disorders not elsewhere classified (84%), bipolar disorders (84%), and schizophrenic and paranoid disorders (77%). At the other end of the spectrum, the categories with highest rates as multiple diagnoses were alcohol use disorders (87%), psychosexual disorders (86%), other substance use disorders (86%), mental retardation (85%), and substance-induced organic mental disorders (74%).

Specific intercategorical associations were examined next for patients receiving more than one diagnosis in Axis I. Table 3 displays through a triangular matrix the numbers of patients presenting the various bicategorical combinations of diagnoses. Alcohol use disorders, which was the category appearing with the largest number of multiple diagnoses, was highly associated with three other categories. In fact, 119 of the 444 patients with alcohol use disorder (or 27% of them) were additionally diagnosed as having other substance use disorder, 118 (27%) additionally had major depression, and 63 (14%) had a coexisting adjustment disorder. With regard to the 317 patients diagnosed with other substance use disorder, 64 (20%) also presented with major depression, and 43 (14%) were found to have adjustment disorders as an additional diagnosis. Of the 68 patients presenting with mental retardation, 21 (31%) exhibited an additional diagnosis of other disorders of childhood and adolescence, and 16 (24%) were found to have a comorbid adjustment disorder. Dysthymic disorder was diagnosed in 261 patients; 80 (31%) of them also presented with major depression, and 36 (14%) experienced an anxiety disorder. Of the 533 patients with anxiety disorders, 64 (12%) of them were also diagnosed with major depression. Similarly, of the 25 patients with somatoform disorders, 6 (24%) received an additional diagnosis of major depression. Among the 29 patients with psychosexual disorders, 7 (24%) had an additional diagnosis of major depression, and 6 (21%) concomitantly presented with dysthymic disorder. With regard to the 24 patients with impulse control disorders not elsewhere classified, 7 (29%) of them additionally presented with alcohol use disorder. Finally, of the 126 patients with non-mental-disorder condi-

Table 2. Distribution of Axis I Categories as Single Versus Multiple
Diagnoses

Axis I diagnostic categories	Single diagnosis		Multiple diagnoses		Total
	n	%	n	%	n
Mental retardation	10	14.7	58	85.3	68
Other disorders of childhood and adolescence	176	58.3	126	41.7	302
Senile and presenile dementias	151	88.3	20	11.7	171
Substance-induced organic mental disorders	13	26.0	37	74.0	50
Organic brain syndromes	69	67.0	34	33.0	103
Alcohol use disorders	60	13.5	384	86.5	444
Other substance use disorders	44	13.9	273	86.1	317
Schizophrenic and paranoid disorders	186	77.2	55	22.8	241
Psychotic disorders not elsewhere classified	161	84.3	30	15.7	191
Bipolar disorders	172	83.9	33	16.1	205
Major depression	921	72.2	354	27.8	1,275
Dysthymic disorder	90	34.5	171	65.5	261
Other minor affective disorder	72	65.5	38	34.5	110
Anxiety disorders	374	70.2	159	29.8	533
Somatoform disorders	10	40.0	15	60.0	25
Dissociative disorders	2	50.0	2	50.0	4
Psychosexual disorders	4	13.8	25	86.2	29
Factitious disorders	3	100.0	0	0.0	3
Impulse control disorder not elsewhere classified	8	33.3	16	66.7	24
Adjustment disorders	363	69.0	163	31.0	526
Psychological factors affecting physical condition	2	33.3	4	66.7	6
Non-mental-disorder condition (V codes)	36	28.6	90	71.4	126

tions (V codes), 28 (22%) additionally had an adjustment disorder.

Next, the association of Axis I diagnostic categories with a positive diagnosis of personality disorder in Axis II was investigated.

Table 3. Cross-Tabulation of Axis I Categories for Patients Having Multiple Diagnoses

Axis I diagnostic categories	1	2	3	4	5	6	7	8	9	10	11	12	13	14	15	16	17	18	19	20	21	22	23
1. Mental retardation	X	21	1	0	9	2	5	6	2	0	1	1	2	2	0	0	0	0	2	16	0	1	0
2. Other disorders of childhood and adolescence	21	X	1	1	2	13	18	1	2	1	33	9	3	9	2	0	2	0	0	14	0	19	0
3. Senile and presenile dementias	1	1	X	1	2	3	1	3	0	1	7	1	0	0	0	0	0	0	0	2	0	0	0
4. Substance-induced organic mental disorders	0	1	1	X	2	22	9	1	2	0	3	0	0	1	0	0	0	0	1	4	0	2	0
5. Organic brain syndromes	9	2	2	2	X	9	4	1	0	X	2	0	6	30	0	0	0	0	0	5	0	2	0
6. Alcohol use disorders	2	13	3	22	9	X	119	23	18	15	118	27	6	30	3	0	1	0	7	63	1	11	2
7. Other substance use disorders	5	18	1	9	4	119	X	21	3	13	64	26	11	18	0	0	3	0	1	43	0	10	4
8. Schizophrenic and paranoid disorders	6	1	3	1	1	23	21	X	3	0	2	0	0	2	0	0	1	0	0	0	0	0	1
9. Psychotic disorders not elsewhere classified	2	2	0	2	0	18	3	1	X	0	1	1	0	0	0	0	1	0	0	1	0	0	1
10. Bipolar disorders	0	1	1	0	X	15	13	0	0	X	X	0	2	1	0	0	1	0	0	1	0	0	0
11. Major depression	1	33	7	3	2	118	64	2	1	X	X	80	3	64	6	1	4	0	4	3	1	14	0
12. Dysthymic disorder	1	9	1	0	0	27	26	0	1	0	80	X	2	36	4	0	6	0	0	6	1	5	1
13. Other minor affective disorder	2	3	0	0	6	6	11	0	1	2	3	2	X	11	1	0	3	1	1	0	1	3	0
14. Anxiety disorders	2	9	0	1	30	30	18	2	0	1	64	36	11	X	3	0	0	0	0	3	1	4	1
15. Somatoform disorders	0	2	0	0	0	3	0	0	0	0	6	4	1	3	X	0	0	0	2	1	0	0	0
16. Dissociative disorders	0	0	0	0	0	0	0	0	0	0	1	0	1	0	0	X	0	0	0	0	0	0	0
17. Psychosexual disorders	0	2	0	0	0	1	3	1	1	1	4	6	3	0	0	0	X	0	0	3	0	1	0
18. Factitious disorders	0	0	0	0	0	0	0	0	0	0	0	0	0	0	0	0	0	X	X	0	0	0	0
19. Impulse control disorder not elsewhere classified	2	0	0	1	0	7	1	0	0	0	4	0	1	0	2	0	1	0	X	1	0	2	0
20. Adjustment disorders	16	14	2	4	5	63	43	0	1	1	3	6	0	3	1	0	3	0	1	X	0	28	1
21. Psychological factors affecting physical condition	0	0	0	0	0	1	0	0	0	0	1	1	0	1	0	0	0	0	0	0	X	0	0
22. Non-mental-disorder condition (V-codes)	1	19	0	2	2	11	10	1	0	0	14	5	3	4	0	1	1	0	2	28	0	X	3
23. Unspecified /defer/no diagnosis	0	0	0	0	0	2	4	1	0	0	0	1	0	1	0	0	0	0	0	1	0	3	X
Axis I diagnostic categories	1	2	3	4	5	6	7	8	9	10	11	12	13	14	15	16	17	18	19	20	21	22	23

Table 4 exhibits for each Axis I diagnostic group the frequency of patients presenting an Axis II personality disorder. Across Axis I categories, 14% of all patients were diagnosed with a personality disorder. The diagnostic groups presenting the highest frequencies of personality disorder were those corresponding to somatoform dis-

Table 4. Distribution of 4,141 Patients by Axis I Category and Presence of Axis II Personality Disorders

Axis I diagnostic categories	n	Presence of personality disorder	
		n ($n = 577$)	% of Axis I
1. Mental retardation	68	7	10.3
2. Other disorders of childhood and adolescence	302	17	5.6
3. Senile and presenile dementias	171	1	0.6
4. Substance-induced organic mental disorders	50	3	6.0
5. Organic brain syndromes	103	6	5.8
6. Alcohol use disorders	444	80	18.0
7. Other substance use disorders	317	79	24.9
8. Schizophrenic and paranoid disorders	241	6	2.5
9. Psychotic disorders not elsewhere classified	191	10	5.2
10. Bipolar disorders	205	7	3.4
11. Major depression	1,275	75	5.9
12. Dysthymic disorder	261	53	20.3
13. Other minor affective disorder	110	20	18.2
14. Anxiety disorders	533	45	8.4
15. Somatoform disorders	25	9	36.0
16. Dissociative disorders	4	0	0.0
17. Psychosexual disorders	29	6	20.7
18. Factitious disorders	3	0	0.0
19. Impulse control disorder not elsewhere classified	24	4	16.7
20. Adjustment disorders	526	50	9.5
21. Psychological factors affecting physical condition	6	1	16.7
22. Non-mental-disorder condition (V-codes)	126	4	3.2
23. Unspecified/defer/no diagnosis	242	94	38.8

orders (36%), other substance use disorder (25%), psychosexual disorders (21%), dysthymic disorder (20%), other minor affective disorders (18%), and alcohol use disorder (18%).

The distribution of Axis I diagnostic groups across the four DSM-III personality disorder clusters is displayed in Table 5. The first cluster, "odd," including paranoid, schizoid, and schizotypal personality disorders, accounted for 7% of all personality diagnoses. The second, "dramatic," encompassing histrionic, narcissistic, antisocial, and borderline personality disorders, accounted for 45% of all personality disorders. The third, "anxious," including avoidant, dependent, compulsive, and passive-aggressive personality disorders, represented 19% of the personality diagnoses. The fourth cluster, "miscellaneous," including atypical, mixed, and other personality disorders, constituted 30% of the personality disorders. When compared against the above base rates, some Axis I categories were noticeably associated with certain personality disorder clusters. Alcohol use disorders and other substance use disorders were both associated with the dramatic personality cluster. Anxiety disorders and dysthymic disorder were associated with the anxious personality cluster. Other minor affective disorders (cyclothymic, atypical bipolar, and atypical depressive disorders) were associated with the miscellaneous personality cluster.

Finally, an attempt was made to explore the clinical utility of comorbidity patterns through the appraisal of their impact on clinical disposition. To this effect, the distributions in terms of outpatient versus inpatient disposition of the various Axis I diagnostic groups, qualified as single versus multiple diagnosis, and with versus without personality disorder were studied. The results are shown in Table 6, which presents the number and percentage of cases that were hospitalized for each of the four diagnostic patterns and each Axis I diagnostic category. Only the 2,639 patients admitted to either inpatient or outpatient care at WPIC on completion of their initial evaluation were considered here (not so those patients referred to facilities outside WPIC, for whom the final inpatient versus outpatient disposition was uncertain). For the case of multiple Axis I diagnoses, the overall number of patients is different from the sum of patients in individual diagnostic categories due to the fact that some patients had more than one diagnosis.

Focusing attention on inpatient disposition, it can be determined that this was the disposition for 59% of the patients across diagnostic groupings. The dispositional impact of single versus multiple Axis I diagnoses and of the presence of personality disorders were not clear or consistent across patients. However, interesting dispositional patterns appeared when the distributions for individual Axis I diagnostic

Table 5. Distribution of Patients by Axis I Category and Axis II Personality Disorder Clusters

					Personality disorder clusters					
	Odd		Dramatic		Anxious		Miscellaneous			
Axis I diagnostic categories	n ($n = 41$)	Row % (7.1)	n ($n = 257$)	Row % (44.5)	n ($n = 108$)	Row % (18.7)	n ($n = 171$)	Row % (29.6)		
1. Mental retardation	1	14.3	1	14.3	2	28.6	3	42.9		
2. Other disorders of childhood and adolescence	2	11.8	7	41.2	6	35.3	2	11.8		
3. Senile and presenile dementia	1	100.0	0	0.0	0	0.0	0	0.0		
4. Substance-induced organic mental disorders	0	0.0	2	66.7	0	0.0	1	33.3		
5. Organic brain syndromes	2	33.3	1	16.7	1	16.7	2	33.3		
6. Alcohol use disorders	1	1.3	53	66.3	7	8.8	19	23.8		
7. Other substance use disorders	2	2.5	50	63.3	1	1.3	26	32.9		
8. Schizophrenic and paranoid disorders	1	16.7	1	16.7	1	16.7	3	50.0		
9. Psychotic disorders not elsewhere classified	4	40.0	1	10.0	1	10.0	4	40.0		

		n	%	n	%	n	%	n	%
10.	Bipolar disorders	0	0.0	4	57.1	1	14.3	2	28.6
11.	Major depression	4	5.3	32	42.7	20	26.7	19	25.3
12.	Dysthymic disorder	2	3.8	13	24.5	19	35.8	19	35.8
13.	Other minor affective disorder	1	5.0	6	30.0	4	20.0	9	45.0
14.	Anxiety disorders	2	4.4	13	28.9	21	46.7	9	20.0
15.	Somatoform disorders	0	0.0	4	44.4	2	22.2	3	33.3
16.	Dissociative disorders	0	0.0	0	0.0	0	0.0	0	0.0
17.	Psychosexual disorders	0	0.0	3	50.0	1	16.7	2	33.3
18.	Factitious disorders	0	0.0	0	0.0	0	0.0	0	0.0
19.	Impulse control disorder not elsewhere classified	1	25.0	2	50.0	0	0.0	1	25.0
20.	Adjustment disorders	4	8.0	21	42.0	11	22.0	14	28.0
21.	Psychological factors affecting physical condition	0	0.0	1	100.0	0	0.0	0	0.0
22.	Non-mental-disorder condition (V codes)	1	25.0	1	25.0	0	0.0	2	50.0
23.	Unspecified/defer/no diagnosis	12	12.8	41	43.6	10	10.6	31	33.0

Note. Odd includes paranoid, schizoid, and schizotypal personality disorders; dramatic includes histrionic, narcissistic, antisocial, and borderline personality disorders; anxious includes avoidant, dependent, compulsive, and passive-aggressive personality disorders; miscellaneous includes atypical, mixed, and other personality disorders.

categories were examined. Inpatient disposition was highly associated with single Axis I diagnoses of organic brain syndromes and psychotic disorders not elsewhere classified, and with multiple diagnoses separately involving anxiety disorders and adjustment disorders. Other disorders of childhood adolescence were significantly associated with inpatient admission when personality disorders were absent. Alcohol use disorders were closely connected with hospitalization when they were both combined with other Axis I disorders and free of a personality disorder.

DISCUSSION

We have attempted to elucidate patterns of psychiatric comorbidity in a large population presenting for care and assessed with a semistructured procedure. Perhaps most importantly, this design allowed the conduct of a naturalistic study on a fresh and broad patient population, seen in a regular clinical setting before institutionalization took place.

A number of interesting patterns were detected. Regarding frequent comorbid conditions in Axis I, one of the principal patterns found was the co-occurrence of substance use disorders, particularly those alcohol-related, on one hand, and major depression and impulse control disorder, on the other hand. The association with major depression has been often reported in the literature (e.g., Famularo, Stone, and Popper 1985; Khantzian and Treece 1985; Schuckit 1983b; Weiss, Mirin, Michael, et al. 1986), while this has not been the case for the association with impulse control disorder. Another important and broadly based form of comorbidity was that noted between major depression and several neurotic-like conditions such as anxiety disorder, dysthymic disorder, somatoform disorder, and psychosexual disorder. Of these, the association with anxiety disorder has been prominently reported and discussed in the literature (e.g., Barlow, Di Nardo, Vermilyea, et al. 1986; Weissman and Merikangas 1986). Also noteworthy is the association found between mental retardation and other disorders of childhood and adolescence, a widely recognized pattern as pointed out by Sigman (1985) and one in line with the recent relocation of mental retardation from Axis I to Axis II in DSM-III-R (American Psychiatric Association 1987). Mental retardation was also associated with adjustment disorders, a finding much less frequently reported and one that again speaks to the contrast between the relatively stable mental retardation and co-occurring episodic or incidental conditions.

With respect to Axis I–Axis II comorbidity, associations with personality disorders were found for alcohol and other substance use, dysthymic, other minor affective, anxiety, somatoform, and psycho-sexual disorders. Except for the latter, the Axis I categories listed above have been reported to co-occur with personality disorders (e.g., Koenigsberg, Kaplan, Gilmore, et al. 1985). Regarding associations with specific forms of personality disorder, we found that other substance use disorders are particularly associated with the dramatic personality cluster (histrionic, narcissistic, antisocial, and borderline personality disorders). This association is in line with reports relating substance abuse to antisocial personality disorder (Vaglum and Vaglum 1985). We also found that anxiety disorders and dysthymic disorder were significantly associated with the anxious personality cluster (avoidant, dependent, compulsive, and passive-aggressive personality disorders) and that other minor affective disorders (cyclothymic, atypical bipolar, and atypical depressive disorders) were noticeably associated with the miscellaneous personality cluster (atypical, mixed, and other personality disorders). These associations were not apparent in our review of the literature and represent promising new perspectives for future research. It should be noted that the fact that the study was based on initial patient evaluations limited the depth of the appraisals of personality disorder. This limitation may be responsible for the relatively low rate of this diagnosis (14% across the board). Most Axis II diagnoses were "deferred," suggesting the need for more extensive assessments. Systematic explorations of personality markers and the wider use of multiple informants should be useful in this regard.

The impact of comorbidity on clinical disposition appeared to be intricate. Multiple diagnoses in Axis I were associated with inpatient care in the case of three conditions (alcohol use, anxiety, and adjustment disorders), which may be seen phenomenologically as neurotic. On the other hand, two diagnostic categories, organic brain syndromes and psychotic disorders not elsewhere classified, tended to lead to hospitalization when present as single diagnoses. Interestingly, these two diagnoses involve serious disorders (organic, psychotic) ranked high in commonly accepted illness hierarchies such as that described by Foulds (1976). Furthermore, they are not well-defined or understood conditions; they are potentially life-threatening in some cases. On all of these bases, they often require close supervision and prompt assessment. Given that the first three diagnostic categories (alcohol use, anxiety, and adjustment disorders) having an inpatient weight as multiple diagnoses involve less serious disorders and are less potentially lethal in an immediate sense, a severity dimension seems to influence the impact of single versus multiple diagnoses on inpatient disposition.

The presence or absence of Axis II diagnoses did not have a

Table 6. Distribution of Inpatients by Clinical Disposition and by Axis I Category as Single Versus Multiple Diagnosis, and With Versus Without Personality Disorder (PD)

Axis I diagnostic category	Axis I single without PD		Axis I single with PD		Axis I multiple without PD		Axis I multiple with PD	
	n	%	n	%	n	%	n	%
1. Mental retardation	8	75.0	0	—	37	67.6	4	50.0
2. Other disorders of childhood and adolescence	122	76.2	5	60.0	84	64.3	6	16.7
3. Senile and presenile dementias	140	97.1	1	100.0	18	88.9	0	—
4. Substance-induced organic mental disorders	7	100.0	0	—	14	92.9	1	100.0
5. Organic brain syndromes	50	98.0	2	100.0	20	75.0	1	100.0
6. Alcohol use disorders	6	16.7	12	58.3	164	73.8	23	60.9
7. Other substance use disorders	13	61.5	5	80.0	110	72.7	24	54.2
8. Schizophrenic and paranoid disorders	145	81.4	3	33.3	106	76.5	0	—

	n	%	n	%	n	%	n	%
9. Psychotic disorders not elsewhere classified	112	95.5	2	50.0	18	77.8	1	100.0
10. Bipolar disorders	119	78.2	0	—	19	78.9	2	100.0
11. Major depression	653	60.2	17	76.5	210	55.2	20	55.0
12. Dysthymic disorder	31	19.4	9	22.2	85	34.1	14	35.7
13. Other minor affective disorder	37	51.4	4	25.0	9	33.3	5	60.0
14. Anxiety disorders	227	9.7	11	9.1	68	27.9	16	37.5
15. Somatoform disorders	1	0.0	0	—	5	40.0	2	50.0
16. Dissociative disorders	0	—	0	—	2	100.0	0	—
17. Psychosexual disorders	3	0.0	0	—	13	61.5	1	100.0
18. Factitious disorders	3	100.0	0	—	0	—	0	—
19. Impulse control disorder not elsewhere classified	3	66.7	1	100.0	10	60.0	0	—
20. Adjustment disorders	199	46.7	18	22.2	83	72.3	10	50.0
21. Psychological factors affecting physical condition	1	0.0	0	—	2	0.0	0	—
22. Non-mental-disorder condition (V codes)	10	0.0	1	0.0	35	40.0	1	0.0

consistent impact on hospitalization decisions. Nevertheless, whenever such an impact was noticeable (as in the case of other disorders of childhood and adolescence and alcohol use disorders), this was connected to the absence of Axis II disorders. These are examples of situations where more diagnoses appear to detract from rather than contribute to hospitalization decisions.

The complexity of the results obtained raises the question of the nature of comorbidity. Does this refer essentially to combined conditions not anticipated in existing diagnostic systems? Does it primarily reflect a predisposition established by certain syndromes to the development of other conditions? The first question is answered positively for some cases in new standard diagnostic systems, such as the draft of the 10th revision of the International Classification of Diseases (ICD-10) (World Health Organization 1987), which includes a mixed anxiety and depressive disorder. The second option served as a basis for setting hierarchical exclusionary criteria in DSM-III, although they have been challenged in several cases (Boyd, Burke, Gruenberg, et al. 1984). A prospective, longitudinal approach to the study of comorbid conditions, particularly in naturalistic clinical settings, should clarify their interactive unfolding and, therefore, their descriptive validity as well as their impact on clinical decisions and utilization of care.

Chapter 12

Syndrome and Symptom Co-Occurrence in the Anxiety Disorders

Peter A. Di Nardo, Ph.D.
David H. Barlow, Ph.D.

Most diagnostic systems make use of exclusionary criteria that specify that certain diagnoses are not permitted in the presence of another disorder or class of disorders. This rule serves the practical purposes of assigning a single diagnosis to a case for purposes of assignment to treatment or formation of research groups in studies on the validity of diagnostic categories. The *Diagnostic and Statistical Manual of Mental Disorders*, Third Edition (DSM-III) (American Psychiatric Association 1980) and related systems, such as the Feighner criteria (Feighner, Robins, Guze, et al. 1972) and the Research Diagnostic Criteria (RDC) (Spitzer, Endicott, and Robins 1978a), make extensive use of such exclusions.

In DSM-III, anxiety disorders were excluded in the presence of a number of other specific disorders or classes of disorders. For example, affective disorders occupied a higher position than anxiety disorders, so a diagnosis of major depression excluded a diagnosis of panic disorder if, in the clinician's judgment, the panic disorder was "due to" the major depressive episode. Within the anxiety disorders, there also existed exclusionary rules. For example, a diagnosis of generalized anxiety disorder was automatically excluded by the presence of panic disorder. These examples illustrate the distinction made in DSM-III between "essential features" and "associated features" of a disorder. Generalized, chronic anxiety was an essential feature of generalized anxiety disorder, but an associated feature of panic disorder. When chronic anxiety occurred in the presence of panic disorder, it was considered to be a part of the panic disorder rather than an independent, coexisting syndrome.

These exclusionary rules have been criticized on a number of grounds. First, the few studies that have critically examined the hierarchical systems on which the exclusionary rules are based have not provided strong support for the assumptions underlying the hierarchies. In a community study, Boyd, Burke, Gruenberg, et al. (1984) found that when DSM-III diagnoses were assigned without exclusionary restrictions, the presence of any disorder increased the probability of the presence of other disorders that would normally be excluded. For example, the presence of major depression greatly increased the probability of having panic disorder, supporting the assumption that panic is often associated with major depression. Boyd, Burke, Gruenberg, et al. also noted that the presence of any DSM-III disorder was associated with an increased probability of having any other DSM-III disorder, regardless of whether the disorders are related in the exclusionary rules. Using data from the Present State Examination, Sturt (1981) demonstrated that patients with infrequently occurring symptoms or syndromes tend to show a high number of other symptoms or syndromes. Sturt interpreted these results not necessarily as support for any specific hierarchical system, but as evidence of a more general tendency for the presence of any given symptom to be associated with the presence of several other symptoms.

Second, the exclusion of diagnoses leads to a loss of information that is potentially important in understanding relationships among the disorders and in identifying dimensions of pathology that underlie the categories. There is evidence that the presence of additional syndromes may delineate homogeneous subgroups within a major diagnostic category that have different patterns of familial aggregation, course, or response to treatment. In a family study of depression, Leckman, Weissman, Merikangas, et al. (1983) showed that the presence of panic attacks in depressed patients was associated with an increased family prevalence of other anxiety disorders, depression, and alcoholism. In view of these considerations, several investigators have suggested modifications in the exclusionary rules in DSM-III. In response to these suggestions, DSM-III-R (American Psychiatric Association 1987) has eliminated many automatic exclusions and replaced others with decision rules that are based on case-by-case consideration of the relationships among the various symptom clusters in a given patient.

Similarly, several investigators have focused their attention on the DSM-III anxiety disorders and have critically evaluated the hierarchical assumptions underlying this class of disorders (Barlow, Di Nardo, Vermilyea, et al. 1986; Spitzer and Williams 1985c). In considering these hierarchical assumptions, Spitzer and Williams distinguish between "associated features" of a disorder and "coexisting complications" of a disorder. Consistent with DSM-III, associated features are symptoms that are typical aspects of the clinical picture of a particular disorder. In the presence of that disorder, the associated symptomatology would not warrant a separate diagnosis. For example, phobic avoidance of dirt is a typical feature in patients with obsessive thoughts about contamination, so a separate diagnosis of simple phobia is not warranted in such cases of obsessive-compulsive disorder. Similarly, in our work, we have found that fear and avoidance of heights or enclosed places, sufficient to meet the criteria for simple phobia, are often reported by agoraphobics. These symptoms usually prove to be an associated part of the agoraphobic symptomatology because these situations represent the unavailability of an escape route in case of a panic. In these examples, the diagnosis of simple phobia is excluded because the phobia is directly related to the content of the obsessive-compulsive or agoraphobic syndrome. Similarly, chronic anxiety or tension in the presence of a specific phobia or panic disorder may prove to be an associated feature of the phobia or panic disorder. This would be the case if the chronic anxiety is related to the phobia itself, such as a patient with social phobia who worries about the next social encounter or a patient with panic who is constantly fearful about the possibility of experiencing another attack. In both of these cases, a separate diagnosis of generalized anxiety disorder would not be warranted.

Unlike an associated feature, a coexisting complication, as defined by Spitzer and Williams (1985c), is a symptom or symptom cluster that is concurrent with the symptoms of another disorder, but that is not a typical feature of that disorder. For example, a patient at our clinic reported long-standing problems with anxiety, worry, and tension, and also reported a specific fear of the sight of blood, which was precipitated when he witnessed a particularly gruesome suicide. The patient met the criteria for generalized anxiety disorder, but was also given an additional diagnosis of simple phobia because his fear of blood was not related to his generalized anxiety. In work at our clinic, we have also identified cases in which generalized anxiety disorder can be meaningfully assigned as an additional diagnosis in the presence of other anxiety disorder diagnoses (Barlow, Di Nardo, Vermilyea, et al. 1986; Di Nardo, O'Brien, Barlow, et al. 1983). Based on DSM-III-R criteria, generalized anxiety disorder should be assigned as an additional diagnosis when the patient reports chronic anxiety symptomatology in which the focus of apprehensive expectation is on multiple situations other than the anxiety disorder itself. A patient who meets the criteria for panic disorder but who also reports chronic and excessive worry about financial matters and child rearing would be given an additional diagnosis of generalized anxiety disorder. The determination of whether a symptom is an associated feature or a coexisting complication of another disorder is based on the specific content of the symptomatology, so this decision is made on a case-by-case basis. Many of these suggestions have been incorporated into the DSM-III-R anxiety disorder categories.

These suggested guidelines often result in multiple anxiety diagnoses. It is often necessary to assign one diagnosis as the primary diagnosis for purposes of treatment planning or for studies on the discriminant validity of diagnostic categories. When multiple diagnoses are assigned, the disorder that is responsible for the greatest interference with the patient's functioning is given primary status (see Blashfield, Chapter 4, for a broader consideration of primary versus secondary diagnoses). In the case of generalized anxiety disorder and simple phobia above, the blood fear was sufficiently severe to warrant a separate diagnosis, but because the patient's chronic anxiety was interfering with a number of areas of functioning, generalized anxiety disorder was assigned as the primary diagnosis.

At the State University of New York at Albany, Center for Stress and Anxiety Disorders, we developed the Anxiety Disorders Interview Schedule (ADIS) (Di Nardo, O'Brien, Barlow, et al. 1983), a structured interview protocol designed to permit differential diagnosis among the anxiety disorders. The interview also assesses affective disorders and screens for psychotic symptoms and substance abuse. The interview protocol also includes the Hamilton Anxiety Rating Scale (HARS) (Hamilton 1959) and the Hamilton Rating Scale for Depression (HRSD) (Hamilton 1960), with items grouped according to content to permit simultaneous rating of anxious and depressive symptomatology. In reliability studies on the ADIS, we used the stringent criterion of an exact match on primary diagnosis between independent interviewers (Barlow 1985). Using guidelines for interpreting kappa suggested by Spitzer and Fleiss (1974), the ADIS shows high reliability for social phobia (.905); satisfactory reliability for agoraphobia with panic (.854), obsessive-compulsive disorder (.825), and panic disorder (.651); and fair reliability for generalized anxiety disorder (.571) and simple phobia (.558). The ADIS is also designed to gather information beyond that required for establishing the basic diagnostic criteria. The interview assesses the degree and range of avoidance and provides detailed anxiety symptom ratings. This information permits comparison of anxiety symptoms across diagnostic categories.

Since 1982, we have used the ADIS to diagnose and collect data on a large number of patients who presented at our clinic. Although we could reliably assign patients to a single anxiety disorder category, we also noted that many patients satisfied the basic criteria for more than one anxiety disorder. Also, many patients met the criteria for an affective disorder. Using the guidelines described above, we systematically recorded the presence of these coexisting disorders and gathered additional interview and psychometric data to permit a detailed description of symptom and syndrome comorbidity in the anxiety disorders.

We recently presented diagnostic and psychometric findings on a preliminary sample from this group (Barlow, Di Nardo, Vermilyea, et al. 1986). In this chapter, we will present data from 292 patients diagnosed using DSM-III criteria (with modifications discussed above). We will first focus on syndrome comorbidity among the anxiety disorders, examining the distribution of hierarchy-free diagnoses in the sample. Then, we will examine the evidence concerning the distribution of specific symptoms across the anxiety disorders. Specifically, we will consider how depression, panic, generalized anxiety, somatic symptoms, and social fears cut across all of the anxiety disorder categories, and how these symptoms may be used in a dimensional analysis of anxiety.

Syndrome Comorbidity

Table 1 presents the distribution of primary diagnoses within our sample, and the percentage of females within each diagnostic group. As can be seen from the table, agoraphobia and panic disorder are the most common disorders in the sample, accounting for 29% and 23% of the sample, respectively. With the exception of agoraphobia without panic, obsessive-compulsive disorder is the least frequently occurring anxiety disorder. These figures are consistent with earlier reports (Barlow, Di Nardo, Vermilyea, et al. 1986; Di Nardo, O'Brien, Barlow, et al. 1983) on the relative frequencies of the anxiety disorders. The relatively small percentages of major depressive disorder and dysthymic disorder in our sample may reflect the specialized nature of our clinic.

Although our sample is predominantly female, the sex distribution is not equal across the diagnostic categories. Females account for 66% of the total sample and a similar percentage (67%) of panic disorder. However, they make up 82% of those with agoraphobia, 77% of those with dysthymia, 74% of those with simple phobia, and 70% of those with major depression. There are slightly more females (57%) with generalized anxiety disorder and there are slightly more

Table 1. Distribution of Primary Diagnoses and of Females in Each Diagnosis

	Agoraphobia with panic		Agoraphobia without panic		Social phobia		Simple phobia		Panic disorder		Generalized anxiety disorder		Obsessive-compulsive		Major depression		Dysthymia	
	n	%	n	%	n	%	n	%	n	%	n	%	n	%	n	%	n	%
Distribution of diagnosis	86	29	1	0	48	16	24	8	67	23	31	11	15	5	11	4	9	3
Distribution of females in each diagnosis	70	82	0	0	20	41	18	74	45	67	18	57	7	47	8	70	7	77

Table 2. Number of Additional Diagnoses Among the Anxiety and Affective Disorders

	Primary diagnosis																	
	Agoraphobia with panic (n = 86)		Agoraphobia without panic (n = 1)		Social phobia (n = 48)		Simple phobia (n = 24)		Panic disorder (n = 67)		Generalized anxiety disorder (n = 31)		Obsessive-compulsive (n = 15)		Major depression (n = 11)		Dysthymia (n = 9)	
Additional diagnosis	n	%	n	%	n	%	n	%	n	%	n	%	n	%	n	%	n	%
0	47	55	1	100	28	58	16	67	36	54	17	55	8	53	3	27	2	22
1	27	31			13	27	7	29	20	30	8	26	5	33	5	45	3	33
2	8	9			7	15	1	4	8	12	4	13	1	7	3	27	3	33
3	3	3							1	1	2	6	1	7			1	11
4	1	1							2	3								

males with social phobia (59%) and with obsessive-compulsive disorder (53%). These differences are significant ($\chi^2 = 29.84, p < .0002$).

Table 2 presents the number of additional diagnoses among the anxiety and affective disorders. Among the anxiety disorders, additional diagnoses were assigned in 42% to 47% of the cases, with the exception of agoraphobia without panic (0%) and simple phobia (33%). Among the affective disorders, additional diagnoses were assigned in 75% of the cases. Twenty-nine percent of the anxiety disorder cases received one additional diagnosis, and 11% received two additional diagnoses. Instances of three or four additional diagnoses were rare. When clinicians were permitted to assign hierarchy-free diagnoses, they often elected to assign one additional diagnosis to complete the clinical picture. However, it is clear from these data that a hierarchy-free system does not result in indiscriminant assignment of multiple diagnoses.

Next we turn to the distribution of specific additional diagnoses. Table 3 shows the frequency with which the additional diagnoses were assigned. By far the most commonly assigned additional diagnosis was simple phobia (19%), reflecting the frequency with which independent, specific fears occur in the context of other anxiety disorders. Social phobia, generalized anxiety disorder, and dysthymia were assigned as additional diagnoses in 11% of the cases, while additional diagnoses of agoraphobia with panic, panic disorder, and obsessive-compulsive disorder were relatively rare. Current episodes of major depression appear to be relatively rare in our treated sample, a point to which we will return later.

Table 4 shows the distribution of specific additional diagnoses among the anxiety and affective disorders. This table gives the number of cases in which the additional diagnosis was assigned and the percentage of cases within the specific category that received the

Table 3. Number of Cases in Which Each Additional Diagnosis Was Assigned

	n	%
Agoraphobia with panic	3	1.0
Social phobia	32	11.0
Simple phobia	54	18.5
Panic disorder	6	2.1
Generalized anxiety disorder	31	10.6
Obsessive-compulsive	7	2.4
Major depression	12	4.1
Dysthymia	33	11.3

Table 4. Additional Diagnoses Among Anxiety and Affective Disorders

Additional diagnosis	Primary diagnosis															
	Agoraphobia with panic (n = 86)		Social phobia (n = 48)		Simple phobia (n = 24)		Panic disorder (n = 67)		Generalized anxiety disorder (n = 31)		Obsessive-compulsive (n = 15)		Major depression (n = 11)		Dysthymia (n = 9)	
	n	%	n	%	n	%	n	%	n	%	n	%	n	%	n	%
Agoraphobia with panic	—	—	1	2	1	4	0	0	0	0	0	0	1	9	0	0
Social phobia	8	9	—	—	1	4	11	16	5	16	2	13	1	9	4	44
Simple phobia	20	23	7	15	3	13	10	15	9	29	1	7	1	9	3	33
Panic disorder	0	0	1	2	0	0	—	—	1	3	1	7	2	18	1	11
Generalized anxiety disorder	6	7	2	4	2	8	11	16	—	—	2	13	5	45	3	33
Obsessive-compulsive	3	3	2	4	0	0	1	2	1	3	—	—	0	0	0	0
Major depression	5	6	1	2	0	0	3	4	2	6	1	7	—	—	0	0
Dysthymia	10	12	11	23	2	8	6	9	2	6	1	7	1	9	—	—

specific additional diagnosis. For example, the first entry under agoraphobia with panic indicates that eight (9%) of our patients who received a primary diagnosis of agoraphobia with panic received an additional diagnosis of social phobia. The additional diagnoses are differentially distributed among the primary diagnoses. Simple phobia occurs with greatest frequency in agoraphobia, generalized anxiety disorder, and dysthymia. The additional diagnosis of social phobia occurs most frequently among those with dysthymia, while an additional diagnosis of dysthymia occurs most frequently among those with social phobia. Generalized anxiety disorder, which occurs in 11% of the cases in the total sample, occurs much more frequently in the affective disorder cases (45% and 33% of the cases of major depression and dysthymia, respectively).

It should be reiterated that additional diagnoses reflect the clinician's judgment that the symptoms are independent of the content of the primary disorder and are of clinical severity. In 16 additional cases in our sample, the clinician assigned "co-primary" diagnoses. That is, the clinician judged that two independent disorders were of equal severity and equally interfering with the patient's life. Table 5 shows the distribution of these co-primary diagnoses and reveals that major depression or dysthymia was the co-primary disorder in half of these cases.

In addition to data derived from the ADIS and the Hamilton scales embedded in the interview protocol, the patients in our sample completed a battery of self-report instruments that assess anxiety and depressive symptomatology. These instruments included the State-Trait Anxiety Inventory (STAI) (Spielberger, Gorsuch, and Lushene 1970), the Fear Questionnaire (Marks and Mathews 1979), the Cognitive-Somatic Anxiety Questionnaire (CSAQ) (Schwartz, Davidson, and Goleman 1978), the Beck Depression Inventory (Beck, Ward, Mendelson, et al. 1961), and the Psychosomatic Symptom Survey (PSSS) (Cox, Freundlich, and Meyer 1975).

Table 6 presents the mean Hamilton depression and anxiety ratings for the diagnostic groups. On the anxiety scale, dysthymia showed the highest ratings, significantly higher than obsessive-compulsive disorder, simple phobia, and social phobia. Simple phobia showed significantly lower ratings than any other group; agoraphobia, major depression, and panic disorder had significantly higher ratings than social or simple phobia. This pattern of anxiety ratings is similar to the pattern reported by Barlow, Di Nardo, Vermilyea, et al. (1986). The affective disorders and agoraphobia with panic are associated with the most severe anxiety, whereas social and simple phobia are associated with lowest levels of anxiety. Only obsessive-compul-

Table 5. Distribution of Co-Primary Diagnoses

Diagnosis	Social phobia	Simple phobia	Panic disorder	Generalized anxiety disorder	Major depression	Dysthymia
Agoraphobia with panic	3	1	—	0	1	0
Social phobia	—	0	1	1	1	1
Simple phobia	—	0	1	0	2	0
Panic disorder	—	—	—	1	2	1

Note. Dashes refer to combinations that cannot occur together or to combinations that are duplicated elsewhere in the table.

Table 6. Mean Hamilton Scores for the Diagnostic Groups

Hamilton Scale	Diagnosis							
	Simple phobia	Social phobia	Panic disorder	Generalized anxiety disorder	Agoraphobia	Obsessive-compulsive	Major depression	Dysthymia
Depression	9.3[a]	15.3[b]	15.5[b]	15.8[b]	16.6[b]	19.3[b,c]	22.9[c]	24.7[c]
Anxiety	14.1[a]	17.8[b]	20.7[c,d]	20.0[b,c,d]	22.0[c,d]	18.9[b,c]	22.0[c,d]	24.2[d]

Note. Means with similar superscripts are not significantly different.

sive disorder differs in that it is associated with low levels of anxiety in the current sample but had one of the highest anxiety levels in the Barlow, Di Nardo, Vermilyea, et al. study. The latter sample included only 6 obsessive-compulsive cases as compared to 15 cases in the current sample, so the current results may be more reliable.

On the Hamilton depression scale, major depression and dysthymia have the highest ratings, significantly higher than all of the anxiety disorders except obsessive-compulsive disorder. Simple phobia has significantly lower ratings than any other diagnostic group. The remaining anxiety disorders have intermediate scores and are not significantly different from one another. Taken together, the Hamilton scales indicate that simple and social phobia are associated with the lowest levels of general anxiety and depressive symptomatology, and the affective disorders are associated with the highest levels. Among the anxiety disorders, agoraphobia and panic disorder are associated with higher levels of anxiety than the other anxiety disorders, while obsessive-compulsive disorder is associated with higher levels of depression.

Table 7 shows the mean scores on the self-report questionnaires for the groups. Because of the small number of patients with dysthymic disorder and major depressive disorder who completed the battery, scores for these groups are not included. An inspection of the table reveals that simple phobia is consistently associated with the lowest scores on measures of state anxiety, trait anxiety, and depression. On the measures of trait anxiety and depression, there are no other differences among the groups. However, generalized anxiety disorder has significantly higher state anxiety scores than either panic disorder or simple phobia.

The groups show somewhat different patterns of scores on the two measures of somatic symptoms—the CSAQ-somatic and the PSSS. On the CSAQ-somatic, simple phobia and obsessive-compulsive disorder have lower scores than any other group, with no other significant differences among the groups. In contrast, panic disorder and generalized anxiety disorder show the highest mean scores on the PSSS, although not significantly higher than obsessive-compulsive or agoraphobia, while simple phobia and social phobia have the lowest mean scores. The PSSS samples a wider variety of somatic symptoms than does the CSAQ-somatic. The different pattern of scores may reflect the broader somatic symptomatology of panic disorder and generalized anxiety disorder, and the tendency of those with social phobia and simple phobia to experience somatic symptoms that are focused on specific situations.

An inspection of the scores on the subscales of the Fear Question-

Table 7. Mean Questionnaire Scores for the Diagnostic Groups

Diagnosis	STAI		CSAQ		Beck	PSSS	Fear Questionnaire		
	State	Trait	Cognitive	Somatic			Agoraphobia	Blood and injury	Social
Agoraphobia with panic	48.77[b,c]	50.62[b]	22.50	20.12[b]	15.85[b]	52.12[b]	21.75[c]	12.94[b]	16.47[c]
Social phobia	51.57[b,c]	57.64[b]	21.46	20.62	15.69[b]	37.85[a]	5.20[a]	6.35[a]	19.95[c]
Simple phobia	33.18[a]	35.18[a]	15.20	12.00[a]	7.70[a]	16.90[a]	7.07[a,b]	6.36[a]	7.43[a]
Panic disorder	46.03[b]	48.80[b]	19.32	20.35[b]	14.48[b]	60.13[b]	7.43[a,b]	10.28[a,b]	12.03[a,b]
Generalized anxiety disorder	58.20[c]	55.67[b]	20.60	19.73[b]	17.27[b]	58.67[b]	4.75[a]	8.38[a]	11.25[a,b]
Obsessive-compulsive	49.75[b,c]	51.58[b]	21.75	16.67[a]	17.00[b]	54.83[b]	11.00[b]	9.71[a,b]	14.71[b,c]
Mean	48.19	50.24	20.57	19.11	15.05	50.73	10.81	9.73	14.02

Note. Means with similar superscripts are not significantly different. STAI = State-Trait Anxiety Inventory; CSAQ = Cognitive-Somatic Anxiety Questionnaire; Beck = Beck Depression Inventory; PSSS = Psychosomatic Symptoms Checklist.

naire indicates that these subscales may be sensitive[1] in identifying the groups for which they are intended, but do not have great specificity. That is, the subscales not only identify the particular phobic group, but also include other groups as well. For example, on the agoraphobia subscale, agoraphobia has significantly higher scores than any other group. However, the scores of patients with obsessive-compulsive disorder, panic disorder, or simple phobia are significantly higher than those with generalized anxiety disorder or social phobia. The relatively high scores of obsessive-compulsive patients may reflect avoidance of situations related to the content of obsessions of contamination or aggression. Agoraphobia also shows the highest scores on the blood and injury subscale, significantly higher than social phobia, simple phobia, and generalized anxiety disorder. On the social fear subscale, social phobia shows the highest mean score, significantly different from panic, generalized anxiety disorder, and simple phobia, but not agoraphobia or obsessive-compulsive disorder. Agoraphobia and obsessive-compulsive disorder are significantly different from simple phobia, generalized anxiety disorder, and panic. Again, the relatively high scores of the nonsocial phobia groups probably reflect the avoidance of social situations that is associated with the symptomatology of these disorders. Given our findings on the coexistence of social phobia with the other anxiety disorders, some of this overlap reflects the existence of an independent social phobia in a number of patients with other anxiety disorders.

On any individual self-report instrument, there is much overlap among the anxiety groups. On instruments on which there are significant differences, these differences reflect general severity of distress. At the conclusion of this chapter, we will consider preliminary evidence on the usefulness of generating profiles based on several self-report instruments to distinguish among the anxiety disorders.

ANXIETY AND DEPRESSION

We turn next to a consideration of depression, both as an additional syndrome in our anxiety disorder sample and as a symptom that cuts across the categories. At first glance, the low number of additional affective disorder diagnoses in our sample contrasts with the reported overlap between anxiety and affective syndromes (e.g., Breier, Charney, and Heninger 1986; Clancy, Noyes, Hoenk, et al. 1978). However, the comorbidity data presented in Table 4 reflect only current

---

[1] If a paper-and-pencil instrument is being used to identify individuals belonging to a particular diagnostic category, sensitivity refers to the instrument's ability to detect *all* individuals belonging to the particular group.

symptomatology in the sample. The picture changes when we consider past major depressive episodes, which are also assessed in the ADIS. Approximately 30% of our anxiety disorder sample reported at least one past episode of depression that met the criteria for major depression. This is somewhat low, but still consistent with results of studies such as that of Clancy, Noyes, Hoenk, et al., who reported that 44% of a sample of anxiety neurotics reported episodes of depression during the course of their anxiety disorder. Looking at the individual anxiety disorders, we see that past episodes of major depression are differentially distributed among the categories. Interestingly, social phobia and generalized anxiety disorder are associated with the highest incidence of a past depressive episode, with 38% and 39% of these groups, respectively, reporting at least one episode. Only 9% of patients with simple phobia reported past depressive episodes. There were past episodes in 20% of the obsessive-compulsive cases and 29% of the agoraphobia cases. The figures for agoraphobia are in contrast with those of Breier, Charney, and Heninger, who reported a 70% lifetime incidence of major depression in a group of agoraphobics.

Given the considerable overlap between anxiety and affective syndromes, there has been considerable interest in describing and assessing aspects of symptomatology that are unique to these two mood states. Current clinical rating scales or self-report instruments designed to measure anxiety or depression overlap considerably. For example, patients with affective disorders tend to score as high on measures of anxiety used at our clinic as anxiety patients, although on the HRSD the affective patients are clearly distinct from all the anxiety groups except obsessive-compulsive disorder. This degree of overlap is not surprising since the two Hamilton scales are similar in content. In fact, we have noted a 70% overlap in the item content of the two scales.

In 1983 we reported on the existence of several items from the Hamilton scales that discriminated anxiety patients from depressed patients (Barlow 1983). Among these items, in addition to suicidal thoughts, were feelings of hopelessness and motor retardation. Riskind, Beck, Brown, et al. (1987) revised the Hamilton scales to discriminate better between anxiety and depression. The scales were administered to patients with either a diagnosis of major depression or of generalized anxiety disorder. To keep the groups as homogeneous as possible, anxiety disorder patients with an additional affective diagnosis were excluded, as were affective patients with an additional anxiety diagnosis.

Items were reassigned after factor analysis and point-biserial correlations with diagnosis. Items were assigned to the new anxiety or depression scales if their highest salient loading was on either the "anxiety" or "depression" factor, as long as this did not conflict with the results of the point-biserial correlation. This allowed for the assignment of 82% of the items. The remaining items were reassigned on the basis of clinical judgment, with redundant items deleted. Riskind, Beck, Brown, et al. (1987) showed that the revised scales had greater sensitivity for generalized anxiety disorder and greater specificity for major depression than the original scales.

Recently, we examined the ability of these revised scales to discriminate among a variety of DSM-III anxiety disorders and affective disorders (McCauley, Di Nardo, and Barlow 1987). The sample included groups of patients with panic disorder, agoraphobia with panic, social phobia, simple phobia, generalized anxiety disorder, obsessive-compulsive disorder, dysthymic disorder, and major depressive disorder. Anxiety patients were excluded if they received an additional diagnosis of either dysthymia or major depression, and depressed patients were excluded if they received an additional anxiety disorder diagnosis. For purposes of comparison, a mixed group of patients with a primary diagnosis of panic disorder as well as an additional diagnosis of either dysthymia or major depression was included.

Table 8 presents means and standard deviations and the pattern of significant differences among the groups on the revised scales. Agoraphobia with panic showed significantly higher HARS scores than any other diagnostic group. Simple phobia, social phobia, and major depression showed the lowest HARS scores, significantly lower than the mixed and panic groups. HRSD scores fall into four distinct levels. Simple phobia showed significantly lower scores than any other group. Social phobia, panic disorder, and generalized anxiety disorder make up the next level. Agoraphobia, mixed, and obsessive-compulsive disorder are in the third level. This is followed by major depression and dysthymia, which show significantly higher scores than any other group. One point of interest in these results is that the affective groups scored lower on the "purified" anxiety scale than two of the anxiety groups and higher on the "purified" depression scale than all anxiety groups, suggesting that the two groups of disorders can be differentiated from one another. Of course, identification of rating scale items that more clearly differentiate between anxiety and depression is only a beginning; independent replications in other centers are needed. In addition, there may be other dimensions along which these two disorders may be distinguished. Preliminary data describing differential attributional styles for anxious and depressed patients are presented later in the section on generalized anxiety, worry, and cognitions.

Table 8. Comparison of Anxiety Disorder and Depressed Groups on Revised Hamilton Anxiety and Depression Scales

Hamilton Anxiety Rating Scale (Revised)

n	Mean	Group	Simple phobia	Social phobia	Major depression	Dysthymia	Generalized anxiety disorder	Obsessive-compulsive	Panic disorder	Mixed	Agoraphobia with panic
20	17.3 ± 3.8	Simple phobia									
19	19.3 ± 4.5	Social phobia									
15	20.3 ± 6.5	Major depression	*								
15	21.0 ± 6.0	Dysthymia	*								
20	21.2 ± 3.3	Generalized anxiety disorder	*								
17	23.4 ± 5.8	Obsessive-compulsive	*								
19	23.7 ± 4.5	Panic disorder	*	*	*						
19	25.3 ± 3.8	Mixed	*	*	*	*	*	*			
18	27.1 ± 4.7	Agoraphobia with panic	*	*	*	*	*	*	*		

Hamilton Rating Scale for Depression (Revised)

n	Mean	Group	Simple phobia	Social phobia	Panic disorder	Generalized anxiety disorder	Agoraphobia with panic	Mixed	Obsessive-compulsive	Dysthymia	Major depression
20	16.3 ± 2.2	Simple phobia									
19	19.9 ± 4.4	Social phobia	*								
19	20.2 ± 2.3	Panic disorder	*								
20	20.3 ± 3.5	Generalized anxiety disorder	*								
18	22.6 ± 3.4	Agoraphobia with panic	*	*	*	*					
19	23.9 ± 3.3	Mixed	*	*	*	*					
17	24.4 ± 4.4	Obsessive-compulsive	*	*	*	*					
15	28.9 ± 6.1	Dysthymia	*	*	*	*	*	*	*		
15	29.9 ± 3.8	Major depression	*	*	*	*	*	*	*		

Note. Asterisk indicates pairs of groups significantly different at .05 level. From McCauley, Di Nardo, and Barlow (1987).

SYMPTOM CO-OCCURRENCE

Although a hierarchy-free approach to diagnosis permits us to record the presence of additional syndromes without exclusionary restrictions, the problems associated with DSM-III cutoffs for determining the presence or absence of a syndrome still remain. As Frances, Widiger, and Fyer (Chapter 3) point out, the degree of syndrome comorbidity is directly related to the thresholds set to determine the presence or absence of criteria for various disorders. A patient may have significant symptomatology in certain areas and still not meet the DSM-III criteria for an additional diagnosis. For example, a patient with generalized anxiety disorder may also have panic attacks, but because the panics do not occur with sufficient frequency, an additional diagnosis of panic disorder cannot be assigned. This results in a loss of potentially useful information. An alternative to a syndrome approach is simply to measure the presence of various symptoms on a continuum and use these data in a dimensional analysis (Blashfield, Chapter 4). In the following sections we will examine data on the existence of panic; generalized anxiety, worry, and cognitions; somatic symptoms; and social fears as dimensions that cut across the DSM-III anxiety disorders.

Panic

Since panic disorder was first described as a separate anxiety state in DSM-III, panic has come to occupy a central position among the anxiety disorders. DSM-III-R has eliminated agoraphobia with panic as a separate category and instead included agoraphobia as a subcategory of panic disorder. This is a reflection of the central etiologic role assigned to panic attacks in the development of agoraphobia.

Panic attacks occur frequently in anxiety disorders and major depression as well as panic disorder (Barlow 1985). According to DSM-III, patients with social phobia and simple phobia can experience panic attacks when exposed to phobic stimuli. The National Institute of Mental Health (NIMH) Epidemiologic Catchment Area (ECA) study showed a high probability for schizophrenics to have panic attacks (Boyd, Burke, Gruenberg, et al. 1984). The distinction between phobic disorders and panic disorder is that in panic disorder the attacks are spontaneous and unpredictable, whereas in phobic disorders the panics have a clear precipitant. In two studies at our clinic, we have examined the nature of panic symptoms in our anxiety patients to determine if panic symptoms vary across the categories, or if panic symptoms are different in spontaneous versus cued attacks. In the first study, Barlow, Vermilyea, Blanchard, et al. (1985) found that among patients with diagnosed anxiety disorders, between 83% and 100% reported at least one panic attack. In almost all patients reporting panics, regardless of primary diagnosis, the panics included four symptoms, sufficient to qualify as a DSM-III attack. However, patients with agoraphobia with panic, panic disorder, and obsessive-compulsive disorder reported significantly greater percentages of the 12 symptoms (85.6%, 83.3%, and 90.2%, respectively) than all other anxiety groups except simple phobia.

To contrast cued and uncued panics more directly, agoraphobic and panic disorder patients were compared with a group of anxiety disorder patients who had never experienced a spontaneous attack (cued group); and another group comprised of patients with social phobia, simple phobia, and generalized anxiety disorder who reported at least one spontaneous attack (mixed group). In this comparison, agoraphobia and panic disorder patients reported a significantly greater percentage of the 12 panic symptoms than the mixed or cued group. Statistical comparisons showed that agoraphobic and panic disorder patients were more likely to report dizziness and fear of going crazy or loss of control than any other group. There were no differences between the groups on severity of symptoms. Because dizziness and fear of loss of control discriminated unpredictable from cued attacks, the authors suggest that these symptoms be considered as defining characteristics of panic disorder.

The second study was designed to investigate further the differences between cued and uncued attacks. Using a revised version of the ADIS to diagnose patients according to DSM-III-R, Sanderson, Rapee, and Barlow (submitted) compared the uncued panic attacks in a group of panic disorder patients with the cued panic attacks in a group of simple phobic, social phobic, and obsessive-compulsive patients. Because patients in all anxiety disorder categories may experience uncued (spontaneous) panic, the ADIS was redesigned so that symptom ratings for simple phobia, social phobia, and obsessive-compulsive disorder were clearly related only to panic experienced on exposure to a phobic stimulus or an obsessive-compulsive thought or action. Results showed that a significantly greater percentage of panic disorder patients reported symptoms of fear of dying or loss of control, paresthesias, dizziness, faintness, dyspnea, unreality, and choking than the other groups.

Taken together, the results of these studies suggest that there are differences in the phenomenology of cued and uncued panic attacks. It is not clear whether the differences reflect actual differences in symptomatology or differences in self-report. In individuals with uncued panics, the lack of clear cues may predispose them to focus internally and make interpretations such as impending death or loss of control. Conversely, phobic patients have a clear situational explanation for their panics and are less likely to become preoccupied with the panic symptoms or to make catastrophic attributions of the panic symptoms.

Recognizing that preoccupation with panic symptoms is often a characteristic of panic patients, DSM-III-R has included chronic fear of the recurrence of panic attacks as one of the criteria of panic disorder. In a preliminary attempt to quantify patients' "fear of fear," Reiss, Peterson, Gursky, et al. (1986) developed the Anxiety Sensitivity Inventory, a self-report instrument designed to assess subjects' beliefs that anxiety experiences will have negative implications such as illness, embarrassment, or loss of control. In a preliminary study, they found that anxiety sensitivity differentiated a group of anxiety disorder patients from a nonclinical sample and that agoraphobics had higher anxiety sensitivity than other anxiety disorder patients.

In an examination of another cognitive factor related to panic, Sanderson, Rapee, and Barlow (1989) recently reported an experimental investigation of the effects of perceived control on panic symptoms. Panic disorder patients inhaled 5% CO_2 enriched air under two different sets of instructions: although both groups were told to expect physical symptoms associated with CO_2 inhalation, one group was told that they could turn off the CO_2 any time they wished, while the other group was told that the CO_2 would continue for a specified period of time. In fact, both groups received CO_2 for the entire period. The results showed that a significantly smaller percentage of patients who believed they had control over the procedure experienced panic attacks (20%) than patients who believed they had no control (80%). Interestingly, there were no differences in physiologic reactivity or somatic reactions between the two groups. These results suggest that the perception of control is a critical aspect of the phenomenology of panic, and that the presence of physical symptoms alone does not necessarily constitute a "panic attack." Given the fact that panic attacks are common among patients with a variety of DSM-III disorders, as well as in nonclinical populations (Norton, Harrison, Hauch, et al. 1985), these findings suggest that a distinction between panic attacks and panic disorder may lie in the attributions or interpretations of symptoms.

Generalized Anxiety, Worry, and Cognitions

Barlow, Blanchard, Vermilyea, et al. (1986) examined the presence of generalized anxiety symptomatology in a sample of 108 patients who had been independently interviewed and diagnosed by two clinicians using the ADIS and who had received a primary diagnosis of anxiety disorder or affective disorder. The severity of symptomatology on each of the four DSM-III symptom areas for generalized anxiety disorder (muscle tension, autonomic hyperactivity, vigilance and scanning, and apprehensive expectation) was rated on a 5-point scale, (from 0 = none to 4 = very severe). Ratings were based only on general anxiety, and the interview questions specifically excluded symptoms experienced during panic attacks. The results showed that a large proportion of patients in all of the anxiety disorder categories received a rating of moderate severity on at least three of the four symptom areas, satisfying the inclusion criteria for generalized anxiety disorder. The criteria had been met for the last year in 68% of those with agoraphobia, 58% of those with social phobia, 43% with simple phobia, 71% with panic disorder, 100% with obsessive-compulsive disorder, and 66% with major depression. Severity of symptomatology did not differentiate generalized anxiety patients from other anxiety patients. Symptom duration did differentiate among some of the anxiety disorders, with generalized anxiety patients reporting symptoms for more than one-half of their lives, while panic patients reported such symptomatology for less than one-sixth of their lives.

Sanderson and Barlow (1986) examined the extent to which excessive worry was distributed across the anxiety disorder categories. In DSM-III, excessive worry was one possible symptom of generalized anxiety disorder, but in DSM-III-R excessive or unrealistic worry focused on two life spheres as a defining feature of generalized anxiety disorder. A group of patients were interviewed using the ADIS, and all responded to the question, "Do you worry excessively about minor things?" Again, the questions were structured so that concerns about the symptoms of another anxiety disorder were specifically excluded. The following percentages of patients in each category responded positively to the question: agoraphobia, 50%; obsessive-compulsive disorder, 60%; panic disorder, 40%; simple phobia, 50%; and social phobia, 40%. These results indicate that excessive worry is a symptom that appears in all of the anxiety disorders.

Some of the findings reported by Sanderson and Barlow (1986) have implications for the DSM-III-R reformulation of generalized anxiety disorder. The most common spheres of worry reported by this group of patients were family, money, work, and illness. Clinicians making independent judgments could reliably identify these spheres of worry (82% agreement) and could agree on the excessive and/or irrational nature of the worry (88% agreement). When DSM-III and DSM-III-R diagnoses were compared, 22 of 23 patients who met the DSM-III criteria for generalized anxiety disorder also met the DSM-III-R criteria. That is, these patients reported at least two spheres of excessive worry and continuous tension and anxiety for at least 6 months.

There may be other cognitive dimensions that characterize the anxiety disorders and that may be useful in distinguishing anxiety disorders from other classes of disorders, particularly depression. A number of investigators (e.g., Beck and Emery 1979) have described maladaptive cognitive patterns that are hypothesized to be specific to anxiety disorder patients. In an early study on a group of anxiety neurotics, Beck, Laude, and Bonhert (1974) described the typical cognitive pattern as one in which the patient has an exaggerated expectation of personal harm such as illness or injury, humiliation, or rejection. On the basis of clinical observations, the authors concluded that the degree of anxiety is directly related to the patient's estimate of the likelihood of harm and the beliefs about the potential severity of harm. Their sample was diagnosed according to DSM-III and included a mixture of patients with panic, phobic, and generalized anxiety symptomatology, so it cannot be determined if the cognitive pattern described is specific to generalized anxiety disorder or is characteristic of the entire group.

The issue of whether anxiety and depression are associated with distinctive patterns of maladaptive cognitions has been addressed by Beck and his colleagues (Beck 1976; Beck and Emery 1979). They hypothesized that both anxious and depressed individuals attach unrealistically high probabilities to negative outcomes. However, in anxious individuals, these expectancies are attached to specific events; in depressed individuals negative expectancies are more general and global. In addition, anxious individuals are hypothesized to attach higher likelihoods to positive events than depressed individuals. In a test of this model, Beck, Riskind, Brown, et al. (1986) asked patients with generalized anxiety disorder and major depressive disorder to fantasize various outcomes of personally relevant problems. While both groups placed a high probability on negative outcomes, depressed patients attached higher probabilities to negative outcomes than did anxious patients. In addition, anxious patients attached higher probability to positive outcomes. The anxious patients had higher expectancies for a positive outcome to the problem than a negative outcome; the reverse was true for depressed patients.

In a similar study, Heimberg, Vermilyea, Dodge, et al. (1987) compared the attributional styles of dysthymic, anxious, and normal subjects. The results showed that those with dysthymia demonstrated global and stable attributions of negative outcomes and that similar attributions were characteristic of anxious patients with depressive symptoms. Nondepressed anxious patients and normals, on the other hand, showed similar attributions for negative outcomes. In other words, if anxious patients are not also depressed, their attributions for negative outcomes are normal. For attributions of positive outcomes, the dysthymic patients differed from the nondepressed anxious patients, but not the depressed anxious patients. The nondepressed anxious subjects saw themselves as more responsible for positive outcomes and predicted greater success at controlling future positive outcomes.

In a follow-up study, Heimberg, Klosko, Dodge et al. (1989) compared the attributional patterns of dysthymic patients, normals, agoraphobic patients, panic disorder patients, and social phobia patients to determine if different attributional patterns could be found among the various anxiety disorders. In this study, subjects' scores on the Beck Depression Inventory (Beck, Ward, Mendelson, et al. 1961) were used as a covariate, so that the effects of the patients' level of depression on attributional patterns could be statistically controlled. While the level of depression contributed substantially to attributional style, the analysis of covariance revealed differences in attributional styles among the anxiety disorders. Among the anxiety disorders, the social phobic patients showed the highest level of helplessness. They were more likely than agoraphobic patients to believe that the causes of negative outcomes were stable and were less likely to attribute positive outcomes to personal qualities. This attributional pattern is particularly striking in view of the fact that the social phobic patients were significantly less depressed than the other two anxiety groups. Panic disorder patients, although more depressed than normals, were no more helpless than normals, nor did they show a greater tendency toward self-blame. Panic disorder patients also showed different attributional patterns than agoraphobic patients: panic disorder patients believed that the causes of negative outcomes were more restricted and had a stronger belief in their ability to cope with such events. These attributional differences are also striking in view of the clinical similarity of the two syndromes. Heimberg, Klosko, Dodge, et al. (1989) suggested that these attributional differences may be related to the development of the avoidance behavior that differentiates between panic disorder and agoraphobia.

These findings are of particular interest because they suggest that certain cognitive patterns can discriminate between anxiety and depression and that, within the anxiety disorders, cognitive dimensions that are independent of depressive symptomatology can be used to discriminate among the disorders.

Somatic Symptoms

Because physiologic arousal is a major component of fear and anxiety, it is not surprising that all anxiety disorders are accompanied by some degree of somatic symptomatology and that the degree of somatic symptomatology may differentiate among the specific anxiety disorder categories. For example, patients with panic disorder are characterized as having extreme sensitivity to and fear of somatic symptoms because such symptoms have been associated with panic attacks. In an empirical examination of the degree of somatic symptoms among panic disorder patients, Hoehn-Saric (1981) found that on a variety of self-report measures, panic patients could be distinguished from generalized anxiety disorder patients by the predominance of somatic symptoms. In a study conducted at our clinic, Barlow, Cohen, Waddell, et al. (1984) compared groups of panic disorder and generalized anxiety disorder patients on a variety of self-report and psychophysiologic measures. Panic disorder patients scored higher than generalized anxiety disorder patients on the somatic subscale of the CSAQ, but not on the cognitive subscale. On the psychophysiologic measures, panic patients showed significantly higher electromyograph activity than generalized anxiety disorder patients, as well as a tendency to have higher heart rates.

King, Margraf, and Ehlers (1986) compared somatic symptomatology in a group of female patients who met the DSM-III criteria for panic disorder or agoraphobia with panic attacks and a group of nonanxious controls. These investigators were interested not only in comparing somatic symptomatology in the two groups, but in determining how many of the panic patients would also meet the symptom criteria for somatization disorder. To do this, they constructed a questionnaire, the Self-Report Inventory for Somatic Symptoms, to assess somatization symptoms and visceral sensitivity. The scale also contains a checklist of 37 physical symptoms that make up the DSM-III symptom criteria for somatization disorder. Results showed that the panic patients had higher levels of somatization symptoms, gastrointestinal awareness, and cardiovascular awareness. Twelve of the 44 panic patients met the symptom criteria for somatization disorder. It would be of interest to replicate this study using a sample of patients with a variety of anxiety disorder diagnoses to determine if somatic sensitivity and somatization symptoms are a general characteristic of the anxiety disorders or are specific to certain categories such as panic. Also, the study should be replicated on male patients to determine if this pattern is gender related.

One question that is relevant to the discussion of somatic symptomatology is the relationship between self-reports and objective measures of physiologic processes. There is general agreement among investigators in this area that self-reports and physiologic activity are not highly correlated (Ray, Cole, and Raczynski, 1983). For example, those patients with the highest reported cardiovascular symptomatology may not be the patients with the highest heart rates. However, McLeod, Hoehn-Saric, and Stefan (1986) have suggested that low correlations of this type do not necessarily mean that subjects cannot detect changes in arousal levels. To determine if clinically anxious patients are accurate in perceiving changes in physiologic arousal, McLeod, Hoehn-Saric, and Stefan compared self-reports and psychophysiologic measures of heart activity, skin conductance, electromyograph, and blood pressure in a group of generalized anxiety disorder patients under conditions of rest and of psychological stress. Although there were no correlations between self-reports and physiologic measures during rest or stress periods, the investigators found parallel directional changes in self-reports and physiologic measures of heart rate and skin conductance on exposure to stress. They concluded that patients could accurately perceive the direction, but not the degree, of changes in these physiologic responses. This study provides an effective methodology for examining the relationship between self-reports and psychophysiologic measures. Further studies are needed to determine whether the ability to perceive the direction of physiologic changes differentiates other anxiety patients from nonanxious controls, and whether this ability is differentially distributed among the anxiety disorder categories.

Social Fears

Social phobia can be distinguished reliably from other anxiety disorders (Di Nardo, O'Brien, Barlow, et al. 1983) and from avoidant personality disorder, a closely related syndrome (Turner, Beidel, Dancu, et al. 1986). The results of our comorbidity analysis show that social phobia occurs as an independent additional diagnosis in 11% of the cases.

Although social phobia is easily identified as an independent anxiety syndrome, self-report measures of social fears do not readily distinguish social phobics from the other anxiety disorders. In our sample, those with social phobia had the highest mean score on the social fear subscale of the Fear Questionnaire, but not significantly higher than those with agoraphobia or obsessive-compulsive disorder. This suggests that social fear and avoidance are common symptoms among the anxiety disorders.

To examine more closely the distribution of social fears in an anxiety disorder sample, Rapee, Sanderson, and Barlow (in press) compared the responses of social phobic patients, agoraphobic patients, panic disorder patients, generalized anxiety disorder patients, and simple phobia patients to the social phobia section of the ADIS. Results showed that a high proportion of patients in all categories reported social fears; 75% of generalized anxiety disorder patients reported concerns of being observed or humiliated, and 50% of agoraphobic and panic patients reported fears of being observed. At least 80% of the patients in each category reported slight fear in at least one social situation, and more than 50% in each category reported moderate fear in at least one social situation. Social phobic patients reported anxiety in a larger number of social situations and greater impairment associated with the social fears than the other groups. These investigators suggest that the difference between social phobia and other anxiety disorders on this specific anxiety feature may be quantitative rather than qualitative.

CONCLUSION

In this chapter, we have examined comorbidity from two perspectives. We have examined the distribution of additional diagnoses among the anxiety disorders, and we have considered several symptoms that cut across the categories and permit differentiation among the categories. This is a preliminary attempt, and our discussion has remained largely at the descriptive level. Systematic studies are needed to determine if the presence of additional syndromes or specific symptoms increases the discriminant validity of the diagnostic system. For example, it will be important to determine if the presence of additional diagnoses identifies subgroups within any particular category that are homogeneous with respect to clinical or psychometric characteristics, course of illness, or treatment response.

Foa, Grayson, Steketee, et al. (1983) demonstrated that the presence of depressive symptomatology has treatment implications for obsessive-compulsive disorder. Our experience suggests that the presence of additional anxiety syndromes also may have important treatment implications in certain cases. For example, an agoraphobic patient in one of our treatment groups also presented with a distinct blood and injury phobia. This complicated our treatment program, which focused on graduated exposure to situations involving travel and shopping. When confronted with a phobic object, such as a dead squirrel in the road during her driving practice, she experienced the low heart rate and hypotension associated with blood and injury fears. Similarly, when confronted with blood or even verbal descriptions of injury, this patient would occasionally faint (something agoraphobic patients almost never do). In this case, the blood and injury fear had to be treated before substantial progress could be made in the exposure treatment of the agoraphobic syndrome.

The categorical and dimensional approaches to description of the anxiety disorders are not incompatible (Barlow 1988). The categories are defined by the convergence of several dimensions; while a single dimension may be the central defining feature of a category, it may be more accurate to conceptualize patients in a category as having a similar profile on several dimensions. For example, panic disorder is characterized as having high levels of symptomatology on the somatic and panic dimensions, but low levels on worry and avoidance. Even though these profiles may be generally accurate for the patients in a given category, important variations may exist among the patients in the group, and these differences can only emerge with consideration of hierarchy-free additional diagnoses or symptom dimensions.

In a study examining the relationship between the dimensional and categorical approaches to the anxiety disorders, McCauley, Di Nardo, and Barlow (1988) employed cluster-analytic techniques to group patients according to scores on a variety of self-report instruments. Several dimensions that appeared central in defining these groups of patients emerged. Anxiety, depression, somatic symptoms, specific fears, and interference with functioning were dimensions that varied independently among the clusters. In a discriminant function analysis comparing cluster membership and diagnostic category, McCauley, Di Nardo, and Barlow (1988) found that there were coherent relationships between the statistically derived clusters of patients and the patterns of coexisting diagnoses these patients had received. For example, one cluster of patients was characterized by very high levels of somatic symptomatology. This group was made up largely of patients with coexisting panic disorder and generalized anxiety disorder syndromes, indicating that the additional diagnosis of generalized anxiety disorder delineates a distinctive subgroup of panic disorder patients. A similar study by Turner, McCann, Beidel, et al. (1986) also demonstrated the usefulness of such statistical techniques in examining the relationship between empirically derived groupings of patients and the DSM-III anxiety categories. The results of such studies clearly illustrate the complementary nature of the categorical and dimensional approaches, and the potential contribution each can make to descriptive psychopathology. Studies explicating these relationships, particularly as they change over time in a given individual, will form the basis for DSM-IV and the tenth revision of the World Health Organization's International Classification of Diseases (ICD-10), due to appear in the early to mid-1990s. Attempts to project specific combinations of categorical and dimensional approaches to anxiety disorders that might be useful in the next decade based on emerging data are now being made (e.g., Barlow 1988).

Chapter 13

Clinical Evidence of Comorbidity: A Critique of Treated Samples and Longitudinal Studies

David J. Kupfer, M.D.
Linda L. Carpenter, B.A.

F OR SEVERAL KEY reasons, this multidisciplinary volume on comorbidity in anxiety and mood disorders is timely. Nosologic advances and increased interest in objective measures are now stimulating researchers to be more precise in their descriptive work on clinical features. Second, the growing epidemiologic data bases juxtaposed to the data bases from longitudinal studies represent inevitable areas for consensus research. The need for consensus does not denote a necessity for agreement on results or data interpretation. Rather, the need is for agreement on research strategies, definitional terms, and boundaries of domains to be investigated. Examining and interpreting comorbidity issues represents constructive effort toward such agreement.

This volume also raises the question of how knowledge about comorbidity can be used to improve research on biology and treatment in psychiatry. Comorbidity need not be considered a confound-

Portions of this chapter were previously presented at the Conference on Symptom Co-Morbidity in Anxiety and Mood Disorders, Sterling Forest Conference Center, Tuxedo, New York, September 28–30, 1987.

Supported in part by National Institute of Mental Health grants MH-30915 and MH-29618.

ing factor or a complication. One distinct advantage of comorbidity is that it allows us to investigate the influence of one disease on the course of the other. Comorbidity and co-occurrence also provide an opportunity to examine both biologic and clinical relationships between various symptom clusters. Attention given to comorbidity may further our understanding of how controlled and uncontrolled treatment trials influence the course of a disease over time. With these goals in mind, we will first review and contrast the findings of Hirschfeld, Hasin, Keller, et al. (Chapter 18) with the results we obtained in a similar investigation with a sample of recurrent depressive patients. We will then turn our attention briefly to several issues raised by Di Nardo and Barlow's work (Chapter 12) on signs and symptoms in anxiety disorder.

Comorbidity of Depression and Alcoholism

Hirschfeld, Hasin, Keller, et al. (Chapter 18) compared 289 primary depressives to 79 depressives with concurrent alcoholism and found the alcoholics were older; more likely to be separated, divorced, or widowed; and more likely to be males. The two groups were well matched with regard to baseline clinical characteristics. Index episodes lasted an average of 76 weeks (median, 31 weeks), mean ages at onset were about 30 years, median number of prior depressive episodes were equal to one, and the intake Hamilton (Hamilton 1960) score for depression severity for both groups was about 26. Using the Research Diagnostic Criteria (RDC) (Spitzer, Endicott, and Robins 1978a) definition of recovery, these researchers found no significant difference between the groups in time to recovery from the intake major depressive episode. Furthermore, the level of severity of alcohol consumption did not affect the time to recovery. When time to relapse after recovery was examined, they again found the primary depressive patient to be similar to the alcoholics. However, a plot of Global Assessment Scale scores over time revealed that the alcoholics did not show as rapid or steady an improvement as the primary depressive patients. This finding was linked to poorer psychosocial functioning among the alcoholics, particularly in the area of relationships with spouse or mate.

One question that arises is whether the same differences would be found in a sample that is more homogeneous with regard to diagnosis. Since the patients in the Hirschfeld, Hasin, Keller, et al. (Chapter 18) study had experienced a median of only one prior depressive episode, it is unclear how many of these patients would go on to develop recurrent depression. We were able to isolate groups of patients based on RDC assessments at screening for our protocol.

Patients presented in their third or greater episode of recurrent major depressive disorder, with the immediately preceding episode occurring no more than 2½ years prior to the onset of the index episode (protocol described in detail elsewhere by Frank, Kupfer, Jacob, et al. 1987). All previous depressive episodes must have required psychiatric treatment or resulted in significant functional impairment, with a minimum of 10 weeks of remission between the previous and index episodes. From this population of recurrent depressive patients, we derived a group of 191 who had never met probable or definite criteria for schizophrenia, schizoaffective disorder, panic disorder, generalized anxiety disorder, Briquet's disorder, antisocial personality disorder, alcoholism, obsessive-compulsive disorder, phobic disorder, or unspecified functional psychosis. This group of primary depressive patients was compared to a group of 19 patients whose presenting episode or previous episode of major depression also received a probable or definite diagnosis of alcoholism.

Clinical characteristics for these groups are presented in Table 1. Although there is a trend toward greater male representation among

Table 1. Clinical Characteristics

	Alcoholics ($n = 19$)	Patients with primary depression ($n = 191$)
Sex (Male/female)	37%/63%	20%/80%
Mean age at screening (years)	38.2 ± 9.6	39.6 ± 10.8
Mean age at onset of first depressive episode (years)	26.8 ± 9.9	27.1 ± 10.3
Mean duration of index episode (weeks)	26.7 ± 16.0	24.0 ± 18.2
Mean number of previous episodes* Median	4.7 ± 2.7 4	6.4 ± 6.3 4
Mean baseline HRSD total score (17-item version)	21.9 ± 5.6	22.0 ± 4.5
Mean baseline Hopkins (SCL-90) Global Symptom Index	1.3 ± 0.7	1.3 ± 0.6

	Absent		Probable or definite		Absent		Probable or definite	
RDC subtype diagnoses	n	%	n	%	n	%	n	%
Endogenous	1	6	17	94	17	9	174	91
Agitated	14	74	5	26	168	88	23	12
Retarded	13	72	5	28	158	83	33	17
Psychotic	19	100	0	0	189	99	2	1
Incapacitating	13	72	5	28	180	94	11	6

*$p < .05$.

the alcoholics than among the primary depressive patients, the majority of patients are females in both groups. The two groups are similar on a number of counts: mean age about 39 years at screening, mean age at onset about 27 years, approximately 25 weeks' duration of the index episode, baseline Hamilton Rating Scale for Depression (HRSD) score at 22, and a baseline Hopkins Global Symptom Index (GSI) score at 1.3 (Derogatis, Lipman, and Covi 1973). With regard to subtype diagnoses, only the incapacitating subtype classification was more often given to patients in the alcoholic group. The only significant difference in the clinical features we examined was in the number of previous depressive episodes. Here the group with primary depression had a higher mean, but when median values were considered, both groups looked the same. Baseline symptom profiles indicated that patients with comorbid alcoholism were experiencing more hypersomnia (31% versus 12%, $p = .03$), more weight gain (13% versus 2%, $p = .03$), and less diurnal variation (13% versus 44%, $p = .02$) than their primary depressive counterparts.

Several outcome measures were employed, and these are shown in Table 2. The first variable involved the relative progress of the two groups at a particular point in time. The number of patients who completed a 16-week regimen for acute treatment of the index episode was compared to the number who terminated for various reasons, including nonresponse to imipramine, noncompliance, and intolerable side effects. There was approximately the same percentage of completers and noncompleters from the alcoholic group as there was from the group of primary depressive patients. Next we examined the patients from each group who were categorized as "normal re-

Table 2. Outcome Measures

	Alcoholics ($n = 19$)	Patients with primary depression ($n = 191$)	p
Completed 16 weeks of acute treatment	16 (84%)	167 (87%)	NS
Normal response to acute treatment (within 8 weeks)	1 (5%)	61 (37%)	.017
Mean % change over 16 weeks	59.7 ± 26.4	71.4 ± 24.3	.08
Completed continuation treatment	10 (53%)	104 (54%)	NS
Mean days until maintenance therapy began	306.6 ± 66.8	265.6 ± 57.5	.034

sponders" to acute treatment. Criteria for normal response type were defined by a computerized algorithm as follows: HRSD score ≤7 at 8 weeks and at 16 weeks, with a greater than 50% change in HRSD score from baseline to 16 weeks; other completers could be categorized as "slow responders" or "partial responders" based on similar criteria involving HRSD scores at various points in the course of the 16 weeks (Frank, Jarrett, Kupfer, et al. 1984). The primary depressive patients were significantly more likely to show normal (more rapid) response than the alcoholics. While 37% of the primary depressive group recovered from the index episode within 8 weeks after treatment was initiated, only 5% of the alcoholic group recovered in this time period.

Another outcome measure we examined took into consideration a more sustained remission after acute symptoms had subsided. Once a patient met criteria for recovery and remained stable for an extensive period of time, the patient was assigned to one of five experimental cells for maintenance therapy. To make it to this maintenance phase, the patient must have received all of the following for 20 consecutive weeks: (1) a steady medication dose, (2) a continuing score on the Raskin Scale for Depression (Raskin, Schulterbrandt, Reatig, et al. 1969) of ≤5, and (3) an HRSD score of ≤7. We found the same percentage from each group made it to this point in the protocol. These stringent criteria for recovery were met by 53% of the alcoholics and 54% of the patients with primary depression. But when we considered the amount of time it took to achieve this level of recovery, we found the alcoholics required significantly more days ($p < .03$) to reach the maintenance phase of the protocol.

The evidence from our analyses suggests that alcoholic comorbidity does not affect the ultimate probability of recovery from recurrent depression, but it does appear to slow the rate of improvement during the course of treatment. Patients with concurrent alcoholism are not less likely to survive treatment, but they are less likely to progress as rapidly as patients with primary depression. The primary recurrent depressive patients that we studied became asymptomatic more quickly and achieved a stable remission sooner than the alcoholics. The comorbid group did eventually "catch up" with them, the final result being an equivalent percentage from each group meeting criteria for recovery.

That a differential rate of response was observed in our sample and not in the one studied by Hirschfeld, Hasin, Keller, et al. (Chapter 18) may be attributable to the characteristics of each population. The majority of our alcoholic patients were females, not males. Rounsaville, Dolinisky, Barbor, et al. (1987) reported that alcoholic females with major depression showed a more favorable recovery from their alcoholism than did male alcoholics. It may be that gender composition of the two samples complicates the interpretation of results obtained from each.

Our groups had shorter index episodes and a greater number of previous episodes of depression. Since the RDC definition for alcoholism was used to formulate groups, and since level of symptom severity was the basis for recovery in both investigations, it is unlikely that methodological variations contributed greatly to the discordant findings. Perhaps the recurrent quality of depressive disorder in our population is the key factor. Perhaps the patients studied by Hirschfeld, Hasin, Keller, et al. (Chapter 18), many of whom were experiencing their first episode of major depression, had less endogenous depressive features than our population of recurrent patients. Since one cannot ascertain from the available data set how many of the patients in their sample will develop a recurrent depression, we cannot yet conclude that comorbidity retards recovery in just patients with a history of multiple episodes and not in those who suffer from a single-episode disorder. It would be worthwhile to reexamine the Hirschfeld data with this distinction in mind.

Other researchers (Keller, Klerman, Lavori, et al. 1984; Keller, Lavori, Lewis, et al. 1983) have also linked comorbidity to longer recovery time in major depression. These findings, coupled with those discussed in this chapter, raise a number of interesting strategy questions. For example, should depressed patients with concurrent alcoholism (or comorbidity related to another psychiatric disorder) be treated in a different fashion? Should greater treatment emphasis be placed on psychosocial interventions? Perhaps there has been an overemphasis on symptoms as the sole measure of clinical change and long-term course. Other factors such as personality pathology, family history of affective and other psychiatric disorders, and biologic indicators of depression would be fruitful areas for investigation as well. Clearly, there is a need for more diagnostic homogeneity in the groups to be analyzed so potentially confounding variables such as gender and type of major depression can be scrutinized. Research on comorbidity in depression has only begun to elucidate issues needed to understand pathogenesis.

COMORBIDITY OF DEPRESSION AND ANXIETY

In this volume, Di Nardo and Barlow (Chapter 12) discuss a major investigation that examines signs and symptoms of anxiety disorders. Their rich data base represents an opportunity to examine assessment and perhaps follow-up. The cross-sectional view within an episode provides an intensive picture of symptomatic delineation in a large cohort of individuals. Nevertheless, the data base does not allow a perspective of individuals over a sequence of episodes or even throughout the entire length of a single episode.

There are inherent limitations of a setting that is an outpatient specialty clinic for anxiety. If the sample were taken from a general assessment facility or a community-based population, a different picture of symptom comorbidity in anxiety disorders might emerge. However, given a specialized sample of patients such as that described by Di Nardo and Barlow (Chapter 12), one can envision an opportunity for long-term follow-up that may improve generalizability. It would be extremely useful to learn about the eventual course of psychopathology in the 292 patients so accurately described in Chapter 12.

RECOMMENDATIONS FOR FUTURE RESEARCH

Di Nardo and Barlow (Chapter 12) also discuss the need to establish potential relationships between symptom dimensions and categorical diagnoses. As recently concluded in a report from the MacArthur Foundation, there is a "vast armamentarium of methodologic tools, which are unused, underutilized or misused, available to help resolve many different problems in psychiatric research" (Kraemer, Pruyn, Gibbons, et al. 1987, p. 1105). Specifically, in the area of comorbidity research, it is recommended that a greater emphasis be placed on exploratory data analysis, procedures that "enhance the recognition of patterns in data sets to generate hypotheses and [on] description and estimation of effects" (p. 1105).

Concern expressed earlier about the shortcomings of "standard" clinical practice in the treatment of depression (Kupfer and Freedman 1986) is relevant to comorbidity research. The obvious advantages in including such uncontrolled treatment studies as part of collaborative investigations are that large data bases may be derived, and broad regional and socioeconomic class representation is more easily achieved. However, the opportunity to generalize findings, and even to examine differences across various treatment centers, would be enhanced if precise information were always collected on the incidence and types of comorbidity, be it medical or psychiatric.

Although the studies discussed above have not integrated biologic research strategies into their designs, a next logical step would be to incorporate biologic correlates in the comorbidity "matrix." Clearly, the results obtained from our population of recurrent depressed patients call for further analysis of the neuroendocrine and sleep data we have collected from these individuals. The Hirschfeld, Hasin, Keller, et al. (Chapter 18) longitudinal investigation would be enhanced by the availability of biologic data at several time points, and even data from one point in time would greatly benefit the work of Di Nardo and Barlow. Finally, it is hoped that in the future, researchers will seek to include such measures in the early design phase of prospective investigations.

Chapter 14

Somatization: The Most Costly Comorbidity?

Robert Kellner, M.D., Ph.D.

S OMATIZATION HAS BECOME a frequent topic in the research literature (Barsky 1979; Ford 1983; Kellner 1986; Kirmayer 1984; Lipowski 1986; Mayou 1976), and current textbooks contain separate
sections on somatoform disorders (Cloninger 1986a; Nemiah 1980).
The topic is of special interest for this volume because a case can be
made for somatization being the most prevalent comorbidity of anxiety and depression as well as the most costly one.

The present chapter is divided into three parts: first, a brief
overview of the nature of somatization and its comorbidity with
anxiety and depression; second, the prevalence of somatization in the
community and in medical offices and clinics; and third, the implications of comorbidity for psychiatry and psychology.

THE NATURE OF SOMATIZATION AND COMORBIDITY

The term *somatization* was first used by Steckel (1943), who defined it
as a bodily disorder that arises as an expression of a deep-seated
neurosis, a method by which the body was translating into physiologic language the mental troubles of the individual. Since then there
have been numerous theories on the nature of somatization, including its being a defense mechanism, such as a method of denial,
displacement, or rationalization or an attempt at conflict resolution
(Kellner 1986). In the last two decades the term *somatization* has also
been used to describe the presentation of somatic symptoms that are
not caused by physical disease or tissue damage, although specific
physiologic changes can be detected in some of these symptoms by

special techniques (Kellner 1985). An example of this usage is the trend to label observer-rating and self-rating scales that measure the number and severity of somatic symptoms as scales of somatization (Derogatis, Lipman, Rickels, et al. 1974).

For the purposes of the present overview, I have chosen a definition of *somatization* that is in accord with the criteria from the *Diagnostic and Statistical Manual of Mental Disorders* (DSM-III-R) (American Psychiatric Association 1987) for the undifferentiated somatoform disorder (and with slight variations for other somatoform disorders). Somatization indicates "one or more physical complaints, e.g., fatigue, loss of appetite, gastrointestinal or urinary complaints" and either "appropriate evaluation uncovers no organic pathology or pathophysiologic mechanism (e.g., a physical disorder or the effects of injury, medication, drugs, or alcohol) to account for the physical complaints" or "when there is related organic pathology, the physical complaints or resulting social or occupational impairment is grossly in excess of what would be expected from the physical findings" (p. 267). The term does not include conversion symptoms and does not include psychosomatic disease in which tissue damage occurs such as peptic ulcers, ulcerative colitis, and bronchial asthma.

For the purposes of this chapter, the emotional or psychic components of anxiety and depression are labeled *cognitive* anxiety or cognitive depression, whereas the bodily manifestations or complaints are labeled *functional somatic symptoms* (FSS). FSS are bodily symptoms that cut across diagnostic categories: they can occur in normal individuals as well as in patients with psychiatric disorders, affective disorders, and anxiety disorders, and are the bodily symptoms of patients with somatoform disorders (somatization disorder, undifferentiated somatoform disorder, and hypochondriasis) of the DSM-III-R. Thus FSS are the symptoms of somatizing patients as defined in the previous paragraph.

There are numerous differences among the symptoms in these categories. For example, symptoms of patients with somatization disorders include conversion symptoms (such as paralysis or loss of voice). This disorder may be genetically distinct from the other disorders (Arkonac and Guze 1963; Cadoret 1978). Some of the etiologic factors in somatization—including those that determine whether distress is expressed in cognitive (psychic) terms or as somatic complaints—are briefly addressed here; the topic has been discussed in detail elsewhere (Kellner 1986, 1988a). The term *hypochondriacal concern* (or *hypochondriacal reaction*) indicates an unrealistic fear or a false belief of having a disease—a meaning that is in accord with the classifications of the DSM-III-R.

When more than one psychiatric syndrome coexists, it is often impossible to determine with certainty the relationship of the two syndromes. In many cases it is a matter of the observer's judgments. For example, when depression and somatization are present, this may be an occurrence of true comorbidity, which means that two independent disorders coexist and may reinforce each other; or somatization may be an integral part of the depressive disorder and be merely one of its manifestations. In the next several sections I shall discuss the coexistence of somatization and depression and anxiety, the reasons for such coexistence, and which of the above relationships are common phenomena.

Summary of Definition of Terms

Since the terms used in the literature on somatization resemble each other and tend to be confusing, particularly for the reader who is not acquainted with the literature on somatization, a summary of the definitions as used in this chapter is presented.

Somatoform disorders. A group of disorders listed in the DSM-III-R. In these disorders the patients have bodily symptoms in the absence of a physical disease.

Somatization disorder. One of the somatoform disorders listed in DSM-III-R. It is similar to Briquet's syndrome, and its essential features are multiple somatic complaints (at least 13) beginning usually before the age of 30. The disorder has a chronic fluctuating course.

Somatization. A term that has been used to describe a subconscious process by which the patients translate emotional distress into bodily complaints. A more recent usage is the presentation of somatic symptoms in the absence of disease, regardless of the diagnostic category. The latter definition has been adopted for this chapter. Somatization can occur in various psychiatric disorders, including anxiety, depression, and somatoform disorders.

Functional somatic symptoms (FSS). The symptoms of somatizers as defined in the previous paragraph.

Hypochondriacal concern or hypochondriacal reaction. An unrealistic fear or false belief of having a disease.

The Coexistence of Somatic Symptoms With Anxiety

There are numerous studies in which the investigators examine the incidence of somatic symptoms in various anxiety disorders. One of the early studies was by Miles, Barrabee, and Finesinger (1951), who found the following percentages of somatic complaints in psychiatric patients with anxiety neurosis: palpitation, 90%; tires easily, 78%; breathlessness, 75%; rest unsatisfactory, 75%; trembling, 70%; shakiness, 70%; faintness, 70%; headaches, 65%; sweating, 62%; paresthesia, 25%; and sighing, 20%. In another early study, Wheeler, Williamson, and Cohen (1958) compared patients with anxiety neurosis (and included apparently the same diagnostic categories as in the Miles, Barrabee, and Finesinger study); their figures of somatic symptoms were similar to those found by Miles, Barrabee, and Finesinger, and a control group of random normal subjects had substantially lower figures. Numerous subsequent studies have shown that patients with anxiety disorders show an invariably higher prevalence of somatic symptoms than a random group of nonpatients.

The second body of research that links somatic symptoms to anxiety comes from correlational studies. Regardless of whether the study is done with psychiatric patients, medical patients, or normal subjects, there is a robust association between cognitive anxiety and somatic symptoms (Kellner 1986).

The third kind of evidence comes from outcome studies with antianxiety drugs. In double-blind drug trials with psychiatric patients suffering from anxiety, there is a parallel reduction of overt cognitive symptoms of anxiety with those of somatic symptoms. This reduction occurs with the drug as well as with the placebo. Antianxiety drugs, however, reduce somatic symptoms more than the placebo does. This reduction occurs also with antianxiety drugs that are known to have effects only on the central nervous system and have no direct effects on peripheral physiologic activity. Thus some centrally acting antianxiety drugs reduce somatic symptoms either indirectly by reducing cognitive anxiety or by decreasing anxiety as well as simultaneously inhibiting centers that regulate the activity of the autonomic (predominantly sympathetic) nervous system. Or perhaps both effects can occur.

The fourth kind of evidence that demonstrates the coexistence of somatic symptoms with fear and anxiety, as well as pointing to a causal relationship, comes from psychophysiologic research (discussed below).

The Coexistence of Somatic Symptoms With Depression

The literature on depression and somatic symptoms is parallel to that of anxiety and somatic symptoms. The evidence for the association of depression with somatic symptoms has been consistent in numerous clinical studies (Cadoret, Widmer, and Troughton 1980; Katon 1982;

Katon, Kleinman, and Rosen 1982). Somatizing patients are more depressed than normals, and depressed patients have consistently more somatic symptoms than nondepressed subjects. When somatizing patients are compared to patients with physical disease who have similar somatic symptoms, depression is higher in the somatizing patients (Kellner 1986). Correlational studies show a consistent and robust association of cognitive depression and somatic symptoms regardless of whether the studies were carried out in depressed patients, medical patients, or normals (Kellner, Slocumb, Wiggins, et al. 1985).

In drug trials with depressed patients, there is a parallel decrease of cognitive depression and of somatic symptoms in the placebo group as well as in the group treated with an antidepressant drug. This process is analogous to the effects of antianxiety drugs in drug trials of anxiety disorders (Kellner 1988a).

There are several differences between the bodily symptoms of depressed patients and anxious patients. Depressed patients have more conspicuous vegetative symptoms (such as anorexia, loss of weight, and impairment of libido), whereas some other bodily symptoms, particularly those caused by sympathetic nervous system over-activity, are more characteristic of anxiety (such as tachycardia, sweating, and symptoms induced by hyperventilation). Other symptoms, such as abdominal discomfort and various sensations in the chest, tend to occur in both classes of disorders. Since anxiety and depression coexist in many patients, vegetative symptoms as well as symptoms of sympathetic overactivity tend to occur both in depressed and anxious patients.

Other evidence of the relationship of somatization to anxiety and depression comes from studies with somatization disorders; patients with this disorder tend to be substantially more anxious and more depressed than normal controls. The relationship of somatization to anxiety has been found in studies with personality disorders. An exception is antisocial personality traits; these are negatively correlated with cognitive anxiety but are positively correlated with somatic anxiety (somatization) (Cloninger 1986a; Cloninger, Martin, Guze, et al., Chapter 27).

There are also differences in the literature between psychophysiologic studies on anxiety and depression. There is considerably less laboratory research on the physiologic changes that occur with changes in depressive mood than in anxious moods. Changes in depression are more difficult to induce in experimental subjects than changes in anxiety, which can be induced by various experimental stressors.

Stress, Distress, Physiologic Changes, and Somatic Symptoms

Several studies have shown an association between peripheral physiologic activity and somatic symptoms. For example, contraction of striated muscle is associated with tension headaches (Fujji, Kachi, and Sobue 1981; Malmo and Shagass 1949; Sainsbury and Gibson 1954). The electromyographic (EMG) potentials of painful muscles in various parts of the body are higher than those of control muscles (Malmo and Shagass 1949; Sainsbury and Gibson 1954), and some patients with lower back pain have elevated EMG levels in paravertebral muscles (Dolce and Raczynski 1985), particularly when emotionally stressed (Flor, Turk, and Birbaumer 1985). Other examples of physiologic activity inducing somatic symptoms in response to stress are contractions of smooth muscles in the alimentary tract. In normals as well as in patients with functional abdominal complaints, including those with irritable bowel syndrome, contractions tend to coincide with somatic discomfort (Latimer 1983).

Adaptation processes in the central nervous system, such as those producing augmentation or reduction in neuronal firing, influence the degree of peripheral physiologic changes (Grings and Dawson 1978), as well as the frequency of somatic symptoms (Petrie 1967). Individuals have a characteristic pattern of physiologic responses to stress (Anderson 1981), and in some individuals the response remains similar regardless of the kind of stressor used (Lacey 1950; Lacey and Lacey 1958; Lacey, Bateman, and Van Lehn 1953). The idiosyncrasy of physiologic responses probably explains, in part, the differences among individuals in the form taken by recurring functional somatic symptoms.

Stress, such as distressing life events, can induce anxiety, depression, and somatic symptoms. Some individuals appear to respond to stress with predominantly somatic symptoms, whereas others respond predominantly with psychic symptoms or both (Kellner, Pathak, Romanik, et al. 1983).

In patients who complain primarily of somatic symptoms and who are morbidly anxious, somatic symptoms correlate highly with physiologic changes, whereas in normal subjects and in morbidly anxious ones who have predominantly psychologic symptoms, bodily feelings correlate poorly with physiologic changes (Tyrer 1976). Processes other than physiologic changes must influence the perception and report of bodily symptoms in the latter group. Some patients have somatic symptoms that are not associated with detectable physiologic changes. Either there are somatic symptoms that are not caused by changes in peripheral physiologic activity (and in these individuals symptoms are caused by some other mechanisms) or the standard physiologic measures are inadequate to detect subtle physiologic changes that induce these symptoms.

Interaction of Depression, Anxiety, and Somatic Distress

The coexistence of anxiety and depression is discussed throughout this volume and will not be discussed here. Since anxiety and depression coexist in most patients, it is difficult to tease out whether somatization is the consequence of anxiety, depression, or both.

In a study in which more than 300 neurotic psychiatric outpatients with various diagnoses of anxiety disorders and depressive disorders participated, self-rating scales of somatic symptoms were administered (Kellner, Simpson, and Winslow 1972). When the remaining correlations were partialed out, the coefficient of anxiety with somatic symptoms was + .34, and depression with somatic symptoms + .15. The findings suggest that the somatic symptoms tended to be somewhat more strongly associated with cognitive symptoms of anxiety than with those of depression. The study also showed large differences between the ratios of somatic to cognitive symptoms: a few patients who were severely anxious and severely depressed had only a few somatic symptoms; conversely, some patients who rated their somatic symptoms as severe rated their anxiety or depression as only moderate.

So while there is consistent evidence of an association among anxiety, depression, and functional somatic symptoms, as well as evidence that a person has more somatic symptoms at times of stress, anxiety, or depression than at other times, other factors apart from the severity of the cognitive distress will play a part in whether a patient will perceive and report somatic symptoms (Kellner 1988a).

Other Factors Influencing Somatization

Apart from genetic predisposition in somatization (Bohman, Cloninger, and von Knorring 1984; Sigvardsson, Bohman, von Knorring, et al. 1986), several other factors listed below will influence the number and severity of somatic symptoms in people who are physically healthy.

Some types of somatization in adults are associated with stressors in the person's early environment (Bohman, Cloninger, and von Knorring 1984). There is evidence that learning of attending to bodily sensations occurs in childhood (Apley, Keith, and Meadow 1978). The effects on the development of somatization from social class and education (Kellner 1986; Srole, Langner, Michael, et al. 1962) and from culture and subculture (Escobar, Burnam, Karno, et al. 1987; Kirmayer 1984) have been amply demonstrated. People from less developed cultures, lower socioeconomic classes, and lower educational attainments have a tendency to express distress in somatic terms rather than in psychological terms.

Among the other learning processes, the important ones appear to be selective perception of bodily sensation (Kellner 1986; Pennebaker 1982), habitual attention to one part of the body, and the improved skills acquired by learning to perceive (Ádám 1967). Such learning tends to produce amplification of symptoms (Barsky 1979), whereas in others suppression of bodily percepts is likely to cause minimization or denial of bodily sensations (Mayou 1976).

Whether somatic sensations will be attended to or ignored depends to a large extent on the intensity of the somatic symptoms and the attitude toward the symptoms. Distressing somatic symptoms alone are likely to induce fear of disease or the false belief of having a disease. For example, more patients with chronic peptic ulcers believe that they have also another disease or are convinced that they have a disease such as cancer (Stenbäck 1960). When patients fear disease or are convinced that they have a disease, bodily sensation may become the focus of their attention (Kellner, Abbott, Winslow, et al. 1987). One of the sequences in the reinforcement of somatization as well as in a common hypochondriacal reaction (meaning the acquisition of fear of disease or false belief of having a disease) is first the experience of new somatic symptoms at times of anxiety or depression (Kellner, Pathak, Romanik, et al. 1983). Being concerned about disease, the patient attends to bodily sensations and notices these more than previously. The perception of more bodily symptoms leads to an increase in anxiety, with an increase in autonomic activity inducing more somatic symptoms. These elements may become linked, and by frequent repetition the sequence becomes overlearned and the chain becomes predictable (Kellner 1985).

There is evidence to suggest that both the inhibition of emotions and the inhibition of emotional expression by overt behavior are associated with physiologic arousal (Grings and Dawson 1978; Pennebaker 1985). Among other factors that were found to be associated with somatization were hostility and alexithymia (a difficulty in expressing emotions in words) (Lesser, Ford, and Friedman 1979; Nemiah and Sifneos 1970; Shipko 1982). There is extensive literature on somatization disorder (as well as on Briquet's syndrome), and family studies suggest that there is a genetic predisposition (Cloninger 1986a). There is no single theory that can explain somatization; its etiology is not only multifactorial but exceedingly complex (Ford 1983; Kellner 1986; Kirmayer 1986; Mayou 1976), and its link to anxiety and depression is consistently observed.

Various social reinforcers have been reported in the literature, for example, disability insurance (Better, Fine, Simison, et al. 1979), compensation litigation after injuries (Balla and Moraitis 1970), and iatrogenic factors. Misdiagnosis and inappropriate treatment of somatization by a physician appear to play a substantial part. Patients with functional somatic symptoms report ominous and frightening diagnoses from their physicians more often than patients with similar symptoms who had a physical disease (Burns and Nichols 1972). Uncontrolled studies suggest that many chronic somatizing and hypochondriacal patients had received multiple diagnoses from various physicians and were treated for functional somatic symptoms as though they had a physical disease (Kellner 1986). In such cases it appears that an iatrogenic induction or reinforcement of the belief of being ill had occurred.

Various studies suggest the following intricate interaction and comorbidity of somatization with anxiety and depression. Anxiety and depression can be precipitating events for somatization because both disorders can cause distressing somatic symptoms. They can serve as maintaining factors because bodily symptoms are evaluated in a fearful or pessimistic way at times of anxiety and depression (Kellner, Pathak, Romanik, et al. 1983). Somatic symptoms in turn may aggravate anxiety and depression because fears and false beliefs about bodily sensation can make a person more anxious and depressed, thereby establishing a vicious cycle.

PREVALENCE AND BURDEN ON THE COMMUNITY

The prevalence of somatization depends on the diagnostic criteria (Kessell 1960). About 80% of healthy individuals experience somatic symptoms in any one week (Kellner and Sheffield 1973; Pennebaker, Burnam, Schaeffer, et al. 1977; Reidenberg and Lowenthal 1968), making somatic symptoms a normal experience even in physical health.

In most studies of primary care in which patients presented with somatic complaints for which no physical cause was subsequently detected, the proportion of these patients ranged from 10% to 30% (Kellner 1965; Kessel 1960; Shepherd, Cooper, Brown, et al. 1966). In specialty clinics these proportions were found to be even higher (Kellner 1986). There is a tendency for the proportion of somatic symptoms diagnosed as either physiologic or innocuous to increase with an increase in thoroughness of the evaluation and diagnostic sophistication of the attending physician. Conversely, the lower prevalence in primary care facilities is determined by the nature of the study; the diagnosis of minor physical disease is often made on clinical grounds without meticulous laboratory confirmation.

In a general medical facility, many of the functional somatic symptoms get a diagnostic label such as migraine headache, gastritis, or hypoglycemia, when the same complaint in a specialty clinic, after thorough investigation, would have been regarded as benign and recorded as such. The exclusion of substantial physical disease, however, does not necessarily mean that no physical cause for the symptom exists. It can be difficult, sometimes impossible, to distinguish by means of conventional diagnostic methods whether symptoms are caused by transient tissue pathology (Mayou 1976) such as muscular sprains, edema of connective tissue or mucosae, or a viral infection; by physiologic overactivity or minor conversion symptoms (Merskey 1989), or by other mechanisms. Once substantial physical disease has been excluded, special investigations that might determine the exact cause of an apparently benign symptom would be time consuming, expensive, and therefore uneconomical; they are of only little clinical value because the knowledge that they yield seldom determines the nature of treatment or makes prognosis more accurate.

In a study of DSM-III categories in primary care in England, 26% of the patients presented with somatization as defined by the authors: these patients sought medical help for somatic manifestation of psychiatric illness and did not present cognitive symptoms of psychiatric disorders (Bridges and Goldberg 1985). This suggests that somatization is a common presentation of distress even in Western cultures.

Most physicians are rightly concerned with physical diagnosis and often ignore or fail to recognize an emotional disorder in their busy practice. There is evidence that patients with panic disorder, somatization disorder, and major depression will be treated for somatic concomitants of the disorder, and the true nature is not recognized. Goldberg and Blackwell (1970) are psychiatrists; one worked as a primary care physician (general medical practitioner) for the duration of the study and the other interviewed the same patients to make a psychiatric diagnosis. The workload was divided equally. The psychiatrist who acted as the primary care physician needed to exclude physical illness and to plan treatment. Because of his overly busy schedule, he missed a large proportion of psychiatric disorders that his colleague, working at a more leisurely pace and without the responsibility for physical diagnosis, had detected.

The consequences of misdiagnosis can be ineffective and even harmful treatments. For example, there is substantial evidence that patients with somatization disorder, as well as neurosis in general, are more prone to surgical operations than other patients (Cohen, Robins, Purtell, et al. 1953; Ulett and Gildea 1950). Patients with panic disorders are sometimes misdiagnosed for years and treated for somatic manifestations of the disorder (Katon 1982; Noyes 1987).

Another facet that might account for the large percentage of patients with somatization is the relationship of anxiety and depression to psychophysiologic disorders. Some psychophysiologic disorders, such as irritable bowel syndrome (Latimer 1983), abnormal esophageal motility (Clouse and Lustman 1983), minor and inconspicuous manifestation of hyperventilation (Lewis 1959; Lum 1976; Pfeffer 1984), the fibrositis-myalgia syndrome (Goldenberg 1986; Hudson, Hudson, and Pliner 1985), as well as their incomplete and atypical manifestations, are all associated with depression and anxiety. Emotional disorders tend to aggravate these syndromes as well as making physical disease more difficult to bear, often leading to more requests for medical treatment (Kellner 1986).

The burden on the community is formidable. Somatization is an important matter of public health. It it a common cause of absenteeism, and a large part of the physician's time and effort is spent in investigating and treating patients with functional somatic complaints. The cost of somatization has been conservatively estimated as $20 billion, one-tenth of the total medical costs to the country, and this figure does not include psychiatric treatment, disability payments, and time lost from work (Ford 1983).

Thus, somatization may be the most costly comorbidity and yet has been neglected by physicians, psychiatrists, and psychologists. Physicians are not interested in somatization because of the nature of their training; patients with functional complaints are dismissed as the worried well or neurotic who do not merit the same care as people with physical disease. During medical training only a small fraction of the psychiatric rotation is spent on the management of somatoform disorders, and that training usually consists of one or two lectures, soon to be forgotten. The average medical textbook usually contains a brief chapter on hypochondriasis (Barsky and Klerman 1983) and conversion disorders with sparse and often yesteryears' views on clinical management. Until the advent of psychiatric consultation and liaison service in general hospitals, psychiatrists had scant knowledge of somatizing patients. The experience they did have came from patients who also had other major psychiatric disorders, or they based their conclusions on an unrepresentative minority of somatizing patients who, after years of invalidism, were referred to a psychiatrist as a last resort.

To sum up, the frequently quoted statement that 20% of the average physician's time is spent with the somatic manifestations of emotional disorders is probably a substantial underestimate. The general physician believes that only patients with physical diseases merit effort and care. The physician is frustrated because these patients are regarded as a burden. They do not suffer from a disease but take up precious time and do not respond to standard medical treatment. The training of most physicians is inadequate to deal with a large part of their medical practice, leading to mismanagement and unnecessary suffering.

THE MANAGEMENT OF SOMATIZATION AND SOMATIC COMORBIDITY

Treatments

The neglect of research on the treatment of somatizing patients is in striking contrast with its benefits when applied. The efficacy of treatment had been underestimated for several reasons. Nonpsychiatric physicians found that many somatizing patients were resistant to conventional medical treatments, and psychiatrists formed their own opinions about the poor prognosis from chronic, unrepresentative patients who had been referred to them after many years of failed medical treatments. Early studies of psychotherapy suggested that somatizing patients respond less well to conventional insight psychotherapy than patients with overt emotional symptoms (Rosenberg 1954; Stone, Frank, Nash, et al. 1961). Looking back, it appears that the psychotherapeutic strategies employed in these early studies were inappropriate for somatizing patients. Therapists used a traditional nondirective and analytically oriented treatment instead of addressing the patients' current fears of having a serious disease and helping them to cope with their bodily distress (Kellner 1988b). Research in the drug treatment of somatizing patients has been sparse.

Recent research reveals a picture that is entirely different from the early one. Psychiatric consultation with the patient's physician leads to substantial change in the behavior of somatizing patients, even in a chronic and usually treatment-resistant condition such as somatization disorder (Smith, Monson, and Ray 1986). In controlled studies of psychotherapy, the treated group of somatizing patients reported substantially more relief than the group treated with routine medical care (Draspa 1959; Sjodin, Svedlund, Ottosson, et al. 1986; Svedlund, Ottosson, Sjodin, et al. 1983). Moreover, in most controlled studies of treatment in medicine, the difference between the treated group and control group decreases or vanishes on follow-up. Yet in two of the studies of psychotherapy of these disorders (Sjodin, Svedlund, Ottosson, et al. 1986; Svedlund, Ottosson, Sjodin, et al. 1983), the difference between the groups became progressively greater. Psychotherapy apparently reduced the risk of recurrences. There is also consistent evidence that migraine headache, muscle contraction headaches, and probably also disorders caused by excessive contraction of striated muscle elsewhere are relieved by relaxation training and by biofeedback (Blanchard, Andrasik, Ahles, et al. 1980; Jessup, Neufeld and Merskey 1979; Tarler-Benlolo 1978).

Numerous drug trials have shown that antidepressant and anti-anxiety drugs relieve somatic symptoms in depressed and anxious patients (Kellner 1988b). Controlled studies suggest that psychotropic drugs play an important part in the treatment of psychophysiologic disorders such as irritable bowel syndrome (Myren, Lovland, Larssen, et al. 1984) or fibrositis-myalgia syndrome (Carette, McCain, Bell, et al. 1986; Goldenberg, Felson, and Dinerman 1986), as well as in the atypical variants of these syndromes that are often classified among the somatoform disorders and coexist with anxiety and depression.

What Needs to Be Done

The magnitude of the public health problem can be clearly demonstrated, and there is some knowledge about how the burden can be diminished. The study by Smith, Monson, and Ray (1986) shows that psychiatric consultation with the patients' physician alone leads to substantial changes in the behavior of somatizing patients; this suggests that increased psychiatric consultation may have beneficial and perhaps far-reaching results.

Thomas (1978) carried out a controlled study in a family practice. Patients in whom he did not detect major physical disease were either treated symptomatically in the conventional way or were told that the symptoms were of no serious significance and required no treatment. The outcome in the two groups on follow-up was the same, and the reassured group was saved the cost, side effects, and risks of drug treatment. At follow-up, more than 50% of patients with hypochondriasis will have either recovered or greatly improved after supportive psychotherapy and psychotropic medication (Kellner 1983), indicating that a great deal of unnecessary suffering and unnecessary cost could be saved.

More education in psychiatric diagnosis and knowledge of treatment by general physicians would probably be beneficial, but how to accomplish this goal is at present unknown. The National Institute of Mental Health (1987) has started the D/ART program (depression/awareness, recognition, and treatment), which also aims at the education of primary care physicians in the somatic manifestation of depression. It is unlikely that in the near future medical schools are going to change substantially and will prepare physicians for the treatment of the whole patient, as opposed to the "hole" in the patient. The methods of payment reward costly technical procedures but do not reward listening, empathy, or an opportunity for the patients to learn about their disorders and to learn how to cope. There is now evidence to suggest that third-party limitations on outpatient psychiatric services in somatizing patients cost more in the end (Smith, Miller, Monson et al. 1986). Perhaps psychiatrists and psychologists ought to lecture less to the believers and spend more time attending medical meetings to bring the good news to general physicians and surgeons.

Chapter 15

The Dilemma of Homonymous Symptoms for Evaluating Comorbidity Between Affective Disorders and Eating Disorders

Regina C. Casper, M.D.

R ECENT INTEREST IN forging a link between affective disorders, especially depression, and the so-called eating disorders stems as much from the still open question about the psychopathology associated with the development of anorexia nervosa and bulimia nervosa as from certain similarities in the clinical manifestations and neurobiologic findings between the two conditions.

The notion that anorexia nervosa represented a forme fruste of pubertal melancholia and could be viewed as a solution to pubertal conflict was widely accepted a century ago. Lasègue (1873/1964) described the antecedents to anorexia nervosa in the following way: "A young girl, between 15 and 20 years of age, suffers from some emotion which she avows or conceals. Generally it relates to some real or imaginary marriage project, to a violence done to some sympathy, or

This work was supported by National Institute of Mental Health grants R01-MH-35585-03 and R01-MH-40623-01 and the Nathan and Emily Blum Fund. I am grateful to Andrea Sanders for expert and patient assistance in the preparation of this manuscript.

to some more or less conscient desire" (p. 145). Case reports which followed Gull's (1873) and Lasègue's (1873/1964) publications on anorexia nervosa made it plain that such patients were believed to have lost their appetite: "That mental states may destroy appetite is notorious, and it will be admitted that young women at the ages named are specially prone to mental perversity" (Gull 1873, p. 25). In his letters to Fliess, Freud (1887/1954) considered anorexia nervosa the pubertal variant of melancholia.

The discovery of the first hormonal substances at the beginning of this century led to Simmonds' (1914) publication on pituitary cachexia. The subsequent implication of a deficiency of pituitary hormones in the etiology of anorexia nervosa for several decades put an end to speculations about psychological contributions to anorexia nervosa.

Until quite recently, attempts to classify the psychological components in anorexia nervosa were actively discouraged. The first diagnostic system to include anorexia nervosa (not yet bulimia nervosa)—the St. Louis or Feighner criteria (Feighner, Robins, Guze, et al. 1972)—did not permit the concurrent diagnosis of an affective disorder or of schizophrenia; the presence of either condition invalidated the diagnosis of anorexia nervosa. Anorexia nervosa and affective disorders or schizophrenia thus could not coexist. Long-term follow-up studies (Casper and Jabine 1986; Hsu, Crisp, and Harding 1979; Theander 1983) have supported this claim for schizophrenia, but the relationship between anorexia nervosa and affective disorders is certainly less clear and requires much more careful investigation.

Let us first consider some hypotheses of how depressions and eating disorders may relate to each other: (1) anorexia nervosa displaces primary depressive disorder along a continuum; (2) depressive disorders may predispose, psychologically or physiologically, to the development of eating disorders; (3) eating disorders coexist and may interact with a depressive disorder; and (4) depressive features are common in eating disorders, but do not necessarily reflect a concurrent depressive disorder.

The first notion, that anorexia nervosa displaces primary depressive disorder along a continuum, has been by far the most popular and, considering the number of publications, the most fruitful model. Most studies have collected data trying to support the hypothesis that eating disorders are variants of an affective disorder or represent the phenotype of a depressive disorder diathesis:

(1) Genetic and family studies (Biederman, Rivinus, Kemper, et al. 1985; Cantwell, Sturzenburger, Burroughs, et al. 1977; Gershon, Schreiber, Hamovit, et al. 1984; Rivinus, Biederman, Herzog, et al. 1984; Stern, Dixon, Nemzer, et al. 1984; Strober, Morrell, Burroughs, et al. 1985; Winokur, March, and Mendels 1980);

(2)   Epidemiologic studies, including studies on course and outcome (Casper and Jabine 1986; Hsu, Crisp, and Harding 1979; Hudson, Pope, Jonas, et al. 1983a, 1983b; Keller, Herzog, Lavori, et al. 1986; Lee, Rush, and Mitchell 1985; Theander 1983; Walsh, Roose, Glassman, et al. 1985); and

(3)   Shared biologic and neuroendocrine correlates (Boyer, Hellman, Roffwarg, et al. 1977; Brambilla, Cavagnini, Invitti, et al. 1985; Gerner and Wilkins 1983; Gold, Gwirtsman, Avegerinos, et al. 1986; Gwirtsman, Roy-Byrne, Yager, et al. 1983; Katz, Kuperberg, Pollack, et al. 1984).

Following Altschuler and Weiner's (1985) critical assessment, Halmi (1985) summarized the descriptive and neuroendocrine studies. The incidence of concomitant depression varied from 10% to 50% for restricting anorexia nervosa, from 40% to 80% for anorexia nervosa with bulimia, and from 25% to 70% for bulimia nervosa. Halmi concluded that given the problem of malnutrition and selective eating practices among eating disorder patients, their depressive features and endocrine aberrations could not be attributed to primary depressive disorder. Strober and Katz (1987) have reviewed existing evidence and come to similar conclusions; the authors believe that eating disorders and affective disorders differ sufficiently in family history and biologic correlates as well as in course and outcome, epidemiology, and clinical phenomenology that a single mechanism of causation is unlikely. Thus if evidence from several points of inquiry is critically analyzed, the data indicate that eating disorders and affective disorders occur independently. This does not exclude the probability that a depressive disposition might not be a risk factor for the development of an eating disorder.

THE PROBLEM WITH DEPRESSION ASSESSMENT SCALES FOR EVALUATING DEPRESSION IN EATING DISORDERS

So far surprisingly little critical attention has been given to the problem of which criteria ought to be applied for validating the diagnosis of depression in anorexia nervosa or in bulimia nervosa. A common misperception that has plagued much of the depression research in eating disorders is the tacit assumption that symptom similarity indicates commonality of origin. The existence of symptoms named alike yet carrying different meanings in either disorder—such as anorexia, early morning waking, or weight loss—has added to the diagnostic controversy. I have called these symptoms "homonymous," although I am aware that this use deviates slightly from the original definition. I hope to show that the controversy can be brought closer to a resolution if these symptoms are understood and defined within the context of each disorder's pathophysiology.

Informally, many investigators have disputed the wisdom and legitimacy of using traditional depression rating scales for assessing depression in anorexia nervosa, but as of this writing there are no empirical studies that have looked at this question. Our own group (Eckert, Goldberg, Halmi, et al. 1982) used the Minnesota Multiphasic Personality Inventory (MMPI) (Hathaway and McKinley 1951), the Hopkins Symptom Checklist (SCL-90) (Derogatis, Lipman, Rickels, et al. 1974) as well as the Raskin Mood Scale (Schulterbrandt, Raskin, and Reatig 1974). Piran, Kennedy, Garfinkel, et al. (1985) rated depression based on the self-rated MMPI, SCL-90, and Beck Depression Inventory (Beck 1978), as well as the observer-rated Hamilton Rating Scale for Depression (HRSD) (Hamilton 1967). Walsh, Roose, and Glassman, et al. (1985) assessed depression in bulimia on the basis of interviews with the Schedule for Affective Disorders and Schizophrenia (SADS) (Endicott and Spitzer 1978, 1979) and Research Diagnostic Criteria (RDC) (Spitzer, Endicott, and Robins 1978a). Cooper and Fairburn (1986) considered the Montgomery and Asberg (1979) Depression Rating Scale a "sensitive measure of depression," but they omitted the item for reduced appetite from the score "in view of the difficulty in rating this item in patients with eating disorders" (p. 270). Surprisingly, Weissenburger, Rush, Giles, et al. (1986), who assessed weight changes in depressed outpatients, made corrections for assessing depressed patients by omitting weight loss from the list of criteria for endogenous depression and subtracting the appetite and weight loss items from the Beck and Hamilton scores for calculating total depression scores. To our knowledge, no data exist on how the metabolically induced physiologic symptoms in eating disorders, of which many overlap with the symptoms of depression, distort depression scores on depression rating scales.

As mentioned, most investigators have used depression rating scales without much modification, although many were cognizant that the items scored for "endogenous" symptoms (e.g., weight loss, appetite loss, diminished libido, insomnia, early morning waking), when they occur in anorexia nervosa, are either prime symptoms of the illness, or the result of metabolic changes. Endorsement of these symptoms would be expected to result in inflated depression scores for eating disorders.

The least disputed symptom that is also a necessary prerequisite to the development of anorexia nervosa is pathologic weight loss. Most depression rating scales include one, sometimes two, questions related to weight loss. These questions are included with good reason, since about 45% of unipolar depressed inpatients (Casper, Redmond, Katz, et al. 1985) and about 30% of unipolar depressed outpatients (Weissenburger, Rush, Giles, et al. 1986) suffer conspicuous weight loss.

Another shared term, *anorexia* (or want of appetite), is, as we know now, in most cases of anorexia nervosa a misnomer, except in cachectic moribund patients who may lose their appetite altogether or depressed patients with anorexia nervosa. Nonetheless anorexia nervosa patients often claim loss of appetite, despite their lively interest in recipes and in baking cakes or their dreams about food. Therefore, patients would be expected to endorse a statement about lack of appetite.

What patients actually do, we do not know. Despite some awareness of these predicaments, the problem has not been studied, and we are far from a proposal toward its solution. The reason for such lack of attention may be twofold. Since severity of weight loss is a defining diagnostic criterion for anorexia nervosa, eating disorder rating scales that focus on abnormal eating behavior omit this item and also omit the loss of appetite item to which no credence (see Cooper and Fairburn 1986) is given, despite the patient's verbal assertion to the contrary. Similarly, sleep difficulties, amenorrhea, impotence, low body temperature, and concentration difficulties, which are invariably present albeit to a different degree, are considered secondary to starvation and malnutrition, and therefore not rated on scales tapping abnormal eating attitudes and behavior, the so-called core signs of anorexia nervosa. The eating disorder scales, therefore, do not give any information on how the patient might judge these symptoms.

Tables 1, 2, and 3 contrast some emotional, behavioral, physiologic, and cognitive symptoms in anorexia nervosa with those in major depressive disorder. Tables 1 and 2 show that a dysphoric mood, a fault-finding self-appraisal, obsessional tendencies, and withdrawal from relationships may be found in both depression and anorexia nervosa. Similarly, many physiologic symptoms look alike, especially if a depression is accompanied by severe weight loss. How then can the conditions be distinguished on a merely clinical level? The most obvious difference lies in the patients' ideation, in turn reflected in behavior. While anorectic patients retain a purposeful focus and keen interest revolving around controlling their body shape, which leads, for example, to planning meals, exercising, and improving their appearance, such sense of purpose is generally absent in depressed patients, whose thinking is usurped by failure and gloom, the mood being expressed in posture and demeanor.

The lines are less clearly drawn between depressions with increased appetite (Paykel 1977) and bulimia nervosa. Also the fact that bulimic patients regularly display signs of depression and anxiety, which have been interpreted in many studies as secondary to the bulimic behavior, makes a decision difficult. Table 3 presents certain resemblances between the eating and sleeping tendencies of patients

Table 1. Emotions and Mentality in Anorexia Nervosa Contrasted With
Primary Major Depressive Disorder

Anorexia nervosa	Primary major depressive disorder
Emotions	
Dysphoria	Sadness
Mood of frustrated self-pity	All-pervading gloom
Sympathy-seeking reactive depression	Melancholia
Low self-esteem	Low self-esteem (not invariably)
Capacity for pleasure retained (largely body shape-bound)	Little ability for enjoyment
Cognitive and motivational symptoms	
Rarely expresses depressive concerns or mental pain	Depressive ruminations and morbid concerns: life is a torment
Hypervigilance and quickened thinking	Retardation of thinking processes
Exclusionary interest in pursuit of thinness	Narrowed interest, cannot do things
Eating evokes guilt, sense of failure common	Guilt, doom, personal worry, self-condemnation
Food-related dreams	Impoverished dream life
Thinking and ruminating about food, planning meals for hours	Preoccupation with death and dying, loss of interest in self and others, neglects appearance
Keen interest in appearance	
Heightened obsessionality	Heightened obsessionality
Rigid ritualistic behavior	Detail-preoccupied
Indecisiveness	Indecisiveness
Self-reproach and self-doubt	Self-reproach and self-doubt

with atypical depression and the eating and sleeping patterns of
bulimia nervosa patients.

ON THE NOSOLOGY OF EATING DISORDERS AND PRIMARY MAJOR DEPRESSIVE DISORDER

The task of determining the relationship between the two conditions
is not made easier by the fact that neither depressive disorders nor
eating disorders can be said to fit into homogeneous categories. A
sound data base now supports the differentiation into two types of
anorexia nervosa: the fasting type and the bulimic type (Casper,
Eckert, Halmi, et al. 1980; Garfinkel, Moldofsky, and Garner 1980;
Strober 1981). This distinction, ostensibly based on the style of food
intake used to maintain or to further weight loss, extends beyond

Table 2. Behavioral and Physiologic Symptoms in Anorexia Nervosa and Primary Major Depressive Disorder

Anorexia nervosa	*Primary major depressive disorder*
Behavioral	
Inanition and food refusal	Inanition and lack of appetite
Hyperactivity with purposeful continued exercising	Motor retardation, slowed movements, sometimes
Tense, restless, involved in tasks	Restless agitation
Social withdrawal	Social withdrawal
Paranoid hypersensitivity	Paranoid hypersensitivity
Hoarding of food-related items, dawdle over meals	Disinterested in food or meals
Inflexible eating habits	
Physiologic	
Loss of appetite (avowed)	Anorexia (true)
Weight loss	Weight loss
Emaciation	Emaciation rare
Amenorrhea	Amenorrhea rare
Impotence	Impotence
Insomnia	Insomnia
Early morning waking	Early morning waking
Trouble falling asleep	Trouble falling asleep
Fitful sleep	Fitful sleep
Lowered body temperature	Lowered body temperature
Mask-like facial expression	Dejected depressed mien
Aged appearance	Looks older than age
Rarely ever complains of physical pain; belle indifference to physical discomfort	Complains of physical pain, hypochondriasis
Constipation, other gastrointestinal symptoms rare	Constipation, gastrointestinal symptoms

Table 3. Physiologic Symptoms in Bulimia Nervosa Compared With Symptoms in Atypical Depression

Bulimia nervosa or bulimia in anorexia nervosa and eating binges	*Atypical depression*
Hyperphagia (bulimia)	Increased appetite, hyperphagia
Often vomiting	No vomiting
Weight gain	Weight gain
Fitful sometimes extended sleep	Hypersomnia
Menstrual disturbances	Menstrual disturbances
Sexual interest retained	Intermittent sexual interest
Lethargy	Lethargy

consummatory behavior into personality types. The first personality type is rather inhibited, retiring, sometimes bordering on the schizoid, yet can be thoughtful, considerate with a tendency for being obsessional. The bulimic type tends to have a more outgoing, engaging, affectively labile and impulsive temperament and seems cognitively and behaviorally more easily disorganized. The personality of the so-called normal-weight bulimia nervosa corresponds closely to the bulimic type of anorexia nervosa.

Similarly, depressive disorders have been shown to be heterogeneous. The two broad categories relevant for our discussion are the classic unipolar depressions and the group of depressions with atypical vegetative symptoms (Davidson, Miller, Craig, et al. 1982). The two classes of depression differ sharply with respect to the concurrent physiologic symptoms (as outlined in Tables 1, 2, and 3). Early morning waking and loss of libido, appetite, and weight characterize melancholia, whereas hypersomnia, hyperphagia, and weight gain are not uncommonly found in atypical depressions (Quitkin, Rabkin, Stewart, et al. 1985).

The somatic symptoms in depressive disorder could be ignored if somatic symptoms were uncommon or occurred independently of the depression. However, physical changes and depression seem interrelated. For example, Paykel (1977) and Casper, Redmond, Katz, et al. (1985) have found high positive correlations between severity of depression, appetite loss, weight loss, and loss of sexual interest. Unfortunately, Cassidy, Flanagan, Spellman, et al. (1957) do not comment on the relationship to illness severity.

Moreover, there is a need for a critical evaluation of anxiety rating scales in use for eating disorders because the hypothyroid state, lowered metabolism, and reduced sympathetic tone (especially in acute anorexia nervosa) diminishes physiologic activation (e.g., an increase in heart rate or sweating regarded as part of the dimension of anxiety). We omitted these symptoms when patients were asked to complete the Taylor Manifest Anxiety Scale (Casper, Schlemmer, and Javaid 1987). In the absence of this adrenergic response, the severity of anxiety is probably underestimated in eating disorder patients. Of course, aside from physical symptoms, sometimes behavioral symptoms might have a different connotation in eating disorders. For example, the SCL-90 contains an item "feeling uncomfortable about eating or drinking in public" presumably measuring social phobia, which was, not surprisingly, answered in the affirmative by more than half among chronic anorexia nervosa patients.

The issue is not only how to disentangle the symptoms that may be shared by the affective and eating disorders, but also how to measure them accurately and how to control for these symptoms so that they will not be spuriously counted as signs of anxiety, agitation, or depression in eating disorder patients.

Since we know that depression scales differ in type and number of physical symptoms, the error introduced for estimating depression in eating disorders will differ from scale to scale. As a first step therefore, I examined and compared the number of physical symptoms on depression rating scales in proportion to the total items. I will present data from an ongoing analysis illustrating the responses of eating disorder patients to certain physical symptoms on rating scales in comparison to the response of depressed patients and healthy controls. Lastly, some recommendations will be made, and some of the pitfalls for depression or anxiety research in eating disorders will be mentioned.

PHYSICAL SYMPTOMS ON DEPRESSION, ANXIETY, AND EATING DISORDERS RATING SCALES

Table 4 lists seven rating scales or factor scales that are in wide use for assessing symptoms of depression. About one-fourth to one-fifth of the questions inquire about physical symptoms. For the purpose of this discussion, retardation and agitation are excluded, albeit both are symptoms that can be associated with anorexia nervosa. The Carroll (Carroll, Feinberg, Smouse, et al. 1981) rating scale contains a slightly higher proportion, while the MMPI depression scale includes a considerably lower proportion of physical symptoms. The SCL-90 lists only loss of sexual interest or pleasure under the depression factor; all other symptoms make up "additional" single item scales (Derogatis, Lipman, and Covi 1973). Aside from the SADS, Paykel's (1985) interview is the only scale that assesses extended sleep, increased appetite, and weight gain independently.

Table 5 displays items that cluster on the anxiety factor on the SCL-90. To give an example, "feeling so restless you can't sit still" would be expected to be endorsed by malnourished patients, since starvation and malnutrition might lead to motor restlessness, which may be mistaken as agitation. In addition, many patients with anorexia nervosa, afraid that sitting down accumulates more calories than standing or moving, do not allow themselves to sit down for any length of time; a few even limit time in bed. Conversely, due to the reduction in sympathetic tone, "heart pounding" would not be experienced as easily if the patient becomes anxious.

The two most frequently used eating disorder rating scales displayed in Table 6 list few somatic symptom items: 3 of 40 items on the Eating Attitudes Test (Garner and Garfinkel 1979) or no item on the Eating Disorders Inventory (Garner, Olmstead, and Polivy 1983). A

Table 4. Physiologic Symptoms on Commonly Used Depression Rating Scales

Item	Depression rating scales (total item number)						
	HRSD (24)	BECK Depression Inventory (21)	CARROLL Rating Scale for Depression (17)	MONTGOMERY-ASBERG Depression Rating Scale (10)	MMPI (44)	SCL-90	Paykel interview (36)
Gastrointestinal symptoms	#12 Gastrointestinal (appetite) #11 Somatic anxiety	#18 Worse Appetite	#12 Gastrointestinal (appetite) #11 Somatic Anxiety	#5 Reduced appetite	#2 Good appetite #18 Seldom troubled by constipation #51 Good physical health	#19 Poor appetite #40 Upset stomach #60 Overeating	Anorexia Increased appetite
Weight	#16 Loss of weight A, B,	#19 Weight loss	#17 Loss of weight		#155 Stable weight #153 Well most of the time		Weight loss Weight gain
Sleep	#4, 5, 6 Early, middle, late insomnia	#16 Insomnia and early morning awakening	#4, 5, 6 Initial, middle, delayed insomnia	#4 Reduced sleep	#43 Fitful and disturbed sleep	#44, #64, #66, trouble falling asleep, waking early, restless sleep	Initial, middle, delayed Insomnia Increased sleep
Libido and menstrual function	#14 Loss of libido, menstrual disturbances	#21 Interest in sex	#14 Loss of libido			#5 Loss of sexual interest or pleasure	

Note. HRSD = Hamilton Rating Scale for Depression; MMPI = Minnesota Multiphasic Personality Inventory; SCL-90 Hopkins Symptom Checklist.

Table 5.   Hopkins Symptom Checklist-90 Anxiety Factor Scale

Nervousness or shakiness inside
Trembling
Suddenly scared for no reason
Feeling fearful
Heart pounding or racing
Feeling tense or keyed up
Spells of terror and panic
Feeling so restless you can't sit still
Feeling that familiar things are strange or unreal
Feeling pushed to get things done

Table 6.   Physiologic and Depression Symptoms on Three Commonly Used
Eating Disorder Rating Scales

| | Rating scales | | |
Item	Eating Attitudes Test	Eating Disorders Inventory	Psychiatric Rating Scale for Anorexia Nervosa
Sleep	#20 Wake up early in the morning		
Menstrual function	#23 Have regular menstrual periods		Psychosexual immaturity
Gastrointestinal		#35 Suffer from constipation	
Worthlessness		#41 I have a low opinion of myself #50 I feel that I am a worthwhile person	Exaggerated optimism and cheerfulness
Depression			Depressive mood or behavior

psychiatric rating scale originally developed for the Collaborative Anorexia Nervosa Treatment Study (Halmi, Goldberg, Casper, et al. 1979) rates one item only: psychosexual maturity. Since physical symptoms are taken for granted in the eating disorders, an independent estimation on eating disorder rating scales is generally not considered. Patients, on the other hand, who frequently are unaware that their reduced food intake can result in physical symptoms such as constipation or insomnia may report these symptoms in all innocence when asked on a rating scale, albeit occasionally denial of illness may extend to denial of physical discomfort.

LOSS OF APPETITE AND EARLY MORNING WAKING IN EATING DISORDER PATIENTS COMPARED TO UNIPOLAR DEPRESSED PATIENTS AND CONTROLS

To illustrate the complexity of the problem, we will analyze two symptoms—loss of appetite and early morning waking—that are considered core symptoms of melancholia (DSM-III-R) (American Psychiatric Association 1987). Subjects in the eating disorder group were inhospital patients with anorexia nervosa or bulimia nervosa admitted between 1984 and 1986 to the Michael Reese Eating Disorders and Research Program, and former patients assessed on 8- to 10-year follow-up who had originally participated in the Collaborative Anorexia Nervosa Treatment Study at the Illinois State Psychiatric Institute between 1975 and 1977. All anorexia nervosa patients met Feighner criteria and DSM-III (American Psychiatric Association 1980) criteria for anorexia nervosa. Bulimia nervosa patients met DSM-III-R criteria. The patients' ages ranged from 14 to 35 years. Healthy female controls were sex- and age-matched to the follow-up sample, with a mean ± SD age of 24.3 ± 2.9. The data from the unipolar primary depressed population have been published previously (Casper, Redmond, Katz, et al. 1985). In that study, loss of appetite was obtained as a combined rating, which included HRSD scale item 12, video interview Behavior Evaluation Scale item 32 (Katz and Itil 1974), SCL-90 item 19, and SADS-change item 228. Early morning waking combined ratings from HRSD item 6, SCL-90 item 64, and SADS-change item 226. For the eating disorder group, loss of appetite was self-rated on the SCL-90 item 19 and early morning waking on SCL-90 item 64. Symptom presence was determined for both groups as moderate to severe ratings. Table 7 presents the distribution from loss of appetite and early morning waking in all groups expressed as percentages.

Appetite

The data support the contention that *anorexia* is a misnomer when it is applied to anorexia nervosa, since 58% of patients with acute anorexia nervosa, who were on average 38% underweight for age and height, did not report a diminished appetite. To confirm this observation, we analyzed the same patients' responses to the MMPI statement "I have a good appetite" (item number 2): 48% endorsed this statement. The presence of an appetite, of course, explains why many patients are interested in baking and cooking, a phenomenon not observed in depressive patients with a loss of appetite. Nonetheless, a sizable number (42%) of acute anorexia nervosa patients claimed a poor

Table 7. Frequency of Loss of Appetite and Early Morning Waking in
           Various Groups of Patients and Controls, in Percentages

Group	N	Loss of appetite	Early morning waking
Anorexia nervosa acute	15	42.3	44.8
Anorexia nervosa recovered	32	18.8	25.0
Bulimia nervosa	20	10.0	65.0
Unipolar depression	84	64.6	89.4
Controls (ED)	20	0.0	10.5
Controls (UD)	80	0.0	6.0

Note. Loss of appetite: Hopkins Symptom Checklist; overall $\chi^2 = 138.75$, 5 df, $p < .001$. Early morning waking: Hopkins Symptom Checklist; overall $\chi^2 = 11.63$, 5 df, $p < .02$. ED = eating disorders; UD = unipolar depression.

appetite. We have no definitive data that would verify whether this reflects actual appetite loss. A positive response in 42% of the population is substantial enough to record on a depression scale, especially when compared to the significantly lower incidence of appetite loss in physiologically recovered anorexia nervosa patients whose average weight was in the normal range and to the quite low occurrence of anorexia in bulimia nervosa patients. In accordance with the latter observation, 70% of bulimia nervosa patients reported a good appetite. In normals, loss of appetite was an extremely rare occurrence; no control subject in either control group qualified for loss of appetite. By contrast, two-thirds among unipolar depressed patients reported appetite loss, which has been previously reported to be significantly associated with depressed mood ($r = 53$, $p < .001$) and with anxiety ($r = .53$, $p < .001$) (Casper, Redmond, Katz, et al. 1985). Loss of appetite was significantly more frequent in depressed patients than in acute anorexia nervosa patients.

Sleep

As Table 7 indicates, early morning waking typically terminates sleep in the unipolar depressed patient. A sizable proportion, nearly half among acute anorexia nervosa patients, reported early morning waking; the difference in frequency of early morning waking between depressed and acute anorexia nervosa patients was significant. Almost two-thirds of the bulimia nervosa patients woke early in the morning, which would be the opposite of what we hypothesized (i.e., hypersomnia). It should be noted that the bulimia nervosa patients were hospitalized at the time of testing, their meals supervised, and vomiting prevented by bathroom supervision. Bulimic patients tend to use conditions where access to food is limited as an opportunity to induce weight loss and to eat less, below their recommended intake for weight maintenance. Thus prevented from being bulimic, patients actually might have undernourished themselves.

The Eating Attitude Test contains a statement that presumably inquires into early waking but is formulated somewhat differently. When we analyzed the responses to item 20, "Wake up early in the morning," affirmative responses were consistently 10% to 30% higher than responses to early morning waking on SCL-90 item 64. In all likelihood, many of the subjects interpreted the statement as merely descriptive of the time of waking, instead of an inquiry into spontaneous waking in the early hours. The high affirmation rate that we observed in controls (36%) would support this explanation.

Clinically, it is well known that unlike the depressed patient who awakes to oppressive worrying, the patient with acute anorexia nervosa appears lively and animated after waking and often exercises or cleans the house. This difference suggests that anorexia nervosa patients feel different than depressed patients on waking. We therefore analyzed the responses to the MMPI statement (item 3) "I wake up rested and refreshed." Nearly as many acute anorexia nervosa patients (87.5%) as control subjects (90%) stated they woke up rested and refreshed. The number was slightly less for recovered anorexia nervosa patients (76.4%). Less than half of the bulimia nervosa patients (42.1%) woke up refreshed, suggesting that early morning waking in this group feels qualitatively different from that of acute anorexia nervosa patients. Indeed, the frequency of early morning waking in bulimic patients did not differ statistically from the incidence in depressed patients.

Depressive Feeling in Eating Disorder Patients

The question arises how depressed acute anorexia nervosa patients feel. Most studies have found, on average, mild to moderate depression scores (Eckert, Goldberg, Halmi, et al. 1982; Strober 1981). Depression scores in our patient groups were similar: The mean Beck Depression Inventory total score was 14.9 ± 12.1 for acute anorexia nervosa, 11.8 ± 11.1 for recovered patients, and 14.3 ± 12.3 for bulimia nervosa patients, compared to 2.5 ± 2.8 in controls. The large variance in the patient groups suggests that there might be subgroups of more or less depressed patients, for whom an estimation of the contribution of the physical symptoms may be important.

Despite the overall moderate depression scores, two-thirds

among acute anorexia nervosa patients stated on the Beck Depression Inventory that they felt blue or sad and that they cried more frequently; the same items were endorsed by 50% of the bulimia nervosa patients and 10% of the control subjects. Thus ratings of depressed mood or sadness probably ought to be the first step in reaching a differential diagnosis and may be the most reliable indicator of whether or not depressive feelings exist in eating disorders. It would then be crucial not only to obtain a measure of the intensity of the mood disturbance, as is done on most depression rating scales, but also to determine whether these feelings are continuously present, day and night, or whether patients can be cheered up in reaction to pleasurable events.

Another issue that I will briefly examine is whether other symptoms, such as anxiety, which contribute to the dimension of depression, need to be taken into consideration. The experience of anxiety might also be affected by the physical changes associated with eating disorders.

An Example of Problems With Anxiety Ratings in Eating Disorder Patients

Table 5 displays the statements included in the anxiety factor of the SCL-90. Instead of using acute patients, we analyzed the responses of 19 chronic anorexia nervosa patients with a desirable mean body weight for age and height: 80.6 ± 14.0% of ideal body weight, Metropolitan Life Insurance tables (1964). Mean anxiety scores for chronic anorexia nervosa patients (1.14 ± 1.0) and bulimia nervosa patients (1.14 ± .7) significantly differed from those of recovered anorexia nervosa patients (.79 ± .7) and controls (.4 ± .4). An item-by-item analysis revealed significant between group differences for "suddenly scared for no reason," "feeling fearful," and "feeling tense or keyed up." For "suddenly scared for no reason," chronic anorexia nervosa patients showed the highest scores (2.1 ± 1.6). On "feeling fearful," bulimia nervosa patients attained the highest scores (2.8 ± 1.5). For "feeling tense or keyed up," anorexia nervosa and bulimia nervosa patients showed similar scores of 3.1 ± 1.2 and 3.3 ± 1.7, respectively. "Feeling so restless can't sit still" showed the most pronounced difference of all items, with chronic anorexia nervosa patients rating the highest (2.7 ± 1.4). By contrast, scores for "heart pounding or racing" did not differ statistically; furthermore, not the chronic, but recovered anorexia nervosa patients had the highest scores, thus confirming our prediction that adrenergic activation may be sluggish in underweight eating disorder patients. The data suggest that malnutrition and weight loss may affect heart rate and motor activity in opposite ways.

Chapter 16

Comorbid Anxiety Disorders in Childhood-Onset Depressions

Maria Kovacs, Ph.D.

A S MANY CHAPTERS in the present volume illustrate, there is a substantive literature on the admixture of depression and anxiety as symptoms, syndromes, or disorders among adults. The bulk of this literature underscores that it is common for symptoms of depression and anxiety to exist in combination with one another. There are also data that suggest that individuals who suffer from one of these disorders may be particularly likely to manifest the other one as well (for reviews, see Breier, Charney, and Heninger 1985a, b; Stavrakaki and Vargo 1986). The meaning of such observations has, however, been widely debated. Much of the controversy has focused on whether depression and anxiety can indeed coexist as separately diagnosable disorders, and, if so, what the implications are for nosology and clinical management.

Although reliable data on psychiatric comorbidity among depressed children and adolescents are only beginning to accumulate, there are several reasons why this age group should be addressed in a volume that is devoted primarily to adults. First, recent work on depressive disorders among adults suggests that younger age-at-onset (alone or in combination with some anxiety disorders) signifies

Preparation of this chapter was supported by Grant No. MH-33990 from the National Institute of Mental Health, Health and Human Services Administration, and a grant from the W. T. Grant Foundation. Appreciation is expressed to Judith Marsh, Ph.D., for helpful comments on a previous version of this chapter.

greater genetic or psychosocial transmission (e.g., Price, Kidd, and Weissman 1987). Therefore, insofar as affectively disturbed juveniles probably suffer from a form of depression that has a strong familial component, a better understanding of it may be of import for all ages. Second, it has long been believed that certain childhood disorders may predispose individuals to later psychiatric disturbance. For example, separation anxiety has been viewed as a possible precursor of agoraphobia (Gittelman and Klein 1984, 1985). Therefore, knowledge about depression and anxiety in the pre-adult years is pertinent to a better understanding of these phenomena among adults. Finally, the notion that depression and anxiety exist on a continuum (dimension), rather than being categorically distinct, owes much to Bowlby's (1973, 1980) work on the consequences of separation in infants and children.

The purpose of the present chapter is to summarize the data on the coexistence of anxiety and depression among juveniles. In line with the literature on adults, studies with clinical samples or with nonreferred but psychiatrically evaluated subjects will be the focus. To retain further a degree of parallelism with the literature on adults, both symptom co-occurrence and diagnostic comorbidity will be addressed. Then the importance and implications of these data will be discussed.

Symptom Co-Occurrence

It has long been recognized that symptoms of depression and anxiety often coexist among psychiatrically disturbed youths (for example, see Hoehn-Saric, Maisami, and Wiegand 1987; Rutter, Tizard, and Whitmore 1981). In fact, as far back as the 1960s, it had been proposed that depression is one specific disorder that rarely occurs in a pure form in children (Glaser 1968; Toolan 1962). Instead, because of developmental factors, the presentation of depression was said to be "masked" by symptoms and behaviors that would not be typically associated with mood disorder. Although acting-out behaviors were the most frequently cited masking symptoms (or depressive equivalents), symptoms of anxiety were also implicated. School phobia, for example, had been mentioned as one of the symptoms that masks depression in children (Glaser 1968). A variety of other phobias and physical complaints were viewed as depressive equivalents as well (Renshaw 1974).

Frommer (1968) was one of the first to provide a coherent clinical description of various symptom aggregations among depressed children. Her sample consisted of 4- to 16-year-olds who were referred for treatment and whom she diagnosed as "having depressive illness." Based on clinical experience, she delineated three types of symptom patterns: uncomplicated depression, enuretic or encopretic depression, and phobic depression. Of the 190 depressed cases, 33% were of the phobic type, who were distinguished from the rest of the children by a high prevalence of anxiety and clinging behavior.

More recently, the co-occurrence of symptoms of depression and anxiety have been documented both through standardized psychiatric evaluations and paper-and-pencil questionnaires completed by young patients themselves. Using a semistructured psychiatric interview, the Kiddie Schedule for Affective Disorders and Schizophrenia (K-SADS) (Chambers, Puig-Antich, Hirsch, et al. 1985) to gather data from the parents about their children and from the young patients about themselves, Puig-Antich and Rabinovich (1986) studied 80 prepubertal youngsters who met Research Diagnostic Criteria (RDC) (Spitzer, Endicott, Robins 1978a) for major depression. A very high proportion of these children had symptoms of anxiety. Clinically notable phobia (as symptom) was reported for 48%; separation anxiety (as symptom) was present among 59% of them; and 11% had obsessive-compulsive features. However, significant symptoms of anxiety were just as prevalent among 43 comparison cases who had "nondepressed emotional disorder."

Geller, Chestnut, Miller, et al. (1985) described 59 children (aged 5 to 16 years) from their pharmacologic study who had had major depression. The cases were diagnosed according to the *Diagnostic and Statistical Manual of Mental Disorders* (DSM-III) (American Psychiatric Association 1980). The investigators sought to assess the prevalence of symptoms, including anxiety, which are listed in the DSM-III as associated features of major depression in children. Using the K-SADS as the semistructured interview and a severity cutoff score on the pertinent K-SADS item, 71% of the sample was found to have separation anxiety.

The conclusion of Puig-Antich and Rabinovich (1986) that the basic difference between depressed and anxious children is the presence of depressive symptoms (not the manifestations of anxiety) echoed the opinion of Hershberg, Carlson, Cantwell, et al. (1982). From a series of psychiatrically referred 7- to 17-year-old children, the latter authors selected two diagnostic groups: 28 cases with "affective disorder" and 14 children with "anxiety disorder." Clinical ratings revealed that the two groups did not differ in the prevalence of symptoms of anxiety. However, salient depressive symptoms were more likely among the affectively ill children as compared to the anxious children.

The strategy of contrasting groups was also used by Stavrakaki, Vargo, Boodoosingh, et al. (1987). From among a sample of consecutive child psychiatric admissions, they selected subjects (aged 6 to 16 years) with the DSM-III diagnoses of some type of anxiety disorder ($n = 33$) or depression ($n = 51$). Cases with Axis I conditions, as well as cases with the phenomenologically pertinent adjustment disorders, were included. The analyses of self-rated scales completed by the children, parents, and clinicians revealed that depressive disorders and anxiety disorders were essentially *discrete* conditions.

In line with the previously noted studies, Stavrakaki, Vargo, Boodoosingh, et al. (1987) also found that the severity ratings of depressive symptoms discriminated the best between the depressed and anxious groups. That is, the depressed children were concurrently anxious, whereas the anxious children did not seem to be concurrently depressed. Taken together with the finding that anxious children were younger, the authors hypothesized that anxious children may eventually become depressed adolescents or adults.

Finally, symptom co-occurrence has also been documented in diagnostically heterogenous samples of juveniles as well as among children and adolescents who come to clinical attention because of some type of anxiety disorder. For example, Norvell, Brophy, and Finch (1985) studied 30 children (mean age, 11½ years) in a state-supported inpatient facility. The clinical diagnoses included dysthymic disorder, overanxious disorder, conduct disorder, and attention-deficit disorder, as well as other conditions. The depression and anxiety scales, completed by the young patients, were found to be highly intercorrelated, suggesting a "significant relationship between anxiety and depression" (p. 152). Using a different approach and a clinically homogeneous sample, Kolvin, Berney, and Bhate (1984) described 51 school-phobic children, aged 9 to 14 years. Contrary to the reports of others on the low prevalence of depressive symptoms among children with various types of anxiety disorders, these authors reported that 45% of their sample was "unequivocally depressed" based on having at least two depressive symptoms.

DIAGNOSTIC COMORBIDITY

The question of whether depression and anxiety can coexist as disorders has been approached both from a dimensional and a categorical perspective (for example, see Frances, Widiger, and Fyer, Chapter 3; Stavrakaki and Vargo 1986). According to the dimensional or unitary perspective, these syndromes are not separate disorders. Instead, they derive from a common underlying psychopathologic process and are merely different phases of it. But, according to the categorical viewpoint, disorders of depression and anxiety are discrete conditions with different etiologies and clinical course. Therefore, the concept of comorbid anxiety and depressive disorders (as separate entities) is only viable from a categorical standpoint.

The likelihood of detecting the coexistence of such presumably different psychiatric disorders in the same individual is influenced by the existing diagnostic system. In a hierarchical classification system, for example, disorders that are secondary to, or the "result" of another presumably more severe condition would escape detection. In DSM-III, this is particularly the case when certain anxiety and depressive disorders coexist. It is important to note, therefore, that in the studies to be described, the hierarchical exclusion of certain anxiety disorders was not followed.

Two groups of investigators have reported relevant data using nonclinical samples. As part of their work on the familial transmission of depressive illness among adults, Weissman and her collaborators have examined the prevalence of psychiatric illness in the offspring of the probands. In one study, the family-history method of data collection was used to estimate the rates of psychiatric disorders (by DSM-III criteria) among the 6- to 17-year-old children of 133 depressed parents and the children of 82 normal community controls (Weissman, Leckman, Merikangas, et al. 1984). Major depression ($n = 14$) and separation anxiety disorder ($n = 11$) were the most frequent disturbances among the total of 194 children. It was also noted that 8 children had "major depression and any anxiety disorder." Thus 8 of 14 or 57% of the youths with depressive disorders had comorbid anxiety disorders.

In a subsequent study, the children of 91 of the previously studied families (56 depressed probands and 35 normals) were reexamined using direct, semistructured interviews with both the parent about the child and the child about him or herself whenever possible (Weissman, Gammon, John, et al. 1987). The resultant information was used by diagnosticians to provide best-estimate diagnoses. Among the 220 offspring who ranged in age from 6 to 23 years, those who had a depression also had various comorbid psychiatric disorders, with "anxiety disorder" (42%) having been the most frequent.

In one of their recent studies, Kashani, Carlson, Beck, et al. (1987) examined the prevalence of depression and its associated features in a community sample of 150 adolescents, aged 14 to 16 years. Using semistructured interviews, trained clinicians conducted home-based assessments by interviewing the parents about their children and the youngsters about themselves. Based on DSM-III criteria and the study's additional requirement for functional impairment, 12 youngsters (8%) were diagnosed with depressive disorders (7 with both major depression and dysthymia and 5 with dysthymia). All of these youths had other diagnoses, yielding a 100% rate of comorbidity. Comorbid anxiety disorder was the most prevalent, with 9 (75%) of the 12 depressed cases having received this additional diagnosis. Despite the small size of the community sample, this study is important because it provides an estimate of comorbidity for a nonselected, nonpatient population. It is also notable that the rate of comorbid anxiety disorders among the depressed cases is even higher than the rates found in patient samples.

Information on clinically referred, depressed 8- to 13-year-old youths has been reported by Kovacs, Feinberg, Crouse-Novak, et al. (1984a), based on an ongoing, longitudinal, nosologic study of the depressive disorders in childhood. To gather diagnostic information from both parents and children, a standardized semistructured interview was utilized. The sample consisted of youngsters whose index (initial) episode of depression met DSM-III criteria for major depressive disorder, or dysthymic disorder, or adjustment disorder with depressed mood. In their initial report on the clinical presentation of the first 65 study cases with the various types of depressions, the authors noted both a very high rate of overall psychiatric comorbidity, and that about one-third had some type of anxiety disorder.

The problem of comorbidity of anxiety and depression was explored in greater detail in a subsequent report, which used data from a larger portion of the sample (Kovacs, Gatsonis, Paulauskas, et al. 1989). As before, the diagnoses were based on DSM-III criteria. Among the first 104 depressed cases who were enrolled in the study, 41% had one or more anxiety disorders that were contemporaneous with their index episodes of depression. Separation anxiety was the most frequent comorbid anxiety disorder (31%), followed by overanxious disorder of childhood (16%). Although phobic disorders, obsessive-compulsive disorders, panic disorders, and atypical anxiety disorders were also found in conjunction with the index episodes of depression, they were manifested by only 7 of the 104 children.

The comorbid anxiety disorders tended to aggregate with the major affective disorders. That is, children with major depression or dysthymia were found to be three times more likely to have comorbid anxiety disorders as compared to youngsters who had adjustment disorder with depressed mood. Moreover, children who had comorbid anxiety disorders were generally younger when they developed their depressions as compared to the youngsters who did not have coexisting anxiety (Kovacs, Paulauskas, Gatsonis, et al. 1988).

An alternative way to examine the co-occurrence of anxiety and depressive disorders among juveniles is to study samples that were identified as having some type of anxiety disorder as the diagnosis of interest. Rapoport, Elkins, Langer, et al. (1981), who reported on the presentation and outcome of adolescents who had obsessive-compulsive disorder, collected clinical and neurobiologic data on nine youths who had primary obsessive-compulsive disorder (by DSM-III criteria). The authors reported that *all* cases (100%) had a positive lifetime history of major depressive disorder, which typically occurred a couple of years after the onset of the obsessive rituals.

Using a different method of case selection, Alessi, Robbins, and Dilsaver (1987) evaluated 61 consecutively admitted adolescent patients to determine if panic disorder and depressive disorder coexisted among them. They found that 10 (16%) of 61 cases met RDC for definite panic disorder. Additionally, 7 (70%) of those 10 cases had an accompanying depressive disorder.

Bernstein and Garfinkel (1986) evaluated 26 adolescents (aged 9 to 17 years) who were referred to their School Phobia Clinic. Based on the results of a semistructured interview, 18 cases met DSM-III criteria for an affective disorder (major depression or adjustment disorder with depressed mood), and 16 youths had some type of anxiety disorder (mostly separation anxiety). The overlap between depressive and anxiety disorders was evidenced by the fact that 13 children met criteria for both, yielding a 50% rate of comorbidity in this series of referrals.

In a similar vein, Last, Hersen, Kazdin, et al. (1987) reported on the clinical characteristics of 69 youngsters who were referred to their Anxiety Disorders Clinic. The children met DSM-III criteria for some type of anxiety disorder based on the results of semistructured interviews. In this sample of youths who had separation anxiety disorder and/or overanxious disorder as the primary diagnoses, 33% also met diagnostic criteria for major depression. Similar rates of comorbidity were reported by these investigators for a slightly different-sized but apparently overlapping sample, which consisted of cases of separation anxiety disorder or school phobia (Last, Francis, Hersen, et al. 1987).

DISCUSSION

The available data suggest that, both as symptoms and as disorders, depression and anxiety among children and adolescents frequently coexist. Up to about 70% of youngsters with a diagnosable depressive disorder appear to have clinical manifestations (symptoms) of anxiety. From approximately 30% to 75% of them have comorbid anxiety disorders. Interestingly, the association between depression and anxiety was readily detectable irrespective of the nature of the sample—that is, whether subjects were identified because of some type of high-risk versus low-risk status; through community-based surveys; via having an inpatient status; or because of having been referred to a general psychiatric clinic or to a depression or anxiety specialty clinic.

There appears to be considerable variability in the reported rates of *symptoms* of anxiety among depressed youths (from 11% to 71%). This variability is likely to reflect several factors. First, particular symptoms may have different baseline distributions. For example, pathologic obsessions or compulsive rituals are probably far less prevalent than separation anxiety, therefore suggesting that symptom-specific rates may not be directly comparable. Second, the prevalence of various symptoms may be age dependent. Thus for any given symptom, the age distribution of the sample could affect the results. Third, some of the variability in the reported rates may reflect that, as compared to a syndrome, individual symptoms are probably assessed with lower reliability.

The comorbid *diagnosis* of interest among depressed youngsters is usually reported as the presence of any anxiety disorder, with rates from about 30% to 75%. Surprisingly, a similar portion of youths (33% to 100%), who come to attention because they have anxiety disorders, suffer from simultaneous depressive illness. Rates of comorbidity for this pair of disorders therefore seem comparable to one another, irrespective of whether the number of diagnosable depressed or the number of diagnosable anxious cases serve as denominators.

Nonetheless, the substantial variability in the rates across studies suggests caution in interpretation. Undoubtedly, just as in the investigations of symptom co-occurrence, methodological factors probably contributed to the variability in the results. For example, studies have differed in the manner in which clinical data were gathered, in the process of diagnosis, and in the choice of diagnostic systems, all of which could explain some of the variability in the rates of comorbidity.

It is also notable that the information on diagnostic comorbidity and on symptom co-occurrence seem to differ from one another. Studies in which depressed children were compared to anxious children on the prevalence and severity of *symptoms* have consistently reported that the depressive symptoms were the best discriminators. Depressed children tended to be anxious, whereas anxious children did not tend to be depressed. Several factors could account for the contradictory results, including diagnostic specificity, age range of the samples, and sample sizes. First, studies of the rates of depressive *disorders* among anxious patients typically used diagnostically specific and homogeneous samples. The cases were restricted mostly to those with separation anxiety disorder (school phobia), panic disorder, or overanxious disorder. In contrast, in the symptom-prevalence studies, the cases could have "any" anxiety disorder. The resultant differences could therefore mean that depression is more likely to aggregate with some anxiety disorders than with others. Second, studies of the anxiety disorders generally used adolescent patients, which could also account for the high likelihood of depressive disorders among them. In comparison, in the investigations of symptom co-occurrence, the subjects ranged in age from early childhood to adolescence and the specific age distributions of the depressed and anxious cases may not have been sufficiently well matched. Third, compared to the studies of depressed cases, the findings on anxious patients may be less reliable because they have been generally based on smaller sample sizes.

Although the published data are not sufficiently convincing to estimate the true rate of comorbidity, the more conservative figures suggest that at least 30% to 50% of youngsters with a depressive disorder may suffer from a contemporaneous anxiety disorder. The significance of the foregoing information can only be fully appreciated in light of the base rates of these disorders, both in normal and in clinically referred populations, and for the different age groups. Epidemiologic data on the depressions in the pre-adults years, which are just beginning to accumulate, suggest that although the rates are low in normal samples, they gradually rise as a function of age: rates of 1.8% among 9-year-olds and 4.7% among 14- to 16-year-olds have been reported (Kashani, Carlson, Beck, et al. 1987; Kashani, McGee, Clarkson, et al. 1983). The rates of affective disorders are considerably higher among clinically referred or inpatient youths (27% to 50%) (Carlson and Cantwell 1979; Friedman, Clarkin, Corn, et al. 1982). On the other hand, because operational diagnostic criteria for the anxiety disorders in childhood are relatively recent (Gittelman 1986), the base rates of these conditions are yet to be reliably determined. Clinical experience would suggest, however, that the prevalence of anxiety disorders among juveniles would at least equal (and perhaps exceed) the rate of depressions.

Given the presumably high prevalence of these diagnoses in clinical samples, it can be assumed that some portion of the observed comorbidity of anxiety and depression in patient populations is due to chance association. At the same time, however, the high likelihood of this combination of diagnoses among depressed youngsters, as compared to other combinations—for example, conduct disorder and depression comorbidity (Kovacs, Paulauskas, Gatsonis, et al. 1988)—suggests a tendency for aggregation. Although neither the etiology nor the nosologic significance of the association between depression and anxiety is well understood, developmental-theory-based research could make some contributions. For example, it appears likely that the occurrence of certain anxiety disorders in conjunction with depression is mediated by the person's age. There is some evidence, among others, that panic disorder is rare among 8- to 13-year-old depressed youngsters (Kovacs, Gatsonis, Paulauskas et al. 1989) but is much more common among adolescents (Alessi, Robbins, and Dilsaver 1987). Delineation of the concomitant psychological and biologic mechanisms and their developmental progressions would therefore be worthwhile.

The question still remains as to whether the co-occurrences of depressive and anxiety disorders are "real" or whether they are artifacts of the current diagnostic system. Klerman (Chapter 2), for example, noted that psychiatric comorbidity has become an issue because of recent methodological and diagnostic changes in the United States. Furthermore, he, as well as others (Frances, Widiger, and Fyer, Chapter 3) underscored that the multiaxial system of the DSM-III and the encouragement to provide multiple diagnoses even on the same axis have increased the awareness of psychiatric comorbidity. In contrast to the DSM-III, a strictly hierarchical diagnostic system would discourage multiple concurrent diagnoses.

There are at least two factors that suggest that comorbidity of psychiatric disorders has been observed before and is not attributable solely to the DSM-III. As already mentioned, as far back as the 1960s, workers in the area of childhood depression had already described the complex clinical presentation of such youths. In fact, the concept of "masked depression" (Glaser 1968; Toolan 1962) helped to establish the existence of comorbidity as a clinical phenomenon, which otherwise would have been obscured by the hierarchical diagnostic practices of the times. Furthermore, as Klerman (Chapter 2) has noted, the distinction between primary and secondary disorders over one's lifetime, which also predates the DSM-III (as advocated by the St. Louis school), also represents one way to account for multiple disorders shown by the same patient. Finally, information on the evolution of comorbid psychiatric conditions among depressed children suggests that the various disorders have distinct onset-and-recovery patterns (Kovacs, Gatsonis, Paulauskas, et al. 1989; Kovacs, Paulauskas, Gatsonis, et al. 1988). Such patterns would not emerge if comorbidity were solely an artifact of the diagnostic system.

Assuming therefore that at least some portion of the observed comorbidity of depressive and anxiety disorders is real and not artifactual, the remaining question is: why are these phenomena important? Do they have some significance for the clinician who treats such youths? Do they provide an avenue for a better understanding of the evolution of these conditions among adults?

From a clinical viewpoint, there is some evidence that among depressed youngsters with a comorbid anxiety disorder, the anxiety disorder declares itself relatively early and that its effects on the course of the depression depend on other clinical features (Kovacs,

Gatsonis, Paulauskas, et al. 1989). In the absence of pertinent data, it is not known whether, and to what extent, psychotherapeutic treatment that focuses on one of the disorders would help to alleviate the other one as well. However, differential diagnosis should be particularly important if pharmacotherapy is being considered. Although this issue also requires empirical verification, it is possible that, just as among adults, the tricyclic antidepressants may ameliorate the depression and certain symptoms of anxiety among children as well, whereas the anxiolytic agents would be of little value for the depression itself (e.g., Fawcett and Kravitz 1983; Klein 1980).

The implications of childhood-onset comorbid disorders for the patients' later clinical course are not known. It is yet to be established, for instance, to what extent "comorbidity" and "overall clinical severity" overlap as possible prognosticators. It would be particularly useful to know if youngsters with comorbid anxiety and depression are at higher risk for later disturbances than other depressed youths. It would also be informative to have data on the relative prognostic values of both of these diagnostic entities. The results of ongoing longitudinal studies should eventually provide information in this regard.

The fact that separation anxiety disorder is the comorbid condition that has been reported most frequently among depressed youths is of interest. From the perspective of Bowlby (1973, 1980), the co-occurrence of separation anxiety and depression is entirely predictable, although he would probably frown on diagnosing them as separate disorders. According to Bowlby's theory, the presence of pathologic anxiety and depression in school-age youths and adolescents could implicate real or imagined disruptions in significant attachment bonds. In turn, understanding the quality of these youths' attachments may not only provide clues as to their future interpersonal relationships and clinical course, but also could point to potentially useful treatment approaches. Therefore, one research priority should be the development and operational description of psychotherapeutic interventions suitable for such early-onset disorders, which could be then subjected to controlled treatment-outcome trials.

Chapter 17

Alcohol Abuse/Dependence and Comorbid Anxiety and Depression

Roger E. Meyer, M.D.
Henry R. Kranzler, M.D.

M ANY ALCOHOLICS PRESENT to treatment with symptoms of anxiety, depression, and/or irritability. In this context, it is difficult to establish a clear cause-and-effect relationship (in either direction) between the psychopathologic symptoms and drinking behavior. Prior to the introduction of the *Diagnostic and Statistical Manual of Mental Disorders*, Third Edition (DSM-III) (American Psychiatric Association 1980), most mental health professionals explained drinking behavior in the alcoholic on the basis of preexisting psychopathology, and/or psychodynamic factors (Knight 1937; McCord and McCord 1960). Personality theorists concluded that Minnesota Multiphasic Personality Inventory (MMPI) (Hathaway and McKinley 1951) profiles of alcoholic patients across treatment samples indicated that alcoholism was caused by underlying personality or other psychiatric disturbance (Costello 1981; Skinner and Jackson 1978). In DSM-I and DSM-II (American Psychiatric Association 1952, 1968), alcoholism was listed among the personality disorders.

In contrast, over the past 20 years, data from laboratory studies of chronic alcoholic intoxication (Mendelson and Mello 1966; Nathan, O'Brien, and Lowenstein 1971) and from long-term longitudinal studies of individuals who became alcoholic (Kammeier, Hoffman, and Loper 1973; Vaillant 1983) have emphasized psychopathology as a consequence of chronic intoxication. Chronic intoxication is associated with an increase in symptoms of anxiety, depression, and belligerence rather than a decrease in negative mood states (Mendelson and Mello 1966; Nathan, O'Brien, and Lowenstein 1971). These data do not support a strictly "functional" view of drinking behavior. Vaillant has proposed that all of the psychopathology observed in alcoholics results from alcoholism, rather than serving as its cause. His own studies and those of Kammeier, Hoffman, and Loper failed to confirm the presence of specific antecedent psychopathology in individuals who later became alcoholic.

In general, the simple notion of alcoholism as cause *or* result of psychopathology does not adequately address the heterogeneity of the disorder. In a review, Meyer (1986) described at least six potential areas of relatedness between comorbid psychopathology and alcoholism. First, certain psychiatric disorders may serve as risk factors for the development of alcoholism. Second, coexisting psychopathology may affect the course, symptomatic manifestations, prognosis, and treatment response of alcoholic patients. Third, chronic intoxication is associated with increased symptoms of anxiety, depression, and irritability that should not merit a separate psychiatric diagnosis. Fourth, acute alcohol withdrawal is associated with symptoms of anxiety and irritability. Fifth, psychiatric symptoms (depression, insomnia, anxiety, irritability), unrelated to the presence of other DSM-III-defined psychiatric disorders, may persist through a variable period of "protracted abstinence." Sixth, there may be a *meaningful* relationship between intrapsychic and intrafamilial conflicts in relationship to alcohol consumption. Recent data also suggest that specific mood states may become conditional stimuli for alcohol craving (N. Cooney, personal communication, 1989). Finally, there are certain psychiatric disorders that occur in alcoholic patients with no greater frequency than in the general population. In this latter circumstance, it is difficult to establish a relationship between these disorders and the development of alcoholism, except on the basis of chance occurrence.

Since the introduction of DSM-III, there have been a number of published reports on the prevalence of other Axis I and Axis II psychiatric disorders in alcoholic patients (Hesselbrock, Meyer, and Keener 1985; Penick, Powell, Othmer, et al. 1984; Schuckit 1985). As described elsewhere in this volume, DSM-III and DSM-III-R (American Psychiatric Association 1987) encourage the use of multiple diagnoses where separate categories of disorder exist. However, the mere presence of symptoms of anxiety, depression, or irritability does not constitute a diagnosable DSM-III-R condition. Among alcoholics, symptoms of anxiety, depression, or irritability may be related to the diagnosis of alcohol abuse or alcohol dependence, certain alcohol-related organic mental conditions, or the presence of another diagnosable Axis I or Axis II disorder.

Antisocial personality disorder (ASP) is the psychiatric condition that is most prevalent among male alcoholic patients across a variety of studies. The prevalence of ASP varies with the characteristics of the sample, as well as diagnostic criteria employed. The reported prevalence of ASP among alcoholics has ranged from 16% to 49% (Cadoret, Troughton, and Widmer 1984; Hesselbrock, Meyer, and Keener 1985; Penick, Powell, Othmer, et al. 1984). It is not clear that the DSM-III criteria for ASP represent a single personality type (Gunderson 1983). Studies that have employed DSM-III criteria have resulted in substantially higher rates of ASP than those using other diagnostic systems. Moreover, investigators employing the National Institute of Mental Health (NIMH) Diagnostic Interview Schedule to establish a DSM-III diagnosis of ASP (Hesselbrock, Meyer, and Keener 1985) reported a higher prevalence of this disorder than researchers who have utilized other diagnostic instruments (Schuckit 1983b, 1985). Individuals with ASP report dysphoric moods and demonstrate impulsive behavior rooted in sensation-seeking attitudes (Brantley and Sutker 1984). They also have poor and unstable object relations and generally have a history of underachievement, despite normal to above-normal intelligence (Brantley and Sutker 1984). Data from a longitudinal study by Robins, Bates, and O'Neill (1962) offer compelling evidence that conduct disorder identified in young boys is highly correlated with both adult antisocial behavior and alcohol abuse.

Based on results from Swedish adoption studies (Cloninger, Bohman, and Sigvardsson 1981), Cloninger, Reich, Sigvardsson, et al. (1988) postulated that certain heritable temperament traits that are associated with adult antisocial disorder may serve as a significant risk factor for the development of alcohol dependence. Alcoholic individuals with these personality traits may represent a genetically distinct subtype. Cloninger (1987a) found that these individuals have distinctive profiles in a personality inventory that he developed. They show higher scores on "novelty seeking" and lower scores on "harm avoidance" and "reward dependence" than do other alcoholic patients. He has characterized this type of alcoholism as male-limited (type 2), since he has found that it is passed on from fathers to sons and is not affected by the family environment (Cloninger, Bohman, and Sigvardsson 1981). Cloninger's type 2 alcoholics, like alcoholics with comorbid ASP in other studies (Cadoret, Troughton, and Widmer 1984; Hesselbrock, Meyer, and Keener 1985), have an earlier onset and more rapid course associated with the development of alcohol dependence, as well as a higher prevalence of psychosocial disabilities than those alcohol-dependent individuals without ASP. Rounsaville, Dolinsky, Babor, et al. (1987) reported that a concomitant diagnosis of

ASP is also associated with a poorer outcome measured at 1 year posttreatment. Schuckit (1985), using more restrictive criteria for the diagnosis of ASP, has reported that subjects with a diagnosis of primary ASP and secondary alcoholism have a poorer prognosis than primary alcoholics.

There appears to be a growing appreciation that ASP (variously defined) constitutes a risk factor that may affect the development, symptomatic picture, course, and prognosis of a subtype of alcoholism. Comorbid symptoms of anxiety, dysphoria, depression, and irritability in individuals with this subtype of alcoholism may become manifest on the basis of alcohol dependence or, in some cases, on the basis of the personality disorder. The absence of generally effective treatments for ASP complicates the treatment of those alcoholics who suffer this comorbidity. Standard alcoholism treatment programs may vary in efficacy, depending on the percentage of patients they serve who have comorbid ASP (Rounsaville, Dolinsky, Babor, et al. 1987; Schuckit 1985).

DEPRESSION

Because of the frequency with which clinicians have observed depressive symptoms in alcoholic patients in treatment, there has long been research interest in the comorbidity of alcoholism and affective disorder (Jaffe and Ciraulo 1986). The Washington University group has emphasized the distinction between primary and secondary depressive disorder (Guze, Woodruff, and Clayton 1972). Primary depression exists in the absence of other significant psychopathology or physical illness; secondary depression arises in the context of other psychopathology, including alcoholism.

Weissman, Myers, and Harding (1980) studied the co-prevalence of affective disorders and alcoholism in a community sample, using the Research Diagnostic Criteria (RDC) (Spitzer, Endicott, and Robins 1978a). Among respondents with a lifetime diagnosis of alcoholism, 44% also had a lifetime diagnosis of major depression and 15% had a diagnosis of minor depression. This finding is in contrast to data from the NIMH Epidemiologic Catchment Area (ECA) study (Robins, Helzer, and Przybeck 1986), which used DSM-III diagnostic criteria to study prevalence rates of psychiatric disorders in community samples. Robins, Helzer, and Przybeck found that the relative risk of depression among those diagnosed with alcohol abuse/dependence was 2.5 for males and 2.9 for females, which represents only a modest elevation. For those who had current alcohol use disorders, only 2% of men and 13% of women had a concurrent diagnosis of major depression or dysthymia. The discrepancy between these studies may have resulted from the fact that the ECA data were derived from five sites, and at a later point in time than were the data obtained from a single community by Weissman, Myers, and Harding (1980). Furthermore, although both studies employed structured interviews, they used different diagnostic criteria.

The significance of differing diagnostic criteria and/or different assessment instruments on the comorbidity of depression and alcohol abuse was demonstrated in an adolescent community sample by Deykin, Levy, and Wells (1987), and in an adult clinical sample by Keeler, Taylor, and Miller (1979). Deykin, Levy, and Wells found that by using three rather than four criteria for major depressive disorder, as is stipulated by DSM-III, the prevalence of depression in an adolescent sample was doubled. This is relevant to the present discussion since in this study subjects who reported a history of alcohol abuse were almost four times as likely to have a history of major depressive disorder (i.e., four criteria) as those who had no history of alcohol abuse. In the adult sample of recently detoxified alcoholics, Keeler, Taylor, and Miller (1979) found rates of depression that varied from 8.6% to 66%, depending on whether a clinical interview, depression rating scale, or self-administered instrument was employed. These methodological issues may explain some of the observed variability in estimates of comorbidity.

Using data from a national survey, Midanik (1983) was able to examine the relationship between alcohol problems (social consequences, loss of control, and alcohol dependence) and depressive symptoms (as distinguished from depressive disorders). Men were more than twice as likely to report alcohol problems, whereas women were more than twice as likely to report depressive symptoms. The association between alcohol problems and depressive symptoms was similar for both sexes, with nearly 4% of respondents reporting both. However, among those reporting alcohol problems, women reported rates of depressive symptoms nearly double those of men. Among alcohol problems, alcohol dependence was most highly correlated with depression score.

Before discussing depression in clinical samples of alcoholics, it is important to acknowledge the role that comorbidity plays in bringing patients to treatment. Woodruff, Guze, and Clayton (1973) compared alcoholics who had sought outpatient treatment with a sample of their untreated, alcoholic relatives. They found a much higher prevalence of depression among alcoholics in psychiatric treatment, suggesting that comorbid depressive symptoms may be an important determinant for treatment-seeking behavior. Murray, Gurling, Bernadt, et al. (1984) made similar observations.

In general, female alcoholics are more likely than males to be depressed and to suffer from primary depression with secondary alcohol abuse/dependence (Hesselbrock, Meyer, and Keener 1985). Nevertheless, depressive symptomatology in the alcoholic male or female probably has multiple causes, including the toxic effects of alcohol, as well as personality disorders that may antedate the use of alcohol. Depressive symptoms that are present in many patients during drinking and during acute withdrawal clear over time in most individuals (Dorus, Kennedy, Gibbins, et al. 1987), but some alcoholics continue to report symptoms of dysphoria and depression as long as a year after treatment was initiated (Pottenger, McKernon, Patrie, et al. 1978; Rounsaville, Dolinsky, Babor, et al. 1987). Unfortunately, there are no reliable methods to distinguish which depressive symptoms on admission will turn out to be associated with major affective disorder. As a general rule, most clinicians delay decisions regarding antidepressant treatment until the period of subacute withdrawal symptomatology is passed (i.e., after 2 to 3 weeks of abstinence) (Kranzler and Liebowitz 1988; Schuckit 1979).

Data on the relationship between mood and drinking behavior are variable, depending on the specific mood state, the dose of alcohol consumed, and the duration of drinking (Mayfield 1979). Among bipolar patients, periods of heavy drinking tend to occur during mania rather than during depression (Mayfield and Coleman 1968; Reich, Davies, and Himmelhoch 1974). Mossberg, Liljeberg, and Borg (1985) followed a cohort of 12 male alcoholics over a 6-month course after inpatient treatment. Eleven of the subjects developed periods of mood changes lasting 1 to 3 weeks. Seven subjects relapsed, all in connection with periods of mood disturbance. Of these 7 subjects, 5 relapsed after "hyperactive" mood disturbance, and 2 relapsed after "depressive" mood disturbance. These authors concluded that for alcohol-dependent subjects, labile mood, but not specifically depressed mood, may be important in terms of relapse.

It is not certain that altering depressive symptoms will alter pathologic drinking patterns. Rounsaville, Dolinsky, Babor, et al (1987) reported that depressed, male alcoholics had a poorer outcome than did male alcoholics without any other psychopathology, whereas among female alcoholics the converse was true. The data on females represent a replication of the findings of Schuckit and Winokur (1972). Since onset of depression in the female alcoholics studied by Rounsaville, Dolinsky, Babor, et al. generally preceded the onset of alcoholism, it is possible that drinking was initiated to self-medicate symptoms. These investigators did not determine the degree to which treatment for depression affected outcome at 1 year. Pottenger, McKernon, Patrie, et al. (1978) advocated aggressive treatment of depression among alcoholics because they saw it as contributing to continued alcohol consumption. However, data on the use of antidepressant drugs in the treatment of depression in alcoholics are not clear-cut (Ciraulo and Jaffe 1981). Ciraulo, Alderson, Chapron, et al. (1982) reported that recently detoxified alcoholics clear imipramine more rapidly than matched controls—so rapidly that plasma levels achieved at usual therapeutic dosage may not be adequate. Their data suggest that future studies on the use of antidepressants in alcoholic patients should ensure adequate blood levels.

Alcohol use in patients in treatment for depression is also relevant here because a substantial percentage may be drinking heavily, thereby potentially affecting their response to pharmacotherapy. Although in one outpatient sample, only 3 to 139 patients with unipolar primary affective disorder were also found to be alcoholic, another 3 alcoholic patients had secondary depression (Woodruff, Guze, Clayton, et al. 1979). Murray, Gurling, Bernadt, et al. (1984) studied 371 psychiatric inpatients to assess the prevalence of heavy drinking (more than eight drinks daily). Greater than 20% of patients with bipolar depression, minor depression, or bipolar mania reported this level of consumption. Heavy drinking was less common among patients with anxiety disorders (13%) and major depression (12%).

At this juncture, it appears that some alcoholics (particularly females) have a history of major depressive disorder that antedates the development of alcohol-related problems. Furthermore, both male and female alcoholics may develop depressive symptoms in the context of chronic intoxication, in acute withdrawal states, and during a period of protracted abstinence. The cognitive impairment consequent to the toxic effects of ethanol (Becker and Kaplan 1986) and the metabolic disturbance that appears to alter the disposition of antidepressant drugs (Ciraulo, Alderson, Chapron, et al. 1982) may each complicate the response of alcoholic patients to standard antidepressant treatment. Future studies of depression and its treatment in the alcoholic should seek to identify the presence of a separately diagnosable affective disorder; the level of cognitive function; family history of affective illness; careful intake and outcome histories of alcohol use and dependence and of depressive symptomatology; and assessment of life stress and social supports. Biologic indices that have been studied in affectively ill, nonalcoholic subjects will be affected by a recent history of alcohol consumption, thereby limiting the usefulness of the dexamethasone suppression test, studies of biogenic amines and their metabolites, and studies of sleep parameters in alcoholic patients.

Anxiety Disorders

It has long been known that alcohol in modest doses reduces anxiety levels in laboratory paradigms of performance anxiety in normal subjects (Mayfield 1979). There has also been a tradition in clinical practice and theory to attribute alcohol consumption to its tension-reducing properties (Cappell and Herman 1972). Anxiety is a component of the alcohol withdrawal syndrome, and the standard pharmacologic treatment of this disorder includes the use of a decreasing dosage of benzodiazepines (Sellers and Kalant 1976). Following acute withdrawal, many patients complain of a subacute set of symptoms that may include persistent insomnia and anxiety (along with depression and dysphoria). Begleiter and colleagues have gathered electrophysiologic evidence for the existence of altered brain function after acute withdrawal, which they have termed *protracted abstinence* (Begleiter, DeNoble, and Porjesz 1980; Begleiter and Porjesz 1977; Porjesz and Begleiter 1985). In the early weeks after acute withdrawal, alcoholic patients also manifest nonsuppression in the dexamethasone suppression test (Khan, Ciraulo, Nelson, et al. 1984), a blunted thyrotropin-releasing hormone response to thyroid-stimulating hormone (Loosen, Prange, and Wilson 1979), and other biologic abnormalities. The relationship between these abnormalities and the presence of anxiety or other symptoms in detoxified alcoholics remains to be clarified.

While symptoms of anxiety are common during periods of heavy drinking (Schuckit 1985) and detoxification (Mossberg, Liljeberg, and Borg 1985), the prevalence of diagnosable anxiety disorders in community samples of alcoholics has been low. Weissman, Myers, and Harding (1980) found that 9% of their sample also had a lifetime diagnosis of generalized anxiety disorder, whereas 3% were phobic. Robins, Bates, and O'Neill (1962) reported that no men and only 2% of women met criteria for alcohol abuse/dependence and phobia concurrently. Data from the ECA do not include the diagnosis of generalized anxiety disorder.

In clinical samples of alcoholics, the prevalence of anxiety disorders is variable. Schuckitt (1985) found a few cases of primary anxiety disorder among 577 alcoholics being treated at a Veterans Administration hospital. Hesselbrock, Meyer, and Keener (1985) reported a lifetime prevalence of 10% panic disorder and 27% phobic disorder among 321 male and female alcoholic inpatients, with both disorders more common in females. Mullaney and Trippett (1979) found that nearly two-thirds of the alcoholics they studied had phobic symptoms of a moderate to disabling degree. Bowen, Cipywnyk, D'Arcy, et al. (1984) reported that 44% of 48 alcoholic inpatients had anxiety disorders, including 6 with agoraphobia, 10 with recurrent panic attacks, and 11 with generalized anxiety disorder.

As with depressive symptoms (Midanik 1983), there appears to be an association between anxiety symptoms and alcohol dependence. Stockwell, Smail, Hodgson, et al. (1984) observed a temporal relationship between phobic symptoms and alcohol dependence in a sample of 24 hospitalized alcoholics who concurrently suffered from a phobic anxiety state. Most patients reported that their fears of a social situation predated their drinking problems, but that their fearfulness increased during bouts of heavy drinking. Schaefer, Sobieraj, and Hollyfield (1987) identified a significant relationship between anxiety symptoms and severity of dependence. Similarly, Smail, Stockwell, Canter, et al. (1984) and Roelofs (1985) related the development of panic and anxiety symptoms among alcoholics to the development of alcohol dependence.

The problem of comorbidity of alcoholism and anxiety disorders has also been examined in studies of alcohol use among anxious patients. Among 62 patients diagnosed with anxiety neurosis, Woodruff, Guze, and Clayton (1972) diagnosed 15% as alcoholic and an additional 10% as heavy drinking. Bibb and Chambless (1986) diagnosed 13% of a group of 254 outpatient agoraphobics as alcoholic. Alcoholic agoraphobics were significantly more likely to have self-medicated with alcohol and to have begun drinking in an effort to self-medicate. Nevertheless, in this sample, agoraphobia was primary in only 56% and onset was coincidental in 13% of patients. The psychological treatment of anxiety symptoms has become a part of many alcoholism treatment programs. Patients are taught relaxation strategies that do not rely on medication. The use of benzodiazepines or other sedatives is contraindicated by the high prevalence of cross-dependence between these drugs and alcohol. Meyer (1986) provided a rationale for the use of buspirone, a novel anxiolytic, in the treatment of persistent anxiety in alcoholics. An open trial by Kranzler (1987) provided pilot data that support the usefulness of buspirone for the reduction of craving in anxious alcoholics. In the treatment of panic disorder, as in the treatment of depression in alcoholics, attention needs to be paid to imipramine pharmacokinetics. The use of monoamine oxidase inhibitors may be complicated by serious side effects in this population (R. Schottenfeld, personal communication, 1989).

DISCUSSION

Data on the prevalence of specific affective and/or anxiety disorders in alcoholic patients support the general premise that these Axis I disorders (in contrast with ASP) can explain only a limited amount of the variance in course and treatment outcome, *where all patients are exposed to the same general alcoholism treatment program*. They also suggest the possibility, however, that the heterogeneity of alcoholic patients can be characterized by the variability of comorbid psychopathology. There is a need to address the treatment of comorbid psychiatric disorders as one also proceeds with standard alcoholism treatment (McLellan, Luborsky, Woody, et al. 1983). In this context, outcome is best described in multidimensional terms that include measures of alcohol dependence, psychopathology, and other relevant psychosocial data collected at treatment intake and at follow-up.

Apart from diagnosable affective or anxiety disorders, specific evanescent mood states may themselves become associated with relapse in a manner that is highly specific for the individual. Marlatt (1985) interviewed relapsed alcoholics to identify what precipitated their return to drinking. Of 70 patients, 38% reported that negative emotional states were determinants of relapse. This category of precipitant was the most commonly identified by these patients. N. Cooney (personal communication, 1989) has recently completed pilot work that suggests that the elicitation of anxiety or depression results in craving in alcoholic subjects more reliably than does the mere presence of alcohol-related cues. It is possible that in alcoholics who do not meet criteria for DSM-III-R anxiety or mood disorder, specific mood states may serve as conditional cues for alcohol consumption. We believe that this work represents a promising area of investigation.

The clinical research literature in the alcohol field has matured enormously in the context of DSM-III and DSM-III-R. It is no longer tenable to describe all alcoholics in a unidimensional way, to consider all alcoholics as identical, or to presume that all psychiatric symptomatology is etiologically related to the development of the disorder. Because symptoms of depression and/or anxiety may be attributable to alcohol dependence, it is also critical for clinicians and clinical investigators to obtain an adequate alcohol- and drug-use history in patients who present for the treatment of anxiety or affective disorders. As a model that acknowledges the complexity of the interactions, the concept of comorbidity related to alcoholism has substantial utility and represents an important improvement over models that have simply attempted to explain alcoholism on the basis of coexisting or antecedent psychiatric or personality disorder.

Chapter 18

Depression and Alcoholism: Comorbidity in a Longitudinal Study

Robert M. A. Hirschfeld, M.D.
Debbie Hasin, Ph.D.
Martin B. Keller, M.D.
Jean Endicott, Ph.D.
Joanne Wunder, B.A.

THE SIGNIFICANCE OF co-occurring mood disorder and one or more nonaffective diseases in an individual patient has assumed increasing interest among clinical investigators. Of particular interest are the questions: Does this co-occurrence reflect a link in their respective etiologies, or is it simply chance? Even if two or more disorders are independent, does their co-occurrence influence response to treatment, prognosis, or clinical course? To answer these kinds of questions, the nature of the relationship between the disorders must be articulated.

The most widely used approach to this relationship has been the primary-secondary distinction, originally proposed by the Washing-

Completed with the participation of these investigators from the Clinical Studies of the National Institute of Mental Health Collaborative Program on the Psychobiology of Depression: G. L. Klerman, M.D. (Chairperson) (New York); R. M. A. Hirschfeld, M.D. (Co-Chairperson) (Washington, DC); M. B. Keller, M.D. and P. Lavori, Ph.D. (Boston); J. A. Fawcett, M.D. and W. A. Scheftner, M.D. (Chicago); W. Coryell, M.D., N.C. Andreasen, M.D., Ph.D., J. Haley, and P. Wasek, B.A. (Iowa City); J. Endicott, Ph.D. and J. E. Loth, M.S.W. (New York); and J. Rice, Ph.D. and T. Reich, M.D. (St. Louis). Other contributors include: P. J. Clayton, M.D., J. Croughan, M.D., M. M. Katz, Ph.D., E. Robins, M.D., R. W. Shapiro, M.D., R. L. Spitzer, M.D., and George Winokur.

ton University group in St. Louis (Robins and Guze 1972) and Munro (1966) in England. Both groups defined a secondary depression as a depression occurring after the onset of another, nonaffective psychiatric or medical illness. The primary-secondary distinction was codified in the Feighner criteria (Feighner, Robins, Guze, et al. 1972).

The distinction does not convey information about etiology; it simply describes the chronological order of the expression of the disease states. In fact, it is not even necessary for the illnesses to co-occur during the index episode or in the past. It is only necessary that each illness has occurred at some point during the individual's lifetime. Its nosologic utility has been demonstrated in many investigations (Guze, Woodruff, and Clayton 1972; Winokur and Black 1987; Winokur, Black, and Nasrallah 1988), although in some samples it has not been found to be discriminatory (Andreasen and Winokur 1979; Grove, Andreasen, Winokur, et al. 1987).

Studies of the course of secondary depression have attempted to examine the differences between primary and secondary depression and to determine if the subtype has predictive utility. In many instances, it had been hypothesized that the course of secondary depression would be worse than that of primary depression, due to the impairment or complications of the primary nonaffective disorder. Others have hypothesized that the course of a secondary disorder would be influenced by and follow the course of the primary disorder (Andreasen and Winokur 1979).

Although the chronology of onset of a nonaffective disorder and an affective disorder may not predict course and outcome of a current affective disorder, the *co-occurrence* of two disorders may. Many of the studies of secondary depression do not specify whether the nonaffective primary disorder is current, and therefore may be examining purely depressed subjects whose psychiatric histories include episodes of nonaffective illness. Thus a different approach to the relationship between affective and nonaffective disorders is the concept of comorbidity. Comorbidity requires the co-occurrence of two (or more) disease states. The order of onset of each disease is not critical. However, the two (or more) diseases must both be present during the index episode for co-occurrence.

When considering the comorbidity of affective and nonaffective disorders, alcoholism is often mentioned in reference to depression. The association of alcoholism and depression is very common; studies have reported that from 28% to 59% of alcoholics experience depression (Weissman, Pottenger, Kleber, et al. 1977). One assessment of a community sample determined that 2.6% of the respondents were currently alcoholic; of these, 15% were currently depressed (Weissman and Myers 1980). Many studies of secondary depression have found that alcoholism is the most common primary disorder in the patients studied (Grove, Andreasen, Clayton, et al. 1987; Guze, Woodruff, and Clayton 1972).

The familial co-occurrence of alcoholism and depression is also high, and the possibility of a genetic link between the two disorders has been examined. One family study (Merikangas, Leckman, Prusoff, et al. 1985) determined that relatives of probands with depression and alcoholism had increased risk of alcoholism alone and alcoholism with major depression when compared to relatives of probands with depression only. Depressives without alcoholism did not transmit alcoholism, and probands with depression and alcoholism transmitted both alcoholism and depression. The authors concluded that alcohol and depression are probably transmitted independently in families, and the occurrence of relatives with both diagnoses is to be expected by chance. This finding was supported by Grove, Andreasen, Clayton, et al. (1987), whose proposed model of transmission asserted that relatives of patients with secondary depression would exhibit lower rates of primary depression, higher rates of the patients' nonaffective diagnosis, and higher rates of secondary depression than relatives of patients with primary depression. The mechanism of action of the transmission of the disorders is still under investigation, however.

The high rates of co-occurrence for depression and alcoholism deserve attention. Some investigators have proposed that a depressed premorbid personality type leads to alcoholism, whereby the individual tries to self-medicate the depressive symptomatology with alcohol (Tahka 1966). The course of alcoholism may be secondary to the course of depressive symptoms and episodes (Clark, Gibbons, Fawcett, et al. 1985). However, a contrasting view is that the depressive symptoms of alcoholics are attributed to the chronic intoxication, physical withdrawal symptoms, or life-style of the alcoholic (Clark, Gibbons, Fawcett, et al. 1985; Kielholz 1969; Schuckit 1983a), and thus depression would follow the course of the alcoholism and remit with abstinence (Dave and Wanck 1985). The effect of the comorbidity of alcoholism and depression on the course of depression is, therefore, of clinical interest and was studied by us in a sample of unipolar depressed patients with concurrent alcoholism.

This chapter examines two reciprocal aspects of the comorbidity of depression and alcoholism: (1) the influence of alcoholism on the clinical course of depression and (2) the influence of depression on the clinical course of alcoholism. Our expectation was that each disorder would have an adverse effect on the other. It makes sense that one serious mental disorder will negatively affect another. Data from the Clinical Studies of the National Institute of Mental Health (NIMH) group of patients included those with a diagnosis of current primary nonbipolar depression, and specifically excluded patients with alcoholism. A total of 289 patients met these criteria for current primary major depression (the "primaries").

The primaries were contrasted with a group of 79 patients with major depression who also concurrently met criteria for alcoholism (the "alcoholics"). Of these patients, 66 (84%) were alcoholic before they became depressed (secondary depression). The major depression experienced by this group of alcoholics was uncomplicated by bipolar disorder or dysthymia.

As expected, the male-female ratio differed between the groups: 64% of the primaries were women, whereas 37% of the alcoholics were women. The primaries were somewhat older than the alcoholics; approximately twice as many alcoholics as primaries were separated, divorced, or widowed.

The two groups of patients showed a similar duration of their current episode prior to entry. The mean duration was about 18 months, with a highly skewed distribution and a median duration of about 7 months. Both groups had an average age at onset of major depression of about 30 years and a median number of prior episodes equal to 1. Intake clinical features were very similar for the two groups. The mean Hamilton (1960) depression score extracted from the SADS was 26.2 for the primaries and 25.8 for the alcoholics, denoting fairly severe depression in both groups. The study is described in detail elsewhere (Hirschfeld, Kosier, Keller, et al. 1989).

Time-to-recovery from the point of admission to the study for the two groups was nearly identical. More than 40% of patients in both groups were still in the index episodes 6 months after admission; one-third of each group was still ill at 1 year. Approximately 11% (or 1 in 10 patients) of both groups remained ill after 5 years of follow-up.

A comparison between the two groups at 2 years on the SADS scale scores of endogenous features, depressive features, anxiety features, delusions/hallucinations, and manic features revealed no significant differences between the two groups. Hamilton depression scores for the primaries and for the alcoholics were not significantly different.

Even though there was no overall difference in time to recovery between the two groups, the possibility that heavy drinking may influence the time to recovery was examined. Alcoholic patients were divided into three groups based on their level of alcohol abuse at the time of study admission. Neither mean nor median time to recovery was significantly different for patients with different levels of alcohol abuse, although there was a nonsignificant trend in the expected direction for the median time. Even those whose alcohol abuse was very severe at admission (denoting that the drinking caused gross interference in job or social functioning) did not have significantly longer time to recovery.

Comparisons between the primaries and the alcoholics are similar on time-to-relapse into major depression following recovery from the index major depression. There was little difference between the primaries and the alcoholics in terms of time relapse following full recovery. After 4 years, nearly three-quarters of both groups had had at least one more episode of depression.

When psychosocial outcomes between the two groups were examined, differences did emerge. The Global Assessment Scale (GAS) (Endicott, Spitzer, Fleiss, et al. 1976) assessments, which combine psychopathologic and psychosocial status, did not differ at admission or through 2 months of follow-up between the two groups. By 3 months, differences emerged between the two groups, which were sustained at statistically significant levels throughout the 3 years of follow-up. At 2 years the primaries were functioning well on average with only mild symptoms, whereas the alcoholics had some difficulty in functioning with moderate symptoms.

Global assessments of social functioning made by clinical raters completed at 6-month intervals are parallel to the GAS scores. The two groups were not different in global functioning at admission. By 6 months there were significant differences between the two groups, which persisted throughout the follow-up.

Among the five psychosocial areas assessed using the LIFE (work and household duties, interpersonal relations, sexual functioning, general life satisfaction, and recreation), significant differences emerged in only one area, that of interpersonal relations with spouse through 24 months. On this measure, alcoholics scored significantly worse at index, at 6 months, and at 12 months. After that time, the scores did not differ significantly.

Influence of Major Depression on the Clinical Course of Alcoholism

A total of 127 patients with current comorbid RDC alcoholism and RDC major depression were identified in the clinical psychobiology study. Because there was no sample of nondepressed alcoholics in the clinical psychobiology study, we could not compare the clinical course of alcoholism with and without concurrent depression.

The cumulative probability of a 6-month remission from RDC alcoholism by 2 years was .67. Many remissions occurred early. By 12 weeks, the cumulative probability of remission was .34. At 6 months, the cumulative probability of remission was .37, and at 1 year, .52. Of the 79 patients who remitted, the cumulative probability of relapse by

The University of Iowa relapse rates ranged from 34% to 51% among the secondaries; unfortunately, no rates were reported for the primaries (Winokur, Black, and Nasrallah 1988). These contrasted with our relapse rates for depression for both groups of approximately 40% by 1 year, 60% by 2 years, and 66% by 3 years.

However, three-quarters of the Iowa secondary depression sample had diseases other than alcoholism, including personality disorders, anxiety disorders, somatization disorders, and various medical illnesses. Some of these, perhaps the personality and anxiety disorders, may have caused the relatively adverse course in the Iowa group of secondary depressives. Another possibility is that the mix of depression and alcoholism subtypes (Winokur 1983) may have differed in our respective samples. In addition, 16% of the sample in the present analyses had primary depression with secondary alcoholism, which may account for some of the variation in results.

While the Iowa study and our study yielded partially conflicting findings on clinical course of psychopathology, findings on social functioning were similar. In the Iowa sample, patients with a history of alcoholism had much worse prospective social functioning than did those without the alcoholic history (G. Winokur, personal communication, 1988).

Hesselbrock, Hesselbrock, and Workman-Daniels (1986) retrospectively examined major depression and course of alcoholism. They found that lifetime diagnoses of major depression from the NIMH Diagnostic Interview Schedule (National Institute of Mental Health 1981) were not associated with drinking history milestones in 321 hospitalized alcoholics. However, in a follow-up study of 266 of these patients, Rounsaville, Dolinisky, Babor, et al. (1987) found that major depression was related to poorer outcome on a number of dimensions in men, but was related to better outcome in women. A prior diagnosis of depression was associated with alcohol dependence in a follow-up study of narcotics addicts (Croughan, Miller, Matar, et al. 1982). Berglund (1984) found that depression and depressive symptoms predicted later suicide in a series of 1,312 alcoholics hospitalized in Sweden. Studies of major depression and the course of opiate addiction have produced inconsistent findings (Rounsaville, Kosten, Weissman, et al. 1986; Wood, Othmer, Reich, et al. 1977).

Most individuals who enter alcohol or drug treatment have had fairly severe, chronic difficulties with drinking or drug use. A considerably different picture emerges when the problems are examined in community residents, resulting in different impressions of clinical features and course (Clark 1976; Room 1977). Also, considerably different distributions of potential severity indicators such as quantity-frequency of consumption or numbers of alcohol-related problems are obtained in these two types of samples (Room 1977). The alcoholism of the collaborative patients ranged from quite mild to very severe and, taken as a group, could be seen as intermediate in severity between alcohol patients and community residents with drinking problems.

When planning the inclusion of other variables besides subtype of affective disorder in their analyses, we had expected to identify factors consistently predictive of outcome of alcoholism or drinking problems in the clinical literature. These factors would then be included as predictor variables in the analyses of outcome of the drinking problems of the clinical psychobiology study patients. However, despite the many studies that have followed up treated alcoholics, no demographic or other fairly straightforward variables consistently predicted outcome across studies. This absence of factors seemed attributable to the large variability in samples, length of follow-up periods, assessment procedures, and definitions of outcome.

Chapter 19

Comorbidity and Obsessive-Compulsive Disorder

Donald W. Black, M.D.
Russell Noyes, Jr., M.D.

COMORBIDITY, OR THE co-occurrence of two or more disorders, has generated increasing attention. The concept has been incorporated into diagnosis-related groups (DRGs) and influences hospital reimbursement. More important, psychiatric patients with comorbidity differ from those without, and comorbidity has been shown to affect length of hospital stay, response to somatic treatment, and mortality (Black, Winokur, Bell, et al. 1988; Fulop, Strain, Vita, et al. 1987). As Boyd, Burke, Gruenberg, et al. (1984) have demonstrated, the presence of one psychiatric disorder increases the probability of having another. It is not surprising that obsessive-compulsive disorder (OCD), one of the most distinctive and recognizable psychiatric disorders, often coexists with other disorders such as major depression. Although it has been recognized that obsessions and compulsions may occur along with other psychiatric syndromes, the relationship between them is not always clear. That is, does one syndrome cause the other, or are they merely coincidental? Among the disorders that have been linked to OCD are schizophrenia, major depression, Tourette's syndrome, anorexia nervosa, panic disorder, and obsessive-compulsive personality. The relationship between OCD and these disorders will be explored.

SCHIZOPHRENIA AND OBSESSIVE-COMPULSIVE DISORDER

Schizophrenia and OCD have features in common that have led many authorities to postulate that the two disorders are related. For example, they have similar sex distributions (approximately equal), age of onset (early 20s), and marriage and fertility rates (reduced). Both conditions tend to have a chronic, fluctuating course. Historically, both have responded poorly to treatment, particularly psychodynamic psychotherapy, and response to somatic therapies has been limited. The course and treatment response of both illnesses may now be changing because of the development of effective therapies, such as behavioral and pharmacologic therapy in OCD, but in the past these generalizations have held true.

In addition to demographic similarities, many patients with OCD develop overvalued obsessional ideas that suggest delusional thinking. For example, we recently saw a 38-year-old disabled truck driver with extensive cleaning and checking rituals who felt compelled to describe his rituals in a loud voice as he was performing them, so loud, in fact, that neighbors complained. Although the patient did not wish to yell, he firmly believed that harm would come to his family if he did not announce his rituals in this fashion. While the differentiation between an obsession and a delusion is simple in most cases, it may not always be. Although our patient realized that his ritualistic chanting was unreasonable, his actions indicated a belief to the contrary. Such cases have led Insel and Akiskal (1986) to argue that delusions may arise in the course of OCD that do not signify schizophrenia, but rather an "obsessive-compulsive psychosis." They suggested that the delusion represents a reactive, affective, or paranoid psychosis.

If OCD and schizophrenia are truly related, as many investigators have suggested, then OCD should lead to schizophrenia in a significant number of cases, and an increased prevalence of OCD should be found in relatives of schizophrenic patients. Research has not substantiated either proposition. With minor exceptions, long-term follow-up studies show that between 1% and 10% of patients with OCD develop schizophrenia (Black 1974; Ingram 1961; Lo 1967; Pollitt 1957; Rosenberg 1968; Rudin 1953). After reviewing the available studies, Goodwin, Guze, and Robins (1969) concluded that most of these persons did not originally suffer from OCD; they suggested that had schizophrenia clearly been ruled out in the beginning, obsessional patients would not have had an increased risk for developing schizophrenia compared to the general population. Furthermore, an increased incidence of schizophrenia has not been found in relatives of OCD patients (Brown 1942; McKeon and Murray 1987; Sakai 1967).

On the other hand, obsessive-compulsive symptoms are surprisingly common in samples of schizophrenic patients. Rosen (1957) found that 3.5% of 848 schizophrenic inpatients had obsessive-compulsive symptoms of all types, no different in content from those commonly found in uncomplicated OCD. In the Chestnut Lodge follow-up study, Fenton and McGlashan (1986) reported that 21 (13%) of 163 chronic schizophrenic patients exhibited prominent obsessive-compulsive symptoms. In their study, the group with obsessive-compulsive symptoms had poorer long-term outcome in the areas of social relations, employment, psychopathology, and global functioning. This finding contrasts with earlier reports by Rosen (1957) and Stengel (1945) in which obsessive-compulsive symptoms were associated with better outcome. The discrepancy probably reflects changes in diagnostic practice over the last several decades. Many patients described as schizophrenic by Rosen and Stengel showed prominent depressive features with mood incongruent delusions who might now be considered to have affective disorders, thus explaining the improved outcome. The data from patient samples appear compatible with the epidemiologic findings of Boyd, Burke, Gruenberg, et al. (1984) showing that patients with schizophrenia were 12.3 times as likely to have OCD as were persons without schizophrenia, when a hierarchy-free diagnostic system was used.

In summary, longitudinal studies have not found an increased incidence of schizophrenia either in OCD patients or in their relatives. Consequently, OCD and schizophrenia appear to have little relationship. The former belief that some patients with OCD progressed to develop schizophrenia appears to have been based on diagnostic error. As Lewis (1936) observed:

> The surprising thing here is not that some obsessionals become obviously schizophrenic, but that only a few do so. It must be a very short step, one might suppose, from feeling that one must struggle against thoughts that are not one's own, to believing that they are forced upon one by an external agency. (p. 330)

MAJOR DEPRESSION AND OBSESSIVE-COMPULSIVE DISORDER

Depression frequently complicates OCD. In fact, Goodwin, Guze, and Robins (1969) concluded from a review of 13 studies from seven different countries that depression is the most common complication of this disorder. Subsequent studies have reported similar findings. Rasmussen and Tsuang (1986b) found that in 44 OCD patients, 80% reported dysphoric mood and 75% current or past major depression. Rosenberg (1968) found in his sample that 34% of OCD patients had received treatment for depression. The frequency with which the two syndromes overlap has led some authorities to postulate common neurobiologic mechanisms. OCD patients show sleep and neuroendocrine abnormalities resembling those seen in major depression (Insel, Donnelly, Lalakea, et al. 1983; Insel, Mueller, Gillin, et al. 1984) and many improve with the antidepressant drug, clomipramine (-Mavisakalian and Michelson 1983).

Clearly, many OCD patients seek help only when depressed, and this may exaggerate the prevalence of depression in clinical samples. This is what Kringlen's (1965) data appear to show; 17% had depressive symptoms at the time OCD began, but fully 42% had these symptoms at the time of hospital admission. Confirming an association between the two syndromes in the general population, Boyd, Burke, Gruenberg, et al. (1984) found that, in a hierarchy-free diagnostic system, patients with OCD were 10.8 times more likely to have major depression than persons without OCD.

Depression associated with OCD is often considered primary or secondary, depending on chronology, although the temporal relationship is often difficult to determine. In this diagnostic scheme, a primary disorder occurs first and is followed by another (secondary) disorder. Thus depression occurring after the onset of OCD is secondary. It is presumed that the primary disorder is the underlying one, and the other is derivative. Depression has been observed to develop before, during, or after the OCD (Marks, Hodgson, and Rachman 1975), and the two syndromes may co-vary or be independent. Although longitudinal studies show that depression is a frequent complication of OCD, many patients never suffer from depression. In a retrospective study, Welner, Reich, Robins, et al. (1976) found that transition from obsessions to depression occurred three times as frequently (38% of the cases) as the transition from depression to obsessions (11%). When depressive symptoms preceded obsessions, the prognosis was better. The chronological sequence of depression and obsessions appears to have both theoretical importance and practical clinical utility.

Much of the difficulty in separating OCD from depression lies in the overlap of symptoms in the two disorders, particularly guilt, anxiety, self-doubt, and low self-esteem. Vegetative symptoms, such as weight loss and sleep disturbance, may develop in OCD; rituals involving food and sleep are common. Furthermore, it is difficult to differentiate the ruminations and morbid preoccupations of depressed persons from the obsessional thinking found in OCD. Generally, ruminations are ego-syntonic, appear rational but exaggerated, and are seldom resisted. On the other hand, obsessions tend to be ego-dystonic, irrational, and unrealistic. Whereas the depressive patient tends to focus on past events, the obsessional patient focuses on the prevention of future events.

Obsessions and compulsions are common in depressive illnesses;

in fact, depression with obsessive-compulsive features may represent a subtype of affective illness. Obsessional symptoms were present in 14 (23%) of 61 melancholic patients described by Lewis (1936). In a retrospective study of 398 psychotic depressive patients, Gittleson (1966) found 152 (38.2%) patients with obsessional symptoms. Among these patients, the presence of obsessions was associated with premorbid obsessional personality and obsessional personality in their parents. Gittleson also found that depressive patients with obsessional features attempted suicide less frequently than those without obsessions, even though they did not differ with respect to hopelessness or delusional ideas. However, Videbech (1975) could not verify the protective effect on suicide. Although both Videbech (1975) and Vaughan (1976) found obsessional features more common in agitated than retarded depressions, Kendell and Discipio (1970) found no difference between rates of obsessional symptoms in psychotic and neurotic depressive patients.

The course of obsessions and compulsions in depression appears to parallel that of the primary illness. Obsessional features tend to develop during depression and diminish as the patient improves; if present beforehand, the obsessive-compulsive symptoms worsen during the depression and revert to their original intensity afterward (Marks 1987; Videbech 1975). In a prospective study of 92 patients suffering from depressive illnesses, Kendell and Discipio (1970) found that 20 (21.7%) of 92 inpatients with depressive illnesses had obsessive-compulsive symptoms during an initial clinical interview. They found that, as a group, the depressive patients obtained high scores on the Leyton Obsessionality Inventory (Leyton 1970) and that these increased as the illness worsened. They also observed that obsessional symptoms were rare in mania.

Although depression is common in OCD and may lead to significant morbidity, it probably does not lead to suicide (Coryell 1983). Unfortunately, severe depression in OCD patients may worsen prognosis, as it is reported to interfere with behavioral treatments (Foa 1979; Marks 1981).

TOURETTE'S SYNDROME AND OBSESSIVE-COMPULSIVE DISORDER

One of the most interesting relationships is that between Gilles de la Tourette's syndrome and OCD. Tourette's syndrome is a rare disorder characterized by motor and vocal tics often associated with repetitive touching and imitative behaviors. This syndrome usually begins in childhood and is often characterized by obsessive-compulsive symptoms. OCD and Tourette's syndrome share many clinical features, including early onset, a waxing and waning course, chronicity, and occurrence in the same families. Reports have suggested that up to 90% of Tourette's syndrome patients have obsessions and compulsions (Montgomery, Clayton, and Friedhof 1982; Nee, Polinsky, and Ebert 1982). Frankel, Cummings, Robertson et al. (1986) confirmed this association in a study of 63 Tourette's syndrome patients, approximately half of whom had obsessional features. Likewise, the occurrence of tics in OCD has occasionally been noted (Pauls, Towbin, Leckman, et al. 1986; Schilder 1938). Rasmussen and Tsuang (1986a) reported a 5% incidence of Tourette's syndrome in patients with OCD.

A recent study (Pitman, Green, Jenike, et al. 1987) compared 16 Tourette's syndrome patients with 16 OCD patients and 16 control subjects. Of the 16 Tourette's syndrome patients, 10 (62.5%) also met DSM-III (American Psychiatric Association 1980) criteria for OCD, although only one OCD patient and no control subject met criteria for Tourette's syndrome. These investigators also found more tics in patients who had OCD among their relatives. They concluded that the exclusion of OCD in the presence of Tourette's syndrome called for in DSM-III is not supported by data. Futhermore, Pauls, Towbin, Leckman, et al. (1986) presented data suggesting that a single genetic factor may be manifested as tics in some persons and obsessions or compulsions in others. They observed that penetrance in males weighted toward tics and in females toward OCD.

The link between Tourette's syndrome and OCD has yet to be defined, but evidence to date suggests an underlying commonality, indicated by the overlap in symptoms and in the family history of patients. Frankel, Cummings, Robertson, et al. (1986) have hypothesized a common neurobiologic root, based on suggestive evidence that both disorders might involve a dysfunction in the basal ganglia or limbic system.

ANOREXIA NERVOSA AND OBSESSIVE-COMPULSIVE DISORDER

Eating disorders have historically been viewed as obsessive or compulsive behaviors because they involve obsessional concerns over weight and ritualistic dieting (DuBois 1949; Palmer and Jones 1939). In fact, retrospective and cross-sectional studies have shown that many persons with anorexia nervosa have OCD and that many obsessional patients have a history of anorexia nervosa. Kasvikis, Tsakiris, Marks, et al. (1986) found that, of 280 patients with OCD, 16 (10.6%) of 151 females had a past history of anorexia nervosa. None of the males and none of the agoraphobic controls had the disorder. Compared with nonanorectic cases, those with a history of anorexia were younger, had an earlier onset of OCD, and were more often single. The investigators concluded that anorexia is selectively associated with women who have OCD and not anxiety disorders per se.

Despite the possible association between anorexia nervosa and OCD, the symptoms of the two disorders do not necessarily co-vary over time. In one study, the obsessive-compulsive symptoms of anorectics continued whether or not the subjects regained their normal weight (Cantwell, Sturzenberger, Burroughs, et al. 1977). Nonetheless, obsessive-compulsive traits are common in anorexia (Hecht, Fichter, and Postpischil 1983; Rothenberg 1986; Smart, Beaumont, and George 1976) and are apparently associated with a poorer prognosis (Hecht, Fichter, and Postpischil 1983; Steinhausen and Glanville 1983).

Although some authors have postulated a common genetic diathesis between OCD and anorexia, no family studies have looked at the association. There is an intriguing report, however, of identical female twins, one of whom developed OCD and the other anorexia nervosa, both at age 13 (Hecht, Fichter, and Postpischil 1983).

ANXIETY DISORDERS AND OBSESSIVE-COMPULSIVE DISORDER

OCD has historically been classified as an anxiety disorder because phobias and free-floating anxiety are common in obsessional patients. Although this classification has been debated, phobic patients and OCD patients do, in fact, have many similarities, including avoidant behavior, intense subjective and autonomic response to focal stimuli, and a positive response to behavioral interventions. There is considerable overlap between OCD, phobias, and other anxiety disorders. Kringlen (1965) noted that 73 (80.2%) of the 91 obsessional patients in his series reported phobic symptoms. Of 104 depressed obsessional patients collected by Videbech (1975), 40% reported phobic symptoms. The high prevalence of childhood phobias reported by obsessional patients is more evidence of a commonality between OCD and anxiety disorders. Lo (1967) reported that 35% of 59 obsessional patients had significant phobias in childhood. Videbech (1975) reported that 50% of 104 depressed ruminative patients had significant childhood phobias, as did 25% of 89 obsessional patients studied by Ingram (1961). Using a hierarchy-free diagnostic system, Boyd, Burke, Gruenberg, et al. (1984) found obsessional patients 10.9 and 9.7 times as likely to have agoraphobia and simple phobia, respectively, as those persons without OCD.

We recently saw two patients with OCD who had prominent

phobias, illustrating the overlap of symptoms. The first patient, a 20-year-old college student, had obsessional concerns about his physical appearance and would check himself in a mirror repeatedly throughout the day to make sure that there were no new facial blemishes, spots of shaving cream, or dust on his eyeglasses. He also reported significant discomfort in social situations because of possible scrutiny by others and a fear that someone might detect "something wrong" with his appearance. His social phobia (and possible dysmorphophobia) was clearly related to the OCD.

The other patient, a 38-year-old businesswoman, had obsessional concerns with germs and contamination, and had many cleaning rituals, including hand washing. She recently developed fear of developing acquired immune deficiency syndrome (AIDS), although she was in a monogamous relationship and had no risk factors for the illness. She avoided contact with anyone perceived to be homosexual, or who appeared to have ill health (e.g., gaunt appearance) suggestive of AIDS. Her simple phobia was part of her obsessional illness. These cases illustrate how phobias are incorporated into OCD and how easily the two disorders can be confused.

Rasmussen and Tsuang (1986b) found 27% of 100 obsessionals to have a lifetime history of simple phobia, 18% to have a history of social phobia, 18% to have a history of separation anxiety, and 13% to have a history of panic disorder. On the other hand, Barlow and his colleagues (Di Nardo & Barlow, Chapter 12) studied 108 anxiety clinic patients with various diagnoses, including 6 subjects with OCD. Using a structured interview specifically to diagnose DSM-III anxiety disorders, the investigators found that OCD occurred as an additional diagnosis in patients with agoraphobia, social phobia, and panic disorder. Of the 6 patients with OCD, 3 had one additional diagnosis and the others two additional diagnoses. The authors concluded that, due to the considerable symptom overlap, anxiety symptoms should be evaluated without regard to an exclusionary system such as the one found in DSM-III. Pitman, Green, Jenike, et al. (1987) found that, of 16 OCD patients, 14 satisfied criteria for generalized anxiety, 9 for panic disorder, and 10 for a phobic disorder. In contrast, no control subject had these disorders.

An increased prevalence of anxiety neuroses among relatives of OCD patients has been reported (Rosenberg 1967). However, a population study that demonstrated a considerable overlap between other anxiety disorders and phobias failed to reveal a single case of OCD in family members (Weissman, Myers, and Harding 1978). In a study of 44 patients with OCD, 2 mothers and 3 fathers were found to have other anxiety disorders. Unfortunately, the authors (Rasmussen and Tsuang 1986a) provided no comparison with controls, and the findings do not appear to vary from the expected prevalence in the general population (Robins, Helzer, Weissman, et al. 1984).

Obsessive-compulsive symptoms may identify a subset of panic disorder patients. Mellman and Uhde (1987) reported that 27% of 70 panic disorder patients had significant obsessive-compulsive symptoms. Compared with patients without obsessive-compulsive symptoms, the group with obsessive-compulsive features had an earlier age of onset and were more likely to have a personal and family history of major depression and substance abuse. They also showed poorer outcome following treatment. For these authors, the presence of obsessive-compulsive symptoms in panic disorder suggests the possibility of shared biologic and psychological mechanisms.

OBSESSIVE-COMPULSIVE PERSONALITY AND OBSESSIVE-COMPULSIVE DISORDER

Obsessive-compulsive personality disorder as defined in DSM-III-R (American Psychiatric Association 1987) consists of a number of traits, including perfectionism, preoccupation with details, stubbornness, excessive devotion to work, indecisiveness, overconscientiousness, restricted expression of affection, lack of generosity, and inability to throw out obsolete objects. Clearly, many of these traits resemble symptoms of OCD, but it is important to recognize that obsessive-compulsive personality and OCD do not have a simple one-to-one relationship; OCD is not merely a severe form of obsessive-compulsive personality. Apart from superficial similarities, the disorders are phenomenologically and epidemiologically distinct. For example, OCD patients have ego-dystonic symptoms, whereas obsessive-compulsive traits are usually ego-syntonic, rarely provoke resistance, and are not usually associated with a sense of compulsion. In fact, many of these traits are highly adaptive and lead to great productivity. Many professionals, including physicians (Gabbard 1985), have obsessive-compulsive traits. Pollak (1979) reviewed the literature and concluded that obsessive-compulsive personality and obsessive-compulsive symptomatology can be differentiated statistically through factor analysis.

The concept that a compulsive personality creates a vulnerability for OCD is old. Janet (1908) believed that all obsessional patients had an "anal-erotic" personality premorbidly that predisposed to the disorder and that was characterized by obstinancy, parsimony, and orderliness. Later theorists tended to agree, finding support in traditional psychoanalytic works. According to these views, OCD and anal-erotic character share a common developmental basis. That is, the OCD represents a failure of repression, regression to the anal-sadistic level of libidinal organization, and the use of defenses (e.g., isolation, undoing, reaction formation) against excessive hostility (Freud 1948). Others, including Lewis (1936), have not shared the view of a specific predisposing personality. Another possibility is that the two disorders represent an "obsessive-compulsive spectrum" disorder and that the disorder erupts when the thoughts and actions of the person with obsessional personality become disrupted or distorted. Although this view of a continuum has theoretical support (Bennet 1949; Noyes 1949), it has not been subject to careful study.

Obsessive-compulsive personality appears overrepresented among patients who develop OCD, but other premorbid personality types are also found, and a significant minority of OCD patients have no abnormal premorbid personality traits. Rosenberg (1967) examined 47 obsessional patients and found 25 (53%) had a marked or moderate obsessional personality. Other personality types found included 8 (17%) schizoid, 6 (13%) immature, 2 (4%) hysterical, and 1 (2%) cyclothymic; 5 (11%) had personality disturbances that Rosenberg was unable to classify. In a review of seven studies, Black (1974) found that between 64% and 84% of OCD patients had a history of premorbid obsessional personality traits. Kringlen (1965) reported that 72% of 91 obsessional patients had a history of moderate or marked premorbid obsessional traits, particularly orderliness. When this figure is contrasted with Kringlen's nonobsessional neurotic control patients, 53% of whom had these traits, the figure becomes less impressive. Lewis's (1936) early observations still hold: "They [obsessional traits] are . . . just as commonly found among patients who have never had an obsessional neurosis. . . . The traits are also, of course, common among healthy people. They are, conversely, sometimes undiscoverable in the previous personality of patients who now have a severe obsessional neurosis" (p. 328).

Unfortunately, most of the literature on personality in OCD either is retrospective or was published before the development of operational diagnostic criteria. Little information is available using current definitions of personality traits and disorders. In a sample of 44 patients with OCD, Rasmussen and Tsuang (1986b) found 24 (54.5%) with a DSM-III compulsive personality, 4 (9%) histrionic, 4 (9%) schizoid, 2 (4.5%) dependent, and 11 (25%) with no personality disorder. In a retrospective review of 43 OCD patients, Jenicke, Baer, Minichiello, et al. (1986) found 14 (32.6%) to meet DSM-III criteria for schizotypal personality disorder. The schizotypal patients were younger and had significantly poorer response to treatment than nonschizotypal patients. They further found that the number of DSM-III schizotypal features in the 43 patients had a strong negative correlation with treatment outcome.

As the measurement of personality becomes more refined and as sensitive diagnostic instruments are developed, the relationship of obsessive-compulsive personality disorder and OCD can be better explored. Until such studies are accomplished, it is best to think of obsessive-compulsive personality and OCD as separate but overlapping. In short, many persons with OCD have a history of obsessive-compulsive traits, but most persons with obsessive-compulsive traits do not develop OCD. There is some evidence, however, that they may develop depression (Pollitt 1957).

OTHER SYNDROMES

Significant obsessive-compulsive symptoms and traits have also been reported in other disorders, including infantile autism (Kanner 1948), a disorder arising in early childhood and characterized by impairments in verbal and nonverbal communication, imaginative activity, and reciprocal social interaction. Other symptoms include repetitive or stereotyped body movements, such as spitting or head banging, unreasonable insistence on following routines, and preoccupation with narrow interests, such as being interested in lining up objects. Dysmorphophobia, or body dysmorphic disorder, has also been linked to OCD. This disorder is characterized by a circumscribed nondelusional belief that a certain body part is distorted or malformed. This belief leads to a morbid preoccupation with a minor bodily defect that the patient feels is conspicuous to others (Brotman and Jenike 1984). Recent interest in post traumatic stress disorder (PTSD) has drawn attention to its similarities with OCD. PTSD, which occurs in reaction to a life-threatening stressor, may lead to intrusive, ego-dystonic thoughts that resemble obsessions. Interestingly, Helzer, Robins, and McEvoy (1987) reported that persons with PTSD are 10.1 times more likely to have OCD than persons without PTSD. Trichotillomania, or compulsive hair pulling, has many features in common with OCD. Both disorders are associated with ritualistic behaviors that are distressing and irresistible. The two disorders may in fact be related; trichotillomania is reported to respond to the antiobsessional drug clomipramine (Swedo, Leonard, Rapaport, et al. 1989). OCD has also been linked to several neurologic disorders such as Von Economo's encephalitis, focal or temporal lobe seizures, and the Lesch-Nyan syndrome. Each disorder may be characterized by repetitive behaviors that simulate rituals (Yayura-Tobias and Neziroglu 1983).

OCD can also occur along with other disorders, such as alcoholism, somatization disorder, and antisocial personality, but probably at rates no greater than would be expected in the general population.

FUTURE DIRECTIONS

OCD often coexists with other psychiatric syndromes, such as depression, obsessive-compulsive personality, Tourette's syndrome, and anorexia nervosa. Additionally, obsessive-compulsive symptoms may be found in a variety of psychiatric disorders, including schizophrenia, major depression, and panic disorder. Whether the relationship of obsessive-compulsive symptoms and another syndrome represents a common genetic diathesis or psychodynamic or developmental commonality needs clarification.

Further research will be needed to confirm the existence of comorbidity with OCD in some instances and, where such co-occurrence has been established, to explore the nature of the relationships. If reliable and valid measures of personality show that obsessive-compulsive personality is associated with OCD, then efforts must be made to show that the personality disorder exists premorbidly and, as such, represents a predisposing factor for OCD. Prospective follow-up studies of children whose parents have OCD could provide this information. Because the link with schizophrenia appears doubtful, future studies of patients with carefully diagnosed OCD should show that, if delusions occur, they have a unique quality and are not accompanied by other signs of schizophrenia. Likewise, disorders within the schizophrenia spectrum, including schizotypal personality, should not be found in excess in follow-up or in family studies of OCD.

The link between OCD and Tourette's disorder is clearly established, and the question appears to be whether the disorders show a genetic predisposition or whether they represent distinct genetically determined subtypes. Studies designed to explore the biologic substrates of these illnesses and to seek genetic markers may eventually supply the answer. An association between OCD and anorexia nervosa has not been established. Family and twin studies of both disorders should remove any doubts about this possibility. These studies, involving personal interviews with first-degree relatives, are only now being done. They are an important first step in exploring the range and extent of comorbidity.

Depression that occurs after the onset of OCD influences the treatment and outcome of the primary disorder. The nature and extent of this influence needs to be explored through treatment and follow-up studies in which depressed and nondepressed patients are compared. Like secondary depression that complicates most medical and psychiatric illnesses, it is likely that this depression is caused by the primary illness, follows the course of the primary illness, and has features that distinguish it from primary depressive illness. Family and follow-up studies need to be done to show this.

Chapter 20

Comorbidity of Dysthymic Disorder

James H. Kocsis, M.D.
John C. Markowitz, M.D.
Robert F. Prien, Ph.D.

T HE TERM *dysthymia* refers to chronic or intermittent depressive syndromes with insidious onset at an early age and a fluctuant course throughout adulthood. Dysthymia has been conceptualized either as a chronic mild form of affective disorder, or as more closely related to the personality disorders or "neuroses" (Kocsis and Frances 1987). The *Diagnostic and Statistical Manual of Mental Disorders* (DSM-III) (American Psychiatric Association 1980) defined dysthymic disorder (DD) and placed it in the affective disorders section of this classification. The main criteria for the diagnosis were a chronic, persistent depressed or dysphoric mood of at least 2 years' duration, plus the presence of at least three symptoms from a list of 13 cognitive or behavior symptoms of depression.

DD has received relatively little attention in the research and therapeutic literature, although it appears to be a major public health problem (Canino, Bird, Shrout, et al., 1987a; Karno, Hough, Burnham, et al. 1987; Kashani, Carlson, Beck, et al. 1987; Robins, Helzer, Weissman, et al. 1984; Weissman and Myers 1978). Evidence suggests that DD is a heterogeneous syndrome that is often associated with a variety of other psychiatric or medical conditions (Weisman, Leaf, and Bruce 1987, 1988). Other reports further suggest that some patients with DD respond favorably to antidepressant medication (Akiskal,

---

Supported in part by grant MH-37103 and MH-19069 from the National Institute of Mental Health.

Rosenthal, Haykal, et al. 1980; Kocsis, Frances, Mann, et al. 1985; Kocsis, Frances, Voss, et al. 1988; Rounsaville, Sholomkas, and Prusoff 1980; Schildkraut and Klein 1975). A better understanding of comorbidity between DD and other disorders might improve subclassification of DD and lead to better identification of drug-responsive subgroups. This chapter, therefore, reviews the literature on the comorbidity of DD and presents original data from a recent study conducted in psychiatric outpatients at the Payne Whitney Clinic in New York.

CLASSIFICATION OF DYSTHYMIA

The concept of chronic low-grade depression as an affective illness dates back at least to Kraepelin (1921), who described

> certain slight and slightest colourings of *mood*, some of them periodic, some of them continuously morbid, which on the one hand are to be regarded as the rudiment of more severe disorders, on the other hand pass over without sharp boundary into the domain of *personal predisposition*. (p. 1)

Until recently, however, American psychiatry had been dominated by the psychodynamic school, which viewed chronic depressive and dysthymic states as character neuroses with etiology embedded in early environmental influences. In line with this tradition, DSM-II (American Psychiatric Association 1968) considered chronic and mild forms of depression as a class of the personality disorders and neuroses, whereas other forms of affective disorder were listed under psychotic disorders. More recent classifications have shifted to so-called atheoretical or descriptive terms, for example, intermittent depression in the Research Diagnostic Criteria (RDC) (Spitzer, Endicott, and Robins 1978b). The descriptive approach of the RDC was followed in the next revision of the DSM. Inclusion of DD in the affective disorders section of DSM-III was controversial and represented an important codification of this theoretical shift in the conceptualization of chronic depression (Frances 1980). (For an elaboration on these trends in classification, see Klerman, Chapter 2; and First, Spitzer, and Williams, Chapter 5.)

One problem with the DSM-III definition of DD was the lack of distinction from major depressive disorder (MDD). This overlap may have created an artificially high prevalence of comorbidity between the two diagnoses, a phenomenon termed *double depression* by Keller and Shapiro (1982a). DD differed from MDD in its criterion of at least 2 years' duration (1 year in children), and in severity as defined by number of symptoms. Three of a list of 13 symptoms were necessary for a diagnosis of DD, whereas MDD required the presence of 4 of 8 symptoms (see Table 1). Modifications made in the diagnostic criteria for DD in the revision of DSM-III (DSM-III-R) (American Psychiatric Association 1987) require 2 of a list of 6 associated symptoms. This

Table 1. Symptom Criteria for Major Depressive Disorder and Dysthymic Disorder in DSM-III and DSM-III-R

Major depressive disorder	Dysthymic disorder
DSM-III At least four of the following symptoms have been present nearly every day for at least two weeks: (1) poor appetite or significant weight loss, or increased appetite or significant weight gain (2) insomnia or hypersomnia (3) psychomotor agitation or retardation (4) loss of interest or pleasure in usual activities or decreased sexual drive (5) loss of energy; fatigue (6) feelings of worthlessness, self-reproach, or excessive or inappropriate guilt (7) complaints or evidence of diminished ability to think or concentrate (8) recurrent thoughts of death, suicidal ideation or attempt DSM-III-R At least five of the following symptoms have been present during the same two-week period and represent a change in functioning; and including either (1) or (2): (1) depressed mood	DSM-III During the depressive periods at least three of the following symptoms are present: (1) insomnia or hypersomnia (2) low energy level or chronic tiredness (3) feelings of inadequacy, loss of self-esteem, or self-deprecation (4) decreased effectiveness or productivity at school, work, or home (5) decreased attention, concentration, or ability to think clearly (6) social withdrawal (7) loss of interest in or enjoyment of pleasurable activities (8) irritability or excessive anger (9) inability to respond with apparent pleasure to praise or rewards (10) less active or talkative than usual, or feels slowed down or restless (11) pessimistic attitude toward the future, brooding about past events, or feeling sorry for self (12) tearfulness or crying

(2) markedly diminished interest or pleasure in all, or almost all, activities most of the day, nearly every day

(3) significant weight loss or weight gain when not dieting, or decrease or increase in appetite nearly every day

(4) insomnia or hypersomnia nearly every day

(5) psychomotor agitation or retardation nearly every day

(6) fatigue or loss of energy nearly every day

(7) feelings of worthlessness or excessive or inappropriate guilt

(8) diminished ability to think or concentrate, or indecisiveness, nearly every day

(9) recurrent thoughts of death (not just fear of dying), recurrent suicidal ideation without a specific plan, or a suicide attempt or a specific plan for committing suicide

(13) recurrent thoughts of death or suicide

DSM-III-R
Presence, while depressed, of at least two of the following:

(1) poor appetite or overeating

(2) insomnia or hypersomnia

(3) low energy or fatigue

(4) low self-esteem

(5) poor concentration or difficulty making decisions

(6) feelings of hopelessness

---

revision may or may not alter the comorbidity with MDD. Following suggestions by Akiskal (1983c), DSM-III-R also defined DD subtypes according to age of onset and the temporal relationship of dysthymia to MDD and other psychiatric and medical diagnoses. When reviewing the literature and results of studies on the prevalence and comorbidity of DD, the reader should be aware that the reliability and validity of the DSM-III and DSM-III-R criteria sets for DD remain largely untested.

COMORBIDITY OF DYSTHYMIC DISORDER: A REVIEW OF THE LITERATURE

DSM-III Axis I Comorbidity

Community samples. A major contribution to understanding

the epidemiology and comorbidity of DSM-III disorders has come from the National Institute of Mental Health (NIMH) Epidemiologic Catchment Area (ECA) study (Regier, Burke, and Burke, Chapter 6; Regier, Myers, Kramer, et al. 1984; Robins, Helzer, Weissman, et al. 1984). The ECA was a large-scale collaborative investigation of the incidence and prevalence of psychiatric disorders and associated health care usage at five sites across the United States. Representative community samples in New Haven, Connecticut; Baltimore, Maryland; St. Louis, Missouri; Durham, North Carolina; and Los Angeles, California were individually interviewed using the Diagnostic Interview Schedule (DIS) (National Institute of Mental Health 1981). The DIS is a structured clinical interview that assesses a number of DSM-III diagnoses but not chronic medical disease or most personality disorders (see Burke, Wittchen, Regier, et al., Chapter 36). Thus comorbidity of DD with those disorders was not addressed.

The ECA study found DD in 4% of women, 2% of men, and 3.1% of the overall sample, with prevalence ranging from 2.1% to 4.2% at the five sites (Weissman, Leaf, Bruce, et al. 1988). The rate of DD was significantly higher among women and divorced and separated individuals. There was a sex × age interaction, with the prevalence of DD significantly higher for women 18 to 64 years of age than for women over 65 years old. DD was also disproportionately prevalent among lower-income individuals. Weissman, Leaf, Bruce, et al. found a lifetime comorbidity among DD subjects in the ECA study of 38.9% for major depression, 10.5% for panic disorder, 2.9% for bipolar disorder, 46.2% for anxiety symptoms, 29.8% for substance abuse, and 77.1% for any psychiatric disorder. Dysthymic subjects had an increased risk of having each of the above disorders compared to nondysthymics, were more likely to use health and mental health services, and were more likely to receive psychotropic medication, especially minor tranquilizers. The incidence of prescribed drugs supports the claim that some substance abuse problems associated with DD may be iatrogenic (Weissman, Leaf, and Bruce 1987). Study of a subsample in St. Louis also revealed a high comorbidity of DD (7.8 risk ratio) among the 1% of the general populace suffering from posttraumatic stress disorder (PTSD) (Helzer, Robins, and McEvoy 1987).

Other studies have corroborated that DD is a mental disorder of significant prevalence. Weissman and Myers (1978) had previously found a 4.5% prevalence of RDC intermittent depression in the New Haven community; 87.5% had comorbid RDC diagnoses. An epidemiologic study using a Spanish translation of the DIS found a 5.5% urban, 3.3% rural, and 4.7% overall lifetime prevalence of DD among native Puerto Ricans (Canino, Bird, Shrout, et al. 1987a), a number comparable to the 4.8% prevalence among Mexican-Americans in the ECA study (Karno, Hough, Burnham, et al. 1987). Koegel, Burnam, and Farr (1988) found a 9.3% rate of lifetime dysthymia among homeless respondents in Los Angeles.

In Columbia, Missouri, community sampling by structured clinical interview diagnosed 12 (8%) of 150 adolescents 14 to 16 years old as having DD by DSM-III criteria (Kashani, Carlson, Beck, et al. 1987). All had comorbid diagnoses; primary-secondary distinctions for DD were not made from these cross-sectional data. As a group, these adolescents had a significantly greater number of comorbid diagnoses than their nondysthymic peers. Comorbid diagnoses included anxiety disorder (75%), major depression (58%), oppositional disorder (50%), conduct disorder (33%), drug abuse (25%), and alcohol abuse (25%).

Dysthymic disorder among psychiatric patients.   DD also appears to be common among psychiatric patients, especially those with major depression. It has been noted that the overlap of DD with MDD is to some degree an artifact, inasmuch as the two disorders share similar criteria sets and differ only slightly in number of required symptoms. Two retrospective studies have employed RDC for intermittent depression to examine rates of chronic depression among patients presenting to psychiatric clinics for treatment of major depression. Keller and Shapiro (1982a) found that 26% of 101 patients with MDD also had an underlying chronic depression. Keller, Lavori, Endicott, et al. (1983) later replicated these findings with a 25% prevalence of "double depression" among 316 inpatients and outpatients presenting with MDD. Rounsaville, Sholomkas, and Prusoff (1980) found a 36% rate of chronic intermittent depression among 64 MDD patients admitted to an outpatient medication trial.

Klein, Taylor, Harding, et al. (1988) found 31 double depression patients to have comorbid anxiety disorders (71%), eating disorders (22.6%), and substance abuse (45.2%). Kovacs, Feinberg, Crouse-Novak, et al. (1984a) reported a 43% history of DSM-III DD among 65 adolescents presenting for treatment of depression. Of the DD subjects in a prospective study, 93% had concurrent psychiatric diagnoses: MDD (57%), anxiety disorder (36%), attention-deficit disorder (14%), and conduct disorder (11%) being the most common. DD was not divided into primary and secondary subtypes, although "for a substantial portion of DD cases, the concurrent disorders postdated the onset of the DD" (p. 232). The same investigators (Kovacs, Feinberg, Crouse-Novak, et al. 1984b) also found that 70% of adolescents initially diagnosed with DD alone subsequently developed a major depression during a 7-year follow-up. Akiskal, King, Rosenthal, et al. (1981) subtyped 137 chronically depressed outpatients as (1) late onset (residual of major depression), 28%; (2) chronic dysphorias secondary to an underlying chronic medical and/or nonaffective psychiatric disorder, 36%; or (3) characterological (37%). They found that roughly two-thirds of the latter two subtypes developed a superimposed major depression on mean follow-up of 3 years.

Substance abuse has long been associated with dysphoric underlying mood, and a number of studies have linked it with depression (Himmelhoch 1987; Weissman, Pottenger, Kleber, et al. 1977). Frequently prescribed medications—including benzodiazepines, antihypertensives, and histamine antagonists for peptic ulcer disease—are known to induce organic mood disorders; thus iatrogenic dysthymia secondary to prescribed medication may also be common unfortunately (Weissman and Klerman 1977a). The ECA study is the first, however, to report comorbidity of substance abuse among dysthymic patients: a 29.8% prevalence of substance abuse (versus 15.4% for nondysthymics), a 19% use of minor tranquilizers (versus 7.4%), and a 6.7% use of sedatives (versus 2.7%) (Weissman, Leaf, Bruce, et al. 1988).

Markowitz, Kocsis, and Frances (unpublished observations) recently undertook a study of the prevalence and comorbidity of DD in a sample of unselected psychiatric outpatients. Patients completed the General Behavior Inventory (GBI) (Depue, Slater, Wolfstetter-Kausch, et al. 1981), a scale developed to diagnose dysthymia and cyclothymia. Klein, Dickstein, Taylor, et al. (1989) found the GBI to be sensitive and specific for DD in a psychiatric clinic population. A dysthymia scale score above 22 constituted the criterion for diagnosis of DD on the GBI. Fifty-nine GBI forms were completed, and 17 of these scored positive for DD, a prevalence of 29%. Interviewing a subset of eight GBI-positive and seven GBI-negative subjects by a clinician blind to GBI diagnosis yielded DSM-III diagnoses of DD concordant for all but one subject, a false positive.

To determine the types and prevalence of comorbid psychiatric and medical disorders, a sample of 18 dysthymic outpatients was interviewed by a psychiatrist blind to GBI score using the Structured Clinical Interview for DSM-III—patient version (SCID-P) (Spitzer and Williams 1985d) and the Structured Clinical Interview for DSM-III-R—personality disorders (SCID-II) (Spitzer, Williams, and Gibbon 1986). A comparison group of 23 nondysthymic outpatients was also interviewed. The two groups did not differ significantly in age, sex, or marital status. Axis I diagnoses for the two groups are shown in Table 2. DD patients had an average of 2.6 comorbid Axis I diagnoses and 3.6 total Axis I diagnoses compared to 1.7 total diagnoses for DD-negative subjects ($p < .001$ by Wilcoxon rank sum test).

Fourteen of 18 DD (78%) subjects also qualified for the additional

Table 2. Axis I Diagnoses: Lifetime by SCID-P

Diagnosis	Dysthymic ($N = 18$)	Nondysthymic ($N = 24$)
Affective disorder		
Dysthymic disorder	18	0
Major depression	14	6
Bipolar disorder	0	3
Cyclothymic	1	2
Schizoaffective disorder	0	1
Adjustment disorder	1	0
Obsessive-compulsive disorder	3	2
Hypochrondriasis	1	0
Somatization disorder	1	1
Bulimia	3	1
Panic disorder	6	5
Agoraphobia without panic	1	1
Simple phobia	4	2
Social phobia	3	1
Posttraumatic stress disorder	3	1
Generalized anxiety disorder	1	1
Substance abuse	3	9
Schizophrenia	0	1
Dementia	0	1
Organic mood disorder	0	2
Other	1	1
Total	64	41
Average number of Axis I diagnoses	3.6	1.7

Note: SCID-P = Structured Clinical Interview for DSM-III—patient version.

diagnosis of MDD, which was found more commonly among DD than nondysthymic subjects ($\chi^2 = 9.5$, $p = .002$). As others have noted, similarity in the criteria for DD and MDD seems likely to have created this "comorbidity" and to have artifactually elevated the number of diagnoses found in the DD sample. However, even if DD combined with MDD were considered to be the index diagnosis, the dysthymic subjects still had more comorbid diagnoses on Axis I (mean 2.6), compared to 28 among the 14 nondysthymic cases (mean 2.0) ($p < .004$ by Wilcoxon rank sum). It does appear that the DSM-III diagnosis of DD is quite prevalent among unselected psychiatric outpatients. DD is associated with a range of symptoms and dysfunctions that qualify these patients for comorbid diagnoses on Axis I.

A summary of this review of studies of the comorbidity of DD in psychiatric samples would include the following. First, when an index diagnosis of MDD is present in adults or children, one-quarter to one-third of the patients can be expected also to have a history of chronic depression (RDC intermittent depression or DSM-III dysthymic disorder). Second, when an index diagnosis of DD is present, most patients in clinical settings can be expected to meet criteria for MDD at some point in their course as well. Third, based on our research, DD subjects can be expected to fulfill criteria for larger numbers of additional comorbid Axis I disorders than psychiatric outpatients without DD.

Although comorbid diagnoses can logically be expected to affect treatment outcome in patients with DD, few data have been gathered relevant to the treatment implications of comorbid diagnosis. Keller, Lavori, Endicott, et al. (1983) performed an uncontrolled, naturalistic outcome study of "double depression" (i.e., patients who were diagnosed as having DD and MDD simultaneously). Compared to patients with MDD alone, patients with double depression were less likely to recover completely from symptoms of depression and were more likely to relapse into episodes of MDD.

In contrast to these results is the report of Kocsis, Frances, Voss, et al. (1988), who treated a group of outpatients having diagnoses of DD plus MDD in a 6-week, placebo-controlled trial of imipramine. After 6 weeks, 59% of imipramine subjects and 13% of placebo cases recovered completely. It appears that antidepressant medication, given in adequate doses and duration, can produce substantial recovery rates in DD patients with comorbid MDD. Treatment implications of substance abuse in dysthymic patients were addressed in the open treatment study of Akiskal, Rosenthal, Haykal, et al. (1980), who found that alcohol and sedative-hypnotic abuse predicted poor response to a variety of thymoleptic medications. To our knowledge, the implications of comorbid anxiety disorders, eating disorders, and other Axis I syndromes for treatment response of DD have not been investigated.

DSM-III Axis II Comorbidity

While there is an extensive literature on interactions between personality disorders and episodic MDD, little research to date has addressed comorbidity between personality disorders and DD. The authors of DSM-III stated that DD may accompany borderline, histrionic, and dependent personality disorders. DSM-III-R appended narcissistic and avoidant personality disorders to that list. Koenigsberg, Kaplan, Gilmore, et al. (1985) reviewed chart diagnoses of 2,462 psychiatric patients to find that 34% of the 68 DD patients had Axis II comorbidity: 16% classified as mixed-atypical-other, 6% as borderline personality disorder, and 7% as dependent personality disorder. Kocsis, Voss, Mann, et al. (1986) found a 47% prevalence of personality disorder in a sample of outpatients with DD. Atypical-mixed (13%) and dependent (11%) diagnoses were the most common comorbid Axis II diagnoses.

Perry (1985; Chapter 30) studied the prevalence of DD among patients with borderline, antisocial, mixed personality disorder, and bipolar II patients. All 23 cases with definite borderline personality disorder also met criteria for DD, as did 12 of 14 having only borderline traits. Eleven of 14 antisocial subjects, 9 of 12 patients with both borderline and antisocial personality disorder, and 10 of 19 bipolar II subjects also fulfilled criteria for DD. The association between double depression and borderline personality disorder or borderline trait was significantly greater than that with bipolar diagnosis. Zanarini, Gunderson, and Frankenburg (1989) recently found high prevalence rates for DD among DSM-III borderline (100%, $n = 50$) and antisocial (44.8%, $n = 29$) personality disorder patients.

Table 3. Lifetime Axis II Diagnoses by SCID-II

Diagnosis	Dysthymic ($N = 18$)	Nondysthymic ($N = 24$)
Cluster A		
Paranoid	2	0
Schizoid	0	0
Schizotypal	2	0
Cluster B		
Borderline	3	1
Histrionic	3	7
Narcissistic	1	2
Antisocial	0	0
(Self-defeating)	6	2
Cluster C		
Avoidant	6	0
Dependent	2	0
Obsessive-compulsive	2	2
Passive-aggressive	0	0
NOS (except self-defeating)	3	6
No Axis II diagnosis	2	9
Total	30	20
Average number of Axis II diagnoses	1.7	0.9

Note. SCID-II = Structured Clinical Interview for DSM-III-R—personality disorders.

Results from a study by Markowitz, Kocsis, and Frances (unpublished observations) are shown in Table 3. Sixteen (89%) of 18 patients diagnosed by DSM-III-R criteria as having DD also met criteria for an Axis II diagnosis, compared to 15 (63%) of 24 without dysthymia. The mean number of Axis II diagnoses per patient was significantly higher in the dysthymia group (1.7 versus 0.9, $p = .01$, Wilcoxon rank sum). Dysthymic subjects were more likely to have avoidant personality disorder ($\chi^2 = 6.8$, $p = .009$) and had a trend toward greater likelihood of having any Axis II diagnosis ($p < .10$).

Little attention has been focused on how Axis II disorders affect prognosis and treatment of DD. Studies conducted on inpatients with acute depressive episodes have linked comorbid personality disorders and "neuroticism" to poor treatment response (Charney, Nelson, and Quinlan 1981; Zuckerman, Prusoff, Weissman, et al. 1980). It is unknown, however, whether these personality characteristics affect treatment response in DD. Akiskal, Rosenthal, Haykal, et al. (1980) found that "unstable" personality (passive-dependent, histrionic, antisocial, or borderline as defined by DSM-III) predicted poor response to a variety of thymoleptic medications. These findings suggest that Axis II comorbidity does have relevance to medication responsiveness in DD.

DYSTHYMIC DISORDER AND MEDICAL ILLNESS

General statements exist in the medical and psychiatric literature suggesting that chronic medical illness and physical disability are frequently associated with depression or "demoralization" as psychological sequelae (Cassem 1987; Schildkraut and Klein 1975). Chronic endocrinopathies, diseases of the central nervous system, and severe systemic disorders might also be expected to affect mood. Yet few systematic investigations pertinent to such associations have been reported. A textbook of psychiatry noted "at least mild depression" in 22% to 32% of medical inpatients (Cassem 1987). Robinson, Lipsey, Rao, et al. (1986) reported symptoms of depression in a significant number of post-stroke patients followed for up to 2 years, but specific rates of diagnosis of DD were not reported in these studies. Popkin, Callies, Lentz, et al. (1988) found a 4.0% lifetime prevalence of DD and 24.0% rate for MDD among 38 patients with type I diabetes mellitus without large vessel cerebrovascular disease. The prevalence of DD among these diabetic patients appears no greater than among the general population (Weissman, Leaf, Bruce, et al. 1988). Tan, Kales, Kales, et al. (1984), on the other hand, found a 45% prevalence of DD among insomniac patients. Implications of a comorbid medical diagnosis for response of DD to treatment have not been reported.

CONCLUSION

Data reviewed in this chapter suggest frequent comorbidity of DD with Axis I, II, and III diagnoses. Because of overlapping symptoms, DD may at times pass unnoticed behind the mask of comorbid disorders, leading to misdiagnosis and failure to consider specific treatment (Weissman and Klerman 1977a). There is a need for continued research on the comorbidity of DD and on the implications of comorbid diagnoses for its treatment.

DD may prove to be a heterogeneous, "impure" disorder, a "clinical final pathway" (Klerman 1980) largely defined by its comorbidity. If so, further research may demonstrate subtypes of dysthymia that are *primarily* dysthymic and distinguishable from other chronic dysphorias by their response to treatment interventions. To differentiate dysthymia from chronic major depression and to define clinically useful subtypes of DD, researchers must carefully define symptoms, criteria, duration, and comorbidity in prospective studies of general and, especially, clinical populations.

We would suggest that the presence of Axis I, II, or III comorbidity should not be seen as a contraindication to vigorous treatment of DD. It may be that pharmacotherapy and psychotherapy of DD will also diminish or alleviate concurrent personality disorder, or render physical disorders less disabling and demoralizing. Future research must address such issues.

Section V
Evidence for Comorbidity: Family and Genetic Studies

Chapter 21

Comorbidity for Anxiety and Depression: Review of Family and Genetic Studies

Kathleen R. Merikangas, Ph.D.

COMORBIDITY: DEFINITION AND APPLICATION TO PSYCHIATRY

The term *comorbidity*, introduced by Feinstein (1970), refers to the presence of any additional coexisting ailment in a patient with a particular index disease. Failure to classify and analyze comorbid diseases can create misleading medical statistics and may cause spurious comparisons during the planning and evaluation of treatment for patients. Comorbidity can alter the clinical course of patients with the same diagnosis by affecting the time of detection, prognostic anticipations, therapeutic selection, and post-therapeutic outcome of an index diagnosis (Kaplan and Feinstein 1974).

In psychiatry, comorbidity appears to be the rule rather than the exception. Numerous studies of clinical samples of inpatients and outpatients (Di Nardo and Barlow, Chapter 12; Pfohl, Coryell, Zimmerman, et al. 1986; Roth, Gurney, Garside, et al. 1972) have demonstrated the large proportion of patients who simultaneously meet diagnostic criteria for more than a single disorder, both within Axis I and between Axes I and II of the DSM-III (American Psychiatric

This research was supported in part by Alcohol, Drug Abuse, and Mental Health Administration grants AA-07080 and DA-50348, and Research Scientist Development Award MH-00499. Suggestions of Theodore Reich, M.D., and Neil Risch, Ph.D., are gratefully acknowledged.

Association 1980). Similarly, multiple diagnoses within individual subjects appear to be quite frequent in epidemiologic surveys of the general population in the United States (Boyd, Burke, Gruenberg, et al. 1984) and in Europe (Angst, Vollrath, Merikangas, et al., Chapter 7; Wittchen 1988).

Two major approaches have been employed to classify multiple diagnoses within a single individual: assignment of a primary and a secondary diagnosis based on order of onset; and application of hierarchical diagnostic systems in which one condition is inferred to supercede the other. The former approach is preferable because no preconceived etiologic assumptions regarding the relationships between disorders are necessary. However, the primary-secondary distinction may be difficult to apply to the assignment of retrospectively ascertained lifetime diagnoses, which require accurate determination of the age of onset of disorders that often emerge in an insidious manner (Woodruff, Murphy, and Herjanic 1967). The latter approach has not been applied consistently across studies because of differences in the hierarchical structure of the diagnostic systems employed. Moreover, hierarchical relationships may often belie clinical data. For example, Tyrer (1986a) demonstrated that the DSM-III hierarchical system of ranking of the specific classes of anxiety disorders is both arbitrary and contradictory to clinical findings. The elimination of hierarchical relationships between many of the disorders in the DSM-III-R (American Psychiatric Association 1987) criteria will facilitate the assessment of relationships between two or more disorders. Methods for assessing associations between disorders are described below.

ASSOCIATION BETWEEN ANXIETY AND DEPRESSION

A strong association between depression and anxiety has been noted in the clinical literature throughout the past century by such eminent authorities as Hecker (1893) and Freud (1895). However, the nature and the boundaries of this relationship are still obscure. Despite having detached the syndrome of anxiety neurosis from neurasthenia, Freud argued that the vast majority of cases manifest features of both syndromes. In "On Psychopathology: On the Grounds for Detaching a Particular Syndrome from Neurasthenia under the Description 'Anxiety Neurosis'," Freud remarked that although the pure cases of anxiety neurosis may be the most "marked cases," he noted that "more often, however, symptoms of anxiety occur at the same time as, or in combination with, symptoms of neurasthenia, hysteria, obsessions, or melancholia" (p. 112). Furthermore, he postulated shared etiology for depression and anxiety: "the same aetiological determinant may regularly and simultaneously provoke both neuroses" (p. 112).

Explanations for Associations Between Disorders

The major explanations for an association between two or more disorders are shown in Table 1. Two common methodological biases

Table 1.   Explanations for an Association Between Two or More Disorders

Artifact
  Treatment-seeking bias
  Population stratification

True association
  Causal association
  Common etiology

  Alternate manifestations
  Different stages of same disease

that may lead to spurious associations between disorders are: (1) treatment-seeking bias, known as "Berkson's bias," in which persons with two conditions are more likely to be hospitalized or treated (Berkson 1946); and (2) assessment bias, which may include investigator bias, the lack of discrete diagnostic definitions in which a large degree of symptom overlap exists between two diagnostic categories, or the application of diagnostic hierarchies that may mask an association. Spurious associations between disorders may also occur because of the lack of an appropriate comparison or control group, or by the failure to adjust for confounding factors such as sex or age. For example, population stratification may lead to artifactual associations between diseases; if the sample includes a subpopulation in which there is an increased frequency of two unrelated disorders, the disorders may appear to be associated.

Freud's (1895) observations regarding an association between anxiety neurosis and depression have been confirmed by the results of several recent epidemiologic studies, which have shown that the anxiety syndromes and depression co-occur more frequently than would be expected by chance (Boyd, Burke, Gruenberg, et al. 1984). In addition to the significant degree of comorbidity between depression and anxiety in clinical samples, the association is also found among unselected epidemiologic samples of the population of the United States, Switzerland, Canada, and Germany (Angst, Vollrath, Merikangas, et al., Chapter 7; Boyd, Burke, Gruenberg, et al. 1984; Murphy, Sobol, Neff, et al. 1984; Wittchen 1988). The association between anxiety and depression persists after controlling for sex, age, and race. Furthermore, longitudinal studies have also shown that a significant degree of depression occurs in patients with anxiety neurosis across a decade of follow-up (Noyes, Clancy, Hoenk, et al. 1978). Interestingly, this association has been found irrespective of the location of the threshold for the definition of a case of anxiety and depression.

If a true association exists between two disorders, there are two possible explanations for the association. First, the association could be etiologic in that one disorder causes or leads to the second disorder. That is, the presence of one disorder is a necessary precondition for the expression of the other (Figure 1). In this situation, anxiety could cause depression or the converse.

A second possible explanation for an association is that the two disorders are manifestations of the same underlying etiologic factors (Figure 2). This model proposes that anxiety and depression result from the same etiologic factors. For example, pleiotropic effects of the same genes could lead to anxiety, depression, or a combination of the

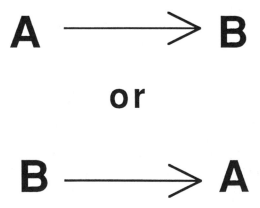

CAUSAL ASSOCIATION

A ⟶ B

or

B ⟶ A

Figure 1. Model that proposes an etiologic, or causal, association in which one disorder causes or leads to the second disorder.

<u>COMMON ETIOLOGY</u>

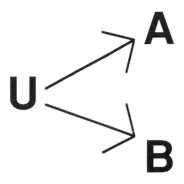

Figure 2.   Model that proposes that two disorders may be manifestations of the same underlying etiologic factor.

two, depending on background genes and the intrinsic and extrinsic environment in which they are expressed.

This chapter will review the evidence from family and genetic studies on the relationship between anxiety and depression. Because these studies span the last decade, during which there has been a rapid evolution of methodology in psychiatric research, the comparability of the data is limited by methodological variation. The major areas of methodological variation concern diagnostic conventions and sampling procedures. Sources of samples in the studies reviewed below include general hospitals, psychiatric hospitals, specialty clinics, private practices, and epidemiologic surveys. Moreover, because several studies have not employed controls with whom comparable procedures to those of probands and their relatives were applied, the morbid risk in relatives of probands must be compared to population base rates that may have been derived from different instrumentation and diagnostic criteria. The control groups in those studies that did employ controls may not be comparative in their selection and characterization. For example, whereas some studies of panic disorder did not exclude controls with major depression (Crowe, Pauls, Slymen, et al. 1980; Noyes, Clancy, Crowe, et al.

1978), other studies employed controls with no lifetime history of any major psychiatric disorder (Weissman, Kidd, and Prusoff 1982). However, despite these methodological differences between studies, several trends that shed light on the possible mechanisms for the association between anxiety and depression emerge.

USE OF FAMILIAL TRANSMISSION DATA TO ASSESS MECHANISMS FOR ASSOCIATIONS

The use of familial transmission data in disease classification was first suggested in the 16th century by a physician named Paracelsus (see Rosenthal 1971). The finding that disorders or subtypes breed true in families constitutes evidence for the validity of these categories. The predictions regarding patterns of familial transmission that derive from the above-cited alternative explanations for an association between anxiety and depression are described below.

Table 2. Causal Mechanism: Predictions From Familial Transmission Data: "Nontransmissible" Association

Proband	Relative
Anxiety	↑ Anxiety only ↑ Anxiety + depression No ↑ depression only
Depression	↑ Depression only ↑ Anxiety + depression No ↑ anxiety only

Table 2 presents the expectations for familial transmission in data if the association between depression and anxiety were attributable to a causal mechanism. If the relationship between anxiety and depression were etiologic, with anxiety causing depression or the converse, the two disorders would be expected to breed true in families. Rather, it would be expected that relatives would manifest an increased risk of the combination of the two syndromes. If anxiety causes depression, relatives of probands with anxiety should have an increased rate of major depression, but *only* in the presence of a lifetime history or concomitant expression of anxiety. Conversely, if depression causes anxiety, rates of anxiety would be elevated among relatives of probands with depression, but *only* in combination with depression. Rates of depression alone should approximate population base rates.

The predictions of the family data for the second possible mechanism for an association between anxiety and depression, that each disorder was a manifestation of similar underlying factors (i.e., genetic or intrinsic versus extrinsic environment or a combination thereof), are shown in Table 3. This model would predict that relatives of probands with pure forms of either disorder should have elevated rates of pure forms of the other disorder as compared to expected population rates. Therefore, relatives of probands with "pure" depression should have an increased risk of pure anxiety, and the converse.

Table 3.   Common Etiology: Predictions From Familial Transmission Data: "Transmissible" Association

Proband Relative	
Anxiety	⤉ Anxiety only ⤉ Depression only ⤉ Both
Depression	⤉ Depression only ⤉ Anxiety only ⤉ Both

Family Studies of Anxiety Neurosis

Table 4 presents the results of family studies of anxiety neurosis as defined by Feighner criteria (Feighner, Robins, Guze, et al. 1972). The studies of Noyes, Clancy, Crowe, et al. (1978) and Crowe, Pauls, Slymen, et al. (1980) demonstrate a high degree of specificity of transmission of anxiety disorders, with a sixfold increase in the risk of anxiety neurosis among relatives of probands with this disorder as compared to that of relatives of controls. In contrast, the risk of depression was not elevated among the relatives of probands with anxiety plus depression in comparison with those of control probands. However, because some of the controls had a history of major depression, this finding is not unexpected.

Studies by Cloninger, Martin, Guze, et al. (1981) and Dealy, Ishiki, Avery, et al. (1981) compared relatives of anxiety neurotics to those of probands with both anxiety and depression. The former study found a twofold increased risk of anxiety neurosis among relatives of probands with anxiety only compared to relatives of probands with both conditions, thereby demonstrating some specificity of transmission of anxiety neurosis. In contrast, the latter study showed no increased risk of anxiety among relatives of anxiety neurotics as compared to relatives of probands with both anxiety and

Table 4. Family Studies: Anxiety Neurosis

| Study | Probands | | | Method | Relatives Diagnosis (%) | |
	N	Diagnosis	Source		Anxiety	Depression
Noyes, Clancy, Crowe, et al. (1978)	112	Anxiety	Treated sample	Family history	18	5
	110	Controls	Surgery department hospital staff		3	4
Crowe, Pauls, Slymen, et al. (1980)	19	Anxiety	Treated sample	Direct interview	31	9
	19	Controls	Hospital staff		4	12
Cloninger, Martin, Guze, et al. (1981)	54	Anxiety	Treated sample	Direct interview	13	8
	12	Depression + Anxiety			6	16
Dealy, Ishiki, Avery, et al. (1981)	62	Anxiety	Advertisement	Family history	14	10
	31	Anxiety + Depression			12	15

depression. The findings of the two studies converge with respect to the risk of depression among relatives, with both studies demonstrating an increased risk of depression among relatives of probands with both anxiety and depression. Taken together, the results of three of the four family studies of anxiety neurotic probands demonstrate specificity of transmission of anxiety neurosis. Moreover, there is no increased risk of major depression among the relatives of probands with anxiety neurosis, thereby providing evidence for separation of the two syndromes. However, the predictions of the causal model versus those of the common etiologic model for the association of anxiety and depression could not be adequately tested because the data were not available in the format presented in Table 2 and Table 3.

Family Studies of Panic Disorder

The studies of probands with panic disorder defined according to Research Diagnostic Criteria (RDC) (Spitzer, Endicott, and Robins 1978a) are presented in Table 5. Similar to the results presented in the former table, the predictions of the causal as compared to the common etiology model could not be assessed because of the lack of classification of probands and relatives into pure disorders versus multiple disorders, and the lack of controls in those studies that did apply this classification. Nevertheless, the increased risk of panic among relatives of probands with panic, and the increased risk of depression among relatives of probands with depression, in all studies indicates that both panic and depression are familial. Cross-transmission of pure panic in probands and pure depression in relatives was found in two of the three studies in which data on cross-transmission could be evaluated (Browning D, Merikangas K, and Weissman M, unpublished observations; Maier, Buller, and Hallmayer 1988). The latter study employed direct interviews of the relatives of probands with panic alone, depression alone, and both depression and panic. This study was the only family study reviewed herein that applied the DSM-III-R criteria, in which no hierarchies regarding comorbid anxiety and depression were applied. If sufficient criteria were present to warrant a diagnosis of an anxiety disorder, the diagnosis was made, irrespective of the temporal association between symptoms of anxiety and episodes of major depression. The authors of this study concluded that although there appears to be some specificity in the familial transmission of panic disorder and major depression, the increased prevalence of major depression beyond population expectations among relatives of probands with panic disorder, and a similar increase in the morbid risk of panic disorder among the relatives of probands with "pure" depression, suggest that there exist some

Table 6.   Family Studies: Phobia

| Study | N | Probands | | Method | Relatives | |
| | | Diagnosis | Source | | Diagnosis (%) | |
					Anxiety	Depression
Munjack and Moss (1981)	68	Agoraphobia	Advertisement	Family history	—	38
	10	Social			—	14
	35	Simple			—	0
Harris, Noyes, Crowe, et al. (1983)	20	Agoraphobia	Self-help group	Direct interview	32	8
	20	Panic	Treated sample		33	4
	20	Controls	Medical illness		15	10

Table 7. Family Studies: Anxiety

Study	Probands				Relatives		
						Diagnosis (%)	
	N	Diagnosis	Source	Method	Anxiety only	Depression only	Anxiety + Depression
Angst, Vollrath, Merikangas, et al. (Chapter 7)	92	Anxiety + depression	General population	Family history	12	28	29
	44	Anxiety only			10	22	29
	91	Depression only			14	25	18
	168	Neither			7	20	6
					Anxiety	Depression	
Noyes, Clarkson, and Crowe (1987)	20	Generalized anxiety disorder	Advertisement	Direct interview	30	7	

One small family study of probands with generalized anxiety disorder (Noyes, Clarkson, and Crowe 1987) compared the relatives of 20 probands with generalized anxiety disorder to data from the previous Iowa family studies (Crowe, Pauls, Slymen, et al. 1980; Noyes, Clancy, Crowe, et al. 1978). Relatives of probands with generalized anxiety disorder had a fivefold increase in generalized anxiety disorder as compared to those of controls or those of agoraphobic probands, and a fourfold increase as compared to those of probands with panic disorder. There was a high prevalence of secondary depression among the probands (70%) and a mild elevation in rates of secondary depression among their relatives with generalized anxiety disorder (20%).

Twin Studies of Anxiety and Depression

Finally, there have been several twin studies that have yielded evidence for the relationship between anxiety and depression. A study of twins in which the proband was ascertained through treatment settings examined the specificity of transmission of the diagnostic categories of pure anxiety, pure depression, and their combination (Torgersen 1985b). No evidence was found for the specificity of transmission or the heritability of either pure neurotic depression or mixed anxiety and depression. In contrast, there was a 3.5-fold increase in both pure anxiety neurosis and mixed anxiety and depression among monozygotic as compared to dizygotic twin pairs. However, the rates were identical for pure anxiety and mixed anxiety and depression among the co-twins of probands with pure anxiety neurosis, thereby indicating a unidirectional lack of specificity of transmission of this disorder. Unfortunately, the small number of twins in this study prohibits the application of statistical models that simultaneously test heritability and diagnostic specificity in the above-cited data.

Two studies of symptoms of anxiety and depression derived from symptom checklists among normal twin pairs recruited from volunteer registries are reviewed in Table 8 (Clifford, Hopper, Fulker, et al. 1984; Jardine, Martin, and Henderson 1984). Data from these studies yield remarkably similar estimates of the heritability of anxiety and depression alone. Moreover, the studies have yielded convergent evidence indicating similar underlying genetic factors leading to the expression of divergent symptom patterns of either anxiety or depression. In a further analysis of the Australian twin data, Kendler, Heath, Martin, et al. (1986) estimated the heritability for each of seven symptoms of anxiety and depression. The range of heritability coefficients was .33 to .77 for anxiety and .33 to .46 for depression. However, caution should be exercised in generalizing from these studies be-

Table 8. Twin Studies of Symptoms of Anxiety and Depression

			Heritability	
Study	N of Twins	Source	Anxiety	Depression
Clifford, Hopper, Fulker, et al. (1984)	1,144	Volunteer registry	.50[+]	.48[+]
Jardine, Martin, and Henderson (1984)	3,810	Volunteer registry	.36	.35

Note. [+] = classical twin method.

cause the assessment of anxiety and depressive symptoms was cross-sectional and based on very few items for each condition.

Implications of Findings

This review of family and genetic studies of anxiety disorders confirms the well-known familial aggregation of these conditions. Furthermore, the twin studies reviewed herein provide evidence that a substantial degree of the transmissibility of these conditions may be attributed to genetic factors. Nearly all studies found a high degree of comorbidity for anxiety and depression in the probands and to a lesser extent in their relatives. However, the lack of consistent methodology precluded an adequate test of the two possible mechanisms for the association that were explicated above.

Studies in which the probands were classified according to the presence of concomitant depression, either primary or secondary to an anxiety disorder, tended to support the explanation that similar underlying factors are involved in the expression of symptoms of either or both disorders among relatives. Families in which probands exhibit prominent manifestations of both anxiety and depression tended to resemble depressed families more than they did families of probands with anxiety disorders alone.

In contrast, families of probands with anxiety neurosis or panic disorder without depression did not tend to have increased familial loading for depression. Most of these studies have applied the RDC or DSM-III diagnostic hierarchies, which exclude a diagnosis of an anxiety disorder if the expression of anxiety is *always* associated with episodes of affective disorders. However, data from the family studies of depression at Yale have demonstrated that patterns of familial transmission of anxiety and depression do not differ for depressed probands with anxiety that is temporally separate or concomitant to depressive episodes (Leckman, Merikangas, Pauls, et al. 1983; Leckman, Weissman, Merikangas, et al. 1984; Weissman, Kidd, and Prusoff 1982). Although this diagnostic convention has now been eliminated in DSM-III-R, most of the family studies reviewed herein have applied this hierarchical exclusion for temporally contiguous presentations of anxiety and depression. Thus most of these data cannot be applied to test the degree of co- and cross-transmission of anxiety and depression to determine whether the association can be attributed to causal mechanisms or to the existence of common etiologic factors.

The consideration of secondary conditions in general has been quite inconsistent across studies. Investigators with an interest in the familial transmission of a particular disorder have only rarely considered the simultaneous presence of additional disorders in both the probands and their relatives. Furthermore, presentation of rates of primary and secondary disorders in both the probands and their relatives is necessary to examine the specificity of transmission of comorbid disorders. This was possible in only a small minority of the family studies examined in this review, such as that of van Valkenburg, Akiskal, Puzantian, et al. (1984) and Maier, Buller, and Hallmayer (1988).

Although the focus of this chapter was primarily on family studies of the anxiety disorders, studies of the families of probands with depression are equally informative with respect to the association between anxiety and depression. Despite the very large number of excellent family studies of depression, data from most studies were not stratified by mutually exclusive categories of major depression with and without anxiety disorders in the probands or their relatives (for a review, see Gershon 1983). The above-cited Yale family study of depression revealed an increased risk of numerous disorders among the relatives of depressed probands with a history of anxiety disorders as compared with those of probands with depression alone (Leckman, Merikangas, Pauls, et al. 1983; Weissman, Kidd, and Prusoff 1982). More recent work that has examined the co-segregation of anxiety and depression in this study suggests that these disorders are manifestations of the same underlying transmissible factors (Merikangas, Risch, Weissman, unpublished observations). However, the lack of probands with pure anxiety disorders limits the comparability of this study to those reviewed above. Such a study is now underway and will permit assessment of the generalizability of the latter findings.

Another family study of major depression has also yielded information on the association between anxiety and the affective disorders (Coryell, Endicott, Andreasen, et al. 1988). The findings provide evidence for a separation between panic disorder and major depression based on differential familial aggregation of anxiety disorders in general and panic disorder in particular among relatives of probands with and without panic disorder. In contrast, relatives of the two groups of probands did not have significantly different rates of affective disorders. When taken together with data on the longitudinal course of depressed patients with and without panic attacks during a single index episode, the findings suggest that panic attacks may represent a severity marker for major depression.

The results of the work of Leckman, Weissman, Merikangas, et al. (1984) and Coryell, Endicott, Andreasen, et al. (1988) on probands with major depressive disorder indicate that concomitant anxiety disorders in depressed probands are associated with increased familial loading of affective disorders. In contrast, the latter study provides evidence for separation of panic disorder and major depression based on increased familial aggregation of anxiety disorders among the relatives of probands with both disorders as compared to those of probands with major depression alone. However, methodological differences, including the lack of a control group, characterization of probands based on a single index episode, and analysis of interviewed relatives only in the latter study, limit the comparability of the findings in the latter two studies of probands with major depression.

In summary, the family and twin studies of anxiety disorders demonstrate a high degree of familial aggregation of anxiety disorders. Relatives of probands with anxiety disorders who manifest prominent affective symptoms tend to exhibit increased morbid risk of anxiety, depression, and their combination. "Pure" anxiety neurosis or panic disorder tends to breed true to a substantial degree. The conclusions of the Maier, Buller, and Hallmayer (1988) study, with which the mechanisms for the association could best be tested, indicate specificity of transmission of panic disorder, particularly the pure form. However, the data also suggest partial overlap in the transmission of panic and depression, thereby indicating some shared etiologic factors. These findings are compatible with Freud's (1895) above-cited observations, which postulate a continuum on which the pure cases of anxiety neurosis may be the most severe form of expression, but which also appear to be the most rare form of this disorder.

Family studies have been shown to be an important mechanism for identifying variable forms of expression of the same etiologic factors for numerous disorders. The application of the family study method to the major psychiatric disorders has provided a wealth of information on the pathogenesis of numerous conditions during the past decades. For the complex human disorders with no clear Mendelian pattern of transmission and generally high population prevalence, family study designs can be applied to address a number of key questions regarding the pathophysiology of these conditions. This review has demonstrated the utility of the application of data on familial transmission of anxiety and depression to identify possible mechanisms for their association.

AREAS FOR FUTURE RESEARCH

There are several areas for future research that are indicated by the results of this review. First, methodology for family studies needs to be standardized across sites and across diagnostic groups of probands. A detailed review of family study methodology is presented by Weissman, Merikangas, John, et al. (1986). Second, diagnostic hierarchies for which there is limited evidence should be eliminated to enable investigators to examine different patterns of familial transmission by secondary and tertiary conditions in probands and their relatives. Third, consistent analytic strategies of primary and secondary conditions need to be established. Fourth, control groups need to be more comparable across studies. There was remarkable inconsistency in the methods of selection of controls as well as the exclusion criteria that were applied in different studies. Fifth, authors should present a table of raw data without age adjustment and stratified by relevant demographic variables in publications of family study data to facilitate standardized analyses of data from several studies. Sixth, statistical methods for analyzing transmission of comorbid disorders need to be developed. Seventh, studies of familial aggregation that systematically examine the source of selection of the probands need to be conducted to identify possible biases that may be related to clinical, epidemiologic, treatment registry samples, and most particularly, samples solicited by advertisement. Finally, longitudinal data on families need to be collected to examine the role of age-dependent expression of disorders, and particularly of comorbid disorders, in patterns of familial aggregation.

Chapter 22

Evidence for Comorbidity of Anxiety and Depression: Family and Genetic Studies of Children

Myrna M. Weissman, Ph.D.

THE FOCUS OF this chapter is on evidence for comorbidity of depression and anxiety disorders in children. The evidence is based primarily on data from family-genetic studies. The purpose is to clarify the relationship between these disorders. Are anxiety and depression etiologically the same disorder with different clinical features? Are they on a continuum of severity? Or are they etiologically different disorders with an overlap in clinical features?

The specific questions relevant to these questions in studying children using family-genetic approaches are: (1) do depression and anxiety disorders transmit between parents and children; (2) do they co-occur within children; and (3) do they continue from childhood to adulthood?

This study was supported in part by Alcohol, Drug Abuse, and Mental Health Administration grants MH-36197 and MH-28274 from the Center for Studies of Affective Disorders; by the John D. and Catherine T. MacArthur Foundation Mental Health Research Network on Risk and Protective Factors in the Major Mental Disorders; by grant #86-213, Child and Adult Depressive Disorders: A Test of Continuities Using Family-Genetic Data, from the John D. and Catherine T. MacArthur Foundation; and by the W. M. Keck Foundation.

Appreciation is expressed to Drs. M. B. Keller, C. Last, A. Kadzin, M. Hersen, W. R. Beardslee, N. Breslau, C. Sylvester, R. J. Reichler, C. L. Hammen, J. Kagan, and H. Orvaschel, who generously provided drafts of their manuscripts.

Inclusion of studies on children in a book on comorbidity of mood and anxiety disorders is quite appropriate because there is increasing evidence that depression and anxiety disorders do occur in children, that the mean age of onset of these disorders is usually in adolescence or young adulthood, and that early onset depressions have high familial loading (Weissman, Wickramaratne, Merikangas, et al. 1984).

Children usually have been excluded from family-genetic, twin, and cross-fostering studies, in part due to real diagnostic problems in their assessment and in part due to the belief that depression did not occur in children. Moreover, most family-genetic studies have originated in adult psychiatry, and there has been less interest in studying children. This situation is changing, and data on the rates and nature of depression and anxiety disorders in children are now becoming available.

DEFINITION OF CHILDREN

Any discussion of psychiatric disorders in children should define what is meant by "children," which is an awkward classification. It can refer to a class of biologic relatives (offspring), to sons or daughters, or to a youthful age group. In family-genetic studies, *children* usually refers to the probands' adult offspring over age 17 years, since younger children have usually not been included in these studies. In this chapter, I will focus on children as the offspring of a proband and as a youthful age group. Data will be presented on minor children, usually ages 6 to 17 years, although the age range varies somewhat in the data presented.

DIAGNOSTIC CLASSIFICATION OF CHILDREN

Anxiety Disorders

Anxiety disorders in the third edition of the *Diagnostic and Statistical Manual of Mental Disorders* (DSM-III) (America Psychiatric Association 1980) have been separated into subtypes for adults and for children. Those anxiety disorders first evident in childhood and adolescence include separation anxiety, avoidant disorder, and overanxious disorder. For adults, anxiety disorders include panic disorder, agoraphobia with and without panic attacks, social phobia, simple phobia, generalized anxiety disorder, obsessive-compulsive disorder, and posttraumatic stress disorder. Although DSM-III includes a separate category of anxiety disorders having their origins in infancy and childhood, except for the explicit requirement that generalized anxiety disorder cannot be diagnosed before age 18, there is no contraindication to diagnosing the other adult anxiety disorders in children.

The revision of the DSM-III, DSM-III-R (American Psychiatric Association 1987), includes some modifications in the anxiety disorders. However, the disorders first evident in childhood do not differ from DSM-III. There is some reclassification of the adult anxiety disorders. Agoraphobia is now a separate disorder. As before, the adult classifications can be applied to children. In DSM-III-R, it is permissible to diagnose generalized anxiety disorder in children.

Depression

In both DSM-III and DSM-III-R, there is no separate category for depression disorders first evident in infancy or childhood. All the adult disorders can be classified in childhood. There are minor criteria changes when used in children. For example, irritability can substitute for depressed mood in children and adolescents. Failure to make expected weight gains can substitute for weight loss. One (not 2) years' duration is required for the diagnosis of cyclothymia or dysthymia in children. Although there are minor differences in the ordering of affective disorders, and they are called mood disorders in DSM-III-R, these changes should not substantially change future considerations of depression or anxiety disorders in children.

There are no published studies on children using DSM-III-R criteria, and only a few are available using DSM-III. For this chapter, most of the diagnoses are based on DSM-III.

Do Depression and Anxiety Disorders Transmit Between the Generations?

Research Strategies

Although family-genetic studies do not yield evidence for the amount of genetic variance contributing to a disorder, the data can provide better understanding of diagnostic heterogeneity. It is quite likely that many of the psychiatric disorders are groups of conditions rather than single entities with different etiologic and modifying risk factors. The use of family data in the absence of specific neuropathologic evidence is one approach to identifying homogeneous diagnostic subgroups. If the diagnostic subgroup under study increases risk of the disorder and "breeds true" within families, potential evidence for the validity of the diagnostic group is suggested. If adult forms of a disorder are related to increased risk of specific disorders in their offspring, this suggests a relationship between the adult and childhood disorders.

Because variation in expression of a particular trait within families is assumed to result from the same latent factor, family studies can yield information on variable expressivity of the gene or genes related to the phenotypic trait. This property of family studies can lead to the development of more precise clinical descriptions of the full spectrum of disorders. Studies of the young children of adult probands can yield information on the transmission of disorders and/or symptoms across generations, on the early signs and childhood forms of the disorder, and on the risk or protective factors that mediate the development of the disorder.

Between-generation studies to determine the relationship of one disorder to another raise questions about the risk of the child's disorder vis-à-vis the parents' diagnoses. For example, if children of parents with depression have increased risk of both depression and anxiety disorder or if children of parents with anxiety disorder have increased risk of both depression and anxiety disorder, this would suggest that anxiety and depression are similar disorders. Alternately, if children of depressed parents have increased risk of depression, but not of anxiety disorder, this would suggest that depression and anxiety are separate disorders. If parents with anxiety disorder have children with increased risk of anxiety disorder and not depression, this would strengthen the theory.

Case-Control Studies

There are several designs for family-genetic studies, and they yield somewhat different information. The case-control design is the most commonly used. A more complete assessment of the design used in family studies can be found in Weissman, Merikangas, John, et al. (1986). With a case-control design, a proband with the illness under investigation is selected for study and is then matched to a control proband (i.e., an individual who does not have the illness under investigation but who is comparable on other characteristics).

Usually the prevalence of the condition among first-degree relatives of the proband is compared to prevalence among the first-degree relatives of controls. In the absence of control groups, the rates of illness among relatives can be compared to population rates. This design requires accurate information on population at risk. In either case, these studies usually have a retrospective cohort design in that the lifetime rates of illness in relatives are obtained on the basis of recall of their lifetime incidence of disorders. As noted before, children under the age of 18 years have traditionally been excluded from these studies.

Top-Down Studies

In family studies of psychiatric disorders, the probands or index cases with the disorder being investigated have nearly always been adults who were selected from treatment settings or from psychiatric or case registries. Family studies which begin with the adult probands and their spouses, and study psychopathology among their offspring as well as other relatives, have been termed *top-down* studies by Puig-Antich (1980).

Bottom-Up Studies

With the increasing interest in childhood psychiatric disorders during the last decade, children have also begun to be defined as the probands in family studies, termed by Puig-Antich (1980) as *bottom-up* studies. Similar to the adult studies, children who serve as probands generally have been selected from treatment settings. Studies that begin with the child or adolescent as the proband, or index case, tend to find very high rates of illness in the child's adult relatives, possibly because of sampling bias. Although the proband is the treated child, it is the parent who brings the child for treatment and who grants permission for the child to be included in the study. Ill parents, or parents sensitized to the effects of the illness because of having several ill family members, may be more likely than well parents to bring their children to treatment and to consent to the child's inclusion in the study.

One method used to control for this ascertainment bias has been to select a comparison control proband group of children with another treated psychiatric illness. The rates of all types of psychiatric illness will also tend to be high in the adult relatives of the child comparison group. However, the types of illness and the magnitudes of the differences in rates between the relatives of the cases and the relatives of the comparison control group can provide more important information than the absolute rates of illness in the relatives.

High-Risk Studies

The high-risk paradigm is a variant of the case-control and the top-down family study (Garmezy and Streitman 1974). The focus is usually limited to the young offspring of ill probands. The proband is a parent. Usually there is no assessment of the proband's first-degree or other relatives, although such an assessment is quite important in understanding transmission of disorders to offspring. In high-risk studies, the offspring are usually studied longitudinally to identify risk factors that are premorbid to, rather than concomitant with, the first onset of the disorder. Such factors may serve to identify vulnerable individuals and permit efforts toward prevention and intervention.

The high-risk design studies have yielded the most data relevant to the topic of transmission of specific disorders between the generations. Data primarily on depressive disorders are now becoming available from these studies.

Evidence From High-Risk Studies

Orvaschel (1983) and Beardslee, Bemporad, Keller, et al. (1983) independently published excellent scholarly reviews of the status of research on parental depression and child psychopathology and reached similar conclusions. Most of the studies included fewer than 40 children and produced a wide range in rates, which the authors attributed to methodological differences between studies. The studies varied by informant (child about self or parent about child); by diagnostic method (symptoms scale or diagnostic interview); by diagnostic criteria; by methods of calculating rates (the family unit or the number of children affected); and by type of affective illness in the parent (unipolar or bipolar).

Although the methodological limitations of the studies conducted at that time were considerable, the findings all pointed in the same direction. The children of affectively ill parents were at a significant risk for developing psychopathology, particularly depression.

Since the publication of these reviews, the methodology of children's studies has improved considerably. There are now at least seven well-designed studies that include children (ages 4 years and older) of parents with major depression or anxiety disorders (see Table 1). Many of these studies are ongoing and have only recently begun to yield data (Breslau, Davis, and Prabucki 1987; Hammen, Gordon, Burge, et al. 1987; Kagan, Reznick, Snidman, et al. 1988; Keller, Beardslee, Dorer, et al. 1986; Orvaschel, Walsh-Allis, and Ye 1988; Sylvester, Hyde, and Reichler 1988; Weissman, Gammon, John, et al. 1987).

More than 350 offspring of depressed parents, 150 offspring of anxious parents, and 400 offspring of controls have been studied. A variety of control groups have been included, most commonly the children of parents never psychiatrically ill. However, children of bipolar and of medically ill parents have also been studied. All these studies have included a structured diagnostic interview of children: Kiddie Schedule for Affective Disorders and Schizophrenia (K-SADS), Diagnostic Interview Schedule for Children (DISC), or Diagnostic

Table 1. Characteristics of Recent High-Risk Studies of Children of Parents With Major Depression and/or Anxiety

Study	Study children Parent diagnoses	N	Control children Parent diagnoses	N	Ages of children (years)	Diagnostic instrument	Family information	Follow-up
Orvaschel, Walsh-Allis, and Ye (1988)	≥1 parent MDD	61	Neither parent ill	45	6–17	K-SADS	History 1st- & 2nd-degree relatives	18 months
Keller, Beardslee, Dorer, et al. (1986)	≥1 parent MDD	72	Neither parent ill	24	6–19	DICA	History & interview 1st- & 2nd-degree relatives	No
Hammen, Gordon, Burge, et al. (1987)	≥1 parent MDD	19	≥1 parent BP	12	8–16	K-SADS	Interview both parents	6 months for 3 years
			≥1 parent CMI	18				
			Neither parent ill	35				
Weissman, Gammon, John, et al. (1987)	≥1 parent MDD	153	Neither parent ill	67	6–23	K-SADS	History 1st- & 2nd-degree relatives	2 years
Breslau, Davis, and Prabucki (1987)	Mother GAD	101	Mother not ill	174	8–23	DISC	Interview mother	No
	Mother MDD	56						
Sylvester, Hyde, and Reichler (1988)	≥1 parent panic	50	Neither parent ill	48	7–17	DICA	No	Yes
	≥1 parent MDD	27						
Kagan, Reznick, Snidman, et al. (1988)	≥1 parent panic	18	Other problems	14	4–7	Direct observation	Interview both parents	No

Note. All studies but Breslau, Davis, and Prabucki used consensus diagnosis. MDD = major depression; BP = bipolar disorder; CMI = chronic medical illness; GAD = generalized anxiety disorder; K-SADS = Kiddie Schedule for Affective Disorders and Schizophrenia; DICA = Diagnostic Interview for Children and Adolescents; DISC = Diagnostic Interview Schedule for Children.

Interview for Children and Adolescents (DICA) (for a review, see Weissman, Merikangas, John, et al. 1986). At least one parent was interviewed. Diagnoses of children were made blindly as to their parents' clinical status. DSM-III criteria were used for the children. Consensus diagnosis was made on all available data.

In all but three studies (Breslau, Davis, and Prabucki 1987; Hammen, Gordon, Burge, et al. 1987; Sylvester, Hyde, and Reichler 1988), family history is available on the child's first- and second-degree relatives, and attention has been paid to the spouse's diagnosis. Four of the studies (Hammen, Gordon, Burge, et al. 1987; Orvaschel 1986; Sylvester, Hyde, and Reichler 1988; Weissman, Gammon, John, et al. 1987) include a follow-up assessment.

The study by Breslau, Davis, and Prabucki (1987) was not designed specifically to estimate familial aggregation of psychiatric disorders, but rather to determine child disability and its effect on families. This study provides some information on relative risk of psychiatric illness in children of depressed mothers. However, because only annual, and not lifetime, prevalence is reported in the Breslau, Davis, and Prabucki investigation, rates are not directly comparable with the other studies.

All of the studies confirm earlier reports that offspring of depressed and of anxious parents are at increased risk of major depression as well as anxiety disorders. A range of diagnoses in children are represented. The rates of any diagnosis in children are quite high and, in studies reporting these data, range from 41.0 to 75.9 per 100 for children of parents with major depression (Table 2).

In children of depressed parents, both major depression and anxiety disorders are transmitted to the children in nearly equal frequency (Table 2). This is also true in the two high-risk studies of the children of parents with panic disorder or generalized anxiety disorder (Table 3). The rates of depression or of anxiety disorders in children of depressed or anxious parents are considerably higher than in children of parents with no psychiatric illness (Table 4).

The range of rates of major depression in children of depressed parents between studies is still wide (15 to 41 per 100), although these variations are not nearly as great as in previous studies (Table 2). The lowest rates in children derive from the Orvaschel (1986) study. As noted before, in the Breslau, Davis, and Prabucki (1987) study, only annual rates of illness are reported, and the parents are mildly ill subjects drawn from a community sample. The highest rates are from the Hammen, Gordon, Burge, et al. (1987) study, which included only 19 children whose mothers had chronic and recurrent depression. Keller, Beardslee, Dorer, et al. (1986) showed that chronicity of depression in parents increased the risk of the disorder in their children.

Table 2. Rates (per 100) of Psychiatric Illness in Children of Parents With Major Depression

| Study | Diagnoses in children | | |
	Major depression	Any anxiety disorder	Any disorder
Keller, Beardslee, Dorer, et al. (1986)	24.0	16.0	65.0
Orvaschel, Walsh-Allis, and Ye (1988)	15.0	20.0	41.0
Hammen, Gordon, Burge, et al. (1987)	41.0	21.0	74.0
Breslau, Davis, and Prabucki (1987)	16.0	21.0	—
Weissman, Gammon, John, et al. (1987)	28.1	39.9	75.9
Sylvester, Hyde, and Reichler (1988)	37.0	44.0	—

Note. All rates are lifetime, except Breslau, Davis, and Prabucki, which are annual.

Table 3. Rates (per 100) of Psychiatric Illness in Children of Parents With Anxiety Disorder

| Study | Diagnoses in parent | Diagnoses in children | |
		Major depression	Any anxiety disorder
Sylvester, Hyde, and Reichler (1988)[a]	Panic	48.0	42.0
Breslau, Davis, and Prabucki (1987)[b]	GAD	11.0	11.0 (GAD) 9.0 (SAD)

Note. GAD = generalized anxiety disorder; SAD = separation anxiety disorder.
[a]Lifetime rates.
[b]Annual rates.

There has been one quite interesting study of the young children (ages 4 to 7 years) of probands with panic disorders using direct observational techniques and a developmental perspective (Kagan, Reznick, Snidman, et al. 1988) (Table 1). Based on observation made

Table 4.   Lifetime Rates (per 100) of Psychiatric Illness in Children of Parents With No Psychiatric Disorder

	Diagnoses in children	
Study	Depression	Any anxiety disorder
Sylvester, Hyde, and Reichler (1988)	9.0	3.0
Weissman, Gammon, John, et al. (1987)	13.4	17.9
Hammen, Gordon, Burge, et al. (1987)	9.0	12.0[a]

[a]Separation anxiety and overanxious disorders.

blindly as to the parental diagnosis, the investigators found that the children of panic probands, as compared to children of controls, were more inhibited behaviorally, were more reluctant to talk to an unfamiliar but friendly examiner, and (in this situation) showed a trend toward sympathetic activation and cognitive stress, as reflected in increased heart rate and cortisol levels. This study suggested that anxiety symptoms may be apparent in the very young offspring of probands with panic disorder. No data on childhood depression are presented.

Evidence From Bottom-Up Studies

The three bottom-up studies (i.e., those that select the child as the proband and examine rates of illness in the child's first-degree relatives) confirm the previous findings about the relationship between depression and anxiety. Puig-Antich and Rabinovich (1986) examined major depression in the relatives of children with major depression, with and without separation anxiety, as well as children with separation anxiety without major depression (Table 5). They found equally high rates of major depression in their adult relatives and no significant difference in rates of depression by proband group.

Table 5.   Lifetime Risk (per 100) of Major Depression in Adult Relatives of Children With Depression and/or Anxiety Disorders

	Diagnosis in children		
	Major depression with separation anxiety (N = 28)	Major depression without separation anxiety (N = 19)	Separation anxiety without major depression (N = 12)
Major depressive disorder first-degree relatives	43	55	39

Note.   Recalculated from data presented in Puig-Antich and Rabinovich (1986).

A second bottom-up family study of 127 relatives of 4 children with overanxious disorder, 8 with separation anxiety, and 11 with major depression found similar rates of major depression in the children's relatives (Livingston, Nugent, Rader, et al. 1985) (Table 6). The rates of panic disorder were elevated in the adult relatives of anxious children. However, it was unclear how many of the children's first- or second-degree relatives were actually assessed in this study. It should be noted that the diagnosis of adult relatives was only by family history. The family history methods usually tend to underestimate illness in relatives.

Table 6. Lifetime Rates (per 100) of Depression and Anxiety Disorders in the Adult Relatives of Children With Depression or Anxiety Disorders

	Diagnoses in children	
Diagnoses in adult relatives[a]	Major depression ($N = 11$)	Separation anxiety or overanxious disorder ($N = 12$)
Major depression	15.5	14.5
Generalized anxiety	5.2	—
Panic	—	11.6

Note. Derived from Livingston, Nugent, Rader, et al. (1985).
[a]Diagnoses by family history in parents, grandparents, aunts, uncles, or siblings.

In the third study, Last, Francis, Hersen, et al. (1987) found extremely high rates of anxiety disorders and major depression in the mothers of 19 children (ages 6 to 17 years) with separation anxiety and 22 with overanxious disorder, as compared to a control group of children with other psychiatric disorders (Table 7). Taken together, these studies in children suggest that depression and anxiety disorders transmit across the generation and are interchangeable.

Table 7. Lifetime Rates (per 100) of Anxiety and Major Depression in Mothers of Children With Anxiety Disorders

	Diagnoses in children		
Diagnoses in mothers	Separation anxiety ($N = 19$)	Overanxious disorder ($N = 22$)	Controls ($N = 15$)
Any anxiety disorder	68.4	86.4	40.0
Major depression	52.6	31.8	26.7

Note. Derived from Last, Francis, Hersen, et al. (1987).

DO DEPRESSIVE AND ANXIETY DISORDERS CO-OCCUR IN CHILDREN?

Understanding the co-occurrence of disorders is useful for clarifying diagnostic problems in transmission, but does not yield much information on the discreteness of disorders unless information on chronology and stability can be obtained. In general, the studies of children on co-occurrence of depression and anxiety report findings similar to those reported in studies of adults. There is a high co-occurrence; chronology is difficult to ascertain but occurs probably equally. In adults, a high co-occurrence of depression, anxiety, and alcohol disorder is reported. In studies of young children, conduct disorder is substituted for alcohol abuse. In older children, both drug and alcohol abuse is reported.

Six studies of children using modern diagnostic criteria report data on the co-occurrence of depression and anxiety disorders in children (Table 8). The studies vary by the type of anxiety or affective disorder studied.

Table 8.   Co-Occurrence of Affective and Anxiety Disorders in Children

Study	Diagnoses in children	Comorbid disorder	%
Kovacs, Feinberg, Crouse-Novak, et al. (1984a, 1984b)	Major depression	Anxiety disorder	33
Kashani, Beck, Hoeper, et al. (1987); Kashani, Carlson, Beck, et al. (1987)	Major depression	Anxiety disorder	75
Weissman, Gammon, John, et al. (1987)	Major depression	Anxiety disorder	55
Puig-Antich (1987)	Major depression	Phobia	48
Puig-Antich (1987)	Major depression	Separation anxiety	59
Bernstein and Garfinkel (1986)	Phobia	Affective disorder	69
Last, Francis, Hersen, et al. (1987)	Phobia	Affective disorder	33

Kovacs and colleagues (Kovacs, Feinberg, Crouse-Novak, et al. 1984a, 1984b) investigated 65 adolescents (ages 8 to 13 years) receiving treatment for a depressive disorder and found high rates of coexisting disorders. Of the children with major depression, 33% had coexisting anxiety disorder. Information on chronology was not available from the cross-sectional data, although the authors felt that the chronology of the other disorders simultaneously or secondarily were equally likely for all but dysthymia, where the early age of onset usually predated the other disorders. Presence of a concomitant anxiety disorder over a 6-year period did not influence remission from or relapse into a new depressive episode.

In a community survey study of 150 adolescents (ages 14 to 16 years) attending public school, Kashani and colleagues (Kashani, Beck, Hoeper, et al. 1987; Kashani, Carlson, Beck, et al. 1987) found that 41.3% had at least one DSM-III disorder. Anxiety, depression, and conduct disorders were the most common. There was high comorbidity between these disorders. Of the 150 adolescents with major depression, 75% had additional diagnoses of anxiety disorders.

In a study of 220 children (ages 6 to 63 years) of depressed and normal parents, Weissman, Gammon, John, et al. (1987) found that 55% of 220 children with major depression had comorbid anxiety disorders.

In a study of 80 prepubertal children with major depression, Puig-Antich (1987) found that 48% had co-occurring phobias; 59%, separation anxiety; and 11%, obsessive-compulsive disorder.

Bernstein and Garfinkel (1986) studied 26 young adolescents with school phobia. They found that 69% met DSM-III criteria for major depression. Children with depression frequently reported anxiety; those with anxiety did not commonly describe major depression, except where the anxiety was severe. In a study of 67 children with separation anxiety (mean age, 9 years) or school phobia (mean age, 14 years), Last, Francis, Hersen, et al. (1987) found that 50% of the children had another anxiety disorder and about 33% had an affective disorder.

DO THE CHILDHOOD DISORDERS CONTINUE INTO ADULTHOOD?

Longitudinal studies, whether or not part of a high-risk design, can yield information on comorbidity. Evidence that there is continuity of a childhood disorder (either anxiety or depression) into adulthood and that disorders are not interchangeable strengthens the evidence for the separation of the disorders. Evidence that the disorders are interchangeable between childhood and adulthood would suggest that they are similar disorders with different manifestations at different ages.

As of this writing, there has not been one published longitudinal study of individuals, first identified as having an anxiety or depressive disorder in childhood, who have been followed to adulthood to determine the natural history, clinical course, or prognostic significance of these childhood disorders and their continuity to the adult disorders. One such study for separation anxiety has just been undertaken by Gittelman-Klein at Columbia University; others for a range of depressive disorders are underway by Kovacs at the University of Pittsburgh and by Rutter at The Maudsley Hospital in London.

Information is available on shorter-term follow-up of children and of retrospective accounts of the childhood of adult patients. In regard to depression, Kovacs, Feinberg, Crouse-Novak, et al. (1984a) studied 65 prepubertal depressed children over 6 years and showed that there is continuity of this disorder. Kandel and Davies (1982, 1986) identified 1,000 15- and 16-year-olds with depressed mood from a high school survey and followed them over 9 years. These investigators found continuity of depressive symptoms (particularly in girls) and high rates of associated social and interpersonal morbidity and drug use. Similar conclusions were reached by Poznanski, Krahenguhl, and Zrull (1976) in a study of 10 youths (mean age, 16.9 years) over 6½ years. They found that 50% of the children were clinically depressed 6½ years later.

Summary of Evidence

Data now available from family-genetic, epidemiologic, and longitudinal studies clearly illustrate the high comorbidity between anxiety disorder and depression in children. The high-risk studies show:

1. Offspring of depressed parents are at high risk for depression and anxiety disorders; that is, their risk for developing these disorders is much higher than that known for children of nondepressed and nonanxious parents.
2. Offspring of parents with anxiety disorders are at high risk for anxiety disorders and depression.
3. The adult relatives of children with depression or with anxiety disorders have high rates of depression and of anxiety disorders.
4. The specificity of these disorders to depression and anxiety is unclear because a host of other disorders are also represented in high-risk offspring.
5. There is a high co-occurrence of depression and anxiety in children, although the chronology of these disorders is not clear.
6. Although there are no data yet available on longitudinal studies of children with anxiety and depressive disorders into adulthood, the shorter-term follow-up studies suggest the continuity and persistence of depression.

Future Research

The findings presented here raise several research issues and point to future directions.

Diagnostic Hierarchies of DSM-III

The high-risk studies thus far have been based on DSM-III criteria. It is possible that the hierarchies of DSM-III could obscure the presence of an existing anxiety disorder in a proband parent because anxiety is not diagnosed in DSM-III if it occurs in the presence of major depression. While this hierarchy has been eliminated from DSM-III-R, the current published data are based on DSM-III. The use of hierarchies could be inadvertently exaggerating the findings on comorbidity because many of the probands may have anxiety disorders that are not diagnosed. In a study that did not use the conventional DSM-III hierarchy and diagnosed anxiety disorder even if it co-occurred with major depression, 87.5% of 56 probands with major depression had some anxiety disorder at some point in their lifetime (Weissman, Leckman, Merikangas, et al. 1984).

Concordance in Diagnosis Between Parents

Since assortative mating for psychiatric disorders is high, any study of children must take into account the diagnosis of the spouse. For example, in the study of 56 probands with major depression, 32.4% of their spouses had a major depression and 44.6% had an anxiety disorder at some point in their life (Weissman, Leckman, Merikangas, et al. 1984).

If a depressed and/or anxious proband is married to a spouse with depression and/or anxiety, then these factors could account for the high rates of depression and/or anxiety in the offspring studied. It is not possible to study these issues from the available data because the comorbid disorders in the proband and the diagnosis of the spouse are often not included in the published findings.

Studies of diagnostically pure proband groups (i.e., depressed patients with no other psychiatric disorders, current or in the past) who are married to a spouse who have similar disorders or who never have had a psychiatric illness are rare. We have such a study underway, but these patients are difficult to locate either in community or clinic samples. When we have attempted to examine the role of illness in offspring, taking into account comorbidity and diagnosis in both parents, we still found equal transmission of depression and anxiety in the offspring (Weissman, Leckman, Merikangas, et al. 1984).

The Specific Anxiety Disorders

Most of the studies look at anxiety disorders without differentiating between the specific types. Further study of the specific anxiety disorders and their comorbidity with depression would be useful. For example, while major depression and anxiety disorders generally co-occur, it is unclear if this is true for all anxiety disorders.

Parent-Child Reports

The discrepancies between parent and child reports of a child's psychopathology should be considered in future analyses. There is considerable agreement that parents and children do not agree on the nature and extent of the children's diagnosis (Weissman, Wickramaratne, Warner, et al. 1987). Although many studies now use best-estimate diagnoses of children based on all available information, there is inconsistency in the published findings. Independent reports of data by parent and by child as well as by a child psychiatrist would be useful in comparing results.

Long-Term Follow-Up

As of this writing, there is not one published study of the continuity into adulthood of depression or anxiety disorders in children. Several studies are underway, and these will help clarify the diagnostic issues.

Familial Aggregation and Discrepancy With Adult Studies

The co-occurrence of depression and anxiety disorders in individuals has been found in studies of adults and of children. The transmission of anxiety and depression across the generations has been shown in samples of children and parents. However, not all family studies of adults have shown the familial aggregation of depression and anxiety disorders (see Crowe, Noyes, Pauls, et al. 1983; Harris, Noyes, Crowe, et al. 1983; Leckman, Weissman, Merikangas, et al. 1983, 1984).

The discrepancy between the adult and children's studies may be due to diagnostic comorbidity and the absence of proband groups with pure anxiety disorders, differences in diagnostic approaches, the small number of studies of anxiety disorders that have included children, and the tentative state of psychiatric diagnosis in children. The familial transmission of anxiety and depression across the ages is still unresolved.

CONCLUSION

The evidence from studies of children lends further support to the comorbidity of depression and anxiety disorders. However, the data are not without problems. For example, studies of sampling from probands with anxiety disorders are small; all the specific anxiety disorders have not been studied; control groups are sometimes lacking; and family history rather than interviews are sometimes used. Most important, the stability of childhood disorders and their continuity to adulthood is unclear. From a research perspective, the importance of understanding affective and anxiety disorders in children should not be overlooked. The model in recent genetic studies has been Huntington's or Alzheimer's disease, both disorders of late onset. Inclusion of children in pedigree studies of these late-onset disorders would be uninformative or even misleading. The child would not have entered the age of risk for the disorder and could be incorrectly counted as unaffected. By contrast, affective or anxiety disorders have quite early onsets (Kashani 1982). Selection of a proband who is an adolescent makes it more likely that the family members will be alive and available for extended pedigree studies; for example, a 14-year-old child will likely have living siblings, parents, and grandparents. With the increasing availability of a genetic map, small nuclear families with at least three affected members will become a powerful tool for understanding linkage of markers for a chromosome to a disorder. If the child is a proband, there is more likelihood of finding sibling pairs and trios for study. The ability to diagnose children accurately will increase the odds of finding these families for study. The clarification of the overlap and distinction between disorders in children will be important in judging who is affected in pedigree studies.

Psychiatric studies of children also provide an opportunity for answering questions about the nature of disorders before the social and economic consequences of illness have occurred. Lastly, studies of first onset may provide information on the sequence of occurrence of disorders and on the factors associated with their onset and may clarify the problem of comorbidity.

Chapter 23

A Twin-Study Perspective of the Comorbidity of Anxiety and Depression

Svenn Torgersen, Ph.D.

S YSTEMATIC STUDIES OF patient populations confirm a common clinical experience: that depressive and anxiety symptoms exist in the same individual (Di Nardo and Barlow, Chapter 12). It might be that the correlation is spurious, that having both anxiety and depressive symptoms increases the probability of being a patient and thereby bringing the individual into a clinical population. However, community epidemiologic studies have shown the same high proportion of mixed anxiety-depressive cases (Boyd, Burke, Gruenberg, et al. 1984).

Longitudinal studies have also demonstated that cases with anxiety may develop into depression, and vice versa (Angst, Vollrath, Merikangas, et al., Chapter 7). However, Hagnell and Gräsbeck (Chapter 8) show in their Swedish longitudinal epidemiologic study that pure anxiety cases seldom turn into pure depressive cases. Correspondingly, pure depressive cases seem also to remain pure depressive cases if they have relapses, in addition to some cases turning into mixed cases. Cases characterized by a mixture of anxiety and other psychiatric symptoms or depression and other psychiatric symptoms seem to be in the same mixed group if they relapse, or they develop into depression. Finally, it is repetitively claimed that antidepressant drugs are therapeutically effective against panic disorder and agoraphobia (Klein 1980). Consequently, there appears to be strong evidence in favor of considering anxiety and depression as part of the same underlying disorder.

However, it might be that this conclusion is premature. Some quite different disorders—might be weakened by the reviewed studies, and then only if the objections about the question of continuity from childhood to adulthood and assortative mating is unimportant. We should be aware of another problem in these studies, namely, the problem of assessing reliably the diagnoses in children. As Weissman (Chapter 22) underscores, the correlation between the assessment from interviews with the parents about the children's symptoms and interviews with the children directly is not high. A false comorbidity as well as a familial relationship between anxiety and depression might result from a blurring of the assessing of emotional states in children.

Merikangas (Chapter 21) has reviewed the family and twin studies dealing with the relationship between anxiety and depression. This chapter considers particularly the mixed anxiety-depressive group. The results of the reviewed family studies are very divergent. Some studies show crossover transmission between pure anxiety, mixed anxiety-depression, and pure depression; others do not.

It seems particularly difficult to find a higher frequency of depression among the relatives of probands with anxiety.

The relatives of mixed cases seem to have either mixed anxiety-depressive disorder themselves, or pure depression, seldom pure anxiety. A higher frequency of pure anxiety is neither uniformly observed among relatives of probands with pure depression.

Therefore, while many interpretations are possible, the review of the family studies may point in the direction of hypothesis three, that the strongest relationship exists between pure depression and mixed cases, while pure anxiety disorders might have another etiology.

SIGNIFICANCE OF TWIN STUDIES

Family studies investigate transmission only within the family generally and cannot study genetic transmission specifically. Twin studies might say more about whether the transmission is genetic or a consequence of common environment. What do twin studies tell?

A questionnaire was sent to more than 3,800 Australian twins from the common population. The results of the study are presented in a number of articles and analyzed according to different genetic models (Jardine, Martin, and Henderson 1984; Kendler, Heath, Martin, et al. 1986). In one of the last published articles (Kendler, Heath, Martin, et al. 1987), the replies to items intending to measure anxiety and depressive symptoms were analyzed for homogeneous or heterogeneous etiology. An advanced multivariate analysis was applied using polychoric correlations. Three "genetic" and three "environmental" factors emerged. The first genetic factor had factor loadings that were high on almost all anxiety and depressive items, and was named the genetic-distress factor. The second genetic factor only loaded on two somatic anxiety items and was called genetic somatic anxiety. The third genetic factor, covering insomnia items, was small and not consistent across sexes. The first environmental factor, which had loadings on both anxiety and depressive items but was higher on the depressive items, was named environmental depression. The second environmental factor loaded mostly on anxiety items and less on depressive items and was named environmental general anxiety. The third environmental factor was again inconsistent insomnia factors.

The main point is that while the environmental factors made a relatively clear differentiation between anxiety and depressive items, the genetic factors revealed a more unspecific anxiety-depressive factor and a small, narrow anxiety factor. The authors' interpretation is that anxiety and depressive features have a common genetic basis, whereas environmental events have a differentiating effect on the development of anxiety and depression. A more straightforward interpretation of the results of the twin study might propose that there exists a common genetic basis for susceptibility to anxiety and depressive feelings, but *in addition* a specific genetic basis for some anxiety experiences. This interpretation is in accordance with their last paper (Martin, Jardine, Andrews, et al. 1988). As to the effect of environmental events, anxiety and depression seem relatively clearly delineated. Furthermore, as the authors rightly admit, what they are studying is not clinical syndromes or disorders, but replies to questions about anxiety and depressive reactions in the general population. To what extent these replies are indications of psychopathology is uncertain and, if so, what kinds of affective or anxiety disorders.

Carey (1987) has commented on their study. By a statistical analysis with simulated data, Carey demonstrated that Kendler and colleagues' approach gives higher estimates of common liability for anxiety and depression compared to competing models of analysis. While not rejecting their methods, he maintains that different approaches have to be tried out before we decide what is the truth: "Who is correct? In today's forum, there is no clear winner" (p. 490).

From the point of view of this chapter, the Australian twin study has not produced a clear decision on whether anxiety and depressive conditions might be the same disorder. If we agree with the conclusions of Kendler and colleagues, we might state: With genetic etiology as the basis for a nosologic classification, anxiety and depressive features are part of the same disorder. If also environmental etiology is considered, they are different disorders. In addition, as suggested by Martin, Jardine, Andrews, et al. (1988), a subgroup of anxiety

Table 2. Diagnoses of Co-Twins of Probands With Major Depression With and Without Anxiety Disorders and Anxiety Disorders Without Major Depression

			Co-twin					
			Major depression without anxiety		Major depression with anxiety		Anxiety disorder without major depression	
Proband		N	n	%	n	%	n	%
Major depression without anxiety	MZ	16	1	6.3	3	18.8	0	0
	DZ	25	2	8.0	2	8.0	2	8.0
Major depression with anxiety	MZ	17	5[a]	29.4	1	5.9	2	11.8
	DZ	34	4[a]	11.8	0	0	4	11.8
Anxiety disorder without major depression	MZ	32	1	3.1	0	0	11	34.4
	DZ	53	2	3.8	0	0	9	17.0

Note. Values are numbers of co-twins in each category. MZ = monozygotic; DZ = dizygotic.
[a] One co-twin has a bipolar disorder.

Table 2 shows an unexpected result: Major depression without anxiety disorder and major depression with anxiety disorder do not breed true. On the contrary, major depression with anxiety disorder is frequent among co-twins of probands with major depression, and vice versa. The frequency is more than two times higher for monozygotic co-twins compared to dizygotic co-twins. For co-twins of probands with anxiety disorder but without concomitant major depression, major depression with or without anxiety disorders is almost absent. Anxiety disorder without major depression is observed among co-twins of probands with major depression with and without anxiety disorder, however, with no higher frequency among monozygotic than among dizygotic co-twins and with a far lower frequency than among co-twins of probands with anxiety disorder without major depression.

What does Table 2 reveal? Major depression with and without anxiety disorders seems to have a similar etiology, probably including genetic factors. Anxiety disorder without major depression, on the other hand, seems to be unrelated to major depression and the mixed type of disorder.

As panic disorder most often has been associated with major depression (Merikangas, Chapter 21), and as anxiety disorders with panic most clearly seem to be genetically influenced (Torgersen 1983), the analysis was also performed restricted to anxiety disorders with panic attacks.

In Table 3, panic disorder, agoraphobia with panic attacks, and generalized anxiety with panic attacks are grouped together in anxiety disorders with panic attacks. Probands and co-twins are then classified according to whether they have major depression with or without panic attacks. The results are similar to what was obtained when all anxiety disorders are included: Major depression with and without panic attacks is relatively often present in the same twin pair. Furthermore, major depression is absent among co-twins of probands with anxiety disorders with panic attacks but without major depression. Moreover, anxiety disorder with panic attacks is almost absent among co-twins of probands with major depression with or without panic attacks. The results are even more clear-cut than when all anxiety disorders were considered. Table 3 shows also that the concordance rate for major depression is much higher when the proband has panic attacks in addition to major depression. When that is not true, the concordance rate among co-twins is very low.

Table 3 indicates a relationship between major depression with and without panic attacks, but no etiologic connection to anxiety disorders without major depression. Furthermore, major depression with panic attacks might seem to be a condition with a stronger

Table 3. Diagnoses of Co-Twins of Probands With Major Depression With and Without Panic and Anxiety Disorders With Panic Without Major Depression

		Co-twin					
		Major depression without panic		Major depression with panic		Panic without major depression	
Proband	N	n	%	n	%	n	%
Major depression without panic MZ	24	2	8.3	3	12.5	2	8.3
DZ	37	2	5.4	2	5.4	2	5.4
Major depression with panic MZ	9	5[a]	55.5	0	0	0	0
DZ	22	4[a]	18.2	0	0	1	4.5
Panic without major depression MZ	18	0	0	0	0	4	22.2
DZ	23	0	0	0	0	0	0

Note. Values are numbers of co-twins in each category. MZ = monozygotic; DZ = dizygotic.
[a] One co-twin has a bipolar disorder.

familial, and possibly genetic, transmission than major depression without panic attacks. This observation is in accordance with the studies of Weissman, Leckman, Merikangas, et al. (1984) and Leckman, Weissman, Merikangas, et al. (1983), which show that relatives of probands with major depression plus panic show a higher frequency of major depression than relatives of probands with major depression without panic disorders.

To sum up, the hierarchy-free analysis of my twin data supports hypothesis three, that mixed anxiety-depression and pure depression have the same etiology, while pure anxiety is another disorder. However, the mixed disorder might be considered as more strongly influenced by genetic and common environmental family factors.

CONCLUSION

Five hypotheses to explain the relationship between pure anxiety disorder, mixed anxiety-depressive disorder, and pure depressive disorder were presented early in the chapter. The first hypothesis indicated that all three disorders were the same disorder; the second, that pure anxiety and the mixed cases were the same; the third, that pure depression and mixed were the same; the fourth, that anxiety and depression were different disorders and the mixed cases were variants of the two; and finally, the fifth hypothesis stated that all three conditions were different disorders.

Although the focus of this chapter is twin studies, results from follow-up and family studies that are presented in this volume were considered. The findings are divergent. Some results from follow-up studies support hypothesis one, others the third hypothesis. The family studies also show results partly supporting hypothesis one, partly hypothesis three, while hypotheses two and four cannot be ruled out. The twin studies also are not clearly conclusive. However, in my opinion, the twin studies tend mostly to support hypothesis three—that pure depression and mixed anxiety-depression are similar disorders, etiologically speaking, while pure anxiety is another disorder. This conclusion especially pertains to the relationship between major depression and panic disorder.

It might seem paradoxical that anxiety and panic attacks symptoms can be associated with major depression, yet major depression is not associated with anxiety disorders and panic disorders. However, symptoms and even groups of symptoms are not the same as disorders. Anxiety symptoms, predominantly panic symptoms, might be a relatively common part of the course of major depression without implying that major depression is a part of the course of anxiety disorders, as the Swedish follow-up study indicates (Hagnell and

Gräsbeck, Chapter 8). Depressive symptoms are frequent in early phases of schizophrenia as well as in the residual phase. The schizo-affective disorder also constitutes a mixture of schizophrenia-like and affective symptoms. Even so, few will argue for an etiologic relationship between schizophrenia and the affective disorders.

It is true that the number of individuals are few in the Norwegian twin study, and the results must be considered preliminary. Larger twin studies are warranted before any firm conclusions can be drawn. In addition, longitudinal studies, follow-up studies, and a close examination of the course of depressive and anxiety disorders—as suggested by the studies of Cloninger, Martin, Guze, et al. (1981); Coryell, Endicott, Andreasen, et al. 1988; and Van Valkenburg, Akiskal, Puzantian, et al. 1984—are necessary. Multiple interviews and inventory techniques have to be used. Then we can see whether there might be important phenomenological differences between the seemingly similar symptoms in the pure and the mixed cases. Perhaps the most promising method would be longitudinal family and twin studies with a variety of interviews and questionnaire techniques.

Evidence for Comorbidity: Biologic Studies

Chapter 24

A Biologic Perspective on Comorbidity of Major Depressive Disorder and Panic Disorder

George R. Heninger, M.D.

T HE ISSUES SURROUNDING the concept of comorbidity in psychiatry are numerous, complex, and not yet fully defined, hence, the need for this volume. However, from the biologic perspective, the central questions may be somewhat more simple. The large questions of diagnostic accuracy at the symptom or syndrome levels, including the central issues of comorbidity versus symptom complexity, have been discussed by other authors in this volume and will not be extensively addressed here. What is of concern from the biologic point of view is the real possibility of true biologic comorbidity that alters the pathogenesis of some syndromes so as to affect diagnosis, prognosis, and treatment. It may be useful to review definitions so that this point can be made more clearly and consistently.

Symptoms:	Any subjective evidence of disease.
Sign:	Any objective evidence of disease.
Syndrome:	Set of symptoms that occur together; the sum of signs of any morbid state.
Morbidity:	A condition of being diseased.
Disease:	Any deviation from the normal structure or function of any part or system of the body that is manifested by a characteristic set of symptoms and signs.
Comorbidity:	The presence of any additional coexisting ailment in a person with a particular index disease.

DISEASE INTERACTIONS DURING PATHOGENESIS

The above definitions do not include the factor of time, and thus they do not explicitly include the concept of pathogenesis. Comorbidity from the perspective of pathogenesis is of immense practical significance, and it has major consequences relative to our logical understanding of the cause and treatment of disease. In most areas of medicine, comorbidity is very common, rather than being an exception. Certainly most practicing physicians, at least those of the secondary and tertiary care level, diagnose and deal with comorbidity in the majority of their patients. For example, every medical student is taught to view comorbidity as a common and frequent medical problem (e.g., unregulated diabetes mellitus and the increased prevalence of low-grade infections).

What is of most interest about comorbidity relative to pathogenesis is the possibility that the temporal sequence of interactions between coexisting diseases can explain significant differences in overall outcome. From a research point of view, the discovery of disease pathogenesis may find one of its best clues in comorbid conditions. A current example of this is human immunodeficiency virus (HIV) infection, which leads to the acquired immune deficiency syndrome (AIDS). Thus, in the discovery of the pathogenesis of AIDS, original observations of an unexplained increased incidence of certain opportunistic infections and neoplasms was the starting point. Only later did the role of HIV infection become apparent as the causative factor in the pathogenesis of the syndrome, leading to the late-appearing opportunistic infections that caused death. In this example, an unrecognized comorbid condition turned out to be the major explanation of the initially observed infections and neoplasms.

In Table 1, the temporal interaction of two disease processes during pathogenesis that leads to comorbidity of secondary infection in AIDS is presented for comparison to a theoretical model of comorbidity of panic disorder and major depression. In the pathogenesis of AIDS and *Pneumocystis carinii* comorbidity, the exposure to *pneumocystis* is universal, since this protozoa can be cultured from all individuals. Also, HIV infection occurs only following transmission of the virus into the body through mucous membranes or more directly into the blood. Once the HIV infection is established, then a variable period elapses before evidence of immunodeficiency is observed. Comorbidity usually exists later in the illness when the HIV impairment of immune function makes the patient vulnerable to opportunistic infections, such as *Pneumocystis carinii* that otherwise would not have been able to establish themselves. The point of this example is that comorbidity exists only at a point in time during the pathogenesis

Table 1. Examples of the Interaction of Disease Processes During Pathogenesis and the Relationships to Comorbidity: A Comparison of AIDS to a Possible Subtype of Major Depressive Disorder

Events in pathogenesis	Healthy subjects	AIDS Patients		
		Early	Middle	Late
Exposure to *Pneumocystis carinii*	yes	yes	yes	yes
Exposure to HIV	yes	yes	yes	yes
HIV infection	no	yes	yes	yes
Immunodeficiency	no	no	yes	yes
Comorbidity: AIDS and secondary infection with *Pneumocystis carinii*	no	no	no	yes
		A Subtype of Major Depressive Disorder		
Exposure to social isolation	yes	yes	yes	yes
Exposure to anxiogenic stimuli	yes	yes	yes	yes
Failure of neuroregulatory systems (panic attacks)	no	yes	yes	yes
Failure of social performance (panic attacks with agoraphobia)	no	no	yes	yes
Comorbidity: Panic attacks with agoraphobia and social isolation related major depression	no	no	no	yes

Note. AIDS = acquired immune deficiency syndrome; HIV = human immunodeficiency virus.

of each disease. By understanding the temporal interaction in the pathogenesis of the two disease states, a more accurate evaluation of etiology is possible. This in turn will lead to more effective prevention and treatment.

In comparison to the comorbidity of secondary infection in AIDS, the possible steps in the pathogenesis of panic disorders and a theoretical type of major depressive disorder are also presented in Table 1. Even though healthy individuals are regularly exposed to periods of social isolation, this exposure does not by itself lead to depression. Similarly, even though healthy individuals are also exposed to anxiogenic stimuli, they do not develop a panic disorder unless there is an impairment of (as yet unknown) neuroregulatory mechanisms. Once there is an impairment of the critical neuroregulatory mechanisms, and the disease progresses, the secondary development of agoraphobia increases social isolation and can reduce social supports. This reduction, in turn, could be a major factor in the development of a comorbid major depressive disorder. In this instance, the comorbidity (similar to secondary infections in AIDS) could be very informative as to the sequence of steps in pathogenesis, which in turn would be important in the design of new treatments. This example is clearly theoretical and is presented only to make the point that understanding temporal interactions during pathogenesis is one of the most important benefits to be derived from the study of comorbidity.

THEORETICAL PERSPECTIVE

In the above examples that illustrate the importance of the interaction of separate disease processes leading to the pathogenesis of a comorbid state, it is critical that the separate biologic processes of each disease can be accurately and repeatedly assessed. In the example of AIDS, both the presence of HIV infection and *Pneumocystis carinii* can be assessed repeatedly with a high degree of sensitivity and specificity at different points in time. With the repeated evaluation of the "biologic markers" for these two separate disease processes, it is possible to piece together the manner in which they combine to produce the final comorbid pathologic condition. Thus the sensitivity and specificity of biologic markers as measures of the processes under study are critical to a reliable evaluation of the processes that are interacting at different points in time to produce the final comorbid clinical diagnosis.

It is quite evident from a careful consideration of the issues raised by other authors in this volume that there are major difficulties in the reliability of defining symptoms, syndromes, or diseases so that they can be quantitatively assessed over time as to their interaction in pathogenesis. Unfortunately, the biologic measures available for application to the study of anxiety and depression are also neither sensitive nor specific, and therefore there is a limit to their usefulness in understanding comorbidity. If sufficiently sensitive and specific measures could be obtained, they would be extremely useful in helping to clarify the various stages of pathogenesis of each illness and the role of that illness in producing comorbidity.

EVALUATION OF BIOLOGIC MARKERS IN PANIC DISORDER AND DEPRESSION

As a first step in working toward a better understanding of the biologic factors involved in pathogenesis and their role in comorbidity, a starting point has often been to assess differences in biologic markers between diagnostic groups. It is important to realize that some of the lack of sensitivity and specificity of the biologic markers could result from inadequate separation of patients into diagnostically pure subtypes. However, a review of the current status of a number of biologic markers for panic disorder and depression may provide information for use in developing methods to study this problem in the future.

The Hypothalamic-Pituitary-Adrenal Axis: Dexamethasone Suppression Test in Major Depressive Disorder and Panic Disorder

The dexamethasone suppression test (DST) has a long and complex history with considerable controversy as to its interpretation and utility. There is little question that there is an abnormality in the regulation of the hypothalamic-pituitary-adrenal (HPA) axis in patients with major depressive disorder, but the methods used to quantify and evaluate this abnormality have been variable and controversial. At present, most investigators (reviewed below) are reporting plasma cortisol values in the afternoon and evening following administration of a 1-mg dose of dexamethasone administered between 9 P.M.and 12 P.M. the day before. The lack of dexamethasone suppression of cortisol below a level of 5 μg per 100 ml of plasma is categorized as nonsuppression. One of the most impressive reports on the utility of this test suggested that genetic subtypes of unipolar primary depressive illness could be distinguished by the DST (Schlesser, Winokur, and Sherman 1979). Familial pure depressive disease was found to have 82% nonsuppression; sporadic depressive disease, 37%; and depressive spectrum disease, 4%. Unfortunately, this robust finding has not been replicated by other investigators (Zimmerman, Coryell, and Pfohl 1986). In addition, false-positive DSTs have been observed in alcohol withdrawal, psychotropic drug withdrawal, acute weight loss, physical exercise, trauma, dehydration, and pulmonary or cardiac disease (Lamberts 1986). Patients with diabetes mellitus are reported to have over a 40% nonsuppression rate (Hudson, Hudson, Rothschild, et al. 1984). Nonsuppression in nondepressed Alzheimer's disease patients ranges from 17% to as high as 80% (Georgotas, McCue, Kim, et al. 1986; McAllister and Hays 1987). Significant rates of nonsuppression are also observed in other psychiatric conditions, with nonsuppression rates as high as 46% in manic disorder, 30% in schizophrenia, and 38% in obsessive-compulsive disorder (Lamberts 1986).

In Table 2, the percentage of patients who were nonsuppressors with a diagnosis of panic disorder is compared to the percentage of nonsuppressors with major depressive disorder. There is a wide range of nonsuppression in panic disorder, half of the studies reporting a range above 18% and the other half below. The rate of nonsuppression in major depressive disorder has ranged between 25% and 82%, with most reviews of the literature reporting the average between 40% and 50%. It is interesting to note in the studies listed in Table 2 that the three studies with concomitant measurements of nonsuppression in panic disorder and major depressive disorder did not find significant differences between the two groups (Avery, Osgood, Ishiki, et al. 1985; Coryell, Noyes, Clancy, et al. 1985; Grunhaus, Flegel, Haskett, et al. 1987). The highest rate of nonsuppression (75%) was observed among inpatients, suggesting that severity of illness or other factors related to general behavioral decompensation is related to nonsuppression of inpatients. Repeated measurements in these patients did not clearly relate to changes in Hamilton depression ratings (Grunhaus, Tiongco, Haskett, et al. 1987). When patients with major depressive disorder alone were compared to patients with simultaneous major depressive disorder and panic disorder at three points during hospitalization, no differences were observed between the two groups (Grunhaus, Flegel, Haskett, et al. 1987). In general, these findings suggest that, in outpatients, patients with panic disorder have less nonsuppression than patients with major depressive disorder; with inpatients, however, the rates are approximately equal. Obviously, there are major differences between the patient samples and the diagnostic thresholds used in the different studies that could contribute to the variability of nonsuppression rates listed in Table 2. However, the data suggest, at least in outpatients, that patients with panic disorder have a nonsuppression rate somewhere between that of normals (approximately 10%) and those with major depressive disorder (approximately 50%).

Even though the DST is the most widely used measure, other abnormalities in HPA axis function have been observed in major depressive disorder and to some degree in panic disorder. It has been quite well established that patients with major depressive disorder have higher serum and urine cortisol levels than controls or patients who are DST suppressors (Rubin, Poland, Lesser, et al. 1987). The HPA axis hyperactivity before dexamethasone administration can account for up to two-thirds of the incidence of DST nonsuppression (Poland, Rubin, Lesser, et al. 1987). This increase in HPA axis activity

Table 2. Dexamethasone Suppression Test in Major Depression and Panic Disorder

	Mean % of patients reported as nonsuppressors	
Study	Major depression	Panic disorder with agoraphobia[a]
Various studies[b]	50[c]	17
Curtis, Cameron, and Nesse (1982)	—	15
Lieberman, Brenner, Lesser, et al. (1983)	—	0
Sheehan, Claycomb, Surman, et al. (1983)	—	12
Whiteford and Evans (1984)	—	29
Bueno, Sabanes,Gascon, et al. (1984)	—	46
Avery, Osgood, Ishiki, et al. (1985)	8	14
Peterson, Ballenger, Cox, et al. (1985)	—	12
Roy-Byrne, Bierer,and Uhde (1985)	—	25
Coryell, Noyes, Clancy, et al. (1985)	16	18
Bridges, Yeragani, Rainey, et al. (1986)	—	13
Judd, Norman, Burrows, et al. (1987)	—	29
Grunhaus, Tiongco, Haskett, et al. (1987)[d]	—	75
Grunhaus, Flegel, Haskett, et al. (1987)[e]	50	56

[a] Median, 18; range, 0–75.
[b] Carroll, Feinberg, Greden, et al. (1981); Carroll (1982); Holsboer (1983); Green and Kane (1983); Shapiro and Lehman (1983).
[c] Range, 25–82.
[d] Inpatients only.
[e] Patients with simultaneous major depression and panic disorder.

is of interest relative to anxiety disorders, since up to 27% of patients with generalized anxiety disorder are nonsuppressors. After successful nondrug behavioral treatment, all of the generalized anxiety disorder patients reverted to suppressors (Tiller, Biddle, Maguire, et al. 1988). This provides evidence that HPA axis function is altered in some patients with anxiety disorders.

In summary, the DST is only sensitive in about 40% to 50% of major depressive disorders, although this may be as high as 70% to 80% in psychotic affective disorders (Arana, Baldessarini, and Ornsteen 1985). Even though the test is highly specific (over 90% in comparison to healthy controls), specificity is considerably reduced when comparisons are made among other medical, neurologic, and psychiatric disorders; depending on the condition, it can drop as low as 30%. The DST has not added much to the prediction of short-term antidepressant response, although some studies using repeated DSTs during clinical treatment find some normalization of the test, usually coinciding with clinical recovery (Baumgartner, Graf, and Kurthen 1986; Peselow, Baxter, Fieve, et al. 1987; Zimmerman, Coryell, and Pfohl 1987). However, peaks of nonsuppression also occurred in over 45% of the patients, irrespective of clinical course (Baumgartner, Graf, and Kurthen 1986). Thus the DST does not appear to be a useful predictor of clinical recovery or relapse. The lack of sensitivity and specificity greatly limits the use of the DST to differentiate disease or pathophysiologic processes leading to the comorbidity of major depressive disorder and panic disorder. At present, it is possible only to estimate that the lower rate of DST nonsuppression in panic disorder relates to the relatively less severe clinical state in the patients sampled. As the panic disorder becomes more severe (e.g., as seen in inpatients), DST nonsuppression rates approach those that are seen in major depressive disorder.

Recent Studies of HPA Axis and Receptor System Function in Major Depressive Disorder and Panic Disorder

In Table 3, similarities and differences between major depressive disorder and panic·disorder are listed for several tests of HPA axis function and receptor system function. When corticotropin-releasing factor (CRF) is administered to patients with major depressive disorder or panic disorder, both diagnostic groups have shown a significantly diminished cumulative adrenocorticotropic hormone (ACTH) response relative to controls (Amsterdam, Maislin, Winokur, et al. 1987; Roy-Byrne, Uhde, Post, et al. 1986). This would suggest a subsensitivity of the CRF receptor systems in the hypothalamus, since at least in major depressive disorder there is an increased cortisol

Table 3.   HPA Axis Function and Alpha-2 Adrenergic Receptor and Beta
Adrenergic Receptor Function in Major Depression and Panic
Disorder, in Comparison to Healthy Controls

Response to test	Major depression	Panic disorder
ACTH response to CRF	Decreased	Decreased
Cortisol response to clonidine	Increased	Increased
Cortisol response to yohimbine	Increased	Increased
Lymphocyte response to mitogen stimulation	Decreased[a]	Normal
Growth hormone response to clonidine	Decreased	Decreased
MHPG response to clonidine	Normal[b]	Increased
MHPG response to yohimbine	Normal	Increased[c]
Plasma melatonin response to nighttime	Decreased	Decreased

Note.   HPA = hypothalamic-pituitary-adrenal; ACTH = adrenocorticotropic
hormone; CRF = corticotropin-releasing factor; MHPG = 3-methoxy-4-
hydroxyphenyleneglycol.
   [a] Dexamethasone suppression test nonsuppressors.
   [b] There is a report of increased MHPG drop following clonidine.
   [c] Only in patients who have frequent panic attacks or have a panic attack following
yohimbine.

response to infused ACTH (Amsterdam, Winokur, Abelman, et al.
1983; Jaeckle, Kathol, Lopez, et al. 1987).

The adrenergic regulation of cortisol secretion is complex. There
is some evidence that the alpha-1 adrenergic receptor system is stimulatory and that the postsynaptic alpha-2 adrenergic system is inhibitory to cortisol release. (The adrenergic receptors have been divided
into subtypes based on the relative responsiveness to different pharmacologic agents.) When the alpha-2 adrenergic agonist clonidine is
administered to patients with major depressive disorder or panic
disorder, both groups show an approximately equal decrease in
plasma cortisol, which is significantly greater than healthy controls for
each diagnostic group (Charney and Heninger 1986a; Siever, Uhde,
and Jimerson 1984). Similarly, when the alpha-2 adrenergic antagonist yohimbine is administered to patients with major depressive
disorder and panic disorder, there is an increase in plasma cortisol
levels in each diagnostic group (Charney, Woods, Goodman, et al.
1987; Price, Charney, Rubin, et al. 1986). An impaired lymphocyte
proliferative response to mitogen has not been found to be associated

with an abnormal DST in depressed patients, but an impaired lymphocyte proliferative response to mitogen was not seen in patients with panic disorder (Surman, Williams, Sheehan, et al. 1986). The growth hormone response to administered clonidine, thought to reflect the sensitivity of postsynaptic alpha-2 adrenergic receptors, is blunted in both major depressive disorder and panic disorder compared to healthy controls (Charney and Heninger 1986a; Charney, Heninger, and Sternberg 1982). The specificity of this test has not been fully developed, but the growth hormone response to clonidine is also blunted in alcohol withdrawal and other conditions involving metabolic abnormalities.

There is considerable evidence that changes in plasma 3-methoxy-4-hydroxyphenyleneglycol (MHPG), a metabolite of norepinephrine, reflect changes in total body norepinephrine turnover as well as that in the brain. Although the amount of MHPG in plasma may only be partly derived from the brain (between 30% and 50%), drugs that decrease norepinephrine turnover in the brain decrease plasma MHPG, and drugs that increase norepinephrine turnover in the brain increase plasma MHPG. Thus, in every instance where brain MHPG changes, plasma MHPG changes proportionally in the same direction. The presynaptic alpha-2 adrenergic receptors located on cell bodies and terminals of noradrenergic neurons act to inhibit cell firing and norepinephrine release when these receptors are stimulated by agonists, such as clonidine. Clonidine has been used as a test of the sensitivity of these receptor systems; when clonidine is administered to healthy controls and patients, there is a decrease in plasma MHPG. It can be seen in Table 3 that, using oral clonidine, MHPG response to clonidine is normal in major depressive disorder but increased in panic disorder (Charney, Heninger, and Sternberg 1982; Siever, Uhde, and Jimerson 1984). One study found that there was an increased MHPG drop following intravenous clonidine in major depressive disorder (Siever, Uhde, and Jimerson 1984). The MHPG response following oral yohimbine is normal in major depressive disorder (Heninger, Charney, and Price 1988), but increased in panic disorder (Charney, Heninger, and Breier 1984). This finding is seen only in patients with frequent panic attacks or in those who have a panic attack immediately following yohimbine administration (Charney, Woods, Goodman, et al. 1987). A possible measure of the beta adrenergic receptor system is the increase in plasma melatonin seen in healthy subjects during nighttime. This increased melatonin level is blunted in major depressive disorder and also in panic disorder (Brown, Kocsis, Caroff, et al. 1985; McIntyre, Norman, Marriott, et al. 1987).

In summary, there does not appear to be a large difference

between major depressive disorder and panic disorder in the abnormality of the responses in five of the eight tests, listed in Table 3. The lymphocytic response to mitogen stimulation was found mainly in patients with abnormal DSTs, and this may account for the differences between the major depressive disorder and panic disorder on this test. Since there is one report of increased MHPG drop following clonidine in major depressive disorder, this test may also not differentiate major depressive disorder and panic disorder.

The only major difference between the two diagnostic groups on the tests listed in Table 3 is the MHPG response to yohimbine, which is limited to a subgroup of panic disorder. The data reviewed in Table 3 suggest that major depressive disorder and panic disorder share a number of abnormalities of neural systems regulating cortisol release, growth hormone release, melatonin secretion, and possibly MHPG response to clonidine and, except for a subgroup of panic disorder patients, possibly the MHPG response to yohimbine. The increased MHPG response to yohimbine is seen only in panic disorder patients with a panic attack following yohimbine, and therefore is not a very sensitive marker (approximately 54% sensitivity) (Charney, Woods, Goodman, et al. 1987). It does appear to be quite specific, however, since the increased MHPG following yohimbine has not been found in other diagnostic groups, including major depressive disorder, schizophrenia, obsessive-compulsive disorder, and generalized anxiety disorder.

Sodium Lactate and Other Provocative Infusion Tests

It has been known for some time that infusion of hypertonic sodium lactate produces panic attacks in vulnerable individuals (Table 4). In patients diagnosed with panic disorder, up to 83% of patients describe panic-like symptoms during these infusions (Liebowitz, Fyer, and Gorman 1984; Liebowitz, Gorman, and Fyer 1985). There have been considerable differences between various studies in the methodology of defining the behavioral end points for panic attacks. With appro-

Table 4. Subjective Reports of Panic Attacks Following Sodium Lactate Infusions, in Percentages

Diagnostic group	Panic attacks
Panic disorder	55–83
Major depression with panic	60–100
Major depression	11–20
Social phobia	7
Healthy controls	0–20

priate controls, the sensitivity of this test approaches the 55% level. It has been reported that in patients with panic attacks that are too infrequent to meet DSM-III (American Psychiatric Association 1980) criteria for panic disorder, the panic attack response rate with sodium lactate is similar to that of patients with frequent panic attacks (Cowley, Dager, Foster, et al. 1987). There have been other reports that sodium lactate increased self-reported anxiety and heart rate equally in patients and controls (Ehlers, Margraf, Roth, et al. 1985).

These discrepancies may reflect differences in patient groups and methodology. When lactate is administered to patients with major depressive disorder with a current or recent history of panic attacks, 60% to 100% of patients are reported to have a lactate-induced panic attack (Cowley, Dager, and Dunner 1986; Dager, Cowley, and Dunner 1987). However, when the test is administered to major depressive disorder patients with a history of panic disorder, the rate of panic attacks is similar to that of patients with social phobia or healthy controls (Cowley, Dager, and Dunner 1987; Dager, Cowley, and Dunner 1987; Liebowitz, Fyer, Gorman, et al. 1987). The subjective experience of panic-like symptomatology during sodium lactate infusion does seem to distinguish patients with panic disorder from those with major depressive disorder. The most interesting finding is that patients with major depressive disorder and panic disorder show response rates similar to those with only panic disorder, indicating that this type of marker may be of use in evaluating the pathophysiology of the two conditions.

There are problems, however, in the use of sodium lactate to stimulate panic-like symptoms. The dependent variable is an end point using a subjective report of symptoms that patients are currently experiencing. That is, patients with panic attacks are only the ones that mainly experience the symptoms, and therefore they are used to reporting these types of symptoms as opposed to the patients with major depressive disorder who are not used to panic experiences. There have not been any large and consistent changes in neuroendocrine or hormonal measures following lactate-induced anxiety (Carr, Sheehan, Surman, et al. 1986). The most important problem in this regard is that panic-like symptoms can be produced in susceptible individuals with a variety of agents, including yohimbine, carbon dioxide, caffeine, isoproterenol, and aspartamine ingestion (Charney, Heninger, and Jatlow 1985; Charney, Woods, Goodman, et al. 1987; Drake 1986; Rainey, Ettedugi, Pfohl, et al. 1984; Woods, Charney, Loke, et al. 1986). To the degree that the compound producing the panic attacks is specific in its mechanism of action, it is possible that information obtained from the use of such agents can be used to understand the neurobiology of the panic attack itself.

Serotonergic Function in Major Depressive Disorder and Panic Disorder

In Table 5 the differences between major depressive disorder and panic disorder across five measures of serotonergic system function are presented. The prolactin response to infusion of large doses of intravenous tryptophan is decreased in major depressive disorder, but is reported to be normal in panic disorder (Charney and Heninger 1986b; Heninger, Charney, and Sternberg 1984). Since tryptophan is a precursor for serotonin, the decreased prolactin response may reflect abnormalities anywhere in the sequence from tryptophan uptake through serotonin release and postsynaptic receptor sensitivity. A more specific test of the system is the use of the serotonin agonist m-chlorophenylpiperazine (MCPP). MCPP produced a normal prolactin response in both major depression and panic disorder; thus the use of the postsynaptic agonist did not demonstrate differences.

Two other measures of serotonergic function can be measured in platelets. Obviously platelets have some difficulties as markers because of the large influence of peripheral metabolic effects on that system. However, it is of interest that platelet serotonin uptake is decreased in major depressive disorder and increased in panic disorder relative to controls (Innis, Charney, and Heninger 1986; Norman, Judd, Gregory, et al. 1986). Also there is evidence that platelet imipramine binding is decreased in major depressive disorder but normal in panic disorder relative to controls (Kafka, Nurnberger, Siever, et al. 1986; Uhde, Berrettini, Roy-Byrne, et al. 1987). Since the imipramine binding is a measure of receptor number connected to the serotonin uptake site, this suggests that there may be some meaningful differences between the two diagnostic groups. Larger studies comparing other diagnostic groups, where these two measures are obtained in the same patients over time and where the effects of treatment are evaluated, need to be conducted.

Table 5. Comparison of Major Depression and Panic Disorder on Measures of Serotonin System Function

Measure of serotonin system function	Major depression	Panic disorder
Prolactin response to IV tryptophan	Decreased	Normal
Prolactin response to IV MCPP	Normal	Normal
Anxiety response to IV MCPP	Normal	Normal
Platelet serotonin uptake	Decreased	Increased
Platelet imipramine binding	Decreased	Normal

Note. IV = intravenous; MCPP = m-chlorophenylpiperazine.

Other Platelet Markers in Major Depressive Disorder and Panic Disorder

Platelets also contain alpha-2 adrenergic receptors and monoamine oxidase type B. Studies of receptor binding in major depressive disorder assessing alpha-2 adrenergic receptor numbers on platelets have been variable, with some studies reporting that major depressive disorder has increased numbers of alpha-2 receptors (Kafka, Nurnberger, Siever, et al. 1986). Other studies have reported no change in panic disorder of platelet alpha-2 binding (Nutt and Fraser 1987). Platelet monoamine oxidase levels have been increased or normal in major depressive disorder, and mixed results have been found of either increased or normal platelet monoamine oxidase activity in panic disorder (Khan, Lee, Dager, et al. 1986; Loosen, Garbutt, and Prange 1987). The use of platelet receptor or enzyme levels as biologic markers in major depressive disorder or panic disorder is problematic because of a large number of factors, such as platelet turnover rate and plasma epinephrine, and cortisol levels that can influence these measures. When correlations are evaluated between platelet and brain monoamine oxidase, individual variations in platelet monoamine oxidase type B activity do not reflect individual variations in either brain cortical monoamine oxidase type B or monoamine oxidase type A activity in patients (Young, Laws, Sharbrough, et al. 1986). Thus there is a considerable problem in the reliability and specificity of the measurement of receptors or enzyme activities in platelets, and this problem greatly reduces the applicability of these techniques to studies of major depressive disorder and panic disorder.

Responses to Thyrotropin-Releasing Hormone and Electroencephalogram Sleep Measurements in Major Depressive Disorder and Panic Disorder

The thyroid-stimulating hormone (TSH) blunting to thyrotropin-releasing hormone (TRH) infusion is not specific for any particular diagnostic group, and its sensitivity is also low (Loosen, Garbutt, and Prange 1987). The prolactin response to TRH is also not abnormal in depressed patients (Unden, Ljunggren, Kjellman, et al. 1987). Therefore the TSH and prolactin response to TRH do not appear to be good measures for distinguishing between panic disorder and major depressive disorder.

There is a large literature (impossible to review here) describing sleep abnormalities in major depressive disorder. Most major depressive disorder patients have more sleep abnormalities than healthy controls. In a study comparing major depressive disorder to major depressive disorder plus panic disorder to panic disorder by itself, all compared to healthy controls, it was found that the major depressive disorder patients were clearly different than the other groups and that the patients who had panic disorder in addition to their major depressive disorder had measures more like the major depressive disorder patients (Dube, Jones, Bell, et al. 1986). The panic disorder patients were not clearly different than the healthy controls. Rapid eye movement latency was reduced in the major depressive disorder patients, and it was intermediate in the mixed group and essentially normal in the panic disorder group. In general these data would suggest that sleep is not very abnormal in panic disorder patients compared to the consistent finding of abnormalities in the sleep of major depressive disorder patients. It is of interest in this regard that major depressive disorder patients show an improvement in their depressive symptomatology following one night's sleep deprivation, but that this improvement is not seen following sleep deprivation in panic disorder (Roy-Byrne, Uhde, and Post 1986). There is some evidence that sleep deprivation may even increase symptoms in panic disorder (Roy-Byrne, Uhde, and Post 1986). The sleep studies do appear to indicate some abnormalities in the major depressive disorder group not shared by the panic disorder group. Sleep symptomatology in patients with both major depressive disorder and panic disorder is somewhere in between. Because of the difficult technology of these studies, repeated measurements during clinical course and treatment have not been fully completed.

Other Possible Biologic Markers in Major Depressive Disorders and Panic Disorder

There is a large literature evaluating the possibility that mitral valve prolapse is related to panic disorder (Shear, Devereux, and Kramer-Fox 1984; Uhde and Kellner 1987) (Table 6). Although most studies find some increased incidence of mitral valve prolapse in panic disorder, there is considerable variability from study to study. In general, most of the literature on this topic finds that the specificity of this

Table 6. Comparison of Major Depression and Panic Disorder on Other Medical and Neurologic Measures

	Major depression	Panic disorder
Mitral valve prolapse	Normal	Increased
Vestibular neurologic findings	Not tested	Increased
Positron emission tomography—blood flow	Not tested	Asymmetry

measure relative to panic disorder is too low to be of much use. The incidence of mitral valve prolapse has not been extensively investigated in major depressive disorder, but generally the abnormality is not as clear as in panic disorder.

The finding of focal neurologic signs usually excludes a diagnosis of major depressive disorder or panic disorder. However, many panic attacks can manifest as focal neurologic symptoms. Therefore, focal neurologic symptoms should not exclude a diagnosis of panic attack (Coyle and Sterman 1986). In patients with panic disorder presenting with dizziness, up to 67% are observed to have abnormalities on otoneurologic examination (Jacob, Moller, Turner, et al. 1985). Even though the abnormalities exist in panic disorder, parallel studies have not been done in a controlled group of major depressive disorders with dizziness; thus the specificity of this marker is not clear. Cerebral ventricular size has not been clearly reported as abnormal in panic disorder or most patients with major depressive disorder (Uhde and Kellner 1987). Both in panic disorder and major depressive disorders the presence of clear changes in cerebral ventricular size often results in the diagnosis being changed to something else. The result is a problem in circular reasoning; studies reporting increased ventricular size exclude patients from a major depressive disorder or panic disorder diagnosis, and thus the claim that this could not be a marker for the excluded disorders is not entirely correct.

One of the more interesting findings relevant to major depressive disorder and panic disorder is the finding of an asymmetry in glucose metabolism in the brains of patients with panic disorder who had panic attacks following lactate. This study requires the use of positron emission tomography and has not been studied in major depressive disorder, so the specificity of this finding has yet to be demonstrated (Reiman, Raichle, Robins et al. 1986).

DISCUSSION

Assuming that the temporal interaction of two disease processes leading to comorbidity is of most importance, the biologic markers reviewed above in major depressive disorder and panic disorder do not appear to have the necessary sensitivity and specificity to be of much use. This conclusion may represent difficulties in the diagnostic purity of the samples studied and the inability of the investigators to delineate subtypes within the diagnostic groups appropriately. It also may represent the lack of specificity of the biologic markers. When marker-positive individuals are compared to marker-negative individuals, either cross-sectionally or longitudinally, no clear differences in disease course or treatment response are seen. It is possible that the markers utilized reflect variable abnormalities in neurobiologic systems that are not directly related to the pathogenesis of a disease process. This possibility is not surprising, since within these broad diagnostic syndromes there may be many biologically pure subgroups.

Specific and different enzymatic defects in brain metabolism could easily lead to similar-appearing clinical pictures (as clearly demonstrated in the field of mental deficiency, where specific genetic enzymatic abnormalities give similar-appearing gross clinical pictures). Hypothetically, subtypes of major depressive disorder or panic disorder could involve a number of neurochemically separate abnormalities that we are not able to evaluate currently. Compared to the sensitivity and specificity of other medical methods of diagnosis, the measurement in major depressive disorder and panic disorder of neuroendocrine variables either at rest or following stimulation, or the measurement of platelet protein levels, are very nonspecific methods. To have the sensitivity and specificity comparable to measures used in other fields of medicine, an exact abnormality within a specifically defined biochemical system of the brain or brain area would need to be assessed. Given that this assessment is not currently possible (and may not be possible in the near future), our ability to develop and utilize specific and sensitive biologic methods for the temporal assessment of the disease process in major depressive disorder and panic disorder appears difficult.

In review of the findings listed in Tables 2 through 6, the following interpretations could be proposed.

HPA Axis and Adrenergic Receptor System Functioning

Since the HPA axis findings in major depressive disorder and panic disorder are not grossly abnormal in comparison to diseases of HPA such as Cushing's syndrome or Addison's disease, the observed DST nonsuppression and blunted response to CRF may represent secondary consequences or adaptive compensations to the stress of the condition. The increased frequency of DST nonsuppression in hospitalized patients with panic disorder suggests that the general stress and behavioral decompensation related to inpatient hospitalization is a major factor in nonsuppression. The lower incidence of DST nonsuppression in panic disorder could easily reflect the less stressed behavioral decompensation of these patients relative to major depressive disorder patients. Future studies would have to control for these nonspecific variables carefully to differentiate the groups.

The blunted ACTH response to CRF and the increased response of cortisol to clonidine and yohimbine seen in major depressive disorder and panic disorder also could be interpreted as nonspecific alterations of the HPA axis in the direction of an overreactivity of a system common to both disorders. The similar blunted growth hormone response to clonidine and the blunted nighttime plasma melatonin response in major depressive disorder and panic disorder may also reflect some nonspecific arousal factors. The one finding that does beckon further investigation is the markedly increased MHPG response to yohimbine seen in panic disorder patients who have frequent panic attacks or panic attack following yohimbine. This MHPG change may point to some specific abnormality in the noradrenergic system in panic disorder.

Provocation Studies

The increased frequency of subjectively reported panic attacks following infusion of sodium lactate, and administration of yohimbine, isoproterinol, caffeine, and other agents in panic disorder patients is not extrememly sensitive, but it may be more specific. Unfortunately, the specificity does not add much information as to the biologic factors involved, since widely differing agents produce the effect. A more parsimonious interpretation would be that the subjective symptomatology is reported as a consequence of unstable neurobiologic systems, which can be provoked by a number of pharmacologic probes.

The use of known provocative tests does not improve our ability to evaluate these processes at different points in time, since the tests are no more sensitive or specific than the clinical diagnosis of symptoms at any point in time. Investigations as to the possible neurobiologic abnormalities that might subserve the abnormal subjective response to these provocative agents are clearly worthwhile. Possibly, with further development of more specific measures, this method will be of more use in the future.

Serotonin System

The abnormalities in the serotonergic system have not been as extensively studied as those in the HPA axis. As with the DST, the patients with major depressive disorder and panic disorder need to be stratified according to severity of illness and inpatient and outpatient status. It is of interest that both platelet serotonin uptake and platelet imipramine binding are decreased in major depressive disorder, and increased or normal, respectively, in panic disorder. Whether the alterations observed in platelets are also present in the brain and could account for the decreased response to tryptophan in major depressive disorder patients remains to be demonstrated. The availability of more specific serotonin agonists for use in the probing of the neuroendocrine system in patients, as well as for treatment of the two conditions should provide improved information on these questions.

The greater abnormality of sleep measures in major depressive disorder compared to panic disorder as with the HPA axis may be related to disease severity. As yet, these measures have not been sufficiently reliable to disentangle the clinical course of patients with panic disorder or mixed panic disorder and major depressive disorder. The other measures, including mitral valve prolapse, vestibular dysfunction, and the positron emission tomography blood flow studies, are not advanced enough to provide reliable markers at this time.

Evaluation of Specificity of Pharmacologic Treatments for Major Depressive Disorders and Panic Disorder

There is not sufficient space here to fully review the specificity of pharmacologic treatments in major depressive disorder and panic disorder, and only the major classes of drug treatments can be mentioned. In general, positive clinical responses in both disorders have been reported for all of the treatments utilized in either condition. Antidepressants such as imipramine and monoamine oxidase inhibitors are useful in the treatment of major depressive disorder and panic disorder. Benzodiazepines (e.g., alprazolam), which are effective in the treatment of panic disorder, have been reported to be effective antidepressants. One of the best types of evidence on nonspecificity of the pharmacologic treatments is the fact that both major depressive disorder and panic disorder respond to the same drugs that alter function of the serotonin system. There have been one or two studies with mianserin and bupropion, which do not appear to be effective in panic disorder, but these studies need replication and further evaluation across different dosages. Electroconvulsive treatment, which is effective in the treatment of major depressive disorder, has not been systematically applied to the treatment of panic disorder; because of medical and social considerations, it probably never will be.

In general, the response to treatment demonstrates more similarities than differences between major depressive disorder and panic disorder. This conclusion suggests two possibilities. One is that the drugs are acting at a superficial level of the pathologic problem to provide compensatory mechanisms for symptom reduction. The alternative is that major depressive disorder and panic disorder are symptomatic manifestations of the same underlying neurobiologic process; therefore, they would be expected to respond equally well to the same treatments. The second alternative would indicate that there is not true comorbidity, but that both disorders represent different

Chapter 25

Interpretative Aspects of Biologic Markers in Psychiatry in Relation to Issues of Comorbidity

Russell E. Poland, M.D.

THE CHAPTER BY Heninger (Chapter 24) clearly illustrates the complexities associated with using biologic markers to understand the relationships among psychiatric disorders. Unfortunately, most if not all biologic markers do not show sufficient sensitivity and specificity for routine clinical use. Rather than address issues associated with each of the markers discussed by Heninger, this chapter will highlight some of the more basic issues associated with the use and interpretation of biologic markers in general and present some real and theoretical examples as illustrations. Most of the illustrations will deal with markers associated with the neuroendocrine system, but the basic principles also should apply to markers associated with other physiologic systems.

METHODOLOGICAL ASPECTS ASSOCIATED WITH THE DEXAMETHASONE SUPPRESSION TEST

One of the most studied biologic markers in psychiatry is the dexamethasone suppression test (DST) response (Carroll, Feinberg, Greden, et al. 1981). Approximately 5% to 10% of normal subjects show

This work was supported by National Institute of Mental Health grant MH-34471, Research Scientist Development Award MH-00534, BRSG funds (S07-RR-05551) awarded by the Biomedical Research Support Grant Program, Division of Research Resources, National Institutes of Health, and by the National Institutes of Health General Clinical Research Center grant RR-00425.

DST nonsuppression/escape, whereas 25% to 75% of patients with major depression show an abnormal response. However, the mechanism(s) underlying the abnormal response is unknown, as is its meaning. Direct and indirect evidence obtained from numerous studies of the hypothalamic-pituitary-adrenal (HPA) axis suggest that there is enhanced driving of central nervous system control over the secretion of corticotropin-releasing factor (Banki, Bissette, Arato, et al. 1987; Gold and Chrousos 1985), resulting in enhanced adrenocorticotropic hormone (ACTH) and cortisol secretion. However, the central neurotransmitter system(s) that underlies the observed pathophysiology is unknown.

It has been suggested that patients showing DST nonsuppression might be more responsive to somatic treatment (Brown, Haier, and Qualls 1980). However, the difference in response to treatment between escapers and suppressors has been inconsistent and modest at best (American Psychiatric Association Task Force on the Use of Laboratory Tests in Psychiatry 1987). In part, methodological issues could account for this, issues relevant to the study of comorbidity.

For example, depending on the dose of dexamethasone (DEX) administered, different groups of escapers and suppressors can be created (Poland, Rubin, Lane, et al. 1985). Figure 1 shows the DST

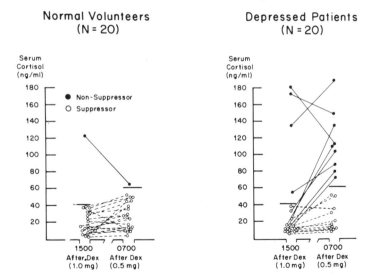

Figure 1. Comparison of two dexamethasone (DEX) suppression tests in normal volunteers and in endogenously depressed patients. For the 1.0-mg test, DEX was administered at 2300 hours and blood was obtained at 1500 hours the following afternoon. For the 0.5-mg test, DEX was administered at 2300 hours and blood was obtained at 0700 hours the following morning. *Closed circles* = DEX escapers; *open circles* = DEX suppressors (Poland, Rubin, Lane, et al. 1985).

response in 20 control subjects and 20 major depressive patients to the standard 1.0-mg DST and a modified 0.5-mg DST. For both forms of the test, DEX was administered the night before at 2300 hours. On the left, serum cortisol was measured in 20 normal volunteers who received both the 0.5-mg and the 1.0-mg DSTs. Nineteen normal subjects showed serum concentrations <40 ng/ml at 1500 hours (16 hours) after the 1.0-mg DST and <60 ng/ml at 0700 hours (8 hours) after the 0.5-mg DST. One normal volunteer was an escaper during both tests. On the right, post-DEX cortisol results for 20 patients with a Research Diagnostic Criteria (RDC) (Spitzer, Endicott, and Robins 1978a) diagnosis of definite endogenous depression are shown. Four patients who showed elevations of serum cortisol concentrations >40 ng/ml at 1500 hours after 1.0 mg DEX (nonsuppressors) also had serum cortisol concentrations >60 ng/ml at 0700 hours after 0.5 mg DEX and were considered nonsuppressors on this test as well. Eleven patients suppressed after both DSTs. However, 5 of the 20 patients who were suppressors based on their 1500-hour serum cortisol concentrations (<40 ng/ml) following the 1.0-mg DEX dose showed 0700-hour serum cortisol concentrations >60 ng/ml following the 0.5-mg DEX dose and would be considered nonsuppressors during the modified DST. Consequently, if one was to perform a treatment study with patients subdivided by pretreatment DST response, the interpretation of the treatment results could be radically different, depending on whether the results of the 1.0-mg DST or the 0.5-mg DST were used to classify the patients as escapers or suppressors.

In addition to the form of the DST, serum DEX concentrations have been found to be lower in subjects who show DST nonsuppression compared with those who show suppression (Lowy and Meltzer 1987). Thus cortisol nonsuppression might not always be a reflection of heightened activity of the central control of the HPA axis, but could be due to insufficient circulating levels of DEX.

To determine the contribution of serum DEX concentrations and HPA activity before DEX administration to the DST response, we measured 24-hour serum cortisol concentration before DEX and serum cortisol and DEX concentrations at 8, 16, and 24 hours after DEX administration (Poland, Rubin, Lesser, et al. 1987). Using a series of discriminant function analyses, we found that both serum DEX and pre-DEX HPA activity contributed to the DST response, but that pre-DEX HPA activity contributed more. As illustrated in Figure 2, approximately one-sixth to one-third of the escapers might have done so due to insufficient circulating DEX concentrations. In contrast, many subjects with elevated 24-hour pre-DEX cortisol concentrations were classified as suppressors. It appears that the standard 1.0 mg-DST might misclassify some patients as escapers due to inadequate

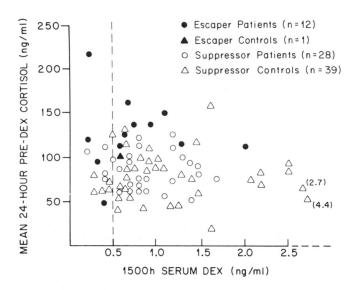

Figure 2.   Bivariate scatter plot of mean 24-hour cortisol concentrations before dexamethasone (DEX) administration versus serum DEX concentrations at 1500 hours for endogenously depressed patients and normal control subjects. *Closed circles* = escaper patients; *open circles* = suppressor patients; *closed triangles* = escaper control subjects; *open triangles* = suppressor control subjects (Poland, Rubin, Lesser, et al. 1987).

serum DEX concentrations, and misclassify some patients as suppressors even though they have elevated pre-DEX HPA activity.

As mentioned in the previous chapter, there are some reports of DST nonsuppression in patients with panic disorder with agoraphobia (Heninger, Chapter 24, Table 2). Whether nonsuppression in this population is due to elevated HPA activity, similar to that observed in many depressed patients, or to insufficient serum DEX levels needs to be addressed. If one is to use the DST as a biologic test for teasing out issues of comorbidity, the methodological aspects of the test need to be refined further. The form of the test administered and DEX metabolism could account for the inconsistent DST results not only in depressed patients, but in patients with panic disorder or generalized anxiety disorder as well (Carson, Halbreich, Yeh, et al. 1988; Tiller, Biddle, Maguire, et al. 1987).

It is worth emphasizing that, methodological aspects aside, a normal DST does not eliminate depression as a core phenomenon in panic and anxiety disorders. Since the sensitivity of the DST is only about 50% for major depression, it is conceivable that panic disorder and generalized anxiety disorder are manifestations of depression, but in a form that is associated only with a normal DST response.

Thus the comorbidity of major depression and panic disorder or major depression and generalized anxiety disorder cannot be resolved using the DST until we better understand more fundamental aspects of this test, as well as other tests of the HPA axis.

NEUROTRANSMITTER HIERARCHIES AND NEUROENDOCRINE RESPONSES

In addition to methodological issues, as illustrated by the DST, another difficulty associated with the use and interpretation of biologic markers is the dearth of information related to the pathophysiologic underpinnings of the markers being investigated. The neuroendocrine system will be used to illustrate this point.

It is now appreciated that secretion of anterior pituitary hormones is prominently regulated by the central nervous system. Small polypeptide and catecholamine hormones are secreted into the portal vessels of the pituitary stalk from neurosecretory cells in the external layer of the median eminence of the basal hypothalamus and are carried to the anterior pituitary to stimulate or inhibit the synthesis of pituitary hormones and their release into the systemic circulation. Various (putative) neurotransmitters (such as dopamine, norepinephrine, serotonin, acetylcholine, gamma aminobutyric acid, and histamine), as well as some recently described central peptides (such as corticotropin-releasing factor, endorphins, bombesin, substance P, and vasoactive intestinal peptide), appear to be involved in the regulation of hypothalamic neuropeptide release. These neurotransmitters and/or neuromodulators may act singly to increase or decrease the secretion of a specific pituitary hormone, but more likely a number of different transmitters are involved in a complex web of interactions, with the final response of the pituitary being determined by their net influence on the secretion of hypothalamic releasing and inhibiting factors into the hypophysial portal blood. Due to this issue of circuitry, it is difficult to know for sure which systems are responsible for an abnormal neuroendocrine response to the administration of a neurotransmitter agonist or antagonist.

For example, it has been reported that the prolactin response to serotonin, or 5-hydroxytryptophan (Heninger, Charney, and Sternberg 1984) and fenfluramine (Siever, Murphy, Slater, et al. 1984) is blunted in depressed patients, suggesting that the serotonin system(s) controlling prolactin secretion is abnormal. It also has been shown that the prolactin response to methadone or morphine is diminished in depressed patients compared to normal control subjects, suggesting an abnormality of the opioid system(s) as well (Extein, Pottash, Gold, et al. 1980; Judd, Risch, Parker, et al. 1982;

Robertson, Jackman, and Meltzer 1984). These results would suggest that both opioid and serotonin systems involved in the regulation of prolactin secretion are abnormal. However, as discussed below, it also is possible that neither of these systems is abnormal or involved in the aberrant prolactin response.

Figure 3 shows a simplified and schematized drawing illustrating the linkage of dopamine, opioid, and serotonin systems, which regulate prolactin secretion. Enhancement of opioid and serotonin neurotransmission stimulates prolactin secretion, whereas increased dopaminergic transmission inhibits its release. As can be seen, both the opioid and the serotonin systems could influence prolactin secretion directly or via stimulation of dopaminergic activity. The abnormal response of prolactin to opioid or serotonergic challenges might be due directly to these systems themselves, or to the abnormal response of the tuberoinfundibular dopamine system to these agents, with the opioid and serotonin systems being normal. Therefore, if panic disorder patients, generalized anxiety disorder patients, and depressed patients all (hypothetically) showed a blunted prolactin response to the administration of a serotonin agonist, one group might have an abnormality of their dopamine system, another an opioid abnormality, and the third a serotonin abnormality. Conversely, both depressed patients and patients with panic disorder might show a normal prolactin response to serotonin agonist administration (Hen-

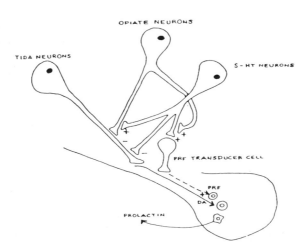

Figure 3. Hypothetical interplay among serotonin (5-HT), opiate, and tuberoinfundibular dopamine (TIDA) neurons in the control of prolactin secretion (Tuomisto and Mannisto 1985).

inger, Chapter 24, Table 5). However, this should not be interpreted to mean that serotonin systems controlling prolactin secretion are normal in both groups. It is possible that one of the groups might actually have both an abnormal serotonin and dopamine system, with the net prolactin response to serotonin stimulation being normal. Due to the complexity and multifactorial control of most physiologic systems, particularly important physiologic systems, the same principles would apply to other biologic markers such as rapid eye movement sleep (REM) latency (Kupfer and Ehlers 1989) or platelet imipramine binding. Without knowing the normal physiology of the biologic markers being measured, inaccurate conclusions easily could be drawn.

COMPENSATORY PHYSIOLOGIC RESPONSES

Another level of complexity associated with the use of biologic markers for addressing issues of comorbidity deals with the attempt by physiologic systems to compensate for an abnormality. This issue has been nicely illustrated at the preclinical level by Downs, Britton, Gibbs, et al. (1987). For this study, adult male rats were injected focally with 6-hydroxydopamine to lesion dopamine systems in the caudate nuclei. One week later the animals were challenged with physostigmine (an indirectly acting cholinergic agonist). Rats were killed 20 minutes after physostigmine, and blood was collected for the measurement of plasma ACTH concentrations by radioimmunoassay. As shown in Figure 4, the 6-hydroxydopamine-lesioned animals showed an enhanced ACTH response to physostigmine compared to the sham-lesioned control animals. Even though the primary insult was on the dopaminergic system, an apparent compensatory cholinergic response occurred.

To illustrate this phenomenon further, I have found that the administration of para-chloroamphetamine (PCA), an amphetamine derivative that selectively lesions serotonin systems (Sanders-Bush, Bushing, and Snyder 1975), also produced animals who showed an enhanced HPA response to physostigmine administration. Adult male rats were treated with saline or PCA and then challenged with saline or physostigmine 7 days later. Thirty minutes after physostigmine administration, the animals were killed and blood was collected for the measurement of plasma corticosterone concentrations. Figure 5 shows that pretreatment with PCA significantly enhanced the corticosterone response to physostigmine. Thus lesions of either dopamine or serotonin systems produce similar neuroendocrine effects associated with the cholinergic control of the HPA axis.

It has been reported that patients with major depression manifest

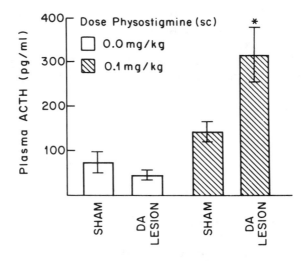

Figure 4. Plasma adrenocorticotropic hormone (ACTH) levels 20 minutes after saline or physostigmine (0.10 mg/kg) in sham and dopamine-lesioned rats. (Modified from Downs, Britton, Gibbs, et al. 1987.)

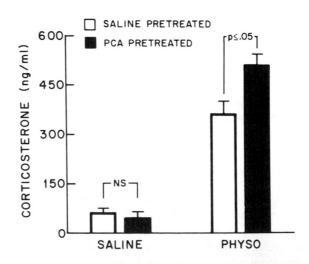

Figure 5. Plasma corticosterone concentrations 30 minutes after saline or physostigmine (PHYSO) (0.25 mg/kg) in saline or para-chloroamphetamine (PCA) (17.0 mg/kg) pretreated rats (R. E. Poland, unpublished).

a heightened sensitivity of REM sleep latency and neuroendocrine responses to cholinergic challenges (Risch, Janowsky, and Gillin 1983; Sitaram and Gillin 1980). It does not appear that patients with generalized anxiety disorder show comparable sensitivity, at least for the generation of REM sleep as determined by the cholinergic REM induction test. This test employs the use of directly or indirectly acting cholinergic agonists to initiate REM sleep when administered 10 minutes after the end of the first REM period (Sitaram and Gillin 1980). Researchers have reported that patients with major depression show a greater sensitivity to REM sleep induction by cholinergic agonists compared to normal controls. Interestingly, this increased sensitivity remains after remission and also occurs in subjects with a family history of affective disorders.

In contrast, patients with generalized anxiety disorder do not show this increased sensitivity to the induction of REM sleep (Sitaram, Dube, Jones, et al. 1984). In addition, patients with a primary generalized anxiety disorder and a secondary depression show a cholinergic REM sleep induction similar to those patients with generalized anxiety disorder alone, whereas patients with a primary major depressive disorder and with a secondary generalized anxiety disorder show responses to the induction test similar to those patients with a major depression alone. Thus this test appears to differentiate depression from anxiety, and it certainly warrants further investigation. However, even if this test eventually is shown to have excellent sensitivity and specificity for separating depression from anxiety, any conclusions regarding comorbidity need to be tempered for the reasons discussed above.

In conclusion, the difficulty with addressing the issue of comorbidity from a biologic perspective is that the available markers are not sufficiently sensitive or specific for a single disorder, and therefore their application to the understanding of comorbidity is limited. Greater attention needs to be paid to methodological issues and to better understanding the physiology of the systems being studied before we can truly understand pathophysiology and apply our findings to issues of comorbidity. In addition, by studying the relationships among biologic abnormalities within subject and patient groups, greater validity can be placed on the interpretation of the results from the individual tests. Further study is definitely warranted for both practical and heuristic reasons.

Chapter 26

Corticotropin-Releasing Factor as a Possible Cause of Comorbidity in Anxiety and Depressive Disorders

Pamela D. Butler, Ph.D.
Charles B. Nemeroff, M.D., Ph.D.

A S THE TITLE of this volume indicates, a number of patients with anxiety disorders exhibit signs and symptoms of depression and vice versa. Prospective and retrospective longitudinal studies described in this volume (Regier, Burke, and Burke, Chapter 6; Angst, Vollrath, Merikangas, et al., Chapter 7; Hagnell and Gräsbeck, Chapter 8) all suggest that the overlap between these two disorders is real and not artifactual.

A question of paramount importance is whether anxiety and depressive disorders share a common etiology and pathogenesis or whether they are distinct disorders that are causally unrelated. Another possibility is that mixtures of the two syndromes (e.g., anxious depression) that differ qualitatively from primary depressive or primary anxiety disorders occur. This dilemma is, of course, analogous to the biologic concept of *parallel* evolution in which similar evolutionary adaptations occur in evolutionarily different biologic structures. One well-known example is the development of long jaws and numerous teeth in animals that feed on fish. This is found in certain fish themselves (garfish) and in crocodiles, birds, and mammals (Young

Supported by National Institute of Mental Health grants MH-42088, MH-40159, and MH-15177.

1962). Investigators are unable to distinguish populations that parallel new developments from those that are descended from each other. In fact, there are a number of examples in medicine in which disorders with different etiologies present with similar symptoms (e.g., Alzheimer's disease and depressive pseudodementia) and, conversely, where the same pathologic process presents quite differently (e.g., syphilis).

Several studies have provided evidence that depression and anxiety disorders may be causally linked in some patients. Epidemiologic studies by Merikangas (Chapter 21) and Weissman (Chapter 22) indicate that these two disorders may indeed share a common etiology. Further, studies by Angst, Vollrath, Merikangas, et al. (Chapter 7) and Hagnell and Gräsbeck (Chapter 8) and others (for a review, see Stavrakaki and Vargo 1986) show that patients with depression are more likely later to develop anxiety disorders than the converse. Thus anxiety may, in some patients, be a precondition or predispose to depression. Indeed, it has been suggested that stress by increasing anxiety may precipitate depression (Lesse 1982).

Parenthetically, it is crucial to note the importance of differentiating between subtypes of anxiety and affective disorders in carrying out and assessing studies on comorbidity. Dealy, Ishiki, Avery, et al. (1981) found that comorbidity occurs more frequently beween panic and depression than between depression and other types of anxiety disorders (e.g., generalized anxiety disorder). Further, Mountjoy and Roth (1982a, 1982b) advocated the position that anxiety and depression can be differentiated on a number of variables, including rating scales, but did not include endogenous depressives in some of their studies.

Biologic findings also indicate a lack of clear differentiation between anxiety and depressive disorders. For example, tricyclic antidepressants are efficacious in treating both panic disorder and major depression (Fyer, Liebowitz, and Klein, Chapter 37), and anxiolytics have been successfully used to treat depressed patients (Amsterdam, Kaplan, Potter, et al. 1986; Dunner, Myers, Khan, et al. 1987; Henry, Market, Emken, et al. 1970). Further, as discussed by Heninger (Chapter 24), a number of the same neuroendocrine abnormalities occur in both depression and panic disorder. From these data, Heninger suggests that there may be a noradrenergic abnormality common to both disorders. However, it is important to note that it is not yet clear whether these similarities are due to a lack of specificity of these biologic markers in differentiating between the two disorders or whether they are indicative of a common etiology.

Briley, Langer, Raisman, et al. (1980) reported that the number of platelet-binding sites for [^{3}H]-imipramine, which in brain binds to presynaptic serotonergic nerve terminals, is markedly reduced in drug-free depressed patients when compared to controls. This finding is particularly striking in elderly depressed patients (Nemeroff, Knight, Krishnan, et al. 1988). Pertinent to the present discussion are recent reports that patients with generalized anxiety disorder or panic disorder have a normal number of [³H]-imipramine binding sites to platelets (Schneider, Munjack, Severson, et al. 1987; Uhde, Berretini, Roy-Byrne, et al. 1987). Data derived from longitudinal studies using biologic markers specific for anxiety and depression should help in understanding the nature of comorbidity. [³H]-imipramine binding to platelets would be a good candidate for use as a marker in such longitudinal studies.

Clearly, a more thorough understanding of the biologic basis of these disorders will be crucial in determining whether anxiety and depressive disorders share a common etiology or whether they are separate clinical entities. Over the years, several biologic theories of depressive and anxiety disorders have appeared. These include biogenic amine theories of depression involving norepinephrine and serotonin (Schildkraut 1965; Schildkraut and Kety 1967; Sulser, Vetulani, and Mobley 1978; for a review, see Jesberger and Richardson 1985) and the hypothesis that benzodiazepines exert their beneficial effect in anxiety disorders by increasing gamma-aminobutyric acid (GABA)-ergic transmission (Costa 1980; Haefely 1984; Tallman, Thomas, and Gallager 1978; for a review, see Shepard 1987) and decreasing serotonergic neuronal activity (Nishikawa and Scatton 1986; Stein, Belluzzi, and Wise 1977; Thiebot, Hamon, and Soubrie 1982; Tye, Iversen, and Green 1979). Increased synaptic availability of norepinephrine has also been implicated in anxiety disorders (Liebowitz, Fyer, McGrath, et al. 1981; Redmond and Huang 1979; Redmond, Huang, Snyder, et al. 1976). Thus both catecholamines and indoleamines have been implicated in the pathophysiology of depression and anxiety. There is, however, still considerable controversy regarding the nature of the involvement of these neurotransmitters in anxiety and depressive disorders, so that it is not yet possible to make a definitive statement regarding the biologic underpinnings of symptom comorbidity in depressive and anxiety disorders based on these data.

Recently, a number of investigators have posited a pivotal role for neuropeptides in psychiatric disorders. The neuropeptide corticotropin-releasing factor (CRF) has been hypothesized to play a role in the pathophysiology of both anxiety and depressive disorders. This peptide, when injected directly into the brains of laboratory animals, produces a number of behavioral effects that are common to both major depression and anxiety disorders. These include sleep disturbances, psychomotor agitation, and appetite loss. CRF also produces a number of the autonomic nervous system alterations seen in patients with panic disorder, generalized anxiety disorder, and posttraumatic stress disorder, and produces the increased startle response seen in generalized anxiety disorder and posttraumatic stress disorder and the decreased libido characteristically seen in depression.

In this chapter, following a review of CRF regulation of the hypothalamic-pituitary-adrenal (HPA) axis, we will present preclinical and clinical evidence suggesting that CRF hypersecretion is involved in the pathogenesis of both anxiety and depressive disorders. While it is clearly premature to make a definitive statement regarding the biologic basis of comorbidity in depressive and anxiety disorders, if the two disorders do in fact share a common etiology, CRF hypersecretion is a plausible candidate.

CRF REGULATION OF THE HPA AXIS

After a more than 25-year attempt, the 41 amino acid structure of CRF was isolated and sequenced by Vale, Spiess, Rivier, et al. (1981) from 490,000 fragments of ovine hypothalami. The intense effort to elucidate the chemical identity of CRF was due both to its seminal involvement in the neuroendocrine response to stress and to its role as the cephalic representative of the HPA axis. Selye (1936) originally described the stress response more than 50 years ago. It consists of an initial alarm reaction in which the animal's resources are mobilized so it can respond to stress, followed by a period of adaptation to continued stress, followed eventually by death if the stress does not cease. During the alarm reaction, adrenocorticotropic hormone (ACTH) is released from the anterior pituitary where it acts on its target organ, the adrenal cortex, causing both increased synthesis and release of corticosteroids into peripheral circulation. The adrenal medulla, an integral component of the sympathetic nervous system, responds by releasing epinephrine and norepinephrine. For this reason, the term *sympathoadrenal response* is often used to describe the organism's response to stress.

We now know that the brain is intimately involved in controlling the release of anterior pituitary hormones. Many years ago, Harris (1948) postulated that a substance produced in the hypothalamus could be humorally transported to the anterior pituitary via a specialized portal system where it could stimulate the secretion of anterior pituitary hormones such as ACTH. There was already anatomic evidence for this specialized circulatory pathway (Popa and Fielding 1930). Indeed, subsequent experiments conducted by Harris and others (for a review, see Guillemin 1980) conclusively demonstrated that the hypothalamus, not the pituitary, is the "master gland" producing hypophysiotropic substances that control release of anterior pituitary hormones (the chemotransmitter portal vessel hypothesis), and that a CRF controlling release of ACTH did in fact exist. Thus the isolation, characterization, and sequencing of CRF as a 41 amino acid peptide by Vale, Spiess, Rivier, et al. (1981) paved the way for understanding neural control of stress responses. CRF indeed appears to be the major physiologic regulator of ACTH secretion. Hemorrhage stress induces a twofold increase in the concentration of CRF in hypothalamo-hypophyseal portal plasma (Plotsky and Vale 1984). Intravenous and intracerebroventricular CRF injections stimulate the release of ACTH from the pituitary (Carsia, Weber, and Perez 1986; Donald, Redekopp, Cameron, et al. 1983; Rock, Oldfield, Schulte, et al. 1984), and immunoneutralization of CRF blocks CRF- and stress-induced ACTH release (Rivier, Rivier, and Vale 1982). As depicted in Figure 1, the effects of CRF on the HPA axis are under stimulatory and

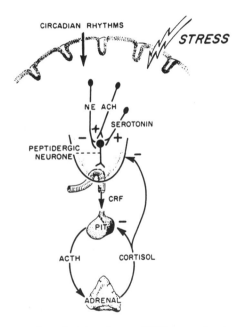

Figure 1. Corticotropin-releasing factor (CRF) secretion into the hypophyseal portal system is under excitatory (+) and inhibitory (−) control by neurotransmitters, which are affected by both stress and circadian rhythms. CRF stimulates adrenocorticotropic hormone (ACTH) release from the anterior pituitary (PIT) gland which in turn causes cortisol to be secreted from the adrenal gland. Cortisol exerts negative feedback at the level of the pituitary and in the central nervous system. NE = norepinephrine; ACH = acetylcholine. (Modified from Martin and Reichlin 1987 with permission from the authors.)

inhibitory control by neurotransmitters and include negative feedback by corticosteroids at pituitary and central nervous system sites.

In accord with its neuroendocrine role in regulating HPA axis activity, CRF-containing neurons are localized in the paraventricular nucleus of the hypothalamus, which projects to the median eminence, the site of the primary plexus of the hypothalamo-hypophyseal portal system (Antoni, Palkovits, Makara, et al. 1983; Liposits, Lengvari, Vigh, et al. 1983; Merchenthaler, Vigh, Petrusz, et al. 1983). Like a number of other hypothalamic release and release-inhibiting hormones originally thought to subserve only neuroendocrine functions (e.g., thyrotropin-releasing hormone, somatotropin-release inhibiting factor, and gonadotropin-releasing hormone), CRF has been found to have a wide extrahypothalamic distribution, which provides the anatomic basis for its role in brain functions, in addition to its regulation of the HPA axis. The extrahypothalamic distribution of CRF is compatible with an involvement in stress responses and emotionality because it is found in a number of forebrain limbic areas such as the central and medial nuclei of the amygdala (Fellman, Bugnon, and Gouger 1982; Merchenthaler, 1984; Moga and Gray 1985), the bed nucleus of the stria terminalis, substantia innominata, septum, preoptic area, and lateral hypothalamus (Chappell, Smith, Kilts, et al. 1986; Merchenthaler 1984; Swanson, Sawchenko, Rivier, et al. 1983). CRF is also found in brain-stem nuclei involved in stress responses and regulation of the autonomic nervous system such as the locus coeruleus, the parabrachial nucleus, and the dorsal vagal complex (Chappell, Smith, Kilts, et al. 1986; Merchenthaler 1984; Swanson, Sawchenko, Rivier, et al. 1983) (Figure 2). Pertinent to the present

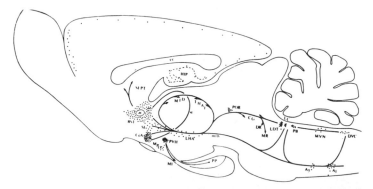

Figure 2. The major CRF-stained cell groups (*black dots*) and fiber systems are illustrated schematically in this sagittal view of the rat brain. Most of the immunoreactive cells and fibers appear to be associated with systems that regulate the output of the pituitary and the autonomic nervous system, with limbic structures and with cortical interneurons. (Reprinted from Swanson, Sawchenko, Rivier, et al. 1983, with permission from S. Karger AG, Basel.)

discussion is the fact that a number of these brain areas are believed to be integrally involved in the pathogenesis of anxiety and depression, and this distribution also places CRF in a position to influence catecholamine neurons, which have long been implicated in both anxiety and affective disorders (Charney, Menkes, Phil, et al. 1981; Jesberger and Richardson 1985; Redmond and Huang 1979; Svensson 1987).

ROLE OF CRF IN ANXIETY AND AFFECTIVE DISORDERS: PRECLINICAL STUDIES

A number of studies have provided evidence concordant with the hypothesis that CRF, by its actions both within the central nervous system and at the pituitary, mediates endocrine and behavioral responses to stress. As will be reviewed below, preclinical studies indicate that CRF integrates centrally mediated electrophysiologic, autonomic, and behavioral responses to stress. A number of these responses are reminiscent of certain of the signs and symptoms of depression and anxiety disorders.

Electrophysiologic studies show that CRF increases neuronal activity in central nervous system areas known to be involved in stress, arousal, and anxiety. Of particular interest are studies that have evaluated the effects of CRF in the locus coeruleus (LC), a brain-stem area containing both CRF and the A_6 noradrenergic cells that projects to almost every region of the neuraxis (Foote, Bloom, and Aston-Jones 1983). The noradrenergic neurons of the LC are involved in the mediation of behavioral activation to incoming stimuli and have long been implicated in the pathophysiology of both depression and anxiety (Redmond and Huang 1979; Simson, Weiss, Ambrose, et al. 1986; Simson, Weiss, Hoffmann, et al. 1986; Svensson 1987). The finding by Valentino and co-workers (Valentino and Foote 1987; Valentino, Foote, and Aston-Jones 1983) that central administration of CRF dose-dependently increases spontaneous discharge rates of noradrenergic neurons in the LC indicates that CRF may be intimately involved in increasing behavioral arousal, orienting the animal toward the external environment, and enhancing the stressful or anxiogenic aspects of the environment. Further, because the LC projects to so many brain regions, activation of noradrenergic neurons in the LC by CRF could be a means of coordinating autonomic and behavioral aspects of the stress response.

Not only does CRF alter firing rates of LC neurons, but it produces a pattern of neuronal excitation in a hippocampal slice preparation (Aldenhoff, Gruol, Rivier, et al. 1983) that prompted the suggestion that if endogenous CRF activates central nervous system neurons that respond to stress, this pattern of neuronal excitation could provide a cellular basis for such activation. Further support for a role for CRF in activating the central nervous system is shown by electroencephalogram changes suggestive of increased arousal in the hippocampus and cortex, which persisted for several hours following low doses of CRF, while higher doses produced seizures in the animals and epileptiform activity, which begin in the amygdala and spread to the hippocampus and cortex (Ehlers, Henriksen, Wang, et al. 1983; Marrosu, Mereu, Fratta, et al. 1987).

CRF mediation of autonomic nervous system responses to stress has been observed in a number of studies. Acting at several central nervous system sites, CRF has been shown to increase sympathetic outflow as evidenced by increased adrenomedullary secretion of epinephrine and norepinephrine with concomitant increases in heart rate, blood pressure, plasma glucagon, and glucose concentrations (Brown 1986; Brown and Fisher 1983; Brown, Fisher, Spiess, et al. 1982; Fisher, Jessen, and Brown 1983; Fisher, Rivier, Rivier, et al. 1982). CRF also inhibits gastric acid secretion by activating the sympathetic nervous system (Konturek, Yanaihara, Yanaihara, et al. 1987; Lenz, Raedler, Greten, et al. 1987). These responses are characteristic of the initial phase of the alarm reaction described by Selye (1936).

CRF also produces behavioral activation that is consistent with its alterations in electrophysiologic and autonomic activity and is similar to the behavior observed in stressed animals. When placed into a familiar nonstressful environment, untreated animals habituate rapidly and go to sleep. In contrast, CRF-treated animals exhibit dose-dependent increases in locomotion, sniffing, rearing, and grooming, which are consistent with increased behavioral arousal (Britton, Lee, Dana, et al. 1986; Britton, Varela, Garcia, et al. 1986; Koob, Swerdlow, Seeligson, et al. 1984; Sutton, Koob, LeMoal, et al. 1982; Tazi, Swerdlow, LeMoal, et al. 1987). These effects appear to be due to a direct action of CRF in the central nervous system because increased locomotion and grooming are seen following central but not systemic administration of CRF (Britton, Varela, Garcia, et al. 1986; Sutton, Koob, LeMoal, et al. 1982) and are not altered by manipulations that decrease HPA axis activity (Britton, Lee, Dana, et al. 1986; Britton, Varela, Garcia, et al. 1986; Eaves, Thatcher-Britton, Rivier, et al. 1985; Morley and Levine 1982). While neither dopaminergic nor opioid neurons appear to be involved in CRF stimulation of locomotor activity (Kalivas, Duffy, and Latimer 1987; Koob, Swerdlow, Seeligson, et al. 1984; Swerdlow and Koob 1985; Swerdlow, Vaccarino, Amalric, et al. 1986), noradrenergic neurons may play a role in CRF-induced locomotion (Imaki, Shibasaki, Masuda, et al. 1987). This is of particular interest because CRF activates noradrenergic neurons in the LC (Valentino, Foote, and Aston-Jones 1983) and increases noradrenergic turnover (Dunn and Berridge 1987). As will be discussed below, CRF interactions with noradrenergic neurons may have implications for both depressive and anxiety disorders.

The effects of CRF in a novel environment provide information about the effects of the peptide in a stressful, aversive environment. When placed into a novel open-field box, control animals rapidly circle the outer squares of the box and then venture into the inner squares (Sutton, Koob, LeMoal, et al. 1982). In contrast, CRF-treated animals did not explore the inner squares but remained in the outer squares either circling the open field, staying close to the floor, or moving slowly backward and forward (Koob and Bloom 1985). The CRF-treated rats also showed decreased rearing and increased grooming and freezing behavior (Britton, Koob, Rivier, et al. 1982; Sutton, Koob, LeMoal, et al. 1982). The increased grooming is of interest because this behavior is seen in stressful situations in the wild and is thought to be a displacement behavior (Hinde 1970). Similarly, Berridge and Dunn (1986) found that, in an unfamiliar environment, CRF, like restraint stress, decreased the duration of time mice spent in contact with novel stimuli; this reaction to novelty may be due to CRF activation of noradrenergic neurons (Berridge and Dunn 1987b). CRF also increased the frequency of stress-induced fighting induced by mild electric footshock, possibly by producing effects similar to those seen at a higher stress level (Tazi, Dantzer, LeMoal, et al. 1987). CRF thus appears to increase sensitivity to the stressful or anxiogenic nature of the environment.

The decreased food consumption and associated weight loss that frequently occur in response to stress may be mediated by CRF. Following intracerebroventricular administration, CRF inhibits feeding in a number of experimental paradigms. In a novel environment, CRF decreased food intake in food-deprived rats (Britton, Koob, Rivier, et al. 1982). CRF also decreased food consumption in a familiar environment following food deprivation (Britton, Koob, Rivier, et al. 1982; Britton, Varela, Garcia, et al. 1986; Krahn, Gosnell, Grace, et al. 1986; Morley and Levine 1982), during free feeding (Gosnell, Morley, and Levine 1983), and following administration of substances known to potentiate feedings, such as muscimol, norepinephrine, dynorphin, and insulin (Levine, Rogers, Kneip, et al. 1983). These decreases in food intake are produced by central nervous system but not systemic administration of CRF and are not affected by manipulations that decrease HPA axis activity (Britton, Varela, Garcia, et al. 1986; Morley and Levine 1982).

Reproductive behavior is also disrupted by stress in a number of species. Both male and female sexual behavior are inhibited in the rat following central injection of CRF (Sirinathsinghji 1985, 1987; Sirinathsinghji, Rees, Rivier, et al. 1983). This inhibition appears to be due to a decrease in gonadotropin-releasing hormone release into portal circulation with consequent inhibition of luteinizing hormone secretion (Petraglia, Sutton, Vale, et al. 1987; Rivier, Rivier, and Vale 1986).

This concatenation of findings indicates that CRF produces neuroendocrine, electrophysiologic, autonomic, and behavioral responses that are similar to those observed during stress and that CRF actually increases the anxiogenic nature of the environment. As stated above, these effects of CRF are reminiscent of a number of the signs and symptoms of anxiety and depression. These include alterations in locomotor activity similar to the psychomotor agitation seen in some depressions and anxiety disorders; increased autonomic activity similar to that commonly seen in patients during panic attacks, in generalized anxiety disorder, and in posttraumatic stress disorder; and the decreased appetite and libido seen in depression and to a lesser extent in anxiety disorders. Further, a number of the effects of CRF are opposite to those observed following benzodiazepine administration: benzodiazepines decrease stress-induced elevations of ACTH and corticosterone (Barlow, Knight, and Sullivan 1979; Lahti and Barsuhn 1975; Torellas, Guaza, and Borrell 1980), stress-induced hypertension (Benson, Herd, Morse, et al. 1970), gastric ulceration (Dasgupta and Mukherjee 1967), and behavioral effects of novelty (Britton and Britton 1981), whereas CRF elicits these stress-like responses.

Further evidence of CRF involvement in anxiety disorders are the reports that CRF produces anxiogenic effects in animal models of anxiety. In one conflict model of anxiety, which has been shown to be sensitive to anxiolytic drugs and treatments that increase neophobia (Britton and Britton 1981), rats were deprived of food for 24 hours and placed in a brightly lit novel open field in the center of which was one food pellet secured to a pedestal. CRF decreased the number of approaches to the food pellet and decreased the amount eaten per approach; these behaviors are consistent with an increase in the aversiveness of the situation and opposite to those seen after benzodiazepine treatment (Britton, Koob, Rivier, et al. 1982). Similarly, in a modified Geller-Seifter conflict test (Cook and Stepinwell 1975), in which a reinforcing stimulus (food) is paired with an aversive stimulus (shock) for part of each trial, CRF produced a dose-dependent decrease in punished (food plus shock) and nonpunished (food and no shock) responding, which was reversed by the anxiolytic chlordiazepoxide (Britton, Morgan, Rivier, et al. 1985). Interestingly, Britton and Koob (1986) also found that alcohol reverses CRF-induced decreases in punished responding; these authors suggested that alcohol may reduce tension by suppressing the activity of brain CRF systems. In accord with the hypothesized involvement of noradrenergic neurons in CRF-induced effects, Cole and Koob (in press) have shown that the noradrenergic antagonist propranolol reverses CRF-induced increases in anxiogenic behavior in a conditioned emotional response paradigm.

In other, nonconflict models of anxiety, which are useful in screening for anxiolytics, CRF also produced anxiogenic effects. CRF decreased active social interaction in a social interaction test of anxiety in rats, which decrease could be prevented by pretreatment with chlordiazepoxide (Dunn and File 1987). CRF potentiated the acoustic startle response (Swerdlow, Geyer, Vale, et al. 1986)—that is, a contraction of the skeletal musculature in response to an intense acoustic stimulus that is enhanced by anxiogenic drugs (Davis and Astrachan 1981) and decreased by anxiolytic drugs (Davis 1979a, 1979b). This CRF-induced potentiation of the acoustic startle response was reversed by pretreatment with chlordiazepoxide (Swerdlow, Geyer, Vale, et al. 1986). Increased startle responses are seen in both generalized anxiety disorder and posttraumatic stress disorder.

These studies support the hypothesis that CRF produces behavioral effects consistent with anxiety or an increased responsiveness to stress, and that this behavioral state can be reversed by classic anxiolytic drugs. While a number of studies have looked at the effects of CRF in animal models of anxiety, there have been no studies as of this writing examining the behavioral effects of CRF in animal models of depression. Indeed, much of the evidence for CRF involvement in depression comes from clinical studies, which will be discussed later in this chapter.

There is growing evidence from preclinical studies showing that endogenous CRF is indeed released under stressful conditions. While central administration of the CRF antagonist α-helical CRF_{9-41} has no discernible effects in nonstressed animals, it suppresses stress-induced increases in autonomic functioning (Brown, Fisher, Webb, et al. 1985; Brown, Gray, and Fisher 1986), reverses stress-induced inhibition of luteinizing hormone secretion and periodic luteinizing hormone pulses in castrated male rats (Rivier, Rivier, and Vale 1986), partially reverses stress-induced decreases in food intake in food-deprived rats (Krahn, Gosnell, Grace, et al. 1986), reverses stress-induced fighting in rats (Tazi, Dantzer, LeMoal, et al. 1987) and restraint-induced decreases in time spent with novel stimuli (Berridge and Dunn 1987a), and decreases defensive-withdrawal behavior in a novel environment (Takahashi, Kalin, Van den Burgt, et al., in press). The antagonism by α-helical CRF_{9-41} of these centrally mediated effects of stress is strong evidence that, besides its endocrine role, endogenous CRF plays an important role in mediating central nervous system responses to stress. This mediation has obvious important implications for a model involving CRF in the pathophysiology of anxiety and depressive disorders. It indicates that alterations in the synaptic availability of CRF in the central nervous system do in fact occur in response to external environmental events, and possibly internal psychological events. These alterations plausibly might play a significant role in anxiety and depressive disorders. Clinical studies demonstrating CRF hypersecretion in depression will be reviewed later in this chapter.

Our group (Chappell, Smith, Kilts, et al. 1986) has reported that both acute and chronic stress produce changes in CRF concentrations in several brain regions. While the above-described studies using a CRF antagonist indicate that endogenous CRF is involved in mediating and coordinating central nervous system responses to stress, this is the first evidence that stress actually alters CRF concentrations in both hypothalamic and extrahypothalamic areas of the brain. The acute stress consisted of 3 hours of immobilization at 4°C, while the chronic stress consisted of exposure to a series of unpredictable stressors for 14 days. The latter regimen of chronic, unpredictable stressors has been shown to produce behavioral and neuroendocrine changes in rats similar to endogenous depression in humans (Katz 1982; Katz and Roth 1979; Katz, Roth, and Carroll 1981). Both acute and chronic stress produced similar changes in CRF-like immunoreactivity (CRF-LI), which may be due to the fact that the chronic unpredictable stress used was designed to circumvent the usual adaptive mechanisms elicited by the intermittent exposure of an animal to a single type of stressor. Exposure to both acute and chronic stress significantly decreased the concentration of CRF-LI in the arcuate nucleus-median eminence and dramatically increased it in the LC. Acute stress also decreased CRF-LI in the medial preoptic area, while chronic stress decreased CRF-LI in the dorsal vagal complex and increased it in the anterior and periventricular hypothalamic areas (Figure 3).

The decrease in CRF-LI in the arcuate nucleus-median eminence following acute and chronic stress is presumably due to the stress-enhanced release of CRF-LI from nerve terminals in the median eminence into the hypothalamo-hypophyseal portal circulation, which activates the HPA. A decrease in CRF-LI in the medial preoptic area following acute stress is interesting because this area contains a large CRF cell cluster (Petrusz, Merchenthaler, Maderdrut, et al. 1985) and is implicated in the stress response (Saavedra 1982; Saavedra, Kvetnansky, and Kopin 1979; Seggie, Uhlir, and Brown 1974). The finding that chronic stress decreased CRF-LI in the dorsal vagal complex is consistent with a role for CRF in the regulation of the autonomic nervous system and its response to stress described above.

Of particular interest is the finding that both acute and chronic

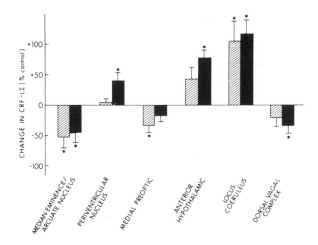

Figure 3. Percentage from baseline of stress-induced changes in corticotropin-releasing factor-like immunoreactivity (CRF-LI) concentration. *Hatched bars* = acute stress; *solid bars* = chronic stress; = significantly different from controls ($p < 5.0$). (Reprinted from Chappell, Smith, Kilts, et al. 1986, with permission from the Society for Neuroscience.)

stress increased the concentration of CRF-LI in the LC. The LC consists almost entirely of noradrenergic neurons, which project throughout the neuraxis (Foote, Bloom, and Aston-Jones 1983), and this structure has been repeatedly implicated in the stress response and arousal functions (Glavin 1985; Korf, Aghajanian, and Roth 1973; Thierry, Javoy, Glowinski, et al. 1968, Weiss, Goodman, Losito, et al. 1981) and in anxiety and depression (Redmond and Huang 1979; Simson, Weiss, Ambrose, et al. 1986; Simson, Weiss, Hoffmann, et al. 1986; Svensson 1987). CRF-positive cells and fibers have been detected in the LC (Swanson, Sawchenko, Rivier, et al. 1983). CRF terminals innervate the LC (Cummings, Elde, Ellis, et al. 1983). As indicated previously, CRF activates noradrenergic neurons in the LC (Valentino, Foote, and Aston-Jones 1983). Thus, because LC neurons project throughout the central nervous system, a stress-induced increase in CRF availability in the LC could be expected to increase noradrenergic activity in a number of brain regions. As will be discussed below, these findings have implications for the pathogenesis of both depression and anxiety disorders because a dysregulation of norepinephrine may be common to both.

We have also reported that the triazolobenzodiazepine anxiolytics adinazolam and alprazolam produce decreases in CRF concentrations in the LC and increases in the hypothalamus (Owens, Bissette, Lundberg, et al. 1987), effects opposite to those of stress. It is tempting to speculate that anxiolytics may exert their effects, at least in part, by decreasing CRF concentrations in the LC. We are currently examining the effects of acute and chronic treatment with anxiolytics and antidepressants on stress-induced alterations in central nervous system CRF concentrations.

It is not clear by what mechanism(s) CRF mediates stress responses in the central nervous system. As indicated above, CRF may do so via interactions with noradrenergic neurons. Evidence consistent with this hypothesis includes: (1) CRF activation of noradrenergic neurons in the LC (Valentino, Foote, and Aston-Jones 1983); (2) reports that CRF increases noradrenergic turnover (Dunn and Berridge 1987); (3) the finding that CRF-induced alterations in both locomotor (Imaki, Shibasaki, Masuda, et al. 1987) and anxiogenic behavior (Cole and Koob, in press) may, at least in part, be mediated by noradrenergic neurons; and (4) our findings that stress increases CRF concentrations in the norepinephrine-rich LC (Chappell, Smith, Kilts, et al. 1986). CRF interactions with serotonergic neurons have not yet been studied.

In conclusion, the results of animal studies provide evidence implicating CRF in the pathophysiology of anxiety and depressive disorders. Administration of exogenous CRF increases the anxiogenic or stressful nature of the environment as seen by its elicitation of neuroendocrine, autonomic electrophysiologic, and behavioral responses similar to those seen in animals exposed to stress. A number of these effects are similar to certain of the signs and symptoms of depression and anxiety, and opposite to those produced by benzodiazepines. Moreover, CRF produces anxiogenic effects in animals, which can be reversed by the anxiolytic chlordiazepoxide. While the clinical studies to be reviewed below indicate that CRF hypersecretion is indeed involved in the pathophysiology of depression, little clinical work has been done examining the role of CRF in anxiety disorders. Studies in which the cerebrospinal fluid concentration of CRF in patients with anxiety disorders is measured would be helpful, as would studies scrutinizing biochemical and behavioral interactions of CRF with neurotransmitter systems believed to be involved in anxiety disorders.

ROLE OF CRF IN ANXIETY AND AFFECTIVE DISORDERS: CLINICAL STUDIES

Although a strong case can be made for the involvement of CRF in the biology of anxiety disorders based largely on preclinical findings, perhaps an even stronger case can be made for CRF involvement in affective disorders.

Because many of the effects of CRF in animals are reminiscent of the signs and symptoms of major depression (e.g., decreased sexual behavior, decreased food intake, psychomotor agitation, and sleep disturbance), we (Banki, Bissette, Arato, et al. 1987; Nemeroff, Widerlov, Bissette, et al. 1984) and others (Roy, Pickar, Paul, et al. 1987) became interested in whether CRF might be involved in the pathophysiology of depression. A further impetus for evaluating the involvement of CRF in depression is that a substantial percentage (40%–70%) of patients meeting DSM-III (American Psychiatric Associaton 1980) criteria for major depression or Research Diagnostic Criteria (RDC) (Spitzer, Endicott, and Robins 1978a) for endogenous depression exhibit hyperactivity of the HPA axis as evidenced by increases in plasma cortisol (Sachar, Hellman, and Roffwarg 1973), cortisol nonsuppression after administration of the synthetic glucocorticoid dexamethasone (Carroll, Feinberg, Greden, et al. 1981; Evans and Nemeroff 1987), and increases in urinary free cortisol excretion (Carroll, Curtis, Davies, et al. 1976). The hypercortisolism is believed to be due to a central rather than a pituitary or adrenal abnormality (Gold and Chrousos 1985). Clearly, hyperactivity of hypothalamic CRF neurons could mediate this effect.

To investigate CRF involvement in the pathophysiology of depression directly, we measured the concentration of CRF in cerebrospinal fluid (CSF) obtained by lumbar puncture from drug-free patients with a DSM-III diagnosis of major depression and in normal controls, schizophrenics, and patients with senile dementia. There was a significant increase in CRF-LI in the depressed patients (Nemeroff, Widerlov, Bissette, et al. 1984) (Figure 4). However, there was no significant correlation between CSF CRF-LI and baseline or postdexamethasone plasma cortisol concentrations (Nemeroff, Widerlov, Bissette, et al. 1984). More recently, we studied a larger group of 54 depressed patients who met DSM-III criteria for major depression, most of whom were melancholic or psychotic, and found that the CSF CRF concentrations of depressed patients were almost twofold greater than neurologic controls or nondepressed psychiatric patients (Banki, Bissette, Arato, et al. 1987) (Figure 5). As in our earlier study (Nemeroff, Widerlov, Bissette, et al. 1984), elevated CSF CRF concentrations did not identify the same patients who were cortisol nonsuppressors. Results from this large patient population showed that CRF hypersecretion is present in about half of hospitalized patients suffering from major depression. This CRF hypersecretion may contribute, at least in part, to hyperactivity of the HPA axis in depressed patients.

CRF also appears to be hypersecreted in suicide victims. There were elevated concentrations of CRF in postmortem CSF of depressed patients who had committed suicide as well as in depressed patients

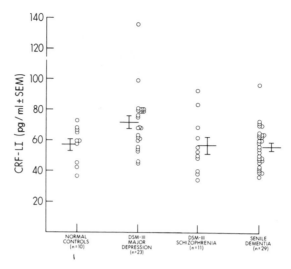

Figure 4. Concentration of corticotropin-releasing factor-like immunoreactivity (CRF-LI) in cerebrospinal fluid (CSF) of normal controls and patients with DSM-III major depression, DSM-III schizophrenia, and senile dementia (DSM-III primary degenerative dementia or multi-infarct dementia, or both). Because the data distribution in the depressed patients were slightly skewed, the data were analyzed by both parametric (analysis of variance [ANOVA] and Student-Newman-Keuls test) and nonparametric (Mann-Whitney U test) methods. By both methods, the CSF CRF-LI concentrations were significantly elevated in the depressed patients when compared to the other diagnostic groups and normal controls ($p < .05$, ANOVA and Student-Newman-Keuls test; $p < .025$, Mann-Whitney U test). (Reprinted from Nemeroff, Widerlov, Bissette, et al. 1984, with permission from the American Association for the Advancement of Science. Copyright 1984.)

who died by means other than suicide (Arato, Banki, Nemeroff, et al. 1986). If CRF is chronically hypersecreted in depressed patients who commit suicide, there should be a concomitant reduction in the density[1] of CRF-binding sites. In support of this, we found a decrease in the density of CRF-binding sites in the frontal cortex of suicide victims when compared to sudden death and homicide victims (Nemeroff, Owens, Bissette, et al. 1988).

Recently, in collaboration with Fink at Stonybrook, we examined whether the increased CSF CRF concentration is a state or trait marker of depression. Prior to electroconvulsive therapy, depressed patients had elevated CSF CRF concentrations. After six electroconvulsive therapy treatments, CSF CRF was not different from controls (Nemer-

---

[1]Drug treatments or pathologic conditions that produce chronic hyper- or hyposecretion of a neurotransmitter into the synapse are frequently accompanied by a compensatory decrease or increase, respectively, in receptor number (i.e., density).

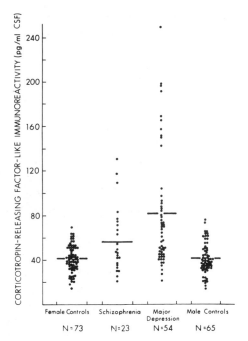

Figure 5. Concentrations of corticotropin-releasing factor-like immunoreactivity (CRF-LI) in cerebrospinal fluid (CSF) of patients with DSM-III schizophrenia, DSM-III major depression, and control subjects with various peripheral neurologic diseases. CSF CRF-LI concentrations were significantly elevated in depressed patients as compared to controls (Student-Newman-Keuls test, $p < .001$) and schizophrenic patients (Student-Newman-Keuls test, $p < .05$). (Reprinted from Banki, Bissette, Arato, et al. 1987, with permission from the American Psychiatric Association. Copyright 1987.)

off, Bissette, and Fink, unpublished observations). This indicates that elevated concentrations of CSF CRF in depressed patients may be a state, rather than a trait, marker.

In contrast to our findings, Roy, Pickar, Paul, et al. (1987) did not find a significant difference in CSF CRF-LI between patients with a DSM-III diagnosis of depression and control subjects. However, depressed patients who were dexamethasone suppression test (DST) nonsuppressors had significantly higher CSF CRF concentrations than DST suppressors, and CSF CRF concentrations were significantly correlated with 4 P.M. post-dexamethasone plasma cortisol concentrations. This patient population at the National Institute of Mental Health was considerably less severely depressed than the patients in our studies. In a small pilot study, Davis, Davis, Mohs, et al. (1984) failed to find a significant difference in CSF CRF concentrations between controls and nine depressed patients. However, there

was a strong positive correlation between ratings of depression severity and CSF CRF concentrations in patients with anorexia nervosa
(Kaye, Gwirtsman, George, et al. 1987).

The difference between these results and ours (Banki, Bissette,
Arato, et al. 1987; Nemeroff, Widerlov, Bissette, et al. 1984) may be
explained by the fact that our patients were largely first-episode,
treatment-responsive patients, and those of Roy, Pickar, Paul, et al.
(1987) had recurrent episodes with multiple drug trials. There are
several likely reasons why we did not find a correlation between
post-dexamethasone plasma cortisol and CSF CRF concentrations. It
is now evident that cortisol secretion involves more than CRF regulation of ACTH secretion. Moreover, CSF concentrations of CRF may
not accurately reflect the CRF concentrations present at the pituitary
corticotroph. Immunoreactive CRF is present in several extra-hypo-
thalamic areas of the human brain (Bissette, Reynolds, Kilts, et al.
1985; Suda, Tomori, Tozawa, et al. 1984), and little is known about the
relative contributions of these areas to lumbar CSF CRF concentrations. While an abnormal DST may well involve CRF hypersecretion
from nerve endings in the median eminence region of the hypothalamus, changes in CRF release from other structures may obscure
changes of CRF secretion in higher brain centers.

In a series of elegant studies, Gold and his colleagues (Gold,
Chrousos, Kellner, et al. 1984; Gold, Loriaux, Roy, et al. 1986) have
observed that depressed patients exhibit an attenuated ACTH response, but normal cortisol response, to intravenously administered
ovine CRF when compared to manic patients, recovered depressed
patients, or normal controls. These findings were almost simultaneously reported by Holsboer and colleagues (Holsboer, von Bardeleben, Green, et al. 1985; Holsboer, Gerken, Stalla, et al. 1987), who
found that patients with a DSM-III diagnosis of major depression had
a diminished plasma ACTH response to intravenous human CRF,
with cortisol concentrations similar to those of normals. This finding
has now been confirmed by our group (Kilts, Bissette, Krishnan, et al.
1987; Nemeroff and Krishnan, unpublished observations). The reduced ACTH response to CRF in depressed patients may be at least
partly due to the hypercortisolism producing normal negative feedback at the level of the anterior pituitary, indicating that the increased
HPA axis activity is due to a suprapituitary site. We have hypothesized that the blunted ACTH response to CRF in depression may be
due to decreased density of CRF receptors on the corticotrophs in
response to chronic CRF hypersecretion.

Gold and Chrousos (1985) have suggested that in early depression there is increased ACTH and cortisol secretion due to hypersecretion of endogenous CRF, but that later in depression the continual

endogenous CRF hypersecretion produces adrenal hypertrophy and increased sensitivity of the adrenal glands to ACTH. Less ACTH secretion would occur in late depression due to continued negative feedback of cortisol on pituitary corticotrophs, but elevated levels of cortisol would continue to be released because of the increased sensitivity of the adrenal. In the study in which we examined the effects of acute and chronic stress on central nervous system CRF concentrations (Chappell, Smith, Kilts, et al. 1986), we found that after chronic stress there was a pattern similar to that hypothesized for late depressed patients: normal plasma ACTH concentrations, increased adrenal weight, and elevated plasma concentrations of corticosterone. In contrast, in acute stress there were increased plasma concentrations of both ACTH and corticosterone and no change in adrenal weights. These findings, taken together, support a role for central CRF in depression. Further support for CRF involvement in the hypercortisolism in depressed patients comes from the finding that continuous intravenous administration of CRF to normal volunteers for 24 hours reproduces the pattern and magnitude of hypercortisolism seen in many depressed patients (Schulte, Chrousos, Gold, et al. 1985).

As indicated previously, the anatomic distribution of CRF provides plausibility for a CRF-norepinephrine interaction (Foote, Bloom, and Aston-Jones 1983), and neurochemical and electrophysiologic data support this contention (Chappell, Smith, Kilts, et al. 1986; Dunn and Berridge 1987; Valentino, Foote, and Aston-Jones 1983). There is abundant evidence that the noradrenergic system is involved not only in anxiety disorders but in the pathophysiology of depression. A catecholamine theory of depression was posited in the 1960s suggesting that a decrease in noradrenergic transmission is responsible for depression and that antidepressants exerted their therapeutic effect by enhancing noradrenergic neurotransmission (Schildkraut 1965; Schildkraut and Kety 1967). This notion was, of course, based on the observations that both monoamine oxidase inhibitors and tricyclic antidepressants increase the synaptic availability of norepinephrine in the brain by preventing amine metabolism or inhibiting reuptake, respectively (Bunney and Davis 1965; Schildkraut 1965), and that reserpine, which depletes monoamines, could precipitate depression (Freis 1954; Muller, Pryor, Gibbons, et al. 1955).

However, while norepinephrine accumulation occurs after acute administration (Iversen and MacKay 1979), 3 to 5 weeks are required for antidepressants to exert their complete therapeutic effect (Oswald, Brezinova, and Dunleavy 1972). Moreover, chronic, but not acute, tricyclic antidepressant treatment decreases the density of brain β-adrenergic receptors (Banerjee, Kung, Riggi, et al. 1977) and decreases the sensitivity of the β-adrenergic receptor-coupled adenylate cyclase system to norepinephrine (Sulser, Janowsky, Okada, et al. 1983). These latter findings of decreased receptor density and second messenger activity in the noradrenergic system have led to a hypothesis opposite to that originally proposed, namely that antidepressants work by decreasing noradrenergic transmission, which suggests that depression may be partly due to increased noradrenergic activity (Sulser, Janowsky, Okada, et al. 1983; Sulser, Vetulani, and Mobley 1978). However, studies assessing the electrophysiologic and metabolic activity of norepinephrine in depressed patients present conflicting data on the nature of the noradrenergic pathology in depression (for a review, see Charney, Menkes, Phil, et al. 1981). Thus while it seems clear that noradrenergic transmission is abnormal in depression, the nature of this abnormality is not yet fully understood.

The involvement of the noradrenergic system in anxiety disorders is somewhat more clear. For example, alpha$_2$-adrenergic antagonists such as yohimbine, which increase noradrenergic activity, produce fear and anxiety in humans, whereas alpha$_2$-adrenergic agonists such as clonidine, which decrease noradrenergic activity, have an anxiolytic effect (Liebowitz, Fyer, McGrath, et al. 1981; Svensson, Persson, Wallin, et al. 1978). Similarly, in animal studies, electrical stimulation of the LC produces fear and anxiety in monkeys, whereas LC lesions have the opposite effect (Redmond 1977; Redmond, Huang, Snyder, et al. 1976). Thus noradrenergic activity appears to be altered in both affective and anxiety disorders.

The evidence presented in this review indicates that CRF hypersecretion may in part underlie the pathophysiology of both of these disorders. The increasing evidence indicating that CRF may activate noradrenergic neurons makes it tempting to speculate that CRF-noradrenergic interactions may be involved in the etiology of these disorders. Several clinical studies have indeed addressed such interactions in depressed patients. Roy, Pickar, Paul, et al. (1987) found that in patients with a DSM-III diagnosis of major depression who were medication-free for at least 2½ weeks, there was a positive correlation between CSF CRF and CSF and plasma norepinephrine concentrations. There were also significant positive correlations between CSF CRF concentrations and urinary outputs of norepinephrine and its major metabolites. Further, Davis, Davis, Mohs, et al. (1984) found a positive relationship between CSF concentrations of CRF and the CSF concentrations of the norepinephrine metabolite 3-methoxy-4-hydroxyphenyleneglycol (MHPG) among depressed patients. In contrast, our group (Widerlov, Bissette, and Nemeroff 1988) found a positive correlation between CSF concentrations of CRF and the serotonin metabolite 5-hydroxyindoleacetic acid (5-HIAA) in depressed patients but no correlation between CSF CRF and MHPG. However, there was an inverse relationship between CSF concentrations of CRF and MHPG in healthy volunteers, leading to the suggestion that a normal inhibitory role of norepinephrine in CRF secretion may be replaced by serotonergic stimulation of CRF release in depression. These studies lend further support to a dysregulation of both noradrenergic and CRF neurons in depression.

The hypothesis that CRF hypersecretion plays a role in affective disorders is an intriguing one. A number of investigators have suggested that early stress or loss can predispose an organism to anxiety and depression in later life (Blazer, Hughes, and George 1987; Lesse 1982). A diathesis stress model fits a role for CRF in depression and anxiety. Gold, Chrousos, Kellner, et al. (1984) have suggested that early stress could alter CRF neuronal functioning (e.g., sensitize CRF neurons), which could predispose the organism to depression when confronted with stressful situations later in life. The notion that anxiety disorders may lead to depression by virtue of continued low self-esteem is not discordant with the notion of a clinical continuum for these two disorders, with CRF hypersecretion and concomitant disruption of other neurotransmitters, such as norepinephrine, being possible etiologic variables. It is also quite possible that if CRF hypersecretion is an etiologic variable in these disorders, it may interact with neurotransmitter systems in a different manner in patients with depression than in patients with anxiety disorders.

Although CRF does appear to be hypersecreted in CSF of depressed patients and to be increased in response to stressful stimuli, it is possible that such hypersecretion may be epiphenomenological rather than causal. Indeed, evidence from electroconvulsive therapy studies (Nemeroff, Bissette, Akilh et al. in press) indicates that CRF hypersecretion is a state-dependent marker that is no longer seen when patients are in remission. The controversy regarding the James-Lange theory of emotion deals with a similar issue. While this theory posits that the autonomic changes that occur during emotion actually produce the feeling of emotion, other theories hold that the converse is true. Clearly, knowing that a variable is state-dependent does not in itself determine its causative role or lack of one. For instance, hypothyroid patients have a thyroid hormone deficiency and high plasma cholesterol levels, both of which are correlated with symptoms of temperature intolerance, lethargy, and fatigue seen in these patients. When treatment with exogenous thyroid hormone brings thyroid hormone and cholesterol levels back to normal, the symptoms also remit. However, only the thyroid hormone deficiency appears to be responsible for producing the symptoms. Similarly, the finding that CRF hypersecretion is a state-dependent variable does not determine its causative role or lack of one in anxiety and depressive disorders.

Although it is, of course, possible that CRF hypersecretion may be an epiphenomenon of anxiety and depressive disorders, a number of the studies reviewed in this chapter do in fact support a causative role. For instance, CRF produces a number of behavioral effects similar to those seen in depressed patients, including sleep disturbances, psychomotor agitation, appetite loss, and decreased libido. CRF hypersecretion could also be responsible for the hypercortisolemia seen in some of these patients. Further, not only are a number of the autonomic nervous system effects of CRF similar to those seen in anxiety disorders, but CRF produces anxiogenic behavior in a number of animal models of anxiety. Perhaps more importantly, the CRF antagonist α-helical CRF_{9-41} reduces stress-induced alterations in eating, sleeping, and sexual behavior, and decreases anxiogenic behavior in animal models of anxiety. This indicates that endogenous CRF may indeed be involved in producing behaviors related to anxiety and depressive disorders. Further preclinical and clinical work is, however, clearly necessary before the role of CRF in these disorders can be fully elucidated.

CONCLUSION

In summary, hyperactivity of CRF neurons in the central nervous system appears to occur in both anxiety and depressive disorders and indeed may play a causal rather than an epiphenomenological role in these disorders. Evidence for a role for CRF in anxiety disorders comes mainly from animal studies showing that CRF produces a number of anxiogenic effects, including effects similar to those seen in animal models of anxiety, opposite to those produced by benzodiazepines, and effects that are reversed by anxiolytics. However, the role of CRF in anxiety disorders in humans is virtually unexplored; examining CSF CRF concentrations in patients with a variety of anxiety disorders would provide information about the role of CRF in anxiety disorders, as would CRF stimulation test data. In terms of affective disorders, there are striking similarities between some of the behavioral effects of CRF in animals and the signs and symptoms of depression. These similarities coupled with the increased CRF concentrations in CSF of depressed patients provide direct evidence that CRF is hypersecreted in depressed patients. The decreased CRF receptor number in frontal cortex of suicides provides impressive support for the CRF hypothesis of depression. If hypersecretion of CRF is indeed involved in the pathology of depression, it would be illuminating to examine the effects of a CRF receptor antagonist in animal models of depression. Finally, the central nervous system distribution of CRF is compatible with a role for CRF in anxiety and depression. In terms of comorbidity, it is tempting to speculate that the data showing a role for CRF in both anxiety disorders and depression indicate that CRF hypersecretion could be a substrate for a common cause of both types of disorders.

Theories of and Perspectives on Anxiety and Depression

Chapter 27

The Empirical Structure of Psychiatric Comorbidity and Its Theoretical Significance

C. Robert Cloninger, M.D.
Ronald L. Martin, M.D.
Samuel B. Guze, M.D.
Paula J. Clayton, M.D.

S OME DIAGNOSTIC CRITERIA have been shown to improve discrimination of different disorders by means of follow-up and family studies (Feighner, Robins, Guze, et al. 1972; Martin, Cloninger, Guze, et al. 1985). However, even when psychiatric cases satisfy the full diagnostic criteria for only a single disorder, they nearly always have some signs and symptoms of two or more psychopathologic syndromes. Furthermore, because of the co-occurrence of features of multiple disorders and other atypical features, approximately 20% of psychiatric cases do not satisfy validated exclusion criteria. Likewise, approximately 20% of psychiatric cases in the general population have been found to satisfy the inclusion criteria for two or more diagnoses in the Epidemiologic Catchment Area (ECA) study (Boyd, Burke, Gruenberg, et al. 1984). When both inclusion and exclusion criteria that have been validated were applied in a treatment sample of psychiatric outpatients, 50% of the treated cases had multiple diagnoses; however, as shown later in this chapter, among the ill relatives

Supported in part by Research Scientist Award MH-00048 and grant MH-31302 from the National Institute of Mental Health, grant AA-03539 from the National Institute of Alcoholism, and a grant from the MacArthur Foundation Network on Risk and Protective Factors in Major Mental Disorders.

of these same cases, only 11% had multiple diagnoses. What is the significance of such psychiatric comorbidity for theories of psychopathology? In other words, what do available observations about psychiatric comorbidity tell us about the pathogenesis of psychopathology?

To interpret the theoretical significance of psychiatric comorbidity, we will first compare the assumptions and predictions about comorbidity that are made by four major theoretical models of psychopathology. The four theories considered here are the Kraepelinian, psychodynamic, sociocultural, and behavioral learning models of psychopathology. Next we will summarize the different classes of causal factors considered in the different theories of psychopathology. Alternative theoretical explanations of the comorbidity of anxiety and depressive disorders will be described as a specific example of causal models of comorbidity.

Given this theoretical background, we will examine the empirical structure of psychiatric comorbidity in two large populations. One study is the Stockholm adoption study of all the adopted children born to single women in Stockholm, Sweden, from 1930 to 1949 (Cloninger, Sigvardsson, von Knorring, et al. 1984). The second study is the Washington University Clinic study in which a random sample of 500 psychiatric outpatients in St. Louis and their family members were given a structured diagnostic interview and followed prospectively over a 6- to 12-year period (Martin, Cloninger, Guze, et al. 1985). These studies provide extensive information about the empirical structure of psychiatric comorbidity and its etiologic basis in samples from both the general population and patients. Using this information, we will discuss tentative answers to key theoretical questions about comorbidity. Is psychopathology comprised of multiple discrete disorders? Alternatively, is there comorbidity that is not explainable by unreliability of assessment methods? If comorbidity is not artifactual, does it have a consistent and stable pattern or structure in different sociocultural groups? If there is a stable structure to observed comorbidity, is it predictable in terms of measurable susceptibility factors or in terms of procedural artifacts of the diagnostic process? What implications do available answers to these questions have for theories of psychopathology, clinical practice, and future research?

Comorbidity in Major Theories of Psychopathology

The discriminating features of four major theories of psychopathology are summarized in Table 1. Other variants of these theories, or combinations of them, have been proposed, but these four models describe the range of perspectives that have been described. Comparison of these different theories will help to define the key theoretical questions related to observations of psychiatric comorbidity.

In the Kraepelinian biomedical theory, psychopathology is entirely comprised of discrete disease entities. Each entity is believed to have specific genetic and neurobiologic antecedents. According to the discrete disease model, comorbidity is an artifact of diagnostic unreliability that arises when categorical diagnoses are based on clinical signs and symptoms that are not sufficiently discriminating. The implication is that different disorders can be distinguished reliably by judicious choice of discriminating features, including the temporal sequence in which symptoms occur and progress. Observed comorbidity in individual cases and their family members is considered to be an artifact of imprecise diagnoses.

A popular extension of the Kraepelinian model allows for a "spectrum" of clinical expression for the same underlying disease (e.g., schizophrenia and schizotypal personality; or manic-depressive disorder and cyclothymic personality). Kraepelin himself advocated the view that each specific disease entity had a spectrum of clinical expression. Despite the range of clinical expressivity, the disease spectra are supposed to be etiologically discrete and clinically mutually exclusive except for unreliable diagnoses.

In psychodynamic theories, psychopathology is comprised of maladaptive response patterns arising as a result of developmental interaction of congenital predisposition and individual experiences. According to these dynamic theories, adaptation or change in response to the challenges of environment and intrapsychic conflicts are mediated by defense mechanisms, such as repression, conversion, and projection (Perry, Chapter 30). The same defense mechanisms may be used by patients with different personality structures, even though there may be moderate correlations between personality and the frequency of use of different defense mechanisms (Perry, Chapter 30). Depending on the type and success of defense mechanisms employed, different patterns of clinical signs and symptoms develop as a result of conscious and unconscious efforts to adapt to various individual (intrapsychic) conflicts and environmental challenges. Accordingly, comorbidity arises as a consequence of the lack of specificity of different defense mechanisms for particular types of personality and its disorders.

According to pure sociocultural theories, behavior patterns are acquired as a result of social learning, which includes imitation of others and conscious symbolic learning of the concepts, attitudes, and values that characterize the culture of a particular population. According to this type of theory, psychopathology arises as a result of

Table 1. Discriminating Features of Four Major Theories of Psychopathology

	Kraepelinian biomedical	Psychodynamic	Sociocultural	Behavioral learning
Disease model	Discrete entity	Maladaptive response pattern	Deviance from social norms	Maladaptive response pattern
Predominant cause	Specific neurobiologic predisposition	Developmental interaction of predisposition and individual experience	Conceptual learning and cognition	Unconscious individual conditioning
Explanation of comorbidity	Diagnostic confusion	Nonspecific defense mechanisms	Nonspecific social influences	Coincidental joint reinforcement of different behaviors

inadequate or inappropriate social learning, producing a deviance from the expected social norm.

Psychopathology can also arise as a result of the encroachment of conflicting cultures on individuals in neighboring areas. The role of cultural relativism in the development of psychopathology has been considered in the work of the cultural anthropologist Frank Boas and his students (e.g., Margaret Mead). Different patterns of social learning are expected to lead to different patterns of behavior, including both normal and abnormal behavior. According to such sociocultural theories of psychopathology, comorbidity is simply a consequence of the nonspecificity of social influences that determine behavior patterns. Such theories provide no reason to expect the existence of any discrete disorders of behavior, or even a pattern or structure to comorbidity that would be the same in different sociocultural groups.

According to behavioral learning models, behavior is learned as an adaptive response to conditioning (i.e., reinforcement schedules of which the individual is not consciously aware). Psychopathology is viewed as the result of inadequate or inappropriate conditioning. As in psychodynamic theories, psychopathology is considered a maladaptive response pattern; unlike the psychodynamic theories, only the individual's experience with reinforcers is considered to be important in the development of psychopathology. According to the behavioral learning perspective, co-occurrence of symptoms is the consequence of coincidental reinforcement of different behaviors, regardless of congenital predisposition.

Causes of Comorbidity in Different Theories

To compare the predictions of different theories regarding psychiatric comorbidity, it is helpful first to summarize the different possible types of causal factors that are central to one or more of these theories. Causal factors for psychopathology are summarized in Table 2 according to dimensions of stability (stable or transient), heritability (heritable or acquired), form (neurobiologic or psychosocial), and specificity (specific or nonspecific). All possible combinations of these various aspects of causal factors are not listed, only those that clarify the similarities and differences between the predictions of the four major theories of psychopathology.

Table 2 lists factors that determine one or more psychiatric disorders. Using anxiety and depression as examples, Table 3 attempts to clarify how such factors can lead to comorbidity. Comorbidity arises if two disorders share at least some antecedents, or if at least one leads to the other. Sharing antecedents subsumes the case in which two diagnoses do not have distinct boundaries (i.e., cannot be reliably

Table 2. Types of Causal Factors in Theories of Psychopathology

A. Stable susceptibility and protective factors
   1. Heritable genetic factors
      a. Specific for single disorders
      b. Nonspecific risk factors
   2. Acquired biologic factors (trauma, toxicity)
      a. Specific
      b. Nonspecific
   3. Familial psychosocial (social learning, conditioning)
      a. Specific
      b. Nonspecific
   4. Nonfamilial psychosocial (individual experience)
      a. Specific (e.g., ballet training and anorexia)
      b. Nonspecific (e.g., low socioeconomic status)
B. Transient precipitative or supportive factors
   1. Genetic (e.g., genes expressed at specific ages like puberty)
   2. Nongenetic biologic factors (e.g., toxins, weight loss)
   3. Psychosocial factors (psychodynamic, sociocultural, conditioning, cognitive)

Table 3. Causes of Psychiatric Comorbidity in Anxiety (A) and Depression (D)

1. Common antecedent factor or factors
   a. No other factors specific for different syndromes
      (X causes A and D with variable probability)
   b. One or more distinct antecedent factors
      (X and Y cause A, X and Z cause D)
2. The development of one syndrome depends on the prior development of the other
   a. Each may predispose to the other
      (A causes D, D causes A)
   b. Only one may predispose to the other
      (A causes D, D does not cause A)

distinguished because of overlapping signs and symptoms).

To discriminate the predictions about comorbidity by the four theories, it is useful to consider predictions about whether (1) psychiatric disorders have discrete boundaries, (2) there are specific genetic and neurobiologic antecedents for different psychiatric disorders, (3) environmental influences that are shared by members of social groups are specific for different psychiatric disorders, (4) environmental influences that are unique to individuals are specific for different psychiatric disorders, (5) psychiatric disorders are viewed as functionally adaptive to experience or only in descriptive terms, and (6) the observed patterns and structure of psychiatric comorbidity is expected to be stable or consistent in different social groups or cultures. The predictions of the four theories about these six questions are summarized in Table 4. If the question is definitely answered affirmatively, a plus sign is listed; if answered negatively, a minus sign is tabulated. In some cases a theory is consistent with either a yes or no answer to a particular question; such ambiguous answers are tabulated with both plus and minus signs. For example, only the Kraepelinian model predicts that psychiatric disorders should have discrete natural boundaries; however, specific developmental or learning events could occur that produce psychiatric disorders that have discrete boundaries, so the other theories are compatible with discrete boundaries.

Overall, the four theories each have a distinct pattern of predictions about these six questions. The sociocultural and behavioral learning models reject the importance of specific genetic and neurobiologic factors, unlike the Kraepelinian and psychodynamic models. The psychodynamic theory predicts that environmental factors unique to individuals have a specific role in the development of different disorders, unlike the Kraepelinian model; accordingly, the psychodynamic and Kraepelinian models are distinguished from one another and the other two learning models. Likewise, the two learning models differ from one another in whether the critical learning is conscious, conceptual, and acquired in social groups (viz., sociocultural model) on unconscious, nonconceptual reinforcement and individually conditioned (viz., behavioral learning model). Therefore, all four theories make distinct predictions about psychiatric comorbidity. With these differential predictions in mind, we can now examine available data to evaluate which, if any, of the theories is consistent with available empirical data about psychiatric comorbidity. Our goal is not to confirm or reject any particular theory because available data may be too limited for that purpose. Rather, the goal is to identify key theoretical questions that must be answered and examine available information to guide future research.

DO PSYCHIATRIC DISORDERS HAVE DISCRETE BOUNDARIES?

The most stringent question about the comorbidity of psychiatric disorders is whether it is even possible to identify natural boundaries between different disorders. Even though all categorical systems of classification assume that it is possible to specify diagnostic criteria that are not arbitrary subdivisions of psychopathology, this basic question remains. Kendell (1982) argued that past psychiatric research has largely failed to demonstrate discontinuity between related psychiatric syndromes, such as schizophrenic and manic psychoses, or other anxiety and depressive neuroses. Kendell emphasized cogently

Table 4. Predictions About Psychiatric Comorbidity of Four Major Theories of Psychopathology

	Kraepelinian biomedical	Psychodynamic	Sociocultural	Behavioral learning
Discrete boundaries	+	+/-	+/-	+/-
Specific genetic and neurobiologic antecedents	+	+/-	+/-	+/-
Specific environmental influences common to social groups	+/-	+/-	+	+/-
Specific environmental influences unique to individuals	-	+	+/-	+
Functionally adaptive to experience	+/-	+	+/-	+
Stable comorbid structure	+/-	+	-	-

Note. + = affirmative; - = negative; +/- = ambiguous.

the importance of determining the presence and location of discontinuity or "points of rarity" in measures of clinical variation that distinguish patients in one disease category from those in other categories. In other words, to distinguish disorders, we need to show that there is minimal overlap in some specific set of clinical symptoms and that cases with an intermediate clinical picture are more rare than pure or typical cases. When such points of rarity are present, separation of patients into clinical groups can be "natural" and precise. However, when there is little separation between overlapping groups, misclassification of individuals is a serious practical problem and raises doubt about the assumption of distinct disorders.

Since 1982, research has provided evidence of the discreteness of a few forms of psychopathology. Cloninger, Sigvardsson, von Knorring, et al. (1984) studied somatization in a complete birth cohort of 859 Swedish adopted women born in Stockholm from 1930 to 1949. Complete medical and psychiatric records for the lifetime of subjects were available because Sweden has a national health insurance program and provides compensation for even brief periods of medical disability. Most sick leaves from work were concentrated in 144 women with recurrent somatic complaints, who were called "somatizers." A discriminant function was derived to distinguish between somatizers and nonsomatizers. Somatizers were distinguished from nonsomatizers by the high frequency of particular complaints: namely, headaches, backaches, and abdominal distress associated with psychiatric disability. The distribution of this discriminant function was examined to determine whether there was a point of rarity separating somatizers from nonsomatizers.

In fact, there was a point of rarity providing a natural boundary between somatizers and others in both the criterion sample and in a replication sample. In later work in a Swedish birth cohort of 807 adopted men, Sigvardsson, Bohman, von Knorring, et al. (1986) extended the earlier findings by showing natural boundaries distinguishing men with cognitive anxiety disorders (comparable to generalized anxiety disorder), somatic anxiety disorders (comparable to somatization disorder), and no anxiety. The distribution of a discriminant function defined by the frequency of bodily pains and somatic illness was trimodal, as shown in Figure 1. The trimodal distribution was confirmed in a replication sample. These findings provide strong support for the separation of somatoform disorders (like somatization disorder) and anxiety disorders (like generalized anxiety disorder) in the third edition of the *Diagnostic and Statistical Manual of Mental Disorders* (DSM-III) (American Psychiatric Association 1980).

In similar studies of the discriminant validity of schizophrenic disorders, Cloninger, Martin, Guze, et al. (1985) showed that schizo-

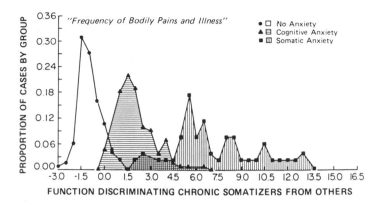

Figure 1.   Trimodal distribution of frequency of bodily pains and somatic complaints in men in the Stockholm adoption study.

phrenia was relatively discrete from other forms of psychopathology. A discriminant function composed of the symptoms characteristic of schizophrenia (auditory hallucinations, delusions of persecution and passivity, other firmly fixed delusions, and the absence of elation) had a bimodal distribution. More specifically, schizophrenics had two or more of these symptoms and nonschizophrenics usually had none; the distribution was bimodal because individuals with only one of the features were relatively rare. Other work cited by Kendell (1982) that had failed to detect this bimodality employed samples with a restricted range (psychotics only) and retained many features that were not individually significant, thereby reducing the likelihood of detecting bimodality.

Despite these successes, studies trying to detect natural boundaries between anxiety and depressive disorders have been unsuccessful. Studies have failed to produce replicable evidence of points of rarity between anxiety and depressive disorders (Kendell 1982). Some separation has been observed in discriminant analyses, but the means of the putative subgroups differ only by about two standard deviations. The weak separation of the anxiety and depressive subgroups is noteworthy because two standard deviations is at the limits of what can be resolved statistically in samples of practical size. By comparison, the difference between the means of the somatic anxiety and cognitive anxiety group in the studies by Sigvardsson, Bohman, von Knorring, et al. (1986) was about four standard deviations. Therefore, methods designed to optimize the discrimination of anxiety and depressive disorders still fail to demonstrate large or replicable differences when the discriminating features are limited to cross-sectional clinical features.

Even the discrimination of cognitive and somatic anxiety disorders was only partial. Figure 1 shows that the groups still overlap partly, so that the disorders can be considered only "relatively discrete." Objective measures of somatic and cognitive anxiety usually have about 25% shared variance (Cloninger 1986b). In other words, there is a basis for defining natural cutpoints between disorders, but some classification errors must be expected. The same limitation applies to the separation of schizophrenia and other psychoses. Accordingly, there is no strong general answer to the question about discreteness of psychopathology because the answer must be qualified (1) in terms of particular sets of disorders and (2) in terms of the degree of separation.

However, failure to detect natural boundaries in some past cross-sectional studies does not prove that natural boundaries could not be demonstrated if longitudinal or etiologic data were used. Nevertheless, available data cast doubt on the simple Kraepelinean assumption that all psychopathology is comprised of discrete, mutually exclusive disorders.

EMPIRICAL STRUCTURE OF COMORBIDITY

To test further predictions of alternative theories of psychopathology, we have examined the observed pattern of comorbidity in a diagnostic and family study of 500 psychiatric outpatients, called the Washington University Clinic study. The diagnostic criteria, which are similar to the Feighner criteria (Feighner, Robins, Guze, et al. 1972), and other procedures used in this study have been described in detail elsewhere (Martin, Cloninger, Guze, et al. 1985). In brief, a random sample of 500 psychiatric outpatients were interviewed in 1967 to 1969 and then independently reinterviewed 6 to 12 years later by psychiatrists using the same interview schedule. A sample of 1,249 of their first-degree relatives were also independently interviewed using the same schedule. The study is a blind and prospective investigation of psychiatric patients and their family members.

Primary diagnoses were distinguished on the basis of chronology from diagnoses with later onset. Final follow-up diagnoses were used in these analyses because the information about lifetime chronology is most complete at the second assessment. First, the observed pattern of association between primary and secondary psychiatric diagnoses was evaluated in the probands (i.e., the psychiatric outpatients) (Table 5). The 500 probands had a total of 612 diagnoses. Of the 500 cases, 50% had no secondary diagnosis. Patients with a primary diagnosis of somatization disorder, antisocial personality disorder, alcoholism, and, to a lesser extent, anxiety disorders (including panic

Table 5. Relative Risk of Proband's Secondary Diagnoses

Proband's primary diagnosis	n of probands	Anxiety		Phobic		Somatization		Antisocial personality		Alcoholism		Drug abuse		Sexual		Mood		Schizophrenic		Organic		Undiagnosed		No second diagnosis		Total
		RR	n	RR	n	RR	n	RR	n	RR	n	RR	n	RR	n	RR	n	RR	n	RR	n	RR	n	RR	n	n
Anxiety	42	—		>81	7	0	0	1.5	1	0.9	6	0	0	0	0	3.3*	30	0	0	0.7	1	0	0	0.3*	10	55
Phobic	3	0	0	—		0	0	0	0	0	1	0	0	0	0	4.8	2	0	0	0	0	0	0	0.7	1	3
Obsessional	7	0	0	0	0	0	0	0	0	0.9	1	0	0	10.6*	1	4.9*	6	0	0	0	0	0	0	0.2	1	9
Somatization	62	0	0	0	0	—		4.0	3	1.6	14	0.5	2	4.0	3	4.5*	49	0	0	0.5	1	0.9	2	0.1	8	82
Antisocial personality	43	1.2	2	0	0	8.1*	5	—	0	3.1	22	6.6*	13	3.8	3	0.82	22	12.7*	2	1.6	3	3.6	6	0.1	7	85
Alcoholism	40	2.6	2	0	0	.1.6	1	0	0	—		0.5	1	1.8	1	3.3*	25	6.4	1	0	2	2.8	3	0.3*	9	45
Drug abuse	6	0	0	0	0	0	0	28.4*	2	3.6	3	—		0	0	1.2	3	0	0	0	0	0	0	0.2	1	9
Sexual	18	11.5*	4	0	0	2.6	1	2.9	1	1.5	5	2.7	3	—		1.3	10	0	0	0	0	0	0	0.3*	5	29
Mood	128	1.8	4	0	0	0	0	0	0	0.8	14	0.6	4	0	0	2.9*	24	0	0	1.3	4	0.2	1	9.0*	105	132
Schizophrenic	40	0	0	0	0	1.6	1	0	0	0.5	3	0.5	1	0	0	2.9*	24	—		3.2	3	0	0	0.6	14	46
Organic	8	0	0	0	0	0	0	0	0	0.8	1	2.5	1	0	0	3.7	6	0		—		0	0	2.4	2	10
Mental retardation	10	0	0	0	0	6.2	1	7.0	1	0.6	1	0	0	0	0	0.4	2	0	0	3.5	1	30.5*	5	0.3	2	13
Undiagnosed	86	0	0	0	0	0	0	0		0.5	6	0.5	2	0	0	0.0*	1	0	0	0	0	—		17.9*	78	87
Not ill	7																							—	7	7
Total	500		12		7		9		8		76		27		8		180		3		15		17		250	612

Note. RR = relative risk. *p < .05.

and generalized anxiety disorders) were significantly more likely to have a secondary diagnosis. In other words, in Table 5 these primary diagnoses have relative risks (or odds ratio) for no secondary diagnosis that are significantly less than 1.0. On the other hand, primary mood disorders (most primary depressions) were significantly more likely to have no secondary diagnoses than were cases with other primary diagnoses.

Depression and substance abuse accounted for most of the secondary diagnoses: specifically 78% of the 362 secondary diagnoses were depression ($n = 180$), alcoholism ($n = 76$), or drug abuse ($n = 27$). Compared to an overall frequency of 29%, secondary depressions were especially frequent in cases with a primary diagnosis of somatization disorder (60%), alcoholism (56%), and anxiety disorder (55%), but were also common in other chronic disorders like schizophrenia (52%). In contrast, cases with a primary diagnosis of antisocial personality were especially likely to have secondary substance abuse (41%), but not secondary depression (26%).

Patients with a primary diagnosis of antisocial personality also had an eightfold increased risk of somatization disorder. In contrast, secondary phobic disorders were diagnosed only in association with primary anxiety disorders. Patients with a primary diagnosis of sexual disorders (homosexuality or sexual deviation) were likely to have a second diagnosis, especially anxiety. Mental retardation was associated with an excess of uncertain diagnoses, but had no specific secondary associations.

Similar patterns of comorbidity were observed in the relatives (Table 6). However, only 11% of the 585 relatives with a primary psychiatric diagnosis had multiple diagnoses. Nevertheless, cases with a primary diagnosis of somatization disorder, antisocial personality, and alcoholism were significantly more likely to have a secondary diagnosis than other cases. Primary anxiety disorders were slightly more likely to have a secondary diagnosis than others, but the difference was insignificant. Primary mood disorders were slightly less likely to have a secondary diagnosis, but this difference was also insignificant.

As in the treatment sample, most of the secondary diagnoses were depression and substance abuse. In fact, these diagnoses accounted for 95% of the 91 secondary diagnoses. Secondary depression was closely associated with somatization disorder, alcoholism, and anxiety disorders; secondary substance abuse was especially closely associated with antisocial personality. Despite the similarity in the types of diagnoses that were comorbid in probands and in relatives, it is most striking that 89% of psychiatric cases among the relatives have only one diagnosis.

Table 6. Relative Risk of Relative's Secondary Diagnoses

Relative's primary diagnosis	n of probands	Relative's secondary diagnoses																								Total
		Anxiety		Phobic		Somatization		Antisocial personality		Alcoholism		Drug abuse		Sexual		Mood		Schizophrenic		Organic		Undiagnosed		No second diagnosis		
		RR	n	RR	n	RR	n	RR	n	RR	n	RR	n	RR	n	RR	n	RR	n	RR	n	RR	n	RR	n	n
Anxiety	41	—	0	0	0	0	0	0	0	1.0	1	0	0	0	0	3.2*	4	0	0	0	0	0	0	0.6	36	41
Phobic	0	0	0	—		0	0	0	0	0	0	0	0	0	0	0	0	0	0	0	0	0	0	0	0	0
Obsessional	2	0	0	0	0	0	0	0	0	0	0	0	0	0	0	28.0*	1	0	0	0	0	0	0	0.1	1	2
Somatization	20	0	0	0	0	—		0	0	6.1*	3	0	0	0	0	50.0*	13	0	0	0	0	0	0	0.0*	7	23
Antisocial personality	58	0	0	0	0	16.5*	1	—		>6.3*	25	>146.1*	8	>16.5	1	10.0*	15	0	0	0	0	0	0	0.0*	24	74
Alcoholism	95	0	0	0	0	1216	1	0	0	—		0	0	0	0	4.4*	11	0	0	12.7	1	0	0	0.5*	82	95
Drug abuse	1	0	0	0	0	0	0	0	0	0	0	—		0	0	∞	1	0	0	0	0	0	0	?	0	1
Sexual	1	0	0	0	0	0	0	0	0	0	0	0	0	—		0	0	—		0	0	0	0	0	1	1
Mood	79	0	0	0	0	0	0	0	0	1.0	2	0	0	0	0	—		0	0	15.4	1	0	0	2.3	76	79
Schizophrenic	12	0	0	0	0	0	0	0	0	3.5	1	0	0	0	0	0	0	—		0	0	0	0	1.0	11	12
Organic	4	0	0	0	0	0	0	0	0	0	0	0	0	0	0	0	0	0		—		0	0	∞	4	4
Mental retardation	7	0	0	0	0	0	0	0	0	0	0	0	0	0	0	0	0	0	0	0	0	0	0	∞	14	14
Undiagnosed	265	0	0	0	0	0	0	0	0	0.1	1	0	0	0	0	0	0	0	0	0	0	—		29.4*	264	265
Not ill	664	—		—		—		—		—		—		—		—		—		—		—		—	664	664
Total	1,249		0		0		2		0		33		8		1		45		0		2		0		1,184	1,275

Note.   RR = relative risk. *p* < .05.

The pattern of association among primary diagnoses in probands and relatives was also evaluated (Table 7). There was a general tendency for an increased risk of the same primary diagnosis in probands and relatives, especially for anxiety disorders, schizophrenia, and mental retardation. In addition, patients with somatization disorder had a fourfold excess of antisocial personality in their relatives compared to other patients. In contrast, probands with primary mood disorders were associated with a decreased risk of relatives with other kinds of psychopathology, including both anxiety and antisocial personality disorders.

Does Comorbidity Have a Stable Structure?

The findings about the structure of comorbidity in the Washington University Clinic study call into question the simple Kraepelinian assumption that all psychopathology is comprised of disorders that are mutually exclusive. In other words, the results of the Washington University Clinic study suggest that particular disorders tend to occur together, and not with other disorders. In view of the importance of these findings, it is essential that we consider whether they are stable and reproducible.

Available data support the generalizability of the findings in the Washington University Clinic study. Specifically, cognitive anxiety disorders like generalized anxiety disorder are positively correlated with nonpsychotic depressions (most chapters in this volume) and type 1 alcohol dependence (Cloninger 1987a) and are negatively correlated with antisocial personality disorder (Cloninger, von Knorring, Sigvardsson, et al. 1986). On the other hand, somatic anxiety disorders like somatization disorder are positively correlated with antisocial personality disorder and type 2 alcoholism (Cloninger 1987a; Cloninger, Sigvardsson, and Bohman 1988). Both these sets of comorbid disorders appear to be independent of risk for manic psychoses (Cloninger, Reich, and Wetzel 1979; Wetzel, Cloninger, Hong, et al. 1980) and for schizophrenic psychoses (Guze, Cloninger, Martin, et al. 1983). Factor analysis of multiple diagnoses among inpatients found independent groups of disorders associated with mania, schizophrenia, and antisocial personality; in other words, mania and schizophrenic disorders were uncorrelated from one another and antisocial personality (Wolf, Schubert, Patterson, et al. 1988).

The reverse relationship of criminality in biologic mothers to somatic and cognitive anxiety disorders in their adopted-away children is summarized in Table 8. The data are from the study of 807 adopted men described earlier in which somatic and cognitive anxiety were found to be relatively discrete disorders (Sigvardsson, Bohman,

Table 7. Relative Risk of Relative's Primary Diagnoses

Relative's primary diagnoses

Proband's primary diagnosis	n of probands	Anxiety		Obsessional		Somatization		Antisocial personality		Alcoholism		Drug abuse		Sexual		Mood		Schizophrenic		Organic		Mental retardation		Undiagnosed		Not ill		Total
		RR	n	RR	n	RR	n	RR	n	RR	n	RR	n	RR	n	RR	n	RR	n	RR	n	RR	n	RR	n	RR	n	n
Anxiety	42	3.6*	10	0	0	1.2	2	0.8	4	1.3	10	0	0	>1	1	0.4	3	0	0	0	0	0	0	1.6	16	1.2	63	109
Phobic	3	7.5	1	0	0	0	0	0	0	0	0	0	0	0	0	0	0	0	0	0	0	0	0	0.4	2	0.6	2	5
Obsessional	7	1.9	1	0	0	0	0	1.3	1	1.6	2	0	0	0	0	2.0	2	0	0	0	0	0	0	1.1	4	0.6	7	17
Somatization	62	1.9	10	0	0	2.0	5	3.6*	21	1.2	16	0	0	0	0	0.6	7	0.5	1	2.0	1	0	0	1.1	40	0.7*	81	182
Antisocial personality	43	0.4	1	0	0	0	0	0.9	3	0.9	5	0	0	0	0	0.6	3	1.4	1	0	0	0	0	0.7	20	1.1	41	74
Alcoholism	40	1.5	4	0	0	0.7	1	0.2	1	1.1	7	0	0	0	0	1.6	8	1.2	1	4.6	1	0	0	0.7	13	1.2	49	85
Drug abuse	6	0	0	0	0	0	0	2.6	1	0	0	0	0	0	0	4.3	2	0	0	0	0	0	0	3.0	5	0.1*	1	9
Sexual	18	0	0	0	0	0.8	5	0	0	0	0	71	1	0	0	4.7*	4	6.9	1	0.8	1	0	0	0	0	0.4	5	17
Mood	128	0.3*	5	2.3	1	0	0	0.4*	9	0.7	25	0	0	0	0	1.5	31	1.1	4	0.8	1	0.9	2	1.0	83	1.3*	220	381
Schizophrenic	40	0.3	1	0	0	0.6	1	0.2	1	0.7	6	0	0	0	0	0.4	3	5.8*	4	0	0	0	0	1.4	27	1.2	59	102
Organic	8	1.4	1	0	0	0	0	0	0	2.8	4	0	0	0	0	1.5	2	0	0	0	0	0	0	0.4	2	1.3	13	22
Mental retardation	10	0	0	0	0	0	0	2.5	4	1.4	4	0	0	0	0	0	0	0	0	10.9*	1	91.6*	5	0.8	7	0.7	17	38
Undiagnosed	86	1.1	7	5.4	1	2.3	6	1.3	11	1.0	15	0	0	0	0	1.0	12	0	0	0	0	0	0	1.1	43	0.9	101	196
Not ill	7	0	0	0	0	0	0	1.9	1	1.1	1	0	0	0	0	3.0	2	0	0	0	0	0	0	1.2	3	0.6	5	12
Total	500		41		2		20		58		95		1		1		79		12		4		7		265		664	1,249

Note. RR = relative risk. *p < .05.

Table 8. Reverse Relationship of Criminality in Biologic Mothers and Somatic and Cognitive Anxiety in Their Adopted-Away Sons in the Stockholm Adoption Study

Criminal conviction in biologic mother	*n* adopted	Risk of anxiety disorder in adoptee (%)	
		Cognitive	Somatic
Yes	49	6	11
No	758	22	6

von Knorring, et al. 1986). This finding suggests that heritable factors that increase risk of somatic anxiety are protective factors for cognitive anxiety, and vice versa (Cloninger 1986b). Because similar findings about patterns of comorbidity of somatic and cognitive anxiety have been obtained in several countries (Cloninger 1986b), the structure of psychiatric comorbidity appears to be stable regardless of sociocultural variation. However, more rigorous cross-cultural studies are needed, with assessment procedures closely standardized.

Is the Structure of Comorbidity Artifactual?

The observed comorbidity of putative categories of psychiatric disorder may be attributable to artifacts of ascertainment, ignorance of optimal diagnostic criteria, and low reliability of assessment. For example, Table 5 shows that most anxiety neurotics in a treatment sample have secondary depressions, but Table 6 shows that anxiety neurotics among relatives seldom do. This association suggests that anxiety neurotics usually seek treatment after they become depressed, and infrequently seek treatment when they are only anxious. Prospective longitudinal studies show that the secondary depressions in anxiety neurotics usually occur after many years of chronic anxiety (Table 9). These ascertainment effects certainly must be considered in interpreting data from treatment samples.

Furthermore, some studies of comorbidity have inflated apparent comorbidity by ignoring exclusion criteria that have been demonstrated to have discriminant validity (e.g., Boyd, Burke, Gruenberg, et al. 1984). Although many of the exclusion criteria in DSM-III were unvalidated, it is ironic that the few exclusion criteria that have been validated would be ignored in much subsequent research. For example, the distinction between primary and secondary depressions has been ignored in some studies of comorbidity despite evidence that their etiology is different (Feighner, Robins, Guze, et al. 1972). Unlike primary depressions, secondary depressions are not familial regardless of the primary diagnosis, including primary anxiety disorders (Cloninger, Martin, Guze, et al. 1981), somatoform disorders (Guze,

Table 9. Natural History of Panic Disorder Among Probands in Washington University Clinic Study

Affected symptom	Age of onset		Mean years
	n	%	
Nervousness	32	100	12.41 ± 6.07
Simple phobias	27	84	18.46 ± 12.99
Social phobias	9	28	18.48 ± 15.81
Palpitations-dyspnea	32	100	20.53 ± 10.72
Panic attacks	32	100	22.30 ± 10.54
Agoraphobia	5	100	22.30 ± 10.54
Obsessions-compulsions	7	16	23.40 ± 8.82
Depressed mood	31	97	28.94 ± 14.26
Depressive syndrome	24	75	31.35 ± 14.15

Cloninger, Martin, et al. 1986b), alcoholism (Guze, Cloninger, Martin, et al. 1986a), or schizophrenia (Guze, Cloninger, Martin, et al. 1983). The studies demonstrating the nonfamiliality of secondary depression that are cited here are especially noteworthy because they are based on the Washington University Clinic study, which is the only study to our knowledge in which there was a wide spectrum of disorders in probands and independent assessment of their relatives. Nonfamilial secondary depressive reactions are also often observed with chronic medical illnesses, particular diseases of kidney that result in severe functional impairment (Hong, Smith, Robson, et al. 1987). These findings suggest that secondary depressions are often demoralization reactions to a wide variety of chronic illnesses and their sequelae, rather than a specific comorbid condition that shares etiologic antecedents with anxiety disorders.

The hypothesis that secondary depression is usually a nonspecific demoralization reaction to chronic impairment also predicts another finding that has been observed about anxiety and depression: the risk of depression in individuals with chronic anxiety disorders is greater than the risk of anxiety in individuals with depressive disorders, even when acute anxiety states that are limited to a single episode of depression are counted as a comorbid disorder. It is very rare for an anxiety disorder to be a chronic residual state following remission of a primary depressive disorder (Cloninger, Martin, Guze, et al. 1981); even when a diagnosis of secondary anxiety disorder appears justified based on retrospective history, examination of earlier medical records nearly always results in a diagnosis of a primary anxiety disorder preceding onset of depression (Cloninger, unpublished data). If anxiety and depression were alternate expressions of the same etiologic factors, there should be an asymmetry in risk. If depression were a more severe form of the same etiologic process, then the risk of anxiety after onset of depression should be greater than the risk of depression after onset of an anxiety disorder. Neither of these expectations is observed. The observed asymmetry casts doubt on both the latter hypotheses and supports a directional relationship in which depression is a nonspecific sequela of chronic disability. Accordingly, current emphasis on the comorbidity of anxiety and depressive disorders may be partly artifacts of the chronicity of anxiety disorders and lack of controls with other chronic medical or psychiatric disorders of comparable levels of functional disability. The findings presented here suggest that anxiety disorders are associated with an increased risk of depression, but to a lesser extent than somatization and substance abuse disorders (Tables 5 and 6).

Some family data have been reported suggesting that patients with mixed anxiety-depressive disorders have an excess of both anxiety and depressive disorders (Merikangas, Chapter 21; Weissman, Chapter 22). In contrast, Torgersen (Chapter 23) finds an asymmetry in the genetic relationship in twins: probands with anxiety disorders less often have co-twins with depression when compared to the risk of anxiety disorders in co-twins of probands with depressive disorders. Furthermore, there is no familial overlap whatsoever between primary anxiety and primary depressive disorders when the temporal sequence of syndrome onset is taken into account (Cloninger, Martin, Guze, et al. 1981), as shown in Table 7. This lack of familial overlap suggests that mixed anxiety-depressive disorders are heterogeneous mixtures of primary anxiety disorders (with secondary depressions) and primary depressive disorders (with coincident anxiety symptoms). Studies that have failed to distinguish the primary psychiatric disorder using validated criteria like those of Feighner, Robins, Guze, et al. (1972) or the Washington University Clinic study (Martin, Cloninger, Guze, et al. 1985) may have inflated the apparent comorbidity of anxiety and depressive disorders because of the use of criteria with less discriminant validity or less reliable assessment methods.

Overall, the comorbidity of anxiety and depressive disorders may have been inflated in some past studies by use of cross-sectional diagnostic criteria with low discriminant validity. Extreme artifactual inflation of comorbidity results when all exclusion criteria are ignored regardless of their ability to discriminate etiologically distinct conditions.

The criticism of the supposed specificity of the comorbidity of anxiety and depressive disorders does not imply that individuals with anxiety disorders do not develop secondary depressions more rapidly or frequently than do others. Rather, the criticism is that available evidence is weak and flawed by procedural limitations, particularly lack of controls with other chronic diseases matched for extent of functional impairment. Until additional controlled studies are conducted, it is premature to draw any conclusions about shared susceptibility factors for anxiety and depressive disorders, whether those supposed susceptibility factors are biologic, social, or cognitive factors. Nevertheless, further research is justified because there are some data supporting the hypothesis that individuals with a specific profile of personality traits (namely, passive-dependent personality) are susceptible to both anxiety and depressive disorders (Cloninger 1986b).

In contrast, the comorbidity of antisocial personality with somatic and cognitive anxiety disorders does not appear to be attributable to procedural artifacts or ascertainment or assessment. First, somatic anxiety and antisocial behavior are markedly different in their clinical form so that the clinical distinction is obvious. Accordingly, the positive association in both individuals and families suggested the possibility of shared etiologic factors, which was later confirmed by adoption studies (Cloninger 1986b). Second, somatic and cognitive anxiety disorders may be difficult to distinguish in some cases, but they have opposite relationships to risk of antisocial behavior. Accordingly, procedural artifacts that reduce the discrimination of somatic and cognitive anxiety disorders may actually attenuate the observed relationship to antisocial personality rather than inflate them, as in the case of anxiety and depressive disorders.

Is the Structure Predictable by Measurable Antecedents?

The available evidence that comorbidity does have a stable structure provides an important clue about the etiology of psychopathology. Many clinicians and researchers have suggested that personality, temperament, or character traits represent stable susceptibility factors for psychopathology. In other words, personality traits represent clinically measurable indicators of individual differences in susceptibility to psychopathology. If so, two key tests are available for this hypothesis. First, antecedent personality traits should be predictive of individual psychiatric disorders, Second, the structure of personality should be predictive of the observed pattern of psychiatric comorbidity. For example, both Kraepelin and Freud thought that personality factors were fundamental to understanding susceptibility to psychopathology. However, Kraepelin thought there were different personality factors underlying each of several specific disorders (e.g., cyclothymic personality was the basic foundation for manic-depressive psychosis and was observable before onset of psychoses and between episodes). On the other hand, dynamic psychiatrists suggest that personality traits are associated with individual differences in characteristic patterns of using ego defense mechanisms, which modify susceptibility to psychopathology in a less specific, but still predictable, manner. That is, dynamic theories predict that there is a stable pattern to comorbidity that is predictable on the basis of personality traits and/or defense mechanisms.

Personality can be viewed as a measure of individual differences in learning because both personality and learning reflect the way behavior is organized as a result of individual experience (Cloninger 1987a, 1987b). Accordingly, social and behavioral learning theories of psychopathology also make predictions about the structure of personality and learning. Pure learning theories classically have rejected the hypothesis that personality has a stable or heritable structure, even though there is consistent evidence that genetic and environmental factors are of roughly equal importance in the development of individual differences in personality traits (Cloninger 1986b, 1987b). Accordingly, pure learning theories consider patterns of behavior to be determined by individual experience alone and do not expect there to be a structure to comorbidity that is stable and heritable regardless of individual experience. For pure learning theories, the only antecedents relevant to later development of psychopathology are experiential. In contrast, dynamic theories hold that the interaction of both neurobiologic predisposition and experiential antecedents is critical to the development of psychopathology. For the classic Kraepelinian model, experiential factors are simply nonspecific triggers of specific neurobiologic susceptibility factors.

Recently, Cloninger described a neurobiologic learning model of personality that is more general than the other theoretical views of personality in the sense that each of the others can be obtained as a restricted case of a more comprehensive conceptual paradigm (Cloninger 1986b, 1987b). This model was based on a synthesis of clinical longitudinal and family studies, psychometric studies of personality structure, and neuropsychopharmacologic and neurobehavioral studies of individual differences in learning and motivation. The model is described in more detail elsewhere, along with peer commentary (Cloninger 1986b, 1987b, 1988). The relevant point for this chapter is that this theory of personality makes many testable predictions about the structure of psychiatric comorbidity.

To understand the predictions about the structure of comorbidity, it is first necessary to understand the structure of personality because personality is hypothesized to modify susceptibility to psychopathology in response to experience. Adaptive personality traits are known to be quantifiable variables that are approximately normally distributed. Factor-analytic studies show that most variability in personality can be accounted for by three independent dimensions, and Cloninger (1987b) has hypothesized three independent neurogenetic regulatory systems that modulate the activation, maintenance, and inhibition of behavior in response to experience. The personality traits that reflect these three systems are called novelty seeking, reward dependence, and harm avoidance, respectively. Each of these three dimensions is bipolar and normally distributed. Individuals who are high in novelty seeking are described as impulsive, exploratory, quick-tempered, and extravagant; those low in novelty seeking are reflective, rigid, stoical, and frugal. Individuals who are high in harm avoidance are fearful, pessimistic, shy, and easily fatigued; those who are low in harm avoidance are daring, optimistic, confident, and vigorous. Individuals who are high in reward dependence are sentimental, warm, persistent, and sensitive to social cues; those who are low in reward dependence are pragmatic, cold, self-willed, and detached.

All possible combinations of deviations on these three factors are empirically observed, as expected according to the hypothesis that these three dimensions are regulated by independent genetic factors. In fact, the characteristics that are expected from the possible combinations of these three adaptive factors correspond to classic descriptions of traditional personality categories (Figure 2). For example, individuals with antisocial personality disorder are defined by their being high in novelty seeking and low in the other two dimensions. In contrast, individuals with passive-dependent (sometimes called "anxious") personality disorder have the reverse configuration of being low in novelty seeking and high in the other two dimensions. Both

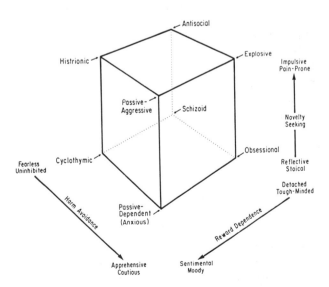

Figure 2. Traditional personality disorders related to the three personality dimensions of novelty seeking, harm avoidance, and reward dependence.

histrionic and antisocial personality disorders are high in novelty seeking and low in harm avoidance, but differ in the reward dependence dimension.

This structural decomposition of personality is useful in understanding the stable structure of psychopathology because specific personality traits are predictors of specific kinds of psychopathology (Cloninger 1986b, 1987a; Cloninger, Sigvardsson, and Bohman 1988; Sigvardsson, Bohman, and Cloninger 1987). In particular, increased susceptibility to somatic anxiety is predicted by high novelty seeking, which is associated with more rapid escape and active avoidance of pain and other forms of aversive stimulation (Cloninger 1988). On the other hand, increased apprehensive expectation or cognitive anxiety is predicted by high harm avoidance, which is associated with sensitivity to passive avoidance and extinction responses to aversive stimulation. Thus individuals with pure somatic anxiety are expected to be high in novelty seeking, but not harm avoidance; individuals with pure cognitive anxiety are expected to be high in harm avoidance, but not novelty seeking. Individuals who are high in both novelty seeking and harm avoidance are expected to have a variety of approach-avoidance conflicts characterized by mixtures of both somatic and cognitive anxiety.

Furthermore, harm avoidance and novelty seeking also modify the risk of impulsive-aggressive behavior, as confirmed by prospective studies in which personality was measured at age 10 and individuals were followed prospectively to age 27 (Sigvardsson, Bohman, and Cloninger 1987). Criminal behavior in general is increased in individuals who are high in novelty seeking. Those who are also low in harm avoidance are particularly likely to commit violent crimes. Accordingly, antisocial or criminal behavior is expected to be positively correlated with high somatic anxiety and negatively correlated with high cognitive anxiety. This is strongly supported by the findings summarized in Table 8.

In addition, high reward dependence is hypothesized to be associated with greater intensity of dysphoric reactions to frustrative nonreward, such as romantic disappointments or failure to receive expected recognition. Moreover, individuals who are high in both reward dependence and harm avoidance are expected to be particularly susceptible to type 1 alcoholism (i.e., alcoholism characterized by binge drinking, loss of control once drinking begins, and guilt about psychological dependence) and rapid development of tolerance and dependence to antianxiety drugs, as supported by longitudinal and family studies of alcoholics (Cloninger 1987a). In addition, these same individuals who are high in both reward dependence and harm avoidance, and their adopted-away biologic relatives, are found to be susceptible not only to type 1 alcoholism, but also cognitive anxiety and dysthymia or neurotic depression (Cloninger 1986b, 1987a).

However, these three adaptive dimensions of personality appear to be independent of schizotypal and paranoid disorders, which seem to involve defects in information processing (Cloninger 1987b). Susceptibility to schizophrenia and schizotypal personality is expected to be independent of individual differences in risk for anxiety, depression, somatization, and substance abuse.

Available data about psychiatric comorbidity strongly support this structural model of personality disorder and psychopathology. However, further research is needed to test the predictions more systematically, as well as to refine and extend the theory. In particular, integrative studies of neurobiology and learning need to be carried out in longitudinal family studies to characterize the interaction of biologic predisposition and experience in the development of psychopathology.

OVERVIEW

Psychiatric comorbidity has a stable structure that appears to be predictable on the basis of antecedent personality dimensions. This does not mean that diagnostic exclusion rules should be indiscriminately ignored; nor does it mean that the many unvalidated exclusion rules of DSM-III should be reified. It is clear that the classic Kraepelinian model must be rejected or modified, but it would be unjustified to ignore exclusion rules that have demonstrated discriminant validity.

It is important to remember that different approaches to classification may be optimal for different sets of disorders. For example, dimensional approaches may be more efficient and powerful in describing personality variation, but types of psychoses may be more accurately characterized in terms of categorical diagnoses. Furthermore, categorical and dimensional approaches to classification can be integrated in a practical and useful manner, as shown elsewhere for nonpsychotic disorders (Cloninger 1986b, 1987a, 1987b).

Much prior work on comorbidity of depression and anxiety has been flawed by inattention to the importance of lifetime chronology. Even more egregious has been the absence of appropriate control groups in studies of the comorbidity of anxiety and depression: chronic medical or psychiatric disorders that are matched for severity and duration of functional impairment should be included to evaluate the specificity of observed relationships. More attention to the comorbidity of somatization, cognitive anxiety, and antisocial behavior would help to broaden traditional perspectives by providing contrast groups of demonstrated utility.

Chapter 28

Psychosocial Factors in Anxiety and Depression

Scott M. Monroe, Ph.D.

D ELINEATING THE IMPLICATIONS of comorbid disorders for theories of anxiety and depression is an exercise of some irony. The task is to examine a literature from which the core information has been elided, or significantly altered, through prevailing diagnostic conventions. This circumstance is because traditional views of these disorders have conceptualized them as discrete, nonoverlapping syndromes. Consequently, we now must reconstruct the missing or distorted data to derive the implications of comorbidity for theories of anxiety and depressive disorders on the one hand, and for classification of these disorders on the other.

In developing the psychosocial perspective on the topic, it is useful initially to place constraints on what is to be considered under the broad heading of "psychosocial." Perhaps the most relevant concept, and the one for which the largest empirical literature exists, is life stress. Owing to prevailing diagnostic practices, however, only a limited number of studies have focused directly on the relationship of life stress to anxiety, depression, and their co-occurrence. These investigations are informative, yet too few in number from which to draw firm conclusions. Given a dearth of primary evidence, it is necessary to enlarge the conceptual scope and to turn to other literatures that bear on the topic. This amplification spans a number of relevant areas of inquiry, ranging from descriptive clinical studies to

The author appreciates and acknowledges the helpful comments provided by Anne D. Simons, John Roberts, and Shari Wade; and by the editors, Jack Maser and Robert Cloninger, on previous drafts of the manuscript. This work was supported in part by National Institute of Mental Health grant MH-39139.

genetic investigations of comorbidity. Utilizing information from both direct and indirect sources provides a broader framework for reconstructing and further understanding how life stress may be related to symptom comorbidity of anxiety and depression.

Following reviews of the literature, the next section of this chapter is devoted to integrating the existing evidence. Major issues from the review to be reconciled with the life stress perspective include (1) severity of disorder, (2) genetic and biologic vulnerability, and (3) chronicity of impairment. A common theme that cuts across these concerns pertains not only to the influence of life stress on comorbid symptoms of anxiety and depression, but equally to the reciprocal influence of psychopathology on psychosocial circumstances, which in turn may exacerbate or color the presenting symptom picture. A variety of methodological and conceptual issues are raised that bear on the task of understanding how risk factors and psychopathology interact in the development of anxiety and depression, and how such interactions over time may be more effectively studied. From this vantage point, it becomes clear that longitudinal changes in stress, depression, and anxiety have important, and previously unnoticed, implications for the existing models of comorbidity of anxiety and depression.

For a review in which life stress plays such a central role, it is essential to delineate the prevailing ideas and strategies underlying the conceptualization and measurement of such an operationally complex construct. This subject comprises several arguments that, while not necessarily unique to the topic of comorbidity, are extremely germane for understanding a life stress perspective. Interestingly, when conceptualizing comorbidity from a life stress viewpoint, particular inadequacies of existing assessment procedures are highlighted more emphatically than in the investigation of either depression or anxiety alone. To appreciate the research performed to date, it is necessary to understand these concerns.

CONCEPTUALIZATION, MEASUREMENT, AND RESEARCH DESIGN CONSIDERATIONS

The idea that the social environment is intimately associated with mental health is one with a long history and wide following (Rosen 1958). Subjective impression and philosophical speculation, however, have only recently been replaced by more rigorous viewpoints. Early attempts to define and operationalize the construct of stress laid the foundation for more systematic exploration of the boundaries and implications of the concept. A brief overview of the development of measurement and of research designs is important for evaluating current research within an informed perspective.

Conceptual and Measurement Developments: Life Stress

Selye's (1936) groundbreaking work on stress in the animal laboratory, and Holmes and Rahe's (1967) innovative translation of the concept into a scale for humans, created a theoretical and methodological context for studying the consequences of stress. Crucial to this enterprise was the recognition that life conditions of different people could be standardized. That is, individual differences in life circumstances could be compared and correlated through such a consensually defined reference system with respect to a variety of adverse psychological and physical outcomes.

The complexities of the task were initially overlooked in the enthusiastic quest for detecting relationships with an assortment of health outcomes. The concepts and methods were quickly adopted by investigators of diverse backgrounds and uncritically applied to a variety of topics. The assessment procedures appeared to be accorded instant validity, having seemingly sprung from the minds of the creators much like Minerva sprung from the brain of Zeus: instantly, fully, and perfectly formed.

The problem was not inherent in the original development of the ideas or procedures, but rather was due to a lack of refinement in thought and method. The complexities of quantifying social experiences that overwhelmed simple approaches to measurement became increasingly impossible to ignore. Fundamental questions arose, including disturbing reports on the basic psychometric properties of the early instruments. The life events self-report checklist of Holmes and Rahe (1967)—the Schedule of Recent Experiences (SRE)—and derivative measures were found to possess poor test-retest reliability (Jenkins, Hurst, and Rose 1979; Monroe 1982a; Paykel 1982). Other questions emerged concerning specific operational procedures designed to reflect recent stress (e.g., adding all events, adding only subtypes of events, using dimensional weights, or only counting specific high-impact experiences) (Monroe 1982c). Conceptually, several theoretical characteristics of life stress began to enlighten discussion (e.g., readjustment, undesirability, exits from the social field, controllability); equally important was the emerging interest in the temporal dimensions of the stress process (including early childhood stressors, current acute stressors, and ongoing chronic stressors). Finally, the definitional criteria for what constitutes an event became an important point of concern. In particular, the self-report checklist format was believed by some to allow too much variability in idiosyncratic inter-pretations of events, thereby undermining the notion of a standard-ized measure (Brown 1981; Dohrenwend, Link, Kern, et al. 1987).

Thus the unidimensional notion of stress slowly gave way to more multidimensional and sophisticated conceptualizations. These newer developments possessed the potential to capture more of the intricacies and virtually infinite arrangements of circumstances in people's ongoing, day-to-day interactions with other persons, places, and things.

Research Design Considerations

Other problems with measurement became apparent when the links between life events and psychiatric disorder began to be viewed skeptically. Since most research was retrospective in design, it was impossible to disentangle confounds between certain types of the events represented in the checklists with the aspects of the disorders under study. For example, SRE checklist items (Holmes and Rahe 1967), such as a change in sleep or a change in recreation, could reflect depressive symptoms or reversals of the cause-and-effect sequence of association (e.g., events bring on disorder, or disorder brings on events) (Dohrenwend 1974). Without attention to distinguishing events from symptoms, or to the relative timing of each, little could be determined about the role of life stress as an etiologic factor.

Another concern highlighted in cross-sectional studies was the tendency for people who had developed some form of disorder to "explain away" or to attribute the occurrence of the disturbance to psychosocial precipitants, irrespective of the underlying validity of the association (Brown 1974). This tendency to palliate a confused psyche with credible explanation could, if left uncontrolled, build more positive, yet specious, findings into the research.

To some extent, these problems could be reduced through the use of prospective designs, wherein more rigorous control over the timing of event occurrence and disorder onset is possible. Yet, without very careful attention to the timing of events and changes in symptoms, many of the problems commonly associated with retrospective de-signs still plague prospective ones (Monroe 1982b). Although new generations of life event checklists have improved on and supplanted the original instruments (Dohrenwend, Krasnoff, Askenasy, et al. 1978; Paykel 1982; Sarason, Johnson, and Siegel 1978), many of the problems with self-report approaches to assessment continue to be evident with either retrospective or prospective research designs (e.g., inability to distinguish events that are consequences of dis-order). Some investigators believe that many limitations are inherent in the self-report format (Brown 1981; Finlay-Jones 1981; Katschnig 1986; Monroe and Peterman 1988), whereas others contend that such approaches, when properly structured, can provide useful information (Oei and Zwart 1986; Zimmerman 1983). In general, the prospective design is a preferred strategy, yet it does not eradicate several of the shortcomings extant with many life event measurement practices (e.g., self-report checklists).

Interview Procedures

With the awareness of the limitations of the original life event measurement procedures, it became clear that the objective underlying the original idea had been lost: to provide a consensually defined or standardized assessment of the dimensions of social experience informative for predicting illness.

Several research groups developed interview-based procedures for assessing life stress (e.g., Brown and Harris 1978a; Paykel 1982). Of these, the most systematic and studied is the Bedford College Life Events and Difficulties Schedule (LEDS) created by Brown and Harris (1978a). Over a number of years, an extensive set of rules and descriptors for standardizing the assessment of life stress has been developed for this system. The definitions of what qualifies as an event, and the rules for assigning particular qualities and dimensions of severity to events, are delineated by an extensive a priori set of rules and examples.

The procedures of the LEDS allow for standardization and replication across individuals. When there is no common set of rules and criteria for defining the events, there is no assurance that comparable experiences have occurred across individuals. With self-report checklists, these crucial standardization components of measurement are left to the idiosyncratic interpretations of the subject (Brown 1981; Brown and Harris 1986). Also in terms of breadth of coverage, the LEDS provides detailed inquiry into the chronic, ongoing stressors of the individual's life, thereby providing a more comprehensive index of day-to-day circumstances.

The foundations of measurement are built on reliability and replicability. Construct and predictive validity comprise an entirely different set of measurement concerns. In this realm, another feature of the LEDS is especially useful. In attempting to derive sensitive measures of stress, Brown and Harris (1978a) adopted an approach labeled "contextual." This terminology reflects the attempt to understand the implications of a life event, not from the eyes of the average individual, but from the vantage point of the individual in whose particular life the event happens. Many features of the person's life context provide useful clues for gauging the impact of such an experience, and this information is used to tailor the ratings of the event to the specific individual's biographical circumstances. For example, the event of bearing a first child will be quite different for a woman with a husband and financial means compared to a recently abandoned and impoverished single mother. It is this component of the approach that brings sensitivity to the standardization of measurement in terms of the likely meaning of the event for the individual (without relying on the methodologically hazardous interpretation provided by the subject).

An extensive literature has evolved using the LEDS (see Brown and Harris 1986). The majority of investigations support the reliability of the instrument over at least a 1-year retrospective time frame (Brown and Harris 1982). For interrater reliability of the event dimensions and their contextual ratings, the approach also rests on firm psychometric grounds (Brown and Harris 1982, 1986; Tennant, Smith, Bebbington, et al. 1979). In terms of validity of the instrument, there is considerable controversy (Brown and Harris 1978b; Tennant and Bebbington 1978).

Opinions on the validity of the LEDS involve two separate issues. First is the question of construct validity: how adequately the system assesses dimensions of life stress. Few direct comparisons have been made between this procedure and others in this respect (cf., Katschnig 1986), yet recent reviews covering the existing work underscore the superiority of the LEDS procedure (Finlay-Jones 1981; Katschnig 1986; Monroe and Peterman 1988). Others offer a conflicting viewpoint (Oei and Zwart 1986; Zimmerman 1983; Zimmerman, Pfohl, and Stangl 1986). Also noteworthy is that the LEDS approach incorporates recent events, as well as ongoing stressors, providing for a more extensive assessment. Furthermore, it has generally been found that using the contextual rating system does provide for control over respondent bias, yet does maintain sensitivity of the measure (Brown and Harris 1986). The majority of the available data at present, then, support the comprehensiveness and sensitivity of the LEDS relative to other measurement systems.

The second validity consideration is more controversial. While there is agreement that the LEDS methodology is a useful predictor of psychiatric problems in general (Bebbington 1986; Brown and Harris 1986), there is significant disagreement about the nature of the particular outcomes predicted. The viewpoints differ with respect to whether or not the LEDS findings pertain to depression in a clinical sense, or to more minor degrees of psychological distress (Bebbington 1986; Tennant, Bebbington, and Hurry 1981a). This concern has considerable implications for understanding the importance of life stress for comorbidity of anxiety and depression. (We will return to it subsequently, but for now we simply wish to outline the basic measurement considerations.)

An additional point is relevant for the study of life stress and comorbidity. The measurement approach must provide *conceptual* breadth to investigate the possibility that different qualities of life stress are related to specific forms, or symptoms, of psychopathology. That is, if the onset of particular disorders are suspected to be at least in part a function of life stress, the procedures must be sufficiently comprehensive to capture adequately the dimensions of theoretical importance for different outcomes. For example, recent work using the LEDS has found that specific types of life events differentially precede the onset of anxiety and depressive disorders (to be reviewed in greater detail subsequently) (Brown and Harris 1986).

Finally, even the best available approaches to measuring life stress are relatively crude. In contemplating challenging tasks for measurement, the translation of an individual's life experiences into a reliable and valid matrix of dimensions and numbers must rank high in difficulty. To this end, it is noteworthy that the LEDS approach is evolving to embrace such intricacies. Refinements in the approach include an expansion of the dimensions covered by the instrument, and procedures for tracking the manner in which life events and difficulties interrelate in the individual's life (Brown, Bifulco, and Harris 1987; Brown and Harris 1986). Adequate methodologies are available, and they are improving, but they remain comparatively primitive in relation to the magnitude of the task assayed.

Social Moderators and Symptom Formation Factors

Over the past decade, increasingly sophisticated models of the stress process have been proposed. These models have been developed on the idea that there are psychosocial factors, in addition to stress, that are related to psychiatric vulnerability. The goal of including these supplemental social features has been to develop more comprehensive models possessing greater explanatory power than those based on stress alone. Thus social moderators are factors that work in concert with stress either to enhance vulnerability to breakdown or to influence the form of symptomatic expression.

The topic of social moderators covers a wide range of considerations. The most common viewpoints suggest that these (1) buffer the effects of stress-induced vulnerability and/or (2) independently create vulnerability (irrespective of stress). A third class of influences posits that social characteristics influence the form of symptoms expressed, but not necessarily the onset of disorder (symptom formation factors)

(Brown and Harris 1978; Prudo, Harris, and Brown 1984). The range of the variables that can be considered under these headings and the operational procedures for measuring them are considerable. The following discussion is restricted to the major variables in current research that may be relevant to the topic of anxiety and depression comorbidity.

Perhaps the most well-known and oft-investigated moderator variable is social support. The term is used to unite a variety of social relationships and behaviors that have been correlated with psychiatric and physical symptoms (Monroe 1989; Monroe and Steiner 1986). Controversy exists concerning the mechanism by which social support operates. For example, is it only effective as a moderator of stress, or do such associations have potential "Main effects" of their own (regardless of stress levels) (Cohen and Wills 1985)? As with the concept of stress, social support is a sufficiently broad notion so that it can easily be confounded with a variety of other factors (e.g., personality) (Monroe and Steiner 1986). In relation to life stress and depression, however, a good deal of evidence has been generated to suggest that the presence of a confiding relationship can buffer the adverse effects of life stress, at least with respect to depression (Brown and Harris 1986).

There is scant direct evidence on the role of social moderators on comorbid anxiety and depression. A similar statement can be made for psychosocial symptom formation factors. Overall, the latter have not received the degree of attention devoted to other social moderators in the general stress and depression literature, yet they possess an inherent attraction for the issue of comorbidity. As will be reviewed subsequently, there are intriguing preliminary findings on the topic.

Summary and Conclusions

The first generation of measures for quantifying life stress were of undeniable initial importance. They set the conceptual and operational stage for studying individual differences in psychosocial stress in the initiation and maintenance of psychological and physical disturbances. Pioneering ventures, although creative, typically are not rigorous. Innovative ideas require method refinement and further conceptual development.

While many of the approaches that have appeared since the inception of life stress measures have proven useful, at present the bulk of the data support the psychometric characteristics of the LEDS. For the study of comorbidity, this measure possesses the content and conceptual breadth to accommodate hypotheses of stressor-disorder specificity and has a preliminary track record on this very issue (to be reviewed subsequently). The approach should not be considered complete, given the complexity of the objective. Yet the LEDS is quite sophisticated compared to current alternatives. The major shortcomings of the LEDS approach concern its labor intensiveness and the costliness of the procedures (Tennant, Smith, Bebbington, et al. 1979). In terms of the hallmarks of science—reliability, validity, and replicability—it appears to be the preferred procedure at present (see Katschnig 1986).

Social moderators and social symptom formation factors provide potentially fertile concepts for studying comorbidity from a psychosocial perspective, yet their application to the literature on comorbidity has been quite limited. The investigator is faced with a variety of measurement approaches for such variables as social support (e.g., Brown and Harris 1986; Cohen and Wills 1985), and it is more difficult to discern at the present stage which dimensions and measures of this concept are most relevant. A similar case exists for the dearth of attention devoted to symptom-formation factors. Yet the intuitive appeal of these notions, along with the limited existing data (to be reviewed), suggest their utility for understanding comorbidity of anxiety and depression.

One final caveat should be offered. There is a tendency for individuals who suffer from psychological or physical disorders to "explain away" the unknown through invoking life stress (Brown 1974). Clinicians and researchers—likewise faced with ignorance of the true initiating circumstances—also may seek solace in false but friendly explanations. Subjectively, life stress is a compelling idea for explaining psychological phenomena and can provide an easy descriptive escape. It is sufficiently amorphous, imprecisely defined, and poorly measured (particularly in relation to contamination with other correlated features of psychopathology) to fit into virtually any explanatory scheme and thereby easily elude falsification. The answer is not to explain away findings from life stress studies based on such tendencies. Rather the point highlights (1) the need to develop objective quantification procedures that capture the essence of individual differences in dimensions of stress; (2) to provide a means to standardize such information across individuals; and (3) to do so without the contaminating biases of either subject or investigator.

LIFE STRESS AND COMORBIDITY

Several lines of evidence suggest the utility of examining comorbidity from a life stress perspective. In this section, sources of indirect evidence are reviewed initially, with the direct evidence from life stress studies on comorbidity following.

Indirect Evidence

The primary goal in reviewing indirect sources of evidence is to select areas of research that are informative for understanding psychosocial factors in relation to comorbidity of anxiety and depression in general. The secondary goal is to examine these literatures for their implications concerning the role of life stress. This approach provides an important backdrop of information against which the relevance of life stress ultimately must be evaluated. Most of the information on the role of life stress, social moderators, and symptom formation factors in comorbidity is indirect or anecdotal, and some information is not supportive of stress as an important explanatory concept.

Descriptive clinical studies. A useful starting point is the descriptive clinical literature. Tyrer (1985, 1986b) has provided the most recent comments and research (Tyrer, Remington, and Alexander 1987) on the less severe forms of anxiety and depression, a topic that has a long history (Slater and Slater 1944). Not only is it difficult to divide minor anxiety and depressive states into discrete categories at one point in time, but, more importantly, only a minority of individuals retain the same diagnoses over time. Observing the longitudinal course highlights the frequent crossing over from one constellation of symptoms to the other.

Similar statements on comorbidity of anxiety and depression are supported for samples of individuals with more severe disturbances (Barlow, Di Nardo, Vermilyea, et al. 1986; Clancy, Noyes, Hoenk, et al. 1978; Dealy, Ishiki, Avery, et al. 1981; Fawcett and Kravitz 1983). Additionally, there is an increasing amount of information on the longitudinal course of these disorders (Breier, Charney, and Heninger 1984; Dealy, Ishiki, Avery, et al. 1981). Especially significant is the finding of temporal independence between periods of anxiety and depression: individuals who display one of the disorders may display the other disorder subsequently, yet not necessarily evidence both at the same time (Breier, Charney, and Heninger 1984, 1985a,b). The crossing-over effect portrayed by Tyrer (1985) for relatively minor psychiatric disturbances appears applicable, then, to some individuals with more severe pathology.

Life stress has been invoked informally to account for such changing presentations over time. Tyrer (1985) posited that, in the general neurotic syndrome, anxiety is the core feature (i.e., it is present even in the absence of major life stress). With the occurrence of stressful life events, new symptoms can emerge (typically depressive), subsequently remitting when the adverse circumstances subside. Although other factors may contribute to the presenting picture (e.g., sex, personality), he contends that these individuals over time "pass, chameleon-like, through different diagnostic hues depending upon the nature of the stresses they encounter" (p. 687).

Overall, this literature suggests a role for life stress for influencing the form of clinical presentation (Tyrer 1986b), although some investigators do not raise the issue (e.g., Breier, Charney, and Heninger 1984). Also, these studies underscore the need to enlarge the perspective on comorbidity from a concurrent focus to one involving the longitudinal or lifetime course of the individual, with the possibility of crossing over from one profile of symptoms to the other.

Cross-cultural research. In keeping with the idea of changing symptom pictures with changing psychosocial circumstances, the cross-cultural literature on psychopathology presents another interesting source of information. Two points are most apparent. First, if indigenous diagnostic practices are portrayed, the opportunity exists to observe "natural" arrangements of comorbid symptom profiles that are not excluded by hierarchical diagnostic conventions. Second, and more directly relevant, cross-cultural variation in comorbid presentations could be related to differences in the psychosocial stressors, social moderators, or symptom-formation factors unique to or characteristic of the different cultures. Restricted variability of important psychosocial processes within a particular culture may preclude detection of broad psychosocial influences on psychopathology.

The most frequently employed diagnostic category in modern China is neurasthenia (with various subtypes) (Kleinman 1986). This is particularly interesting with respect to comorbidity because neurasthenia represents a relatively nonspecific assemblage of psychiatric symptoms (e.g., a mixture of anxiety, depression, and somatization symptoms). Such symptoms are typically arranged hierarchically by DSM-III (American Psychiatric Association 1980) conventions. Of course, neurasthenia has a prominent past in Western (particularly American) nosology, being the historical counterpart to present-day depression in terms of diagnostic popularity (Jackson 1986; Kleinman 1986).

Kleinman's (1986) data suggest considerable overlap of anxiety, depression, and somatization. Applying nonhierarchical DSM-III diagnoses to a sample of 100 locally diagnosed neurasthenic patients, these investigators found 93% met criteria for depression (ranging from major depressive disorder through dysthymia); 69% met criteria for a concurrent diagnosis of anxiety disorder, with 35% qualifying for panic disorder. (Interestingly, the most common subjective description by the patient of the problem was one of anxiety, not depression.) This work is informative for the clear presence of comorbidity, although the temporal progression of the subtypes could not be discerned with confidence (e.g., if panic preceded or followed depression). Furthermore, psychosocial stressors appeared to be strongly associated with these problems, although the evidence provided is based only on descriptive material.

More generally, reviews of cross-cultural studies on depression have emphasized cultural influences on symptom formation: the experiences and expression of depression shift according to cultural boundaries (Marsella, Sartorious, Jablensky, et al. 1985). Although much of the variability in symptoms is attributed to psychological versus somatic expressions, a considerable degree of comorbidity involving depression and anxiety appears to be involved. For example, Kleinman (1986) found that although psychological symptoms of depression and anxiety were not volunteered by the patient to the interviewer (in contrast to the physical symptoms), the psychological counterparts of these symptoms were acknowledged after direct questioning.

More subtle ideas follow from these areas of research in relation to stress and comorbidity. Cultural traditions may not just operate in ways that generate psychosocial stress, they may also profoundly affect the symptomatic expression and experience of the disorder. Kleinman's (1986) work focused on the importance of "local meanings" for interpreting the psychiatric picture (Geertz 1983), and how the cultural ethic plays a role in both forming and filtering the presenting complaints. The manner in which such "threatening" breakdowns (personally and societally) are socially sanctioned, or the relatively undifferentiated schema through which they are processed, may mesh in complex ways with psychosocial parameters. Thus whether these broad cultural forces are best conceptualized as stressors, moderators of stress, or symptom-formation factors is unclear.

Supportive of cultural implications for stressors, moderators, and symptom-formation factors is the work of Prudo, Harris, and Brown (1984) with women from the Outer Hebrides. In studying the symptomatic expression of affective disorder, these investigators overrode the hierarchical rules and paid particular attention to the differentiation and comorbidity of anxiety and depression. Using the Present State Examination (PSE) (Wing, Cooper, and Sartorius 1974b), they found that the form of the disorder, along with its severity and course, were related to the extent the women were integrated into the traditional island culture. Specifically, the less integrated women had lower rates of anxiety disorder but higher rates of depression. In contrast, the most integrated women exhibited the reverse pattern: high rates of anxiety disorder, low rates of depression. Furthermore, the highly integrated women were found to be less likely to remit from their disorder compared to the less integrated women. (Note that this latter point can extend the role of symptom-formation factors to inhibiting recovery or promoting chronicity.) Explaining this social patterning, or social crossing over between anxiety and depression, the investigators suggested that differences in cultural integration produced psychosocial differences in (1) the nature of life stress experienced, (2) moderators of stress, and (3) symptom-formation factors. (The latter findings will be reviewed in greater detail in the section on life stress studies.)

It is noteworthy that the distinction pertaining to cultural integration in this work paralleled a social class distinction in a previous work by these authors in the Camberwell section of London (Brown and Harris 1978a). In the Outer Hebrides and in Camberwell, less integration into the local culture was similar in importance with respect to increasing the risk for depression (via an increased incidence of life stress). Finally, social class differences in the rates of depression, along with differing factor structures of the symptoms of depression across social classes, provide data compatible with the idea that psychosocial factors may influence the incidence *and* patterning of affective symptomatology (Dohrenwend and Dohrenwend 1969; Prusoff and Klerman 1974).

Symptom variability and subtypes of affective disorder. The concept of a syndrome inherently permits variability in the signs and symptoms that define the diagnostic class. Factors underlying such variability in expression of depression have been a topic of debate for more than 50 years (Gillespie 1929; Jackson 1986; Mapother 1926), and in more recent times have received considerable empirical attention. Most generally stated, at one extreme is the view that symptom differences reflect etiologic diffferences; at the other extreme is the view that symptom differences reflect nonetiologic differences (e.g., differences in pathophysiology, personality, or psychosocial factors) (Fowles and Gersh 1979). Stated somewhat differently, this topic concerns the specificity of initiating conditions for distinct disorders (Depue and Monroe 1986).

In terms of life stress, the issue of specificity has received mixed support. While a general level of specificity has been demonstrated with respect to major classes of psychopathology (e.g., the stressors preceding an episode of schizophrenia differ from those preceding an episode of depression) (Brown and Birley 1968), the major issue has centered around the endogenous-nonendogenous distinction in depression. The data thus far have indicated that life stress does not distinguish between these subtypes. For example, a significant proportion of individuals with endogenous symptoms profiles experience antecedent stressors, as does a significant proportion of individuals with nonendogenous profiles (Brown and Harris 1986; Paykel

1982) (cf., Cooke 1981; Matussek and Wiegand 1985).

Yet there are data suggesting psychosocial factors are related to the form of symptoms once an episode has begun (Brown and Harris 1986; Paykel 1982), or to the course of disorder, for endogenous-nonendogenous patients (Monroe, Thase, Hersen, et al. 1985). For example, Brown and Harris (1986) reported that the type of early childhood loss (by death or separation) accounted for the form of depressive symptoms during a clinical episode (endogenous versus nonendogenous). In terms of the longitudinal course of disorder, the occurrence of life events preceding treatment entry predicted a more favorable treatment outcome and maintenance of treatment gains for patients with endogenous profiles; life events preceding treatment entry for nonendogenous patients were not predictive of treatment outcome or follow-up longitudinal course (Monroe, Thase, Hersen, et al. 1985). Thus psychosocial factors have been reported to play a role in moderating the expression of depression at one point in time and longitudinally. Replication of these findings would place such considerations on a firmer foundation.

A variant of this issue, and one that may be most befitting with respect to comorbidity, pertains to the factors that influence the "choice" of symptom focus (or preoccupation) for any particular individual. Not versed in the full range of psychiatric symptoms, operational criteria, or hierarchical rules for classification, individuals with polymorbid symptoms may present with a range of specific foci embedded within a complex of nonspecific psychiatric and physical symptoms. These are the people who, although distressed, do not frequent psychiatric services, but rather present in greater numbers to general practitioners (e.g., Cooke 1981) or to medical specialists. Closer examination of the psychiatric history of these people brings to light the long-standing undercurrent of anxious and depressive symptoms, waxing and waning over time. For example, studying 195 nonpsychiatric, primary care patients, Katon, Vitaliano, Russo, et al. (1987) found a subgroup of patients with panic disorder who tended to focus on somatic symptoms selectively, and who also could be labeled as suffering from hypochondriasis or somatization (Katon 1984). Additionally, these patients were found to have a higher risk of lifetime major depression compared to the nonpanic disorder patients.

Patients with different surface clinical presentations, yet common co-occurring symptoms of anxiety and depression, raise important questions concerning the role of life stress, social moderators, and symptom-formation factors in the initiation, presentation, and maintenance of the symptoms. Although there are no life stress data currently available, work on this topic is again compatible with the findings from the cross-cultural literature: the expression of symptoms varies in relation to stressors, moderators, and/or symptom-formation factors. Findings of this type imply that the issue of comorbidity should be extended to a wider contingent than those who only consult mental health services; this broader grouping may constitute a large portion of symptomatic people detected in community surveys who do not seek psychiatric services (Depue and Monroe 1986; Uhlenhuth, Balter, Mellinger, et al. 1983). Interestingly, it is just such forms of minor psychiatric problems, labeled distress or demoralization, that some investigators believe are the most amenable to explanation within a life stress framework, a point of considerable importance that we will return to subsequently (e.g., Bebbington 1986; Link and Dohrenwend 1980). Taken together, these literatures suggest that psychosocial influences may be related to the variability of symptom expression in minor and major forms of affective disorders.

Multivariate studies of symptoms and classification. A number of investigators have employed multivariate analyses in attempts to clarify classification issues in depression (Blashfield 1984), and many of these studies have implications for comorbidity of anxiety and depression (Gersh and Fowles 1979; Mullaney 1984). In one of the more extensive reviews on the issue of anxiety and depression, Gersh and Fowles (1979) found consistent evidence across a number of investigations for a subgroup of anxious-depressed patients. Descriptively, such individuals have a relatively early onset, chronic course (with a large number of episodes), poor response to antidepressant treatment, and strong suicidal tendencies. They also have been characterized as being relatively *low* on reactivity to stressors during the depression, and relatively *low* on life events preceding their psychiatric problems.

These data are important with respect to the consistency with which the anxious-depressive subgroup has been documented; 40 studies supported such a group (Mullaney 1984). The interpretations of Gersh and Fowles (1979) are at variance with the other evidence reviewed in this section and suggest that life stress may *not* be an important consideration in the development and course of these disorders. These points raise important concerns with respect to the study of life stress with chronic disorders (Depue and Monroe 1986). We address this discrepancy subsequently in formulating the implications of life stress research for understanding comorbidity of anxiety and depression.

Family and genetic investigations. Several recent family investigations have reported that comorbidity of anxiety and depression in the proband predicts an increased rate of lifetime major depression and anxiety disorders among family members (i.e., concurrent or longitudinal crossover comorbidity [Leckman, Weissman, Merikangas, et al. 1983; Van Valkenberg, Akiskal, Puzantian, et al. 1984]), although some controversy exists (Noyes, Crowe, Harris, et al. 1986). These results have implications for conceptualizing the possible role of life stress, particularly from a stance that can incorporate both biologic and psychosocial aspects of vulnerability.

A study by Kendler, Heath, Martin, et al. (1987) provided provocative findings that elaborate on this complex issue. Multivariate genetic analyses, applied to a clinically unselected twin sample (3,798 pairs) that provided self-report measures on anxiety and depression, indicated that genes largely influence the overall level of symptomatology in a *nonspecific* manner. In contrast, the environment possessed effects that predisposed *specifically* to symptoms of anxiety versus symptoms of depression. Compatible with these findings is the idea that particular psychosocial environments, or life stressors, may be specifically related to either anxiety or depression. The specificity of stressor-symptom associations (at least for this sample) must be viewed within the more general context of a strong genetic component predisposing to either form of affective expression.

Such findings open up new lines of investigation for life stress and comorbidity. For example, studying twins longitudinally in relation to life stress and the form of affective disorder would be potentially informative, especially with respect to the hypothesis of increased crossing over of symptoms with changing psychosocial contexts. The degree to which these associations from the work of Kendler, Heath, Martin, et al. (1987) can be extended to clinical populations also remains to be evaluated. Nonetheless, these results indicate that life stress may have specific influences on the form of symptoms expressed within genetically predisposed individuals.

Life stress in relation to anxiety or depression. Most life stress studies and psychiatric disturbances have been on depression (Brown and Harris 1986; Finlay-Jones 1981; Monroe and Peterman 1988), although an increasingly large number of studies have examined life stress in relation to anxiety disorders (Monroe and Wade 1988). At a very general level, the major parallels between the two literatures with respect to a life stress position are (1) the role of recent life stress in bringing about the initiation of the respective disorders and (2) the role of early life stressors during childhood predisposing to the adult disorders (Brown, Harris, and Bifulco 1985; Tennant, Hurry, and Bebbington 1982). These parallels do not necessarily imply that recent or remote stressful circumstances carry similar implications for both forms of disorder, but simply point to common aspects that warrant closer scrutiny for further similarities and differences.

Reviews of the literature on life stress and depression consistently indicate the importance of adverse life experiences preceding the onset of an episode (Cooke and Hole 1983; Finlay-Jones 1981; Monroe and Peterman 1988; Paykel 1982). In particular, much of the relationship is due to single, major events (often signifying loss) and/or serious ongoing difficulties (as measured by the LEDS) (Brown and Harris 1986). While the consensus is strong that such events do precede depression, controversy remains over (1) how important a contributory role life stress plays and (2) the clinical severity of the disturbances that are preceded by events.

Recent reviews of the literature on life stress and anxiety disorders have indicated that: (1) the most consistent affirmative findings are from studies in which panic was a prominent feature of the anxiety disorder studied; and (2) two classes of stressors most consistently precede anxiety disorders (especially agoraphobia): interpersonal conflict and biologic-endocrine events (Monroe and Wade 1988; Tearnan, Telch, and Keefe 1984).

A few studies performed separately on anxiety and depression provide some insight into comorbidity, both independently and in relation to stress. For anxiety disorders, the moderating role of depression has been indicated as an important consideration, at least for hospitalized agoraphobic women (i.e., depression predicted a more favorable course) (Roberts 1964). For depression, the work of Brown and Harris (1978a) is again of interest. Although the individuals in the original Camberwell study were interviewed with the PSE and met the research group's criteria for depression, it is interesting that the subjective report of most patients was that they suffered from "nerves," not depression (Brown and Harris 1978a). Furthermore, depressed women with high levels of anxiety reported severe events that did not entail loss; depressed women without anxiety typically reported loss events. Unfortunately, there were no onset cases of anxiety without depression in the sample. Therefore, no further tests of the stressor characteristics associated with anxiety features (alone or comorbid with depression) were undertaken to explore the specificity of events that predicted the anxiety component.

These findings prompt further inquiry into the possibility of more precise associations between life stress dimensions and distinctive forms of psychiatric disturbance. Existing studies on this issue are reviewed in the next section.

Summary and conclusions. Several fields of study bearing on the topic of comorbidity consistently raise the issue of life stress as an important concern for understanding comorbidity and its implications for anxiety and depressive disorders. Specifically, that the expression of anxiety and/or depressive symptoms may be dependent, at least in part, on life stress considerations (i.e., specific stressors and/or social moderators) or symptom formation factors was a theme that appeared repeatedly in the majority of studies reviewed. The sole exception to this was the finding from the review of anxious depressive patients by Gersh and Fowles (1979), wherein it was suggested that life stress did not play an important part in the provoking or clinical course of anxious depressive patients. To a lesser extent, existing work indicates that other comorbid symptom presentations could be related to life stress and/or social moderators (e.g., somatization) (Katon, Vitaliano, Russo, et al. 1987).

Several issues for the study of life stress in relation to comorbidity were raised, including (1) life stress and comorbidity in terms of cross-sectional presentation *and* lifetime course of the individual; (2) life stress and comorbidity in relation to genetic predisposition; and (3) life stress, comorbidity, and the clinical severity of the psychopathology. These issues will be taken up subsequently, after we attend to the specific studies on life stress and comorbidity.

Life Stress and Comorbidity: Direct Evidence

Comorbidity of anxiety and depressive symptoms has been investigated in only a handful of studies. The findings are generally consistent with the more general information gathered from indirect evidence (already reviewed), yet also point to more specific issues of importance.

A general population study by Cooke (1980, 1981) reported on the association between life events and the co-occurrence of anxiety and depressive symptoms. Four symptom constellations were derived from a principal component analysis, one of which, labeled anxiety-depression, included such features as nervousness, tension, guilt, depressed mood, and crying spells. Life events were assessed for the previous 12 months with a semistructured interview, based on the work of Paykel (1974). Only life events rated as "almost certainly independent" or "probably independent" of the individual's illness were employed, and a total life stress score was computed from consensually derived weights of the amount of upset entailed by the event (Paykel, McGuiness, and Gomez 1976). Symptoms were assessed with a 29-item self-report scale (Cooke 1980). In addition to the anxiety-depression component, there was a component labeled cognitive; another characterized by loss of libido and appetite, fatigue, constipation, and depressed mood; and a final one that included diurnal variation, early awakening, weight loss, agitation, and irritability.

All four component scores were correlated with the total life stress index. Only the component of comorbid anxiety-depression symptoms, however, was significantly related to life stress ($r = .25$ for preonset stress); none of the other component correlations approached significance (e.g., $r < .10$). Moreover, the correlation between life stress and the anxiety-depression component was significantly different from the other three correlations.

Although these findings are suggestive of specificity of life stress for the anxious-depressive symptom complex, there are limitations of this work. First, there was no clear specification of how "onset" timing was determined. Without specifying onset, one does not know which events to include (e.g., pre- or post-onset events) or how chronically symptomatic individuals, so common in such surveys, were handled (Depue and Monroe 1986). Second, the stress index was relatively insensitive in the breadth of dimensions covered, especially with respect to the types of events that have been reported by others to precede depression (e.g., one long-term threat event, or undesirable event scores) (Brown and Harris 1986; Paykel 1982). (This would tend to attenuate the correlations, possibly obscuring associations with other components and possibly decreasing the reported association for the comorbid component.) Third, it is unclear how severe, or clinically relevant, the psychiatric symptoms in the community respondents were. The important point raised by this study is that one common form of psychiatric symptoms in the community is a constellation of anxiety and depression, and that this symptom profile—and not the others reported—was related to life stress.

An investigation by Torgersen (1985a, Chapter 23) provides an interesting perspective on comorbidity in anxiety and depression from a combined genetic and psychosocial perspective. The PSE was used to provide information for lifetime and current symptoms for a nationwide sample of 318 same-sexed twins (who had attended any psychiatric facility in Norway prior to 1975 for neurotic or borderline psychotic states). Diagnostic judgments were made by three judges, each independently diagnosing the twins from a written summary of the case (which contained information from the interview and from psychiatric records). Diagnoses were moderately reliable across the judges for the 150 patients diagnosed with separate anxiety and depressive disorders. The overlap of symptoms, however, was considerable, and a discriminant function analysis was employed (Torgersen 1985b). To create "pure" subtypes, the author used cutoff points on the discriminant-score dimension, yielding three equal-size groups of 50 each: pure anxiety neurosis, pure neurotic depression, and mixed anxiety-depression.

In terms of life stress, differences were found between the groups with respect to precipitating events. Pure anxiety neurotics had more pregnancy or childbirth events, whereas the mixed anxiety-depression and pure depression groups were more often characterized by problems in marriage or love relations, and by losses or threats of loss. (Note the similarities of the specific life events associated with the anxiety and depression groups to those suggested in the reviews of these two literatures discussed previously.) Furthermore, the pure neurotic depressive patients tended to have experienced childhood loss more often.

While intriguing and possessing several important features (e.g., a patient sample of twins), this study's limitations should be kept in mind. There is little information on the manner in which the life stress data were procured. Given the few events reported on, it is likely that the methods were not as comprehensive or sensitive as more state-of-the-art measures; this limitation may help to explain the overall low proportion of patients with any of the antecedent stressors. At most, only about one-third of any group had the particular event, although this was still sufficient to yield significant between-group comparisons. On the other hand, no information was provided on how the relative timing between onset of the disorder and occurrence of the event was determined (an approach that could spuriously inflate event totals, although it is unlikely to do so in a differential manner across groups).

Perhaps most stimulating is the context in which this information can be interpreted within the overall study. In a previous communication, Torgersen (1985b) interpreted the patterning of concordance rates between the monozygotic and dizygotic twins across the three groups to reflect: (1) hereditary factors as most important for pure anxiety neurosis; (2) common childhood environmental factors as most important in pure neurotic depression; and (3) current adult stress as most influential for mixed anxiety-depression. Presumably, the precipitating events varied in the magnitude of their etiologic contribution across the groups, with a strong role played by recent life events for mixed anxiety-depressive neurotics, a lesser role for the pure depressive group (e.g., a symbolic trigger for early childhood loss), and even a smaller absolute role for the pure anxiety group. In summary, while different qualities of life stress distinguished the groups, the importance of these varied in relation to the contribution of heredity to the particular disorder.

Barrett (1979) directly addressed the question of stressor-disorder specificity, comparing life stress experiences for symptomatic volunteers with Research Diagnostic Criteria (RDC) (Spitzer, Endicott, and Robins 1978a) diagnoses of major depressive disorder ($n = 34$), episodic minor depressive disorder ($n = 71$), chronic depressive disorder ($n = 29$), generalized anxiety disorder ($n = 53$), and panic anxiety disorder ($n = 19$). Life events were assessed with Paykel's (1974) 61-item self-report inventory for the 6 months prior to the agreed on onset date of the disorder (with the exception of the chronic depression group, for whom events were reported only for the last 6 months before the study). Initial analyses were performed between the depression and anxiety groups (i.e., each group, respectively, collapsed across its subtypes). Depressive patients were found to have experienced more undesirable and exit life events (life events indicating exits of individuals from the person's social field) compared to the anxiety group (e.g., 57.7% versus 41.7% for undesirable events). These percentages were informally compared to the rate of 16.8% for a nondepressed control group reported by Paykel, Meyers, Dienelt, et al. (1969).

These groups were further partitioned into subtypes and compared with respect to event categories. The panic anxiety group was similar to the major depressive disorder group in the proportion of individuals with such experiences (i.e., undesirable events, exit events) during the prior 6 months. In a complementary manner, generalized anxiety disorder and chronic depressive disorder evidenced similar rates of events (yet lower than for the major depression and panic group comparisons). Barrett (1979) speculated that such common features for the anxiety and depressive groups could suggest a common underlying disorder with different presenting symptoms.

Barrett's (1979) study, too, possesses several positive features (e.g., strong diagnostic practices providing subgroup distinctions). While his work does not address the issue of comorbidity in the groups studied (owing to the RDC hierarchy rules), the author is one of the few to attempt to study the general issue of stressor-disorder specificity in relation to anxiety and depression. Furthermore, it is useful to find within the same study results that are compatible with findings from the separate investigations of life stress in relation to these disorders, and to find speculation concerning the role of life stress in the onset of each.

The major limiting factor, however, pertains to the life stress assessment procedures. Although the criticisms previously discussed with respect to self-report life stress questionnaires are applicable, perhaps the most stimulating point involves the conceptual breadth of the measurement procedures. Specifically, there may be other "qualities" associated with the undesirable events that differentially preceded the major depression and panic groups that were not tapped by the methodology employed (i.e., stressor-disorder specificity).

It was noted previously that the early work of Brown and Harris (1978a) alluded to stressor-disorder specificity for anxiety and depression. Depressed individuals in Camberwell with high levels of anxiety tended to have severe events not involving loss. Subsequently, Finlay-Jones and Brown (1981) studied the concept of danger in relation to anxiety disorders and simultaneously elaborated the concept of loss in relation to depression. Most significantly, they also provided data on the characteristics of life stress that predisposed to the separate initiation or comorbidity of anxiety and depression.

The sample for this work was comprised of women consulting (for any reason) a general medical practice in London. The 164 women interviewed (of 220 approached) were characterized as relatively young (aged 16 to 40), unattached (> 80%), and affluent. Assessment interviews were conducted in the subject's home a few days following the consultation. Included were (1) a shortened PSE covering the 12 months prior to the interview; and (2) the LEDS covering the 12 months before the interview (for individuals who had relatively stable asymptomatic or symptomatic histories) or the 12 months prior to the onset of symptoms (with attention to the relative dating of events and onset being determined). All interviews were conducted by a psychiatrist trained in the use of the PSE, the rating of "caseness" of psychiatric disorder, and the LEDS.

Diagnoses were made at weekly meetings by at least four raters (other than the original interviewer) blind to the subjects' social circumstances. For disagreements, consensus judgments were made. Women who were rated as cases had symptoms of "sufficient severity to merit psychiatric attention according to standards generally accepted" in England (Finlay-Jones and Brown 1981, p. 804). Ratings were provided of the predominant syndrome (overriding hierarchical rules): anxiety, depression, mixed anxiety-depression, and other. Forty-five women had an onset of psychiatric disorder in the previous 12 months: 17 "case depression," 13 "case anxiety," and 15 "case depression–case anxiety." Discriminant function scores reliably reproduced the clinical ratings; the PSE/ID/CATEGO computer program reliably reproduced the pure groups, but could not perform the mixed class because of the hierarchical format (Wing 1976; Wing, Cooper, and Sartorius 1974).

In developing the measures of danger and loss, only events previously rated as severe on long-term threat with the LEDS procedures were rated on a 4-point scale. Danger was defined "as the degree of unpleasantness of a specific future crisis which might occur as a result of the event" (Finlay-Jones and Brown 1981, p. 806), while loss spanned deaths or separations, physical health, jobs, careers, material objects, and cherished ideas. Each scale was rated independently, but they were not mutually exclusive. An event could receive high scores on both dimensions, but in general this did not happen. Weighted kappa interrater reliabilities on the 138 severe events ranged from 0.89 to 0.95 for loss and from 0.81 to 0.95 for danger.

The clearest distinction emerged in preliminary analyses for the events rated on the top two levels of the respective 4-point scales, and subsequent analyses were based on severe loss only, severe danger only, and severe loss and danger events. The findings varied slightly depending on the time frame employed (e.g., 3 months versus 1 year prior to onset), but remained essentially congruent throughout. The following discussion is confined to the 3-month period data.

Overall, loss events were found to be much more frequent prior to depression onset (65%) relative to controls (3%) and to anxiety onset (8%); mixed anxiety-depression (47%) was also significantly different than the control and anxiety onset groups, but not from the case depression onset group. Danger events were significantly more common in the period prior to onset for the anxiety group (62%) compared to the noncase controls (8%) and to the depression onset group (24%); mixed anxiety-depression individuals (47%) significantly differed from the controls, but did not differ significantly from the depression or the anxiety groups. Finally, both a severe loss and danger were reported significantly more frequently by cases of mixed anxiety-depression (33%) compared to controls (0%) and anxiety cases (0%); while in the predicted direction, the mixed group was not different from the depression group (12%). Most importantly, controlling for the independence of the events by including only events that were not likely to be related to an insidious onset of symptoms indicated that the findings were unlikely to be contaminated by prior psychiatric functioning.

These findings portray a relatively clear picture of stressor-disorder specificity: events possessing specific characteristics preceded the initiation of specific syndromes. Mixed presentations (i.e., cases of anxiety and depression) were symmetrically found to be preceded by thematically congruent mixed psychosocial circumstances (i.e., stressor characteristics of both danger and loss). A strict specificity conclusion is tainted by the finding of an elevated rate of danger events for the case depression group, especially as more lengthy intervals preceding onset were examined. (Anxiety, however, was unrelated to loss, as a pure specificity position would posit.) The authors provide several interpretations of these findings in support of a strict specificity position. For example, most of the depressed women who had reported a severe danger event subsequently found that the crisis predicted by the event either terminated benignly or was translated into a loss event.

The findings from this study are compelling conceptually and methodologically because of the use of rigorous life stress and diagnostic assessments. The work is procedurally complex, and the sample is small and unrepresentative of either psychiatric patient or nonpsychiatric community groups. These points underscore the need for replication. Criticisms of the work revolve around the question raised previously of how such cases resemble other definitions of clinical affective disorders (e.g., Bebbington 1986). These are important concerns, and they will be taken up again in the final section of the chapter.

Finally, the work of Prudo, Harris, and Brown (1984) is relevant. As noted previously, several social features distinguished women in the Hebrides with respect to the development of anxiety or depressive disorders. In general, similar life event procedures and diagnostic practices were employed as in the investigation by Finlay-Jones and Brown (1981). In terms of events, the type of event experienced was related to the form of symptoms developed: loss of a parent was related to anxiety, and loss of other close relatives to depression. The authors related differences in event effects "backwards" to sociocultural differences influencing attachment styles and sensitivities to particular forms of stress. Because of such individual differences, subjects were thought to be differentially vulnerable to developing an anxiety disorder. While overall rates of disorder were less than those in Camberwell, and the provoking agents (life events and chronic difficulties) were also less frequent in the rural setting, the differences in rates of illness were interpreted to be partially offset by social vulnerability factors. Of additional importance, psychosocial symptom factors in this study (i.e., sensitivity to loss) extended to the *duration* of the disorder once begun, creating a situation in which there was a prolonged inability to recover from the psychiatric disorder following the event (Prudo, Harris, and Brown 1984).

Summary and conclusions. The existing information from direct studies of life stress and comorbidity of anxiety and depression is sparse, but is revealing with regard to specific stressor-disorder associations. It is also methodologically sophisticated in terms of life stress assessments. The findings point to a realm of variables that could contribute to an understanding of onset, symptom formation, and maintenance or remission of comorbid symptomatology at one point in time. Alternatively, these variables may clarify the temporally independent incidence of anxiety and depressive episodes at different points in time in the course of an individual's life.

ISSUES, COMMON THEMES, AND IMPLICATIONS

There are at least three related issues that emerge from the review. These involve (1) the severity of disorders involving comorbid symptoms; (2) the genetic and biologic predisposition to such disturbances; and (3) the chronicity of these symptoms. With respect to life stress and comorbidity, a common theme will be echoed within each section: that psychopathology (syndromal or subsyndromal) can impact the social environment in ways that create increased life stress. Such stress, in turn, can feed back on the primary pathology, either exacerbating the condition or coloring the presentation with co-occurring symptomatology. A life stress perspective affords one useful framework for integrating these issues, as well as for providing insights on other specific concerns involving severity, predisposition, and chronicity.

Life Stress and Severity of Disturbance

The co-occurrence of anxiety and depressive symptoms appears across several levels of severity. In the community, such symptom arrangements, as measured by self-report, were found to correlate with life stress by Cooke (1981) and Kendler, Heath, Martin, et al. (1987). Again in the community, yet diagnosed with more rigorous procedures (i.e., Wing, Cooper, and Sartorius 1974b; Wing, Nixon, Mann, et al. 1977), Finlay-Jones and Brown (1981) found specific associations between events of loss, danger, and loss-danger and the disorders of depression, anxiety, and depression-anxiety, respectively. Finally, the cross-cultural (Kleinman 1986), clinical descriptive (Breier, Charney, and Heninger 1984, 1985a, b), classification (Gersh and Fowles 1979), and family (Leckman, Weissman, Merikangas, et al. 1983) studies attest to such comorbidity within patient samples, each portraying life stress with varying degrees of influence. Central questions, then, concern (1) the comparability of co-occurring symptom profiles across the differing levels of severity; and (2) the relationship of these profiles to life stress.

The question of severity lies at the core of a major controversy in life stress research on depression. It was noted previously that one group contended that life stress predicts relatively severe, clinical forms of depression (Brown and Harris 1978a; Craig, Brown, and Harris 1987). Another group posits that stress-related syndromes are of more mild severity and of lesser clinical importance; consequently, life stress studies are not informative for unipolar depression in clinical populations (Bebbington 1986; Tennant, Bebbington, and Hurry 1981b). Both groups have assembled effective arguments and supportive data. The purpose at present is not to enter into the debate, but to outline the implications of either side for advancing understanding of comorbidity involving anxiety and depression.

The studies reviewed above by those who contend that life stress is related to clinically important disturbances (Finlay-Jones and Brown 1981; Prudo, Harris, and Brown 1984) clearly indicate the potential importance of specificity of stressful circumstances for differentially initiating anxiety, depression, or comorbid disorders. Although numerous questions remain (e.g., the role of genetic and biologic predisposition), it is apparent from this viewpoint that life stress should be an integral component of the research agenda. For present purposes, this perspective need not be discussed further. This is *not* to minimize its importance for understanding symptom comorbidity; the implications should be clear. Rather, the purpose of examining the existing evidence from the opposing perspective—that stress is unimportant for the onset of clinically relevant disturbances—is to point out other complementary issues with respect to the role of life stress in comorbidity of anxiety and depression.

The core of the debate concerns the comparability of depressed individuals who have and have not experienced antecedent life stress. Some believe that the psychiatric sequelae following severe life events are fundamentally different from depressions that arise without antecedent stressors. Empirically, however, distinctions in quality or severity of symptoms between these two groups have not been substantiated. The diagnostic precision of current diagnostic instruments—such as the Schedule for Affective Disorders and Schizophrenia (SADS) (Endicott and Spitzer 1978) or the PSE—is not sufficient to distinguish between the two groups, should they, in fact, be different. Comparisons of endogenous versus nonendogenous patients with respect to prior life stress, or comparisons of depressed patients with and without prior life stress, have not supported the view that event-related disturbances are different in kind or severity (Brown and Harris 1986; Hirschfeld 1981; Paykel 1982).

Comparisons using biologic markers have not indicated that stress is differentially related to the hypothesized biologic versus nonbiologic subgroups (e.g., response to dexamethasone suppression test) (Dolan, Calloway, Fonagy, et al. 1985; Lesser, Rubin, Finder, et al. 1983), although some data are suggestive (cf., Roy, Pikar, Linnoila, et al. 1986). At present, then, it appears that there is currently no reliable method for distinguishing between depressed individuals with these hypothetically different modes of onset and forms of disorder. Individuals who are depressed and report prior life stress appear similar in degree and in the form of their presentation to individuals who are depressed and report no prior life stress.

At a minimum, then, the existing research suggests that the

psychiatric sequelae of exposure to severe adverse events *at least* effectively mimic the clinical syndromes of depression or anxiety, such that one cannot reliably distinguish between the two groups given the resolution power of current procedures. This delicate differential diagnosis becomes even more difficult when attempting to provide lifetime diagnoses covering prolonged periods of time. The resolution of the diagnostic instruments is further compromised by the memory requirements (Bromet, Dunn, Connell, et al. 1986; Zimmerman and Coryell 1985). Overall, this means that psychosocial factors could operate as separate, but as yet indistinguishable, influences within the population of individuals who evidence comorbidity of anxiety and depression.

The interplay between the psychological and biologic influences on symptom comorbidity can be viewed in two different ways. Assuming independence of the psychosocial and biologic forces, a proportion of individuals with comorbidity possess different underlying disorders simply by coincidence. For example, there may be individuals who have a relatively pure depressive episode, but whose clinical picture is colored by psychosocial circumstances that imbue it with significant anxiety features. These individuals would be combined with others in the sample for whom comorbidity is primarily the product of a common neurobiologic diathesis (Breier, Charney, and Heninger 1984, 1985a, b).

The scope of the problem expands ominously when one considers that these two sources of influence—the psychosocial and biologic—may not be independent. It is clear from a variety of studies that depression has significant adverse ramifications for the afflicted individual's psychosocial sphere (Weissman and Paykel 1974). These correlates are commonly viewed as consequences of the illness. Yet there is no reason to assume that such problems cannot create psychosocial circumstances that "fall back" on the primary pathology, and thereby influence the clinical picture. For example, the psychosocial consequences of a depression may contain attributes of, or bring about events heralding, heightened danger (e.g., impaired functioning raising the specter of being fired from work, or having serious marital problems). These stressors may then lead to a significant anxiety component and the development of a comorbid picture. Of course, the converse scenario—of correlates of anxiety disorders leading to depression—is equally relevant and is often discussed as secondary depression (Breier, Charney, and Heninger 1985b). One would expect from such correlated contributions to the symptom picture that life stress substantially influences the composition of samples displaying comorbidity of anxiety and depression, especially for concurrent comorbidity.

In summary, the existing literature on symptom comorbidity of anxiety and depression from a life stress perspective suggests two alternative, yet equally viable, interpretations. First, life stress may be influential for the initiation and symptomatic form of clinically relevant anxiety, depressive, and anxiety-depressive states (Finlay-Jones and Brown 1981). Second, if not of concurrently or longitudinal etiologic importance, life stress and/or symptom formation factors impact the symptom picture in ways that can create clinically confusing, or indistinguishable, pictures with other comorbid disturbances. Most work on comorbidity is based on, and still developing from, the descriptive characteristics of the population of individuals who manifest such symptom arrangements. At the present stage of knowledge, it would seem prudent to understand the manner in which life stress may influence the development or coloring of comorbid disorders.

Genetic Predisposition and Life Stress

Genetic vulnerability depicted by the Torgersen (1985a) and Kendler, Heath, Martin, et al. (1987) studies indicates that some, if not most, predisposed people are biologically different from the nonpredisposed. There are two aspects of this finding that are important for considering the potential role of life stress and for the methods required in future research.

First, and most simply, biologic differences could exist as abstract potential, without readily observable overt manifestations. For instance, the neuroregulatory systems may operate adequately under normal circumstances, yet evidence dysregulation only under specific challenge conditions. If one conceptualizes susceptibility along a continuum of biologic risk, and if life stress is one contributing component to the initiating conditions, then there is an inverse gradient of risk associated with life stress (i.e., the greater the diathesis, the less stress required). Under such conditions, it is important to emphasize that the model for testing the influences of stressful events must take into account the implications of the diathesis. Comparisons along the dimensions of stress should be made on comparably predisposed individuals. (Note that traditional case versus control comparison, without including risk stratification, is not an appropriate design.) Another useful way to achieve this goal is through "within-subject" longitudinal research designs, using the predisposed individual as his or her own control over time (Depue and Monroe 1986).

Few studies have directly addressed this issue. McGuffin, Katz, and Bebbington (1987) compared the frequency of depression in first-degree relatives of 83 depressed patients with and without antecedent life stress (assessed with the LEDS). Although findings varied depending on the criteria adopted for defining illness among relatives, no support was found for greater familial loading in the relatives of probands without life stress preceding the index depression. (For one set of criteria of the three reported for defining depression in relatives, the findings were actually counter to the hypothesis: depressed probands who reported life stress evidenced a greater familial loading of depression.) Although these null findings do not support the diathesis-stress premise, they do exemplify the principle of stratifying individuals along the risk parameters to investigate the potential differential role of life stress (see also Perris, von Knorring, Oreland, et al. 1984).

With specific reference to other aspects of life stress and social moderators, some additional points are noteworthy. For predisposed individuals, minor events may have disproportionate consequences relative to nonpredisposed individuals and may provide a better basis for studying longitudinal relationships (Monroe 1983). In a related manner, major events are relatively infrequent; their effects on symptom change could be obscured statistically by the effects of the more prevalent minor stressors on symptom changes (Depue and Monroe 1986).

The second implication of vulnerability for studying life stress is more challenging theoretically and methodologically. Genetic or acquired biologic differences in predisposition may be more intricate than mere potential awaiting activation. Predisposition may be expressed via relatively unstable neurobiologic regulatory systems, made manifest through ongoing behavioral and psychological concomitants. That is, the vulnerability in underlying biologic systems may be behaviorally apparent on a chronic, albeit subsyndromal or intermittent, basis (Depue and Monroe 1986). As indicated above, this possibility is intriguing because it suggests that, if stress impacts such systems within vulnerable individuals, it may do so at levels less than those required to influence the nonvulnerable.

Methodologically, this view severely complicates the research requirements. A large array of concerns pertaining to cause-and-effect ordering or to confounding are brought to bear within such a model. The fluctuating psychobiologic circumstances may precipitate psychosocial sequelae that simply reflect the effects of increasing psychopathology. Alternatively, the instability may lead to psychosocial circumstances that legitimately predispose to serious exacerbations of the underlying condition (Rutter 1986). Predisposition, then, is not necessarily a static concept, but may wax and wane in accord with variation in the dynamic potential of the separate, and individually variable, biologic and psychosocial risk conditions.

There are many implications of a fluctuating predisposition that is comprised of dynamically interactive components. The psychological and behavior concomitants of relatively minor dysregulation may be manifested as variations in mood and behavior within the normal range, as subsyndromal affective symptomatology. These correlates, in turn, may "sculpt" psychosocial circumstances by heightening the probability of the occurrence of major adverse events. For example, increased social withdrawal and irritability may create a lack of social support and bring about serious arguments or separations from potentially supportive networks (Monroe and Steiner 1986). These latter events may, in turn, conspire to exacerbate the neurobiologic dysregulation and elevate the subsyndromal to the syndromal (Rutter 1986). Depending on the psychosocial climate, the expression of distress may vary accordingly in terms of anxiety and depressive features. (Note that this is similar to the example discussed previously with respect to life stress and different comorbid syndromes, except that the case is extended here to periods of subsyndromal affective instability.) Risk conditions may not simply merge coincidentally, they may gravitate together, conspiring toward sufficient overall conditions for initiation of an episode.

The arbitrary nature of assigning temporal or causal priority to any component of the elaborate system should be emphasized. In the case illustrated above, the movement from subsyndromal to syndromal may never have taken place without the necessary psychosocial circumstances—circumstances that served as both consequences and causes in the developmental scheme. At the present stage of knowledge, consequences of the unfolding process should not be accorded artifact status and summarily dismissed. They may represent one necessary, but insufficient, part of a complex of circumstances required for onset (Meehl 1977).

Redefining consequences of prior processes as intervening variables imposes difficult design and method requirements. For example, it is very hard to dismantle the correlated features and overlap between such variables as personality, life stress, social support, and psychopathology (Monroe and Steiner 1986). Each, however, may be important in nontrivial and unique ways in the developmental system. The challenges to the actual conduct of research implied by a fluctuating predisposition are equally demanding. Partitioning of variance may be as arbitrary as assigning causal priority. To begin to understand how individual components of the process relate to the overall progression, more appropriate indices to estimate the importance for particular variables will be required (see Brown and Harris 1986; Cooke and Hole 1983; Finlay-Jones 1981; Paykel 1982). It is also clear that such work can only be performed with close attention to the temporal ordering of the variables under study (Monroe and Peterman 1988). Retrospective investigations are more susceptible to interpretational problems, but with proper controls can be informative. Prospective designs, which are directed toward the tracking of variables in the process, are ultimately preferred (Depue and Monroe 1986).

A few qualifying points are worth noting. First, to the extent that genetic factors provide a requisite condition for the disorder, the other components of the model are obviously meaningful only in this context. Yet they are still potentially meaningful within the context of genetic factors. As noted previously, the within-subject design may be a more useful method for studying stress shifts under such circumstances; these designs might profit from including less dramatic, but more frequent, life events. The different components in this model, however, continue to promise pivotal influence in terms of the pathologic progression (Monroe and Peterman 1988; Rutter 1986). To the extent that genetic factors are not a prerequisite for some affective disorders, and that the biologic diathesis is not the province of an unfortunate few but is more pervasively inherent in the biology of being human, then the other components of the model are applicable within a more far-ranging context.

Second, life stress is partly determined by a larger matrix of forces. The majority of life stressors are not entirely aleatory experiences. A host of social (e.g., Prudo, Harris, and Brown 1984) and person (e.g., personality) variables predispose to individual differences in life stress. At one level or another individuals are at least accomplices in creating the circumstances that they experience and endure (Monroe and Peterman 1988; Rutter 1986). These wider social influences, too, represent another important part of the multifactorial picture (see Prudo, Harris and Brown, 1984).

Chronicity and Life Stress

The discussion of severity, and especially predisposition, suggests that comorbidity of anxiety and depression may be best characterized by a relatively enduring profile of changing symptoms, not by isolated episodes. The theme is the same: disturbed functioning may precipitate life stressors that can (1) exacerbate the condition, and/or (2) produce other characteristics of the symptom profile (e.g., anxiety versus depressive symptoms). This theme fits well with the chronicity cited by Gersh and Fowles (1979) and others (Stavrakaki and Vargo 1986), and is reminiscent of the characterizations by Tyrer (1985) of individuals who change symptom profiles over time, remain chronically impaired and are refractory to treatment.

This issue raises the question of the "depth" of the vulnerability and the dimensions of the chronicity. Are the individuals with chronic minor psychiatric disturbances the very ones who, under adverse biologic or psychosocial conditions, develop full syndromal disorder (e.g., akin to the vulnerability of dysthymic individuals to major depression; Keller, Lavori, Endicott, et al. 1983)? In this regard, Brown and colleagues (Brown, Bifulco, Harris, et al. 1986) found that individuals with chronic symptoms indeed were more vulnerable under life stress to developing major psychiatric disorders. Stress, then, could be instrumental for the development of major depressions superimposed upon dysthymia (i.e., double depressions; Keller, Lavori, Endicott, et al. 1983). Further work is required to understand the manner in which psychosocial conditions may be related to changes in the longitudinal course, and symptomatic coloring, of the disturbance.

The concerns involving severity, predisposition, and chronicity suggest an interpretation of the one anomalous point from the previous literature review. Recall that the literature on multivariate studies and classification suggested that life stress was not an important factor for understanding the subgroup of anxious-depressive individuals (Gersh and Fowles 1979). Problems with this interpretation can now be presented. First, most of the evidence cited has been anecdotal and not based on optimal measurement practices. Second, the concerns raised above pertaining to biologic predisposition, and to research designs that control for risk levels, are applicable. Major life events may not be the optimal focus for studying the possible consequences of stress with chronically disturbed persons. More sensitive assessment procedures, particularly those incorporating minor yet frequent events, may provide more informative results. (And once again, this approach will require careful attention to the difficult task of attempting to separate and understand causes and consequences of the ongoing psychopathology.)

Since chronicity represents such a strong thread running through several descriptions of the anxious-depressive disorders, delineating the psychosocial conditions operating to *maintain* the disorder is useful for clarifying important distinctions. From a psychosocial perspective, Prudo, Harris, and Brown (1984) found that the social structure and attachment styles of women in the Outer Hebrides fostered chronicity of anxiety symptoms that outlasted initial depressive symptoms. Prolonged life difficulties, secondary chronic dysphorias, and personality disturbances are additional psychosocial circumstances that could contribute to a chronic picture (Depue and Monroe 1986). Such ambient psychosocial circumstances could provide important insights into the factors that inhibit recovery for subtypes of individuals with chronic symptoms of anxiety and depression.

In summary, while characterization of the anxious-depressive group as unresponsive to psychosocial stressors may be valid, there are ways of studying life stress more adequately in chronic populations (e.g., within-group comparisons and more minor stressors). Given the weight of evidence suggesting a role for life stress in comorbid expression of anxiety and depression, it appears premature to rule out such considerations.

CONCLUDING REMARKS

Diverse sources of information suggest that psychosocial factors, especially life stress, social moderators, and psychosocial symptom-formation factors, are important for expanding understanding of comorbidity in anxiety and depression. There are two ways in which these variables may be related to the development of comorbid disorders. First, specific dimensions of life stress, and specific social factors, may be related to specific syndromes. For example, loss events may lead to depression, danger events to anxiety (Finlay-Jones and Brown 1981). Second, even if not germane for the genesis of clinically relevant disorders, life stress and symptom-formation factors appear capable of producing co-occurring symptomatology that colors and complicates the diagnostic picture. This complication means that the pool of individuals who meet clinical criteria and possess comorbid symptomatology is likely to be very heterogeneous.

The focus of the review has been on psychosocial considerations. Clearly, however, such factors do not operate independently of other predispositional variables. Perhaps the major limitation in the existing literature is the degree to which investigators of different perspectives have not incorporated findings from other networks of information. The resulting models and theory are thereby quite limited. This concern is illustrated by the studies of Breier, Charney, and Heninger (1985a, b). Based on their descriptions of comorbidity of anxiety and depression, both concurrently (i.e., both sets of symptoms occurring contemporaneously) and consecutively over the individual's life (i.e., the crossing over from one profile to the other), these investigators suggested two alternative models for conceptualizing the phenomenon: (1) a shared neurobiologic diathesis for both disorders and (2) a specific neurobiologic diathesis for one disorder, which leads to pathophysiologic vulnerability for the other (Breier, Charney, and Heninger 1984, 1985a, b).

In light of the life stress research and the inability to distinguish between stress-related and nonstress-related affective disturbances, these models are incomplete for capturing the complexity of comorbidity of anxiety and depression. In particular, findings on genetic predisposition, along with findings from life stress in relation to anxiety and depression, suggest that different biologic and psychosocial processes produce clinically comparable symptom pictures, and/or that these two risk domains are related in a complex manner over time.

Consequently, several alternatives to, or variants of, the models proposed by Breier, Charney, and Heninger (1984, 1985a, b) may be entertained. For example, there may be a shared neurobiologic diathesis for both disorders that requires specific psychosocial stressors for activation. Or alternatively, a specific neurobiologic vulnerability to one form of disorder may exist, with a psychosocially induced vulnerability to the other disorder. Additionally, of course, specific forms of disorders may be determined by specific psychosocial circumstances (as suggested by the life stress studies). Further permutations of these alternatives may be generated, but the thrust of the discussion remains the same. An enlarged conceptual framework is required for furthering understanding of comorbidity. Furthermore, within such a framework attempts should be made to explain how the predispositional factors operate *together*—temporally and psychobiologically—to produce at least one cluster of sufficient conditions for initiating an episode (Meehl 1977; Weiner 1977).

At a very basic level of describing such an expanded framework, it would be helpful to begin with the inclusion of two other prominent theoretical perspectives that bear on the topic of comorbidity: the cognitive and biologic approaches. It is clear that both cognitive processes and central nervous system neuroregulatory mechanisms are, in part, entrained to environmental input, a large part of which is socioenvironmental. The normal process of adaptation is the integration of, and harmonious interplay between, these three levels of functioning. For instance, common neurobiologic systems have been implicated in depressive and anxiety symptoms (e.g., noradrenergic hyperactivity) (Breier, Charney, and Heninger 1985b); these systems, in turn, may be especially responsive to specific forms of psychological stress (Gray 1982; Weiss, Goodman, Ambrose, et al. 1984; Willner 1985). Similarly, cognitive theory on anxiety and depression holds that thoughts involving hopelessness and loss predispose to depression, whereas danger and threat of loss predispose to anxiety (Beck, Brown, Steer, et al. 1987). It is unlikely that such cognitive activity arises independent of psychosocial circumstances. Overall, psychosocial factors do not operate alone, or independently of other predispositional parameters. These three levels of study provide an integrated psychobiologic perspective for understanding the synthesis of predispositional parameters over time into the processes leading to the onset of disorder.

Noteworthy in this respect are the studies that exemplify this point in a preliminary manner. The research by Torgersen (1985a) is especially informative in this respect. While different qualities of life stress reliably preceded the onset of the three different patient groups (i.e., depressed, anxious, and mixed depressed-anxious), the contribution of the different events was couched in the context of genetic and early development risk parameters. Thus the relationship of life events to anxiety disorders was qualified by the underlying importance of heritability, whereas for the comorbid anxiety-depressive cases, current psychosocial factors were found to be relatively more important.

The complementary findings from the twin study of Kendler, Heath, Martin, et al. (1987), and the life stress study of Finlay-Jones and Brown (1981) raise interesting questions for a model of comorbidity integrating psychosocial, cognitive, and biologic considerations. For example, would the affected twins in the Kendler, Heath, Martin, et al. investigation evidence crossing over of symptoms in tandem with theoretically important shifts in psychosocial circumstances, as suggested by the Finlay-Jones and Brown (1981) work? Alternatively, were the women studied by the latter investigators representative of the normal population, or did they possess a biologic vulnerability that would qualify the conclusions in terms of the spectrum of individuals vulnerable to disorder under such psychosocial conditions? Furthermore, would these women evidence crossing over of symptoms with changing circumstances, or evidence an anxiety baseline, as suggested by Tyrer's (1986b) characterization of the neurotic comorbid group?

Findings from several literatures indicate that a wide array of considerations are brought to bear on the topic of comorbidity of anxiety and depression. Few attempts have been made to integrate and systematize these results from the different perspectives, yet studies that have begun this task provide important insights on the issues involved. The mandate for future inquiry includes a creative blend of thinking from the psychosocial, cognitive, and biologic realms. Within this broadened framework, the concept of stress may help to explain how different levels of vulnerability operate together, over time, to translate the potential of predisposition into the presence of psychopathology.

Comorbidity of Anxiety and Depressive Disorders: A Helplessness-Hopelessness Perspective

Lauren B. Alloy, Ph.D.
Kelly A. Kelly, M.S.
Susan Mineka, Ph.D.
Caroline M. Clements, M.S.

A LONG-STANDING DEBATE has existed in psychiatry and clinical psychology over whether anxiety and depression are distinct disorders (Kraepelin 1883/1981) or states belonging to different parts of a single continuum of affective disorders varying in severity (Eysenck 1960; Lewis 1934, 1938; Mapother 1926). Although anxiety and depressive disorders historically have been viewed as distinct nosologic entities—for example, in the first three editions of the *Diagnostic and Statistical Manual of Mental Disorders* (DSM-I, DSM-II, DSM-III) (American Psychiatric Association 1952, 1968, 1980)—the two syndromes exhibit considerable overlap in their (1) manifest symptomatology (see Angst, Vollrath, Merikangas, et al., Chapter 7; Di Nardo and Barlow, Chapter 12; Dohrenwend, Chapter 10; Garber, Miller, and Abramson 1980; Gersh and Fowles 1979; Grinker 1966; Mendels, Weinstein, and Cochrane 1972; Prusoff and Klerman 1974; Regier, Burke, and Burke, Chapter 8; Roth and Mountjoy 1982); (2) family history (see Leckman, Merikangas, Pauls, et al. 1983; Leckman, Weissman, Merikangas, et al. 1983; Merikangas, Chapter 21; Weissman, Chapter 22; Weissman, Leckman, Merikangas, et al. 1984; but for alternative findings, see Cloninger 1986b; Cloninger, Martin, Guze, et al. 1981); (3) treatment response (see Fyer, Liebowitz, and Klein, Chapter 37; Klein 1980); and (4) hypothesized etiology (see Garber, Miller, and Abramson 1980; Greenberg, Vazquez, and Alloy 1988). Indeed, the recent modifications of the hierarchical exclusion rules for mood and anxiety disorders in the DSM-III-R (American Psychiatric Association 1987) originated in large part as a response to the growing awareness of the co-occurrence or comorbidity among psychopathologic syndromes in general, and between anxiety and depressive disorders in particular.

The existence of symptom co-occurrence and syndrome comorbidity in anxiety and depression, both within single episodes of illness and across multiple episodes within an individual's lifetime, has significant implications for theoretical models of the etiology, course, and remediation of these disorders (Cloninger, Martin, Guze, et al., Chapter 27; Greenberg, Vazquez, and Alloy 1988). Although sophisticated theories of depression and anxiety have been proposed, these models have not taken into account syndrome comorbidity and, with few exceptions (Bowlby 1973, 1980; Beck 1976; Beck and Emery 1985; Garber, Miller, and Abramson 1980; Higgins 1987; Riskind 1989), have not addressed the issue of the relationship between anxiety and depression at all (cf., Greenberg, Vazquez, and Alloy 1988). Thus the purpose of this chapter is to present an integrated theory of some forms of anxiety and depressive disorders that explicitly addresses and, in many cases, predicts the features of comorbidity that have emerged from recent clinical, epidemiologic, and psychopathology studies. We emphasize from the outset that, as detailed below, our theory is *not* meant to deal with comorbidity among *all* forms of depression and anxiety.

In the remainder of this chapter, we present evidence for four phenomena or features of comorbidity between anxiety and depression that we believe should be addressed and explained by any theoretical model of the pathogenesis and course of these disorders. We then describe the basic postulates of a cognitive-behavioral theory of anxiety and depression, the helplessness-hopelessness theory, and show how this theoretical perspective explains and, in many cases, predicts these four comorbidity phenomena. We then briefly review three other cognitive-behavioral theories of depression and anxiety and examine their ability to account for the four features of comorbidity. Finally, we suggest directions for future research designed to test the helplessness-hopelessness perspective that may advance understanding of comorbidity, as well as its implications for common etiologies of some anxiety and depressive disorders.

PHENOMENA OF COMORBIDITY IN ANXIETY AND DEPRESSION

Klerman (Chapter 2) distinguishes between the co-occurrence of symptoms or syndromes within single episodes of illness (*intra-episode comorbidity*) and over the life span of the individual (*lifetime comorbidity*). A review of evidence on both types of comorbidity in anxiety and depression, derived from a variety of clinical, epidemiologic, and psychometric studies, suggests four phenomena that require explanation. However, a caveat is in order. Within psychiatry and clinical psychology, interest in the issue of comorbidity is relatively recent (Klerman, Chapter 2). Investigators have only begun to examine their existing data for symptom or syndrome co-occurrences or specifically to design studies in advance recognizing the problem of comorbidity. Therefore, the evidence supporting some of the four comorbidity phenomena below is still sparse. Additionally, some of the current data on comorbidity of anxiety and depression may be biased by the use of DSM-III hierarchical rules, by which an affective disorder diagnosis automatically excluded an anxiety disorder diagnosis. Thus we view the following four features of comorbidity as tentative and await further evidence for their validity.

Lifetime Comorbidity

The sequential relationship between anxiety and depressive disorders. Many longitudinal studies examining the stability of anxiety and depressive disorder diagnoses have found that anxiety disorders are more likely to precede depressive disorders than the reverse. Regarding changes in diagnostic status, Freud (1926/1959) was perhaps the first to notice that prolonged anxiety states often end in depression. A number of longitudinal epidemiologic studies now support the observation that individuals presenting initially with pure anxiety disorders are more likely subsequently to become depressed than vice versa. For example, Kandell (1974) found that 24% of individuals who had first received an anxiety diagnosis were rediagnosed several years later with a depressive disorder. By contrast, only 2% of those who first received a depressive diagnosis were later rediagnosed with an anxiety disorder. Several other studies reported in this volume have obtained similar results. Angst, Vollrath, Merikangas, et al. (Chapter 7) found that 49% of their cases with pure anxiety disorders went on to develop major or minor depression (either alone or in conjunction with anxiety) in the subsequent 7 years, whereas only 33% of the cases with pure depression later developed an anxiety disorder (either alone or in conjunction with depression). Among individuals who longitudinally manifested both disorders, many more of those with pure anxiety later developed depression (62%), compared to those with pure depression who later developed anxiety (18%). Merikangas (Chapter 21) also reports results from family and genetic studies indicating that anxiety tends to precede depression more often than the reverse. These findings from longitudinal epidemiologic studies are consistent with observational studies of the sequential relationship between anxiety and depression in human and nonhuman primates responding to separation and loss of an attachment figure.

Differential comorbidity between depression and the anxiety disorders. Important differences have been found among the various anxiety disorders with respect to their lifetime or intra-episode comorbidity with depression. Evidence from clinical, epidemiologic, and family studies suggests that individuals who receive the diagnoses of panic disorder, agoraphobia, obsessive-compulsive disorder, and posttraumatic stress disorder are generally more likely to experience depression than are those with generalized anxiety disorder, social phobia, or simple phobia.

A number of clinical studies have reported that larger percentages of those with agoraphobia and panic disorder have personal or family histories of depression than do patients with generalized anxiety disorder, simple phobias, or social phobias. However, Di Nardo and Barlow (Chapter 12) found a high rate of concurrent depression among social phobics. Dealy, Ishiki, Avery, et al. (1981) and Raskin, Peeke, Dickman, et al. (1982) observed that individuals with panic disorder were approximately twice as likely as patients with generalized anxiety disorder to have a history of major affective disorder. In the National Institute of Mental Health (NIMH) Epidemiologic Catchment Area (ECA) project, Regier, Burke, and Burke (Chapter 6) reported that individuals with a major depressive disorder were twice as likely to meet criteria for concurrent panic disorder (18%) than simple phobia (9%). Gardos (1981) found that 52% of agoraphobic and panic disorder subjects, as compared to only 36% of subjects with other types of anxiety disorders, met Research Diagnostic Criteria (RDC) (Spitzer, Endicott, and Robins 1978a) for current or past unipolar depression. Similarly, Breier, Charney, and Heninger (1984) observed that 68% of the agoraphobic and panic disorder patients they studied met criteria for major depressive disorder at some time in their lives. Further, Munjack and Moss (1981) found that agoraphobic patients were significantly more likely than social or simple phobic patients to have family histories of affective disorders (see also Bowen and Kohout 1979).

Several investigators have also reported high rates of depression among individuals with obsessive-compulsive disorder and posttraumatic stress disorder, although these researchers did not explicitly compare the rates of depression in these two disorders with the rates of depression in other anxiety disorders. For example, in summarizing many lines of evidence, Rachman and Hodgson (1980) concluded that obsessive-compulsive disorder is highly associated with syndromal and symptomatic depression. In a pilot study with members of a veterans' center outreach group, Green, Lindy, and Grace (1985) found that 77% of the members who received diagnoses of posttraumatic stress disorder had a history of depressive disorders. These results are comparable to those of Sierles, Chen, McFarland, et al. (1983), who found that 72% of the veterans with posttraumatic stress disorder in their sample had a history of depression.

Intra-Episode Comorbidity

The sequential relationship between anxiety and depressive symptoms. Several lines of evidence suggest that among individuals who experience both anxiety and depressive states, the anxiety symptoms are more likely to precede the depressive symptoms than the reverse. Observational studies of human and nonhuman primates' responses to separation and loss of an attachment figure also suggest a sequential relationship between anxiety and depression within an episode. For example, when infant monkeys are separated from their mothers in the first year of life, most initially display a period of intense agitation characterized by hyperactivity, excessive vocalizations, and a sharp rise in cortisol levels. This initial *protest* phase, as it is often called, is sometimes (but not always) followed within 1 to 3 days by a phase of *despair* or depression, characterized by sharp decreases in play and other social activities and increases in self-directed behavior, such as self-clasping (for reviews of the determinants of the response to separation, see Coe, Wiener, Rosenberg, et al. 1985; Mineka 1982; Mineka and Suomi 1978; Suomi, Mineka, and Harlow 1984). Very similar results have been described by Spitz (1946), Robertson and Bowlby (1952), and Bowlby (1960) in their observations of young human children's responses to prolonged physical separation from their mothers, with the most common pattern being a biphasic protest-despair response. More recently, Bowlby (1980) described the protest response as a prototype for anxiety in adults, and despair as a prototype for depression in adults. Particularly noteworthy for the present purposes is that when protest and despair are both experienced, protest always precedes despair rather than the reverse. It should be noted, however, that protest does not always lead to despair, and that under unusual circumstances, such as after many repeated separations, despair may occasionally occur with very little, if any, protest (Mineka, Suomi, and Delizio 1981).

Bowlby (1980) also reviewed the literature on adult humans' responses to loss through death of an attachment figure, and a similar picture emerges. Typically, a brief period of numbness and disbelief is followed by a phase of yearning and searching for the lost figure, lasting for months and sometimes years, which is then followed by a phase of disorganization and despair. The yearning and searching phase resembles a period of intense anxiety, including pangs of intense pining, spasms of distress, anger, great restlessness, insomnia, and obsessional thoughts about the lost person. Once the loss has been accepted as permanent, the phase of despair, depression, and apathy typically begins.

This sequence of anxiety symptoms followed by depressive symptoms is also described in the human and animal literature on the effects of exposure to uncontrollable aversive events. For example, Wortman and Brehm (1975) argued that when an individual loses control, he or she initially becomes aroused and attempts to restore control and freedom. This reactance phase, which bears some resemblance to anxiety, does not persist indefinitely in the face of repeated exposure to uncontrollable outcomes. With prolonged exposure, the individual gives up and becomes helpless (Seligman 1975). If reactance and helplessness are adequate experimental analogues of anxiety and depression (respectively), this theory, along with findings such as those of Roth and Kubal (1975), are consistent with the sequential nature of the anxiety-depression relationship described here. Similarly, in their studies of experimental neurosis and learned helplessness in cats, Thomas and Dewald (1977) described a pattern of responses to unpredictable and uncontrollable events that most often included agitated, anxiety-type symptoms initially, followed by depressive-type symptoms.

Relative infrequency of pure depression. Cross-sectional studies examining the phenomenology of anxious and depressive states within individual episodes of illness have frequently found that it is more difficult to identify individuals with pure depression than it is to identify persons with pure anxiety (Dobson 1985c). For example, although the overlap between anxiety and depressive disorders has been estimated at 25% to 40% (Klerman 1977), cases of anxiety without significant depression are relatively common, whereas cases of depression in the absence of concomitant anxiety are rare (Dobson 1985c; Dobson and Cheung, Chapter 34; Greenberg, Vazquez, and Alloy 1988). A number of investigators have attempted to identify individuals with high and low levels of concomitant anxiety and depression (e.g., Clements, Alloy, Greenberg, et al., in press; Gotlib and Asarnow 1979; Greenberg and Alloy, in press; Kennedy and Craighead 1979; Miller, Seligman, and Kurlander 1975; Siegel and Alloy, in press). Using predetermined cutoff scores for trait anxiety and depression, these investigators were unable to identify a sufficient number of high-depressed, low-anxious subjects to complete a two-by-two factorial design.

The infrequency of pure cases of depressive disorder is also demonstrated by the rates of concurrent anxiety symptoms and diagnoses among individuals with primary diagnoses of depression. For example, in the World Health Organization study of 572 depressed patients in Canada, Iran, Japan, and Switzerland, anxiety and tension were among the most frequently reported symptoms, occurring in 76% to 100% of the cases across all settings (Jablensky 1985). Overall and Zisook (1980) suggested that anxiety usually accompanies depressed mood in all types of depression. Numerous clinical investigations have reported high levels of anxiety (sometimes in atypical form such as agitation) in a majority of depressed individuals regardless of subtype of depression (e.g., Gersh and Fowles 1979; Grinker 1966; Grinker and Nunnally 1968; Leonhard 1979; Lorr, Sohn, and Katz 1967; Mendels, Weinstein, and Cochrane 1972; Overall, Hollister, Johnson, et al. 1966; Paykel 1972; Prusoff and Klerman 1974; Teja, Narang, and Aggarwal 1971).

In both community and treated samples, individuals meeting DSM-III criteria for a primary depressive disorder also exhibited high rates of anxiety disorders, when investigators ignored DSM-III hierarchical rules. For example, Leckman, Merikangas, Pauls, et al. (1983) reported that 58% of 133 depressed patients in their sample also met criteria for a concurrent diagnosis of agoraphobia, panic disorder, or generalized anxiety disorder. In contrast, Dealy, Ishiki, Avery, et al. (1981) found that only one-third of 93 panic and generalized anxiety disorder patients also met criteria for a secondary affective disorder. In the ECA project, Regier, Burke, and Burke (Chapter 6) report that 43% of individuals with an affective disorder, but only 25% of those with an anxiety disorder, also meet diagnostic criteria for the other disorder during their lifetimes. Among individuals seeking treatment at the Albany Center for Stress and Anxiety Disorders, 90% of those with a primary major depressive disorder also met DSM-III criteria for an additional anxiety disorder, whereas only 17% of those with primary anxiety disorders met criteria for an additional affective disorder diagnosis (Di Nardo and Barlow, Chapter 12, Table 4). Indeed, in summarizing the results of many diagnostic studies, Dobson and Cheung (Chapter 34) argue that an average of 67% of primary depressed patients meet criteria for an additional anxiety diagnosis (range, 42% to 100%), whereas an average of only 30% of primary anxiety patients meet criteria for an additional depression diagnosis (range, 17% to 65%).

Unique and overlapping symptoms in anxiety and depression. Although the syndromes of anxiety and depression show a high degree of comorbidity, some symptoms occur much more often in conjunction with one syndrome or the other, whereas other symptoms are common to both disorders (Garber, Miller, and Abramson 1980). Table 1 summarizes the pattern of overlapping and syndrome-specific affective, behavioral, somatic, and cognitive symptoms.

From a general perspective, there are many studies demonstrating that depressed and anxious persons are more readily discriminated on the basis of the presence versus absence of depressive features than of anxiety features (Costello and Comrey 1967; Gersh and Fowles 1979; Roth, Gurney, Garside, et al. 1972). For example, Downing and Rickels (1974) obtained physicians' ratings of anxiety and depression symptom severity in primary depressed and anxious patients. Whereas depressed patients were rated as high on both types of symptoms, anxious patients received high ratings only on anxious symptoms. Similarly, Di Nardo and Barlow (Chapter 12) report that patients with primary affective disorders score as high as primary anxiety patients on a variety of measures of anxiety, but are distinct from all anxiety patients except obsessive-compulsive patients on the Hamilton Rating Scale for Depression (Hamilton 1960). Emotion theorists (e.g., Izard 1971, 1977; Russell 1980; Tellegen 1985) have suggested that depression and anxiety share affective elements that are typically viewed as characteristic of anxiety (e.g., fear in Izard's model, high negative affect in Tellegen's model), but that depression also contains emotional components pathognomonic of depression (e.g., sadness, Izard; low positive affect, Tellegen). The information processing of depressed and anxious individuals may also be more discriminable for depression-relevant content than for anxiety-relevant material. Greenberg and Alloy (in press) and Greenberg and Beck (1989) found that depressed and anxious subjects (both students and psychiatric outpatients) exhibited enhanced processing of and memory for stimuli with anxiety content, whereas only depressed subjects showed enhanced processing and recall of depressive stimuli.

Table 1. Summary of Symptoms Unique and Common to Depression and Anxiety

Type of symptoms	Unique to depression	Unique to anxiety	Overlap both syndromes
Affective	Severe sadness and despair Low positive affect	Severe fear and tension	Dysphoria/negative affect Crying Irritability
Behavioral	Psychomotor retardation Anhedonia Loss of interest Suicidal acts (and ideation)	Increased activity Behavioral agitation	Decreased activity Lowered response initiation Decreased energy Behavioral disorganization and performance deficits Increased dependency Poor social skills
Somatic	Decreased SNS arousal Decreased appetite Reduced sexual desire	Increased SNS arousal	Restless sleep Initial insomnia Panic attacks
Cognitive	Hopelessness Perceived loss	Perceived danger and threat Uncertainty Hypervigilance	Helplessness Repetitive rumination and obsessions Worry Low self-confidence Negative self-evaluation Self-criticism Self-preoccupation Indecisiveness Poor concentration

Note. SNS = sympathetic nervous system. Although this table bears some resemblance to Table 6.1 of Garber, Miller, and Abramson (1980), we have rearranged the position of some symptoms and added some new symptoms based on more recent evidence of symptom occurrences in the two syndromes.

There are also examples of both unique and overlapping symptoms within each of the major symptom categories: affective, behavioral, somatic, and cognitive. Among affective symptoms of anxiety and depression, general negative affect or dysphoria, crying, and irritability occur equally often in the two disorders (e.g., Derogatis, Lipman, Covi, et al. 1972; Garber, Miller, and Abramson 1980; Izard and Blumberg 1985; Prusoff and Klerman 1974; Roth, Gurney, Garside, et al. 1972; Tellegen 1985; Watson and Clark 1984). The emotions of sadness and fear occur to some degree in both syndromes (Izard and Blumberg 1985), but severe sadness and despair is more frequent among depressed patients, whereas severe fear and tension is more common among anxious patients (Derogatis, Lipman, Covi, et al. 1972; Prusoff and Klerman 1974; Roth, Gurney, Garside, et al. 1972).

Among behavioral symptoms, response disorganization, performance deficits, and poor social skills are common to both syndromes (e.g., Bootzin and Max 1980; Garber, Miller, and Abramson 1980; Mandler 1972; Merluzzi, Rudy, and Krejci 1986; Miller 1975; Sarason 1985; Seligman 1975). Perhaps as a result of their social and behavioral deficits, many depressed and anxious persons show increased dependency on others (e.g., Beck 1967, 1976; Beck and Emery 1985). In addition, depression has a de-energizing effect on behavior, leading to decreased activity, fatigue, and lowered initiation of voluntary responses (e.g., Beck 1967; Garber, Miller, and Abramson 1980; Lewinsohn 1974a; Seligman 1975). Anxiety is also sometimes associated with decreased response initiation and immobilization (e.g., Beck and Emery 1985; Bootzin and Max 1980; Garber, Miller, and Abramson 1980; Jablensky 1985; Mandler 1972), but more typically, anxiety has an energizing effect on behavior, leading to increased activity, motivation, and behavioral agitation (e.g., Beck and Emery 1985; Garber, Miller, and Abramson 1980). Many investigations have indicated that severe psychomotor retardation and suicidal acts and ideation are specific to depression (e.g., Akiskal 1985a; Beck 1976; Benshoof 1987; Derogatis, Lipman, Covi, et al. 1972; Di Nardo and Barlow, Chapter 12; Prusoff and Klerman 1974; Roth, Gurney, Garside, et al. 1972). Loss of interest in activities and social relationships and anhedonia are also uniquely associated with the depressive syndrome (e.g., Costello 1972; Garber, Miller, and Abramson 1980; Klein 1974; Lewinsohn 1974a).

Consistent with the behavioral symptomatology, only depressive patients appear to be somatically hyporeactive, exhibiting poor appetite and reduced sexual desire (e.g., Derogatis, Lipman, Covi, et al. 1972; Prusoff and Klerman 1974). On measures of electrodermal, cardiovascular, and muscular responses, depressive patients exhibit decreased autonomic arousal (for reviews, see Foa and Foa 1982;

Garber, Miller, and Abramson 1980). In contrast, anxious patients show increased sympathetic nervous system arousal, including increased heart rate, skin conductance responses, muscular tension, pains, and dizziness (e.g., Agras 1985; Beck and Emery 1985; Foa and Foa 1982; Garber, Miller, and Abramson 1980; Weiner 1985). Initial insomnia and restless sleep (e.g., Garber, Miller, and Abramson 1980; Roth, Gurney, Garside, et al. 1972) are common to both disorders, although there may be other features that differentiate the two groups' sleep (Akiskal 1985a). Additionally, panic attacks may be common occurrences across depression and the anxiety disorders (e.g., Barlow 1985).

Depression and anxiety share many cognitive features. Both depressed and anxious persons report feelings of helplessness and low self-efficacy (e.g., Bandura 1977; Barlow 1985; Beck 1967; Beck and Emery 1985; Dohrenwend, Chapter 10; Lang 1985; Mandler 1972; Rehm, Chapter 35; Seligman 1975). Both groups are highly self-absorbed and engage in much self-criticism and negative self-evaluation (Beck 1967, 1976; Beck and Emery 1985; Carver and Scheier 1982; Greenberg and Alloy, in press; Greenberg, Vazquez, and Alloy 1988; Pyszczynski and Greenberg 1987; Sarason 1985). Anxious and depressed persons ruminate about their inadequacies and problems, worry about future negative consequences, and experience obsessions and indecision (Beck 1967, 1976; Beck and Emery 1985; Benshoof 1987; Borkovec 1985; Derogatis, Lipman, Covi, et al. 1972; Di Nardo and Barlow, Chapter 12; Prusoff and Klerman 1974; Sarason 1985). Depressed and anxious people are characterized by selective processing of negative information (e.g., Derry and Kuiper 1981; Greenberg and Alloy, in press; MacLeod, Mathews, and Tata 1986; Mathews and MacLeod 1986), interfering thoughts, and difficulty in concentration (Beck 1967; Beck and Emery 1985; Benshoof 1987). In contrast, hopelessness and perceptions of loss are unique to the syndrome of depression (Beck 1967; Beck and Emery 1985; Di Nardo and Barlow, Chapter 12; Garber, Miller, and Abramson 1980; Melges and Bowlby 1969), whereas perceived danger, uncertainty about future outcomes, and hypervigilance are more specifically associated with anxiety (e.g., Beck, Brown, Steer, et al. 1987; Di Nardo and Barlow, Chapter 12; Garber, Miller, and Abramson 1980; Greenberg, Vazquez, and Alloy 1988; MacLeod, Mathews, and Tata 1986).

THE HELPLESSNESS-HOPELESSNESS THEORY OF ANXIETY AND DEPRESSION

Abramson, Seligman, and Teasdale (1978) proposed a reformulated theory of human helplessness and depression that attempted to re-

solve a number of inadequacies associated with the original hypothesis (Seligman 1975). Recently, Abramson and colleagues (Abramson,
Alloy, and Metalsky 1988; Abramson, Metalsky, and Alloy 1989;
Alloy, Abramson, Metalsky, et al. 1988; Alloy, Hartlage, and Abramson 1988) further expanded and revised the reformulated theory and,
for reasons that soon will become clear, referred to this theory as the
hopelessness theory of depression. Unlike most other psychological
theories of depression or anxiety, the hopelessness theory, as we
extend and develop it in this chapter, explicitly addresses the issue of
comorbidity between *some* types of depressive and anxiety disorders.
Moreover, the theory can account for the four phenomena of comorbidity outlined above. In this section and the next, we describe the
hopelessness theory of depression and its predictions regarding the
relationship between anxiety and depression.

Preliminary Concepts

In presenting the hopelessness theory, it is useful to distinguish
among necessary, sufficient, and contributory causes of symptoms
(Abramson, Metalsky, and Alloy 1989; Alloy, Abramson, Metalsky, et
al. 1988). Necessary causes refer to those etiologic factors that must be
present in order for a set of symptoms to occur. Sufficient causes refer
to those etiologic factors that, once present, ensure manifestation of
the set of symptoms. Finally, contributory causes refer to those etiologic factors that increase the probability that symptoms will occur,
but are neither necessary nor sufficient for symptom expression. In
addition to varying in their logical relationships to the occurrence of
symptoms, causes may also be distinguished according to their temporal relationships to symptom onset. Distal causes operate early in
an etiologic sequence, when there is little or no manifestation of
symptoms. Proximal causes, however, operate relatively late in the
causal pathway and may occur immediately prior to or concurrent
with symptoms of the disorder. (For simplicity of exposition, we have
presented the proximal-distal distinction in terms of a dichotomy.
Strictly speaking, however, it is more appropriate to think in terms of
a proximal-distal continuum.)

Current Statement of the Hopelessness Theory
of Depression

The hopelessness theory of depression can be understood best in
terms of these concepts about causes of symptoms. The hopelessness
theory specifies a chain of distal and proximal contributory causes
hypothesized to culminate in a proximal sufficient cause of depression.

A proximal sufficient cause of depression: Hopelessness.
According to the hopelessness theory, a proximal sufficient cause of
depression is an expectation held with high confidence that highly
desired outcomes will not occur or that highly aversive outcomes will
occur, and that no response in one's repertoire will change the likelihood of occurrence of these outcomes. The common language term
hopelessness captures the three core elements of the proximal sufficient
cause featured in the theory: (1) negative expectations about the
occurrence of highly valued outcomes (a negative outcome expectancy); (2) feelings of helplessness about changing the likelihood of
occurrence of these outcomes (a helplessness expectancy); and (3) a
high degree of certainty about both of these beliefs (Garber, Miller,
and Abramson 1980).

It is useful to compare the proximal sufficient cause of depression
featured in the hopelessness theory with the proximal sufficient cause
featured in the original learned helplessness theory of depression
(Seligman 1975). According to the original theory, a proximal sufficient cause of depression was the expectation that one cannot control
outcomes regardless of their hedonic valence or their likelihood of
occurrence. Thus the original theory is seen best as a helplessness
theory of depression. In contrast, Abramson and colleagues (Abramson, Metalsky, and Alloy 1989; Alloy, Abramson, Metalsky, et al.
1988) view only a subset of cases of expected lack of control, those also
involving highly certain negative expectations about the occurrence of
highly valued or important events, as resulting in depression. This
revision makes the hopelessness theory more similar to other cognitive theories of depression (e.g., Beck 1967; Brown and Harris 1978a;
Melges and Bowlby 1969) than was the original theory and, as will
become clear below, is crucial in understanding the theory's specification of the relationship between anxiety and depression.

Abramson and colleagues (Abramson, Metalsky, and Alloy 1989;
Alloy, Abramson, Metalsky, et al. 1988) view expectations about both
the probability of important outcomes and one's ability to influence
the probability of these outcomes occurring as crucial to the development of hopelessness. Although helplessness is a necessary component of hopelessness, it is not sufficient to produce hopelessness. For
hopelessness to develop, helplessness must be accompanied by a
high degree of certainty about the expected occurrence of negative
outcomes (Garber, Miller, and Abramson 1980).

A key prediction of the hopelessness theory is that hopelessness
temporally precedes and is a proximal cause of the symptoms of
hopelessness depression. Alternatively, hopelessness may have no
causal status and may be simply another symptom of depression.
Relevant to this issue, Rholes, Riskind, and Neville (1985) found that
students' initial levels of hopelessness predicted their levels of de-

pression 5 weeks later, over and above the predictive capacity of initial depression (see also Riskind, Rholes, Brannon, et al. 1987). Similarly, in a prospective study, Carver and Gaines (1987) reported that dispositional pessimists were more likely than optimists to develop postpartum depression, when prepartum levels of depressive symptoms were controlled statistically. Although these studies do not establish that hopelessness caused depressive symptoms at a later time, they demonstrate the temporal precedence of hopelessness in predicting change in depressive symptoms.

It is important to emphasize that hopelessness is a proximal sufficient, but not a necessary, cause of depression. The theory explicitly recognizes that depression may be a heterogeneous disorder, and allows for the possibility that factors such as genetic vulnerability, neurotransmitter dysregulation, loss of interest in reinforcers, and other variables also may be sufficient to cause depression. In essence, the hopelessness theory postulates the existence of *hopelessness depression* as a subtype of depression.

Abramson and colleagues (Abramson, Alloy, and Metalsky 1988; Abramson, Metalsky, and Alloy 1989; Alloy, Abramson, Metalsky, et al. 1988) have proposed that hopelessness depressions are characterized by a particular constellation of symptoms: retarded initiation of voluntary responses, sad affect, suicidal acts and ideation, low energy, apathy, psychomotor retardation, sleep disturbance, and difficulty in concentration. Low self-esteem and increased dependency will also be symptoms of hopelessness depression under some circumstances (Abramson, Metalsky, and Alloy 1989). Note that some symptoms hypothesized to occur in the hopelessness subtype of depression are completely overlapping with symptoms currently described as comprising the syndrome of depression in DSM-III-R (e.g., sad affect, lack of energy, psychomotor retardation), whereas others only partially overlap with symptoms currently described as part of the depressive syndrome (e.g., retarded initiation of voluntary responses). Other symptoms included as part of the depressive syndrome in DSM-III-R (e.g., anhedonia, appetite disturbance) are not viewed as being part of the typical hopelessness depression syndrome.

In contrast to symptom-based approaches to the classification of the depressive disorders, etiology figures prominently in the definition of hopelessness depression (for the advantages of defining hopelessness depression in this way, see Abramson, Metalsky, and Alloy 1989. This subtype may cut across existing diagnostic categories of depression (e.g., major depressive disorder, dysthymia) and may even include individuals who currently receive other psychiatric diagnoses (e.g., some individuals currently diagnosed with anxiety disorders). Elsewhere we have elaborated the concept of hopelessness depression and its hypothesized cause, particular symptoms, course, therapy, prevention, and relationship to other subtypes of depression (Abramson, Metalsky, and Alloy 1989; Alloy, Abramson, Metalsky, et al. 1988; Alloy, Clements, and Kolden 1985; Alloy, Hartlage, and Abramson 1988; Halberstadt, Andrews, Metalsky, et al. 1984).

The criticism of tautology has sometimes been leveled at the hopelessness theory due to failure to appreciate that the theory presents a conceptual reorganization of the various phenomena typically associated with the concept of depression. In the usual description of depression, hopelessness is considered a "symptom" (e.g., Beck 1967). In contrast, the hopelessness theory reorganizes the phenomena of depression into a hypothesized causal sequence, giving causal status to some features previously viewed as symptoms (e.g., hopelessness), while maintaining symptom status for others (e.g., sadness) (for a similar account of Beck's cognitive model of depression, see Beck, Rush, Shaw, et al. 1979).

Because hopelessness is a hypothesized cause, its appearance must precede the symptoms of hopelessness depression. Once present, however, hopelessness may persist and coexist with these symptoms. This coexistence should not blur the distinction between the causal status of hopelessness and the symptom status of these resultant phenomena. Analogously, the acquired immune deficiency syndrome (AIDS) virus may temporally coexist with the symptoms it produces. Thus, to avoid tautology in testing the hopelessness theory, it is crucial that hopelessness not be included in measures of the dependent variables to be predicted (e.g., depressive symptoms). Of course, hopelessness may appear as a symptom in other subtypes of depression, but these other subtypes would not be viewed as hopelessness depressions (because the hopelessness was not antecedent).

One hypothesized causal pathway to depression. The hopelessness theory specifies a sequence of events in an etiologic chain hypothesized to culminate in hopelessness and thus the symptoms of hopelessness depression. The hypothesized causal chain begins with the occurrence of negative life events (or nonoccurrence of positive life event) and ends with the production of hopelessness depression symptoms (Figure 1). Each event in the chain leading to hopelessness is a *contributory* cause of depression because it increases the likelihood of, but is neither necessary nor sufficient for, the occurrence of depressive symptoms. In addition, these contributory causes vary in proximity to the occurrence of depressive symptoms. For the sake of brevity, throughout the remainder of the chapter, we will use the

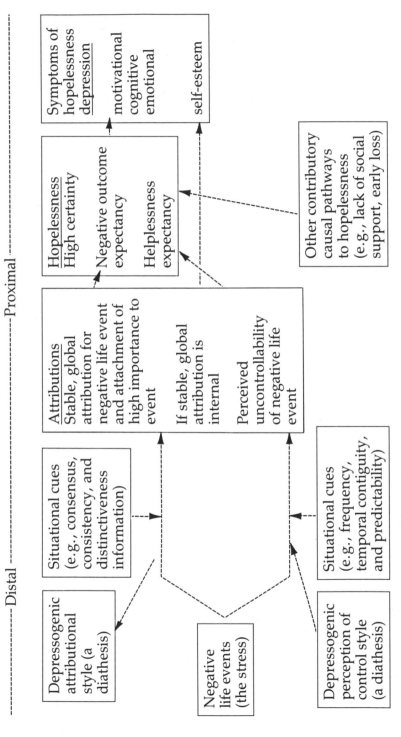

Figure 1. Hopelessness theory of depression.

phrase "negative life events" to refer to both the occurrence of negative life events *and* the nonoccurrence of positive life events. In addition, strictly speaking, the causal chain featured in the current statement of the theory begins with a "*perceived* negative life event."

Proximal contributory causes: Causal attributions for and perceived control over particular negative life events and the degree of importance attached to these events. According to Abramson and colleagues (Abramson, Metalsky, and Alloy 1989; Alloy, Abramson, Metalsky, et al. 1988), once people perceive that particular negative life events have occurred, the degree of importance attached to these events and the causal attributions made for them are important factors in whether or not hopelessness and, in turn, depressive symptoms (specifically, hopelessness depression) develop. Social psychologists have discovered that a major determinant of when people make spontaneous causal attributions is the occurrence of a negative event (e.g., Weiner 1985; Wong and Weiner 1981). This is precisely the initiating event in the causal chain postulated by the hopelessness theory.

In the hopelessness theory, four attributional dimensions are crucial for understanding how negative life events may contribute to the formation of hopelessness: internal-external, stable-unstable, global-specific, and uncontrollable-controllable. The internality dimension describes whether the cause of an event is perceived as due to something about the self (internal) or something about other people or circumstances (external). The stability dimension involves whether the cause is perceived as recurrent or enduring over time (stable) or more transient (unstable). The globality dimension involves whether the cause is perceived as likely to affect many outcomes across a wide range of situations (global) or few outcomes in few situations (specific). The controllability dimension refers to the event rather than the cause of the event, and involves the person's assessment of the degree to which the outcome can be influenced by his or her responses.

In brief, the negative outcome expectancy component of hopelessness (Clements and Alloy, in press) and, in turn, (hopelessness) depressive symptoms are more likely to occur when negative life events are attributed to stable and global causes and viewed as important than when they are attributed to unstable, specific causes and viewed as unimportant. Stable and global causal attributions imply that similar negative events are likely to recur across a wide variety of situations and thus imply a negative future. On the other hand, Clements and Alloy (in press) suggested that the helplessness expectancy component of hopelessness and, in turn, (hopelessness) depressive symptoms are more likely to occur when negative life events are perceived to be uncontrollable (i.e., independent of one's responses) than when they are judged to be controllable (see also Wortman and Dintzer 1978). Viewing past negative events as uncontrollable suggests that similar events in the future will also be beyond one's control. Finally, when negative life events are attributed to internal as well as stable and global causes, hopelessness will be accompanied by lowered self-esteem (Crocker, Alloy, and Kayne, in press; Tennen and Herzberger 1987).

Abramson, Seligman, and Teasdale (1978) demonstrated that the perceived controllability of an outcome is logically orthogonal to its perceived locus of causality. People may make either internal or external attributions for outcomes they perceive as uncontrollable. Similarly, the perceived controllability of an event is also independent of the perceived stability (and globality) of its causes. Events that an individual feels helpless to affect may be attributed either to stable, unchanging factors or to unstable, less recurrent causes that, when they occur, are independent of the person's behavior.

If causal attributions and perceptions of control for negative events modulate the likelihood of becoming hopeless, then it is important to describe what influences the kinds of causal attributions and control perceptions people will form in a given situation. Over the past 20 years, experimental and social psychologists have found that individuals' causal attributions and judgments of control for events are, in part, a function of the available situational information (e.g., Alloy and Tabachnik 1984; Kelley 1967; McArthur 1972). For example, internal, stable, and global attributions for an event are more likely when contextual information suggests that the event is low in consensus (e.g., failing to be promoted in one company while co-workers are promoted), high in consistency (e.g., frequently being passed over for promotions in the company), and low in distinctiveness (e.g., failing to be promoted in other companies as well as this one) (Kelley 1967; Metalsky and Abramson 1981). An event is more likely to be judged uncontrollable if it occurs infrequently, unpredictably, and not in close temporal contiguity to one's responses (Alloy and Tabachnik 1984).

Available informational cues constrain the attribution process by making some attributions for particular life events more plausible than others and some implausible (Hammen and Mayol 1982). Social psychologists have also identified the motivation to protect or enhance one's self-esteem, focus of attention, desire for control, choice, amount of effort, and self-presentational concerns among additional factors influencing attributions and perceptions of control (e.g., Alloy and Tabachnik 1984; Harvey, Ickes, and Kidd 1976, 1978, 1981).

Distal contributory causes: Attributional and control styles.
Abramson, Seligman, and Teasdale (1978) identified individual differences in attributional style as a more distal factor that also may constrain the attribution process and influence the content of causal attributions for a particular event (see also Ickes and Layden 1978). Abramson, Seligman, and Teasdale speculated that some individuals exhibit a general, frequently stable, tendency to attribute negative events to internal, stable, global factors and to view these events as very important, whereas other individuals do not (for a more detailed discussion of the stability of attributional styles, see Alloy, Hartlage, and Abramson 1988). Similarly, Clements and Alloy (in press) hypothesized that individual differences in perception of control styles may serve as a distal contributory factor that modulates people's control perceptions for particular negative life events. Some individuals may possess a greater tendency than others to perceive negative events as uncontrollable. Thus one's explanations for specific negative events experienced are hypothesized to be a joint function of the contextual information surrounding these events and one's attributional and control styles (Alloy and Tabachnik 1984; Metalsky and Abramson 1981).

According to the hopelessness theory, given equivalent situational cues, individuals who exhibit the hypothesized depressogenic attributional and control styles should be more likely than those who do not to attribute particular negative events to internal, stable, global factors and perceive these events as uncontrollable. In this way, the likelihood of forming negative outcome and helplessness expectancies and, consequently, of developing (hopelessness) depressive symptoms increases. In the presence of positive life events or absence of negative life events, however, people exhibiting the hypothesized depressogenic attributional and control styles should be no more likely to develop hopelessness, and therefore depression, than people not exhibiting these styles. This aspect of the hopelessness theory can be conceptualized as a diathesis-stress component (Alloy, Kayne, Romer, et al., in press; Clements and Alloy, in press; Metalsky, Abramson, Seligman, et al. 1982; Metalsky, Halberstadt, and Abramson 1987).

The logic of the diathesis-stress component implies that depressogenic attributional and control styles in a particular content domain (e.g., for interpersonal events) provide "specific vulnerability" (Beck 1967) to hopelessness depression when an individual confronts negative life events in that content domain (e.g., social rejection). The specific vulnerability hypothesis requires a match between the content areas of an individual's depressogenic cognitive styles and the negative life events encountered for hopelessness, and thus hopelessness depression, to occur (Abramson, Metalsky, and Alloy 1989; Alloy, Abramson, Metalsky, et al. 1988; Alloy, Clements, and Kolden 1985; Alloy, Hartlage, and Abramson 1988; Anderson and Arnoult, 1985; Hammen, Marks, Mayol, et al. 1985).

In sum, the etiologic sequence displayed in Figure 1 represents one hypothesized causal pathway to the development of hopelessness depression (for a presentation of the empirical support for the theory, see Abramson, Metalsky, and Alloy 1989). Because the links in this causal sequence are not viewed as necessary for the development of hopelessness, there may be other factors that also contribute to hopelessness, and thus to hopelessness depression (Abramson, Metalsky, and Alloy 1989; Alloy and Koenig, in press).

The Relationship Between Anxiety and Hopelessness Depression: Helplessness-Hopelessness Theory

In our current expansion of the hopelessness theory, the relationship between some anxiety syndromes and one form of depression (hopelessness depression) depends on the interrelation among the three components of hopelessness: helplessness expectancy, negative outcome expectancy, and certainty of these expectations (for a related perspective, see Garber, Miller, and Abramson 1980). According to the theory, an individual who expects to be helpless in controlling important future outcomes, but is unsure about his or her helplessness, will exhibit pure anxiety. With an uncertain expectancy of helplessness, the person believes that future control may be possible, and consequently experiences increased arousal and anxiety, accompanied by intense scanning of the environment for control-relevant cues, enhanced activity, and efforts toward gaining control (i.e., an "aroused anxiety syndrome"). If the person becomes convinced of his or her helplessness, but is still uncertain about the future likelihood of important negative events (or nonoccurrence of positive events), a retarded, "mixed anxiety-depression syndrome" will result. Arousal will decrease, the person will "give up" and become passive or immobilized, but will still worry and ruminate about future outcomes.

Whereas anxiety is caused by helplessness (uncertain or certain), depression (specifically, the hopelessness subtype) occurs when helplessness becomes hopelessness. A person who expects that he or she will be unable to influence the occurrence of important desired outcomes will be anxious, but may hold out hope that these events will occur through other means. If the perceived probability of future negative outcomes becomes certain, then helplessness becomes hopelessness and anxiety should give way to a depressive syndrome characterized by despair, loss of interest, and suicidality. Thus according to the hopelessness theory, the syndromes of anxiety and depression share an expectation of uncontrollability (and possibly, a common control style diathesis, see Figure 1), but differ in their negative outcome expectancies (Garber, Miller, and Abramson 1980).

Complementing the present formulation, a number of theorists have proposed that anxiety is caused by a sense of helplessness (e.g., Beck and Emery 1985; Lazarus 1966, 1968; Lazarus and Averill 1972; Mandler 1972), but depression by a sense of hopelessness (e.g., Arieti 1959; Beck 1967; Brown and Harris 1978a; Melges and Bowlby 1969). Indeed, Darwin (1872/1955) observed that "If we expect to suffer we are anxious, if we have no hope of relief we despair" (p. 176).

FOUR COMORBIDITY PHENOMENA: A HELPLESSNESS-HOPELESSNESS PERSPECTIVE

Here we elaborate on the relationship between anxiety and depression predicted by the hopelessness theory and discuss the manner in which the theory handles the four phenomena of comorbidity outlined above. Although these phenomena are tentative, we believe they provide a heuristic framework for developing the predictions of the helplessness-hopelessness theory with respect to certain patterns of symptom and syndrome co-occurrence.

The Anxiety-Depression Sequential Relationship: Lifetime and Intra-Episode Comorbidity

As discussed above, several lines of evidence suggest that anxiety may be more likely to precede depression than the reverse, both within and across episodes. Such findings are consistent with the helplessness-hopelessness perspective on the comorbidity of anxiety and depression. Individuals exhibiting anxiety and a sense of helplessness, but still maintaining some hope that bad outcomes will not occur, may become convinced for one reason or another that the negative outcomes are inevitable. As they become certain that negative outcomes will occur, they may be expected to develop (hopelessness) depression. This transition from anxiety to depression may be rapid and sudden, or slow and gradual, depending on the nature of the life events encountered and on the attributions made for those events. In addition, experiences with helplessness and anxiety symptoms at one time in life may increase a person's vulnerability to more certain helplessness and even full-blown hopelessness at a later time (such vulnerability may be mediated by maladaptive attributional and control styles). For example, a person who feels helpless to control outcomes at one time, may, when a negative life event occurs at a later time, be more likely to conclude that negative outcomes are inevitable and the future hopeless; at this point (hopelessness) depressive symptoms may develop. Such reasoning may explain the sequential progression from anxiety to depression across episodes of illness in an individual's lifetime.

This explanation for the transition from anxiety to depression is consistent with the common observation that depression often sets in after a major loss has occurred (for a review, see Monroe, Chapter 28), whereas anxiety may have accompanied anticipation or threat of that loss. Indeed, Finlay-Jones and Brown (1981) found that loss events frequently preceded onset of pure depression (65%) or mixed anxiety-depression (47%), but not pure anxiety (8%); "danger events," defined as "the degree of unpleasantness of a specific *future* crisis which *might* occur as a result of the event," more commonly preceded pure anxiety (62%) than pure depression (24%), with mixed anxiety-depression intermediate (47%). Presumably, loss events and individuals' explanations of loss events increase the likelihood that they will become hopeless and therefore depressed, whereas "danger" or "threat" events, with their inherent uncertainty, are likely to promote uncertain helplessness and thus anxiety.

By contrast, the reverse pattern seems less likely to occur. Once individuals become convinced that circumstances are hopeless, bad outcomes (such as a major loss or failure) will already have occurred or be imminent. At that point, depressive cognitive and motivational deficits and despair are likely to interfere with one's capacity to recognize control opportunities and that further bad outcomes are not necessarily inevitable. In other words, once one has developed symptoms brought about by hopelessness, it may be more difficult (although not impossible) to see one's helplessness as uncertain.

The hypothesis-testing strategies of cognitive therapy may be helpful in breaking up depression through precisely this route. By encouraging depressed individuals to attempt some task that they are convinced they are unable to do, they may come to see that, at least some of the time, their responses do exert control over outcomes. An interesting question that stems from the present perspective is whether individuals undergoing cognitive therapy will develop anxiety symptoms when attempting task assignments that they think they are unable to master. From the present perspective, it would seem that some anxiety symptoms would be common, although a full-blown diagnosis of an anxiety disorder would be improbable.

The helplessness-hopelessness perspective is also consistent with the results of observational studies of the intra-episode sequential relationship between anxiety and depressive symptoms within individuals. When an individual anticipates some bad, potentially uncontrollable, outcome, the resulting sense of possible helplessness should provoke anxiety. As long as the individual remains uncertain about the negative outcome and his or her helplessness in controlling it, then a relatively pure anxiety state, characterized by activation, arousal, vigilance, apprehension, and worry, would be expected. If efforts to exert control fail, the individual may become increasingly convinced of his or her helplessness. Certain helplessness accompanied by an uncertain negative outcome expectancy would produce a symptom pattern of mixed anxiety and depression. If the individual becomes convinced of his or her helplessness *and* certain that the bad outcome will occur, hopelessness depression should set in.

This line of reasoning is consistent with observations of human and nonhuman primates' responses to separation and loss. When monkey infants or young children are separated from their attachment figures, the initial phase of agitation (protest) has been seen by some (Kaufman 1973; Kaufman and Rosenblum 1967) as an example of a fight-flight response, drawing attention to the separated infant and increasing the likelihood of reunion. Coe, Wiener, Rosenberg, et al. (1985) summarized research showing that one of the prominent behaviors during this protest phase—vocalizations—occurs only at high levels if the monkey infants are in some proximity to their mother. They suggest that the vocalizations are emitted in an attempt to control the situation; if the infant is isolated, no attempts at control are made. The protest phase has also been described as having parallels to the reactance phase (Wortman and Brehm 1975) that occurs when an organism loses control and senses that its freedom is being threatened (Mineka and Suomi 1978). Here the agitation and arousal are seen as efforts to regain freedom and control.

The protest phase, characterized by these attempts to gain or regain control, is time limited. If the separation persists, some young monkeys and children will return to normal, but others will lapse into a phase of despair or depression. This is most likely to occur if the infant is not adopted during the separation or, in the case of human infants, if no other family members are present during separation from the mother (Bowlby 1973; Mineka 1982; Mineka and Suomi 1978). Such findings are consistent with the helplessness-hopelessness perspective in that despair-depression sets in only after attempts at regaining control have failed (i.e., the hope of reunion with the mother approaches zero and no other familiar replacements for the lost mother are available).

As we have seen, Wortman and Brehm's (1975) integration of reactance and helplessness theory (e.g., Seligman 1975) predicts the biphasic protest-despair response to separation and loss. In addition, however, it predicts that with many repeated exposures to uncontrollable events such as separations, the protest (reactance or anxiety) phase should diminish in duration and intensity, and the organism should more rapidly lapse into despair-depression. This is precisely the pattern of results observed by Mineka, Suomi, and Delizio (1981) in young peer-reared monkeys (1½ to 3½ years old) subjected to repeated separations from each other. Across a series of eight, 3-day separations (interspersed with 4-day reunions), the agitated protest behaviors virtually disappeared, and the depressed behaviors occurred earlier and with much greater intensity. In the terms of the helplessness-hopelessness theory, the young monkeys became increasingly convinced of their helplessness to control the separations and of the inevitability of the separations (i.e., they became hopeless.)

The Differential Comorbidity of Anxiety Disorders With Depression

Previously, we described evidence of differential rates of comorbidity among the anxiety disorders and depression. Specifically, panic disorder with and without agoraphobia, obsessive-compulsive disorder, and posttraumatic stress disorder are more likely than simple or social phobias and generalized anxiety disorder to be associated with depressive symptoms and disorders. The helplessness-hopelessness theory can account for this phenomenon as well.

Within the framework of the helplessness-hopelessness theory, individuals with persistent and pervasive cognitions of helplessness who believe they are chronically helpless in a number of areas of their lives should be more likely than individuals who experience more transient or situation-specific helplessness to be certain of their helplessness and, consequently, to exhibit symptoms associated with mixed anxiety-depression. Further, chronic and pervasive feelings of helplessness should increase one's vulnerability to the development of full-blown hopelessness and the additional consequent depressive symptoms. We suggest that certain anxiety disorders demonstrate greater overlap with depression than do other anxiety disorders as a function of the pervasiveness and certainty of their helplessness. Individuals who experience uncued and unpredictable aversive phenomena such as panic attacks, obsessions, or compulsions should be characterized by more chronic and pervasive feelings of helplessness and thus be more likely to exhibit symptoms of depression as well as anxiety than those whose helplessness is more uncertain and situationally specific.

According to the helplessness-hopelessness theory, cognitions of certain helplessness lead to a mixed anxiety-depression syndrome consisting of a particular set of symptoms described earlier (see also

Table 1 and Figure 2). Certain of these symptoms, such as panic attacks, obsessions, and compulsions, may be so aversive and seemingly uncontrollable as to increase the severity and certainty of the sufferer's helplessness. In this way, we postulate that a vicious cycle may develop in individuals with relatively certain helplessness. The experience of symptoms of a mixed anxiety-depression syndrome intensifies one's sense of helplessness, thus increasing the likelihood of experiencing these symptoms in the future.

Consistent with the helplessness-hopelessness perspective, individuals with obsessive-compulsive disorder, panic disorder, and agoraphobia are characterized by more generalized and certain helplessness than those with simple and social phobias. For example, Bandura (1977) found that simple phobic patients' estimates of their self-efficacy were lowest during encounters with their phobic stimuli and returned to higher levels in other situations. Similarly, Beck and Emery (1985) observed that social phobic patients tend to view themselves as helpless only in specific social situations. By contrast, Mavissakalian and Barlow (1981) reported that feelings of discouragement and helplessness were common in their chronic obsessive-compulsive patients with unpredictable and uncontrollable intrusive thoughts. In addition, Uhde, Roy-Byrne, Vittone, et al. (1985) found considerable variation in the frequency and duration of panic attacks both within and across 38 patients with panic disorder. Indeed, these patients' panic attacks seemed to occur "out of the blue," in no discernible pattern, making the attacks unpredictable. Uhde, Roy-Byrne, Vittone, et al. suggested that this lack of predictability may interfere with the patients' normal coping mechanisms, thereby increasing their feelings of helplessness. Consistent with this suggestion, Rachman and Levitt (1985) found that 50% of their agoraphobic patients reported a decline in their feelings of control during weeks in which they had experienced at least one panic attack. In panic-free weeks, only 22% of the patients reported feeling less in control; 42% indicated feeling efficacious. Only 25% of the agoraphobic patients reported an increase in control during weeks in which they had panicked.

There is reason to expect that individuals with posttraumatic stress disorder would also experience chronic and pervasive feelings of helplessness in a manner similar to that described by Uhde, Roy-Byrne, Vittone, et al. (1985) with respect to persons with spontaneous panic attacks. According to DSM-III-R, one of the characteristic symptoms of posttraumatic stress disorder is the reexperiencing of the precipitating trauma through repetitive nightmares or intrusive memories. In addition, individuals with posttraumatic stress disorder have reported experiencing exaggerated startle responses, panic attacks (Ettedgui and Bridges 1985), and, in rare cases, dissociative states in which the traumatic event is "relived" (American Psychiatric Association 1987).

Although the evidence on the comorbidity between generalized anxiety disorder and depression is equivocal, there are hints that generalized anxiety disorder may be less likely to exhibit comorbidity with depression. We speculate that patients with this disorder are unlikely to get caught in the cycle described above. The symptoms commonly associated with generalized anxiety disorder (e.g., worry) seem to be less noxious than panic attacks, obsessions, or compulsions. They may be more closely linked to specific spheres or domains of functioning (e.g., worry about performance in particular situations), and therefore be less pervasive and unpredictable. In particular, the helplessness-hopelessness perspective predicts that individuals whose generalized anxiety disorder involves apprehensive expectations in only a few, specific domains (i.e., who meet minimal DSM-III-R criteria for generalized anxiety disorder) will be less likely than those with more pervasive worries to be depressed as well. Circumscribed concerns may decrease the generalized anxiety patient's likelihood of becoming certain about his or her helplessness. This will maintain the relatively pure, "aroused anxiety syndrome" and preclude the development of mixed anxiety-depression symptoms characteristic of the shift to certain helplessness.

The Relative Infrequency of Pure Depression

Evidence reviewed earlier indicated that anxiety and depressive symptoms often co-occur and that pure depression (without anxiety) appears to be relatively rare, whereas pure anxiety (without depression) is more common. Such observations are readily accounted for in the helplessness-hopelessness framework. Following the logic of this theory, the cognition of hopelessness is a subset of helplessness cognitions. That is, individuals who are hopeless are, by definition, also certain about their helplessness and may be expected to show a mixed symptom picture of anxiety and depression. Because the reverse is not true (that is, individuals who are helpless are not necessarily hopeless), it is to be expected that pure anxiety, without depression, may be fairly common.

How does the theory account for the small proportion of individuals who appear to experience pure depression without anxiety? One possibility is that a qualitative shift in symptomatology may occur for some individuals once they become hopeless, resulting in the disappearance of anxiety symptoms. In particular, the anxiety symptoms of uncertain helplessness (arousal, agitation, vigilance) should disappear as hopelessness sets in, in part because of the incompatibility of the two sets of symptoms (severe sadness, despair, psychomotor retardation, and suicidal ideation versus arousal, agitation, and vigilance). Alternatively, cases of pure depression without any anxiety symptoms may not be cases of hopelessness depression. If this alternative is correct, then the hopelessness depression subtype is likely to be one characterized by a mixed picture of anxiety and depressive symptoms, and likely not to include cases of depression without anxiety.

Common and Unique Symptoms of Anxiety and Depression

The helplessness-hopelessness theory also suggests why depressive features, rather than anxiety features, better differentiate anxious and depressive patients. Given that hopelessness is a subset of helplessness, then symptoms such as suicidal ideation, severe sadness and despair, and psychomotor retardation would be expected to only occur in individuals who are hopeless and depressed. Both depressed and anxious patients, however, are helpless, and thus one would expect to find symptoms of anxiety in both anxiety disorders and depression.

Previously we described patterns of affective, behavioral, cognitive, and somatic symptoms that appear to be specific to anxiety or to depression, as well as symptom patterns common to both disorders (see Table 1 for a summary). The helplessness-hopelessness perspective, like other cognitive theories of psychopathology (e.g., Beck 1976; Forgus and Shulman 1979; Guidano and Liotti 1983; Ingram 1986), explains the manifestation of individual symptoms as the consequences of particular thoughts or cognitions. Thus the helplessness-hopelessness theory predicts that the specific combination of the three components of hopelessness determines the particular pattern of symptoms exhibited. In turn, the particular components of hopelessness experienced are influenced by the causal pathway presented in Figure 1. Figure 2 summarizes the manner in which the helplessness-hopelessness theory explains the unique symptoms and the overlapping symptoms of anxiety and depression.

According to the theory, when an individual expects that he or she may not be able to influence the occurrence of important future outcomes, but is unsure, a relatively pure, "aroused anxiety syndrome" will result. Uncertainty about one's ability to cope leads one to become fearful and tense (e.g., Beck and Emery 1985; Mandler 1972). Consequently, the future is perceived as dangerous and threatening (Beck and Emery 1985) and one is likely to become hypervigilant, searching the environment for cues relevant to one's control over future outcomes (Beck 1976; Beck and Emery 1985; MacLeod,

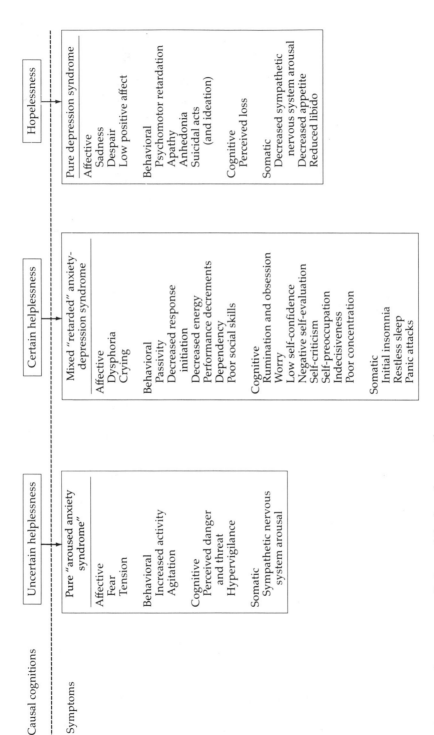

Figure 2.   Symptom predictions of the hopelessness theory.

Mathews, and Tata 1986; Mathews and MacLeod 1986; Sarason 1985). According to the theory, perceptions of possible helplessness and threat also lead to behavioral activation and intensification of efforts to regain control, because one still believes that further efforts may be successful. Numerous studies have documented that increased motivation and action are the initial responses to possible loss of control (for reviews, see Mandler 1972; Wortman and Brehm 1975). Partly as a result of the threatened lack of control and partly in support of or in preparation for the enhanced control-seeking behaviors, sympathetic nervous system arousal increases (Lang 1985) and contributes to the maintenance of the anxiety syndrome.

If a belief of certain helplessness is accompanied by uncertainty about future negative outcomes, a new set of symptoms, characteristic of a mixed anxiety-depression syndrome, should emerge. The expectation of certain helplessness is hypothesized to lead to negative self-evaluation and self-criticism because the sense of personal efficacy has been considered an important determinant of one's self-concept (e.g., Bandura 1977; Seligman 1975; White 1959). The helpless individual may ruminate about his or her powerlessness to affect future outcomes and may become preoccupied with thoughts of personal inadequacies (e.g., Beck 1967; Beck and Emery 1985; Mandler 1972; Sarason 1985). Thoughts of helplessness and preoccupation with personal failure, in turn, are likely to interfere with one's ability to concentrate on other activities or tasks (Pyszczynski and Greenberg 1987; Sarason 1985). Further, those who feel helpless will be indecisive because they believe that all of their actions are doomed to failure and thus that no alternative is the "right one" (Seligman 1975). Inasmuch as they expect that the probability of future negative events is still uncertain, even though they believe that they cannot personally influence whether or not these events happen, worrying and obsessions about possible negative outcomes should also be prominent features of the helplessness-induced, mixed anxiety-depression syndrome.

The cognition of certain helplessness leads to the behavioral symptoms of passivity, decreased energy, and lowered response initiation (Abramson, Metalsky, and Alloy 1989; Abramson, Seligman, and Teasdale 1978; Seligman 1975). The logic of the theory here is straightforward. If a person is helpless and is confident that nothing he or she does matters, then the incentive for emitting active instrumental responses decreases (Alloy 1982; Bolles 1972). Beck (1967) refers to this motivational effect as "paralysis of the will." Consistent with this logic, numerous studies in animals and people have demonstrated that prolonged exposure to positive or negative uncontrollable events produces passivity and deficits in response initiation (e.g., Abramson, Seligman, and Teasdale 1978; Maier and Seligman 1976; Seligman 1975). As a consequence of reduced activity, "giving up," and feelings of inefficacy, helpless people will exhibit performance decrements (Abramson, Seligman, and Teasdale 1978; Seligman 1975) and may depend increasingly on others to carry out tasks that they feel unable to accomplish successfully (Beck 1967; Beck and Emery 1985).

With regard to somatic symptoms, anticipatory worry about possible uncontrollable negative outcomes often leads to difficulty in falling asleep and restlessness during sleep (Bootzin and Engle-Friedman 1987; Bootzin and Nicassio 1978). Panic attacks may develop as individuals feel helpless in the face of possible negative events and fear losing control of even themselves. Helplessness will lead to affective symptoms of general dysphoria, fear of an uncertain future, and sadness about the loss of one's power to influence the course of events. Indeed, experimentally induced helplessness (e.g., by exposure to uncontrollable aversive events) has been found to increase self-ratings of both anxiety and depression (Gatchel, Paulus, and Maples 1975; Gatchel and Proctor 1976; Miller and Seligman 1976).

When a person becomes certain that desired outcomes will not occur or undesired outcomes will occur and that he or she cannot influence the probability of these outcomes, helplessness changes to hopelessness. According to the helplessness-hopelessness theory, hopelessness is hypothesized to lead to a third set of symptoms that are more characteristic of depression (see Table 1) and may reflect intensifications of the affective, motivational, and physiologic processes produced by the helplessness syndrome. The expectation that the future is bleak and without promise should lead to extreme sadness, despair (Abramson, Metalsky, and Alloy 1989; Alloy, Abramson, Metalsky et al. 1988; Garber, Miller, and Abramson 1980), loss of interest, and anhedonia. With no hope for improvement in the future and little enjoyment in the present, one may become suicidal. Several investigators have demonstrated that hopelessness is the best predictor of suicidal ideation and behavior, even controlling for depression (e.g., Beck, Kovacs, and Weissman 1975; Beck, Steer, Kovacs, et al. 1985; Kazdin, French, Unis, et al. 1983; Minkoff, Bergman, Beck, et al. 1973; Petrie and Chamberlain 1983). Similarly, apathy, psychomotor retardation, and autonomic hypoarousal may be due to severe decreases in energy and motivation for initiating voluntary responses (Abramson, Metalsky, and Alloy 1989; Beck 1967).

Consistent with the hypothesis that expectations of hopelessness are specifically related to a "pure depression" syndrome, Beck, Riskind, Brown, et al. (1988) found that psychiatric patients with major depressive disorder had higher mean hopelessness scale scores than patients with generalized anxiety disorder or mixed nonaffective, nonanxiety disorders. In addition, hopelessness was more strongly correlated with self-report and clinician-rated measures of depression than with measures of anxiety. Moreover, the correlations between hopelessness and measures of anxiety became nonsignificant when depression levels were controlled statistically, whereas hopelessness remained correlated with measures of depression after controlling for anxiety levels.

Additional Considerations in Understanding Comorbidity

To this point, we have described only one manner in which anxiety and depression may co-occur simultaneously in an individual from the helplessness-hopelessness perspective: Some symptoms that are usually classified as signs of either anxiety or depressive disorders are, in fact, common to both disorders as a consequence of cognitions of certain helplessness (see Table 1 and Figure 2 and the sections on intra-episode comorbidity above). As Garber, Miller, and Abramson (1980) explained, however, there are several additional considerations in fully understanding the complexity of the comorbidity of anxiety and depression. First, an individual's evaluation of his or her helplessness may shift from uncertain to certain, on a day-to-day or even moment-to-moment basis (for a method to measure daily variability, see de Vries, Dijkman-Caes, and Delespaul, Chapter 40). When that individual judges his or her helplessness to be uncertain, we would expect to see symptoms of "pure anxiety," whereas when the same person believes his or her helplessness is definite, symptoms usually associated with depression should also be exhibited.

In addition, symptoms of both anxiety and depression may occur together but be unrelated. One may be uncertain of one's helplessness and outcomes in one area of life (e.g., financial) while believing in the certainty of one's helplessness and negative outcomes in a different domain (e.g., interpersonal). Another possibility is that a confident expectation of a negative outcome may produce uncertainty about another outcome. For example, feeling sure that losing one's job is imminent may lead to doubt about one's abilities and outcomes in other areas, such as supporting one's family.

In the above cases, we described how different events may lead one to hold different expectancies simultaneously for one's helplessness and probable outcomes. In addition, a single event may produce several possible outcomes, each regarded with a different level of certainty. A person may be certain that some negative outcome will occur and that he or she will be unable to prevent it from occurring, yet be uncertain as to when it will happen or its ultimate consequences. As Garber, Miller, and Abramson (1980) discussed, in each of these cases the person would be expected to exhibit both anxiety and depressive symptoms, with each set of symptoms caused by the relevant cognition of helplessness or hopelessness.

OTHER RECENT COGNITIVE-BEHAVIORAL THEORIES OF ANXIETY AND DEPRESSION

Although many theorists have proposed models of depression or anxiety, few have attempted to account for both phenomena within a single theoretical framework (Greenberg, Vazquez, and Alloy 1988). In this section, we review three other cognitive-behavioral theories of the relationship between anxiety and depression and discuss the ability of these theories to deal with the four phenomena of comorbidity: the sequential relationship, the differential comorbidity of various anxiety disorders with depression, the relative infrequency of pure depression, and the common and the unique symptoms.

Beck's Schema Theory

The most notable existing theory that addresses *both* anxiety and depression is Beck's cognitive theory of the emotional disorders (Beck 1967, 1976; Beck and Emery 1985). Beck argues that anxious and depressed individuals are characterized by maladaptive cognitive schemata containing negative beliefs about the self, the world, and the future. A schema is a cognitive representation in memory that integrates current and incoming information in an internally consistent pattern. Schemata facilitate perception, comprehension, and recall of relevant information, but can also lead to distortion and bias (Taylor and Crocker 1980) because information is assimilated to the content of the schema. For example, information that is incongruent with an existing schema may be forgotten or ignored, or may be distorted in such a way as to make it consistent with the content of the schema.

According to Beck, the negative schema characteristic of *both* depressed and anxious individuals leads to systematic biases and distortions in interpretating self-relevant information when activated by personally significant negative life events (but see Alloy and Abramson 1988). These biased inferences, in turn, lead to the development of symptoms (Alloy, Clements, and Kolden 1985). Depressed and anxious persons both exhibit schema-based distortions in interpreting life events. The two groups can be distinguished, however, by the specific contents of their schemata, and the resulting inferences and symptoms. Depressed individuals' schemata are hypothesized to be organized around themes of personal deficiency, worthlessness, hopelessness, and loss, whereas those of anxious persons are believed to be organized around themes of threat, danger, and uncertainty (Beck 1976; Beck and Emery 1985).

Schema theories, such as Beck's, can more readily account for certain of the four comorbidity phenomena than others. For example, to explain the relative infrequency of pure depression, schema theorists would have to argue that most situations likely to activate depressive schemata are also likely to activate anxiety schemata. Intuitively, this does not seem an unreasonable assumption. Events triggering a sense of loss and hopelessness about certain outcomes may also activate a sense of threat about their consequences, and thus concurrently activate anxiety schemata, producing comorbid depression and anxiety. To explain the relative frequency of pure anxiety as compared to pure depression, schema theorists would have to argue that a variety of events may be able to activate anxiety schemata without the concurrent activation of depressive schemata. Again, this does not seem implausible, as a sense of threat, danger, and uncertainty can more plausibly exist without a sense of loss and hopelessness than the reverse.

The frequently observed sequential relationship between anxiety and depression can also, in a post hoc fashion, be explained by Beck's schema theory. The explanation would require an assumption that certain individuals possess latent schemata for both anxiety and depression, or that certain experiences can change an anxiety schema into a depressive schema. Anxiety schemata are by their very nature anticipatory of uncertain negative outcomes. The contents of threat, danger, and uncertainty are oriented toward what might happen and whether anything can be done about it. Research by Mathews and MacLeod (1986) and MacLeod, Mathews, and Tata (1986) has provided strong evidence that patients with generalized anxiety disorder do indeed show hypervigilance toward threat cues and that their diversion of attention to these threat cues can occur without awareness. By contrast, depression schemata contain beliefs that negative outcomes are inevitable or faits accomplis; that is, they are oriented toward past losses or toward certain future bad outcomes (hopelessness). Logically, a period of uncertainty about possible negative outcomes is likely to precede the actual occurrence of a negative outcome. Therefore, one might expect that an anxiety schema would be activated before the occurrence of a bad outcome. When the person recognizes that a negative event has occurred and is irreversible, then one might expect a depressive schema to be activated. This explanation may account for the frequently observed sequential pattern of anxiety and depressive symptoms in individuals experiencing social stressors such as separation and loss.

Schema theories can also partially account for the longitudinal epidemiologic finding that individuals receiving an anxiety diagnosis are more likely later to receive a depressive diagnosis than the reverse. A severely anxious individual worries about poor performance in a variety of areas and may experience significant interference as a result of the inhibitory effects of anxiety on performance (e.g., Beck and Emery 1985; Mathews and Eysenck 1987). Thus a maladaptive cycle may be established in which concern about possible failure or negative outcomes causes anxiety, and the anxiety state itself actually causes some failures or bad outcomes. As the cycle continues, depressive schemata, which center around the inevitability of failures or bad outcomes, may develop or become activated (cf., Beck and Emery 1985). This cycle would result in the anxiety-depression sequence.

However, given the logic presented thus far, schema theories do not appear to account easily for why depressive diagnoses seldom lead to a subsequent anxiety diagnosis. Above we stated that schema theorists would probably account for the relative infrequency of pure depression by arguing that most situations activating a depressive schema could also be expected to activate a sense of threat and, therefore, an anxiety schema as well. At one level, this explanation seems inconsistent with the observation that depressive disorders rarely turn into pure anxiety disorders. However, perhaps a schema theorist might argue the following: Patients receiving a depressive diagnosis probably have a mixed anxiety-depression symptom picture (given the base rates for pure depressive symptomatology). Therefore, the fact that mixed anxiety-depression rarely ends in pure anxiety simply means that once both depressive and anxiety schemata have been activated, it is unlikely that the depressive schema will become inactive while leaving the anxiety schema active.

To account for the differential comorbidity among the various anxiety disorders and depression, schema theorists could make one of two related arguments. First, Beck and Emery (1985) suggest that the different anxiety disorders are characterized by somewhat different schemata. It follows that some anxiety disorder schemata may more closely resemble, or be more compatible with, depressive schemata than are other anxiety disorder schemata. For example, if depressive schemata were more similar to panic disorder schemata than to phobia schemata, then a particular event activating a panic disorder schema may also activate the depressive schema, whereas the same would not be true of an event activating a schema for simple phobias. Beck and Emery (1985) maintain that the active schema in panic disorder revolves around a sense of "helplessness in the face of serious danger . . . lead[ing] a person to believe that he is trapped in a dangerous situation or is overwhelmed by an internal derangement" (p. 109). The content of this panic disorder schema resembles that of depression (loss and hopelessness). By contrast, the schemata activated in simple phobias are much more specific about the source(s) of danger, generally include the belief that escape would cause the fear to subside, and bear little resemblance to that of depression. Alternatively, over time the experiences associated with certain anxiety disorders (such as panic disorder or obsessive-compulsive disorder) may be sufficiently debilitating to activate depressive schemata concerning hopelessness.

To explain the common and unique symptoms of depression and anxiety, schema theorists would posit that certain symptoms are associated with the activation of anxiety schemata and others are associated with the activation of depressive schemata. The logic of schema-symptom specificity is similar to that discussed above in the helplessness-hopelessness perspective on common and unique symptoms. Anxiety schemata for danger, threat, and uncertainty would be expected to give rise to symptoms of arousal, agitation, and hypervigilance (e.g., Mathews and MacLeod 1986), sometimes intermixed with immobilization (Beck and Emery 1985). Depressive schemata for loss and hopelessness would be expected to give rise to loss of interest in pleasurable activities, extreme sadness and despair, and suicidal ideation (Beck 1967). Both types of schemata might be expected to give rise to negative self-evaluation and self-criticism, symptoms common to both anxiety and depression (Beck 1967, 1976; Beck and Emery 1985).

Bowlby's Attachment-Object Loss Theory

In his seminal three-volume work, Bowlby (1969, 1973, 1980) has written extensively about anxiety and depression as understood from the vantage point of attachment theory. Attachment theory builds on many observations from both the ethological and the psychoanalytic literatures (although it rejects most of the psychoanalytic suprastructure). In the most recent version (1980), Bowlby also incorporates research and theorizing from contemporary cognitive psychology. Because of this link with other cognitive schema approaches to anxiety and depression, it is included here as part of our discussion of cognitive-behavioral theories of anxiety and depression.

Bowlby postulates an evolutionary-biologic protective function for attachment behavior in many higher species. For the young, the chief function of an attachment object is to provide a base of security from which the infant can explore the environment. When confronted with a frightening stimulus, the infant not only withdraws from that stimulus but also retreats toward an attachment object. Because of its function in providing a secure base, separation from an attachment object can, in and of itself, create fear-anxiety and can greatly exaggerate the response to other frightening situations. Thus the commonly observed initial protest response to separation from an attachment object is seen as a prototype for anxiety. Once a young child develops a fear that the terrifying experience of separation may occur again, the child is fairly likely to exhibit separation anxiety and anxious attachment, characterized by excessive clinging and proximity-maintaining behavior.

If a separation persists, protest behaviors gradually wane and are replaced by behaviors characterized by depression, despair, apathy, or withdrawal. Protest behaviors are thought to be adaptive in that they may often have served to increase the probability of reunion after a separation has occurred. As hope of reunion diminishes, the protest decreases and feelings of depression increase. This phase is thought to serve the function of grieving and ultimately of accepting the loss. In discussing these observations, Bowlby notes the parallel with Freud's (1926/1959) last theory regarding the relationship between anxiety and depression. For both Freud and Bowlby, "when the loved figure is believed to be temporarily absent the response is one of anxiety, when he or she appears to be permanently absent it is one of pain and mourning" (Bowlby 1980, p. 27), and "anxiety is the reaction to the danger of losing the object, the pain of mourning the reaction to the actual loss of the object" (Bowlby 1973, p. 29).

As discussed earlier, the biphasic protest-despair response to separation seen in young children has its parallels in the responses of adults to loss of an attachment object through divorce or death (Bowlby 1980). Moreover, Bowlby maintains that early experiences with separation or loss have profound and persistent effects on responses to separation and loss later in life, with later reactions being mediated, in part, by the patterns of attachment behavior (e.g., anxious attachment) that were established early in life. In addition, Bowlby argues that early separation or loss experiences serve to establish cognitive schemata ("structures" or "programmes") for attachment that "become so engrained . . . that they come to operate automatically and outside awareness" (1980, p. 55). Later in life, when a person responds to information regarding a loss, individual differences in these cognitive structures regarding attachment, separation, and loss will determine the nature of that response. Bowlby argues that such individual differences in cognitive schemata are responsible for "disordered variants" of mourning: that is, mourning that does not fit the "normal" prototypical sequence seen in individuals without an early history of loss or in individuals with especially secure attachment relationships. Chronic mourning and absence of grieving are two examples of disordered variants. In this regard, Bowlby likens his theory to that of Beck's discussed above. Bowlby claims that he is somewhat more explicit than is Beck about the early childhood origins of these cognitive schemata.

Because Bowlby's theory addresses anxiety and depression as they occur in response to separation and loss, it does not purport to account for the origins of all cases of anxiety or depression. Nevertheless, it does appear to be able to account for many of the major features of the four phenomena of comorbidity described at the outset of this chapter, at least as they occur in response to separation and loss. For example, the often-observed sequential relationship between anxiety and depressive symptoms is specifically predicted by Bowlby's theory with respect to the expected biphasic response to separation and loss events. The theory does not as explicitly address changes in diagnostic status seen over years. However, because the basic stance is similar to that of helplessness-hopelessness theory on the point that depression occurs as hopelessness regarding reunion sets in, Bowlby's theory would appear to be able to account for such results in much the same way that we did.

Bowlby also appears to be able to explain the relative infrequency of pure depression. Because anxiety precedes depression as a response to actual or threatened separation and loss, people may become anxious about the threat of a loss, but not become depressed if the loss never occurs or if a substitute attachment object is found. As certainty that a loss has occurred sets in, Bowlby (1980) maintains that a mixed anxiety-depression symptom picture should be expected:

> When, however, the effort to restore the bond is not successful sooner or later the effort [the protest-agitation-anxiety symptoms] wanes. But usually it does not cease. On the contrary, evidence shows that, at perhaps increasingly long intervals, the effort to restore the bond is renewed: the pangs of grief and perhaps an urge to search are then experienced afresh. (p. 42)

By the same reasoning, pure depression would be expected to be more rare because of the periodic resurgence of urges to search for and restore the lost object.

Regarding the differential comorbidity of the various anxiety disorders with depression, Bowlby explicitly predicts the relationship of agoraphobia-panic disorder with depression and the lack of relationship of simple phobias with depression. Bowlby does not discuss obsessive-compulsive disorder and therefore does not consider the overlap between this disorder and depression. For Bowlby (1973), agoraphobia (and probably panic disorder, although that term was not in use in 1973) is a "pseudophobia." Whereas simple phobias are characterized by the fear of the *presence* of some object or situation and an urge to avoid or withdraw from that object or situation, agoraphobia or pseudophobia is characterized by fear of "the *absence or loss* of an attachment figure, or some other secure base towards which he would normally *retreat*" (Bowlby 1973, p. 260). Given the central role that disordered attachment relationships (early in life and/or in adulthood) play in the etiology and maintenance of both agoraphobia and depression, it is not surprising that agoraphobia and depression should coexist. Indeed, Bowlby points to a study by Roth (1959, 1960) in which 37% of his agoraphobics reported a bereavement or sudden illness in a close relative as a precipitating event for their agoraphobia. Parkes (1969, 1971) has also shown that panic attacks and other symptoms of anxiety are common among bereaved people. By contrast, simple phobias do not generally arise as a function of disordered attachment relationships or bereavements, and so would not be expected to overlap as often with depression. Bowlby (1973) does, however, argue that some cases of simple phobia in childhood are, in fact, cases of separation anxiety where the object of the fear is mistakenly attributed to an outside object, rather than to separation from the mother per se. He makes an interesting and moderately compelling case for reinterpretation of Freud's case of Little Hans in this vein.

To explain the common and unique symptoms of depression and anxiety, Bowlby's argument would be similar to ours and to that of Beck. Danger or threat of loss should provoke the agitation and arousal characteristic of protest. As certainty of the loss sets in, symptoms of apathy, withdrawal, and hopelessness may be expected to occur. However, Bowlby also predicts that earlier experiences with loss will significantly affect the symptomatology seen in the depressive response phase to a later loss. Here, Bowlby builds on the observations of Brown and Harris (1978a) who found that early loss by death was a vulnerability factor for psychotic depression, whereas early loss by causes other than death was a vulnerability factor for neurotic depression. The suggestion of Bowlby and of Brown and Harris is that early loss by death sets up expectancies or schemata predisposing the person to respond to subsequent losses with the same sense of hopelessness and retardation. By contrast, early loss by causes other than death sets up expectancies or schemata predisposing the person to respond to subsequent losses as though they may be reversible, leading to "despair mixed with angry, perhaps violent protest and . . . to a condition more likely diagnosed as a neurotic than as a psychotic one" (Bowlby 1980, p. 310).

Higgins' Self-Discrepancy Theory

Higgins' (1987) self-discrepancy theory is the most recent cognitive-behavioral theory to address specifically the relationship between anxiety and depression. Self-discrepancy theory is derived from the tradition in psychology of viewing emotional discomfort as a consequence of conflicting or incompatible beliefs. Unlike past theories of belief incompatibility, self-discrepancy theory predicts which types of negative emotions and emotional disorders will be induced by particular kinds of incompatible transient or chronic beliefs. Discrepancies among six different types of self-representations determine individuals' proneness to negative emotional states and disorders. These six self-state representations are described by three domains of the self viewed from two perspectives: (1) one's *actual self* is the representation of attributes that someone (either *oneself* or a *significant other*) believes one possesses; (2) one's *ideal self* is the representation of attributes that someone (*oneself* or a *significant other*) would like one to possess (i.e., hopes, aspirations, wishes); and (3) one's *ought self* is the representation of attributes that someone (*oneself* or a *significant other*) believes one should possess (ie., duties, obligations, responsibilities). The first two self-representations (actual-own and actual-other) are typically denoted as self-concept. The four remaining representations are self-directive standards or guides.

Self-discrepancy theory posits individual differences in motivation to meet particular self-standards and assumes that discrepancies between the self-concept (actual-own self) and particular self-standards reflect particular types of negative psychological situations. Higgins argues that perceived discrepancies between the actual-own self and ideal self (own or other) represent the absence of positive outcomes (i.e., the nonattainment of hopes and wishes). Thus a person who perceives this discrepancy will be vulnerable to dejection-related emotions, such as disappointment, dissatisfaction, and sadness and to more severe depression. In contrast, perceived discrepancies between the actual-own self and ought self (own or other) represent the presence of negative outcomes (i.e., expectation of punishment or disapproval from others). Such discrepancies are associated with vulnerability to agitation-related emotions such as fear, threat, and guilt and to more serious anxiety. In general, the greater the magnitude and accessibility of self-discrepancy, the more the individual will experience the kind of discomfort associated with that particular type of self-discrepancy. The accessibility of a particular self-discrepancy depends both on the frequency and recency of past activation, and the relevance of immediate environmental stimuli to that self-discrepancy.

Although self-discrepancy theory has generated an impressive body of empirical evidence (see Higgins 1987), it does not easily account for the four features of anxiety-depression comorbidity. The theory most readily explains some of the unique and common symptoms of anxiety and depression. Although self-discrepancy theory does not specifically address the particular symptoms likely to be associated with the activation of various self-discrepancies, the theory does specify consequent emotions associated with activation of different self-discrepancies. Discrepancy-specific emotional patterns should be associated with unique sets of behavioral, cognitive, and somatic symptoms. According to the theory, activation of discrepancies between the actual and ought selves leads to the agitation-related emotions of fear, threat, and guilt and thus to associated increases in activity, arousal, and vigilance. In contrast, actual-ideal discrepancy activation leads to dejection-related emotions of disappointment, sadness, and shame and therefore to associated symptoms of hopelessness, perceived loss, loss of interest, and anhedonia. Inasmuch as both types of discrepancies involve failure to meet important self-standards, both may be associated with symptoms common to anxiety and depression, such as negative self-evaluation and self-criticism, self-preoccupation and obsessions, poor concentration, behavioral disorganization and performance deficits, crying, and dysphoria. On the other hand, symptoms of helplessness, passivity, and decreased energy, which are also common to both anxiety and depression, are not so easily explained by self-discrepancy theory. These symptoms are likely to be uniquely associated with the dejection-related emotions and, therefore, to the activation of actual-ideal discrepancies.

Self-discrepancy theory must also explain the relative infrequency of pure depression and relative frequency of pure anxiety. This pattern would result if actual-ideal self-discrepancies are rarely activated without simultaneously activating actual-ought discrepancies, but actual-ought self-discrepancies are frequently activated alone. This difference could occur if most individuals who are vulnerable to depression possess similar ideals and "oughts" (or hopes and obligations), whereas the ideals and oughts of individuals who are less vulnerable to depression are more distinct from one another. For example, if a depression-prone individual views academic achievement as a duty to one's parents as well as a personal ideal, then a failure on an exam would be likely to activate both actual-ideal and actual-ought discrepancies and result in a mixed anxiety-depression response. In contrast, an individual who is not especially depression-prone may perceive school achievement as a responsibility to his or her parents, but wish for athletic success as his or her personal ideal. For this person, failure on an exam would activate only actual-ought discrepancy and thus an anxiety response alone. An athletic failure, in contrast, would activate actual-ideal discrepancy and thus a depressive response alone. However, the reasons why depression-prone people would be more likely to possess similar ideals and duties than other people is not addressed by the theory.

Self-discrepancy theory is also silent about possible determinants of the anxiety symptoms central to the different anxiety disorders (e.g., panic attacks, obsessions and compulsions, phobias) and therefore about the differential comorbidity of anxiety disorders with depression. Differential comorbidity could be explained by assuming either that the overlap between ideals and oughts is greater for some anxiety disorders than others or that actual-ought and actual-ideal discrepancies are more likely to be activated simultaneously for some anxiety disorders than for others. These assumptions are not specified in the theory, however. Finally, self-discrepancy theory does not easily predict or explain the sequential relation between anxiety and depression. Although actual-ought discrepancies might become activated prior to actual-ideal discrepancies in response to negative life events, there is no obvious theory-derived explanation for this sequence.

Comment on Other Cognitive-Behavioral Theories

As discussed above, these three cognitive-behavioral theories address some aspects of the relationship between anxiety and depression and, in this respect, are unusual among contemporary theories of anxiety or depression. Because no one of them was developed with the four phenomena of comorbidity in mind, it is not surprising that they are not able to explain all of these phenomena. However, if future research corroborates the reliability and validity of these four comorbidity features, then future revisions of these theories should take them into account more explicitly.

At present, it appears that Beck's schema and Bowlby's attachment-object loss theories are best able to account for many of the features of comorbidity, although some only in a post hoc fashion. We would urge other theorists to delineate and test these theories more precisely. For example, further development and validation of instruments and tasks for measuring the presence of latent anxiety and depressive schemata could be useful in assessing these theories' accounts of the comorbidity phenomena. In addition, specific predictions of Bowlby's theory about the effects of early childhood separation and loss experiences on anxiety and depressive schemata should be operationalized and tested, ideally with prospective designs. However, rather than giving further detail about the refinement and testing of these three theories, we now turn to future directions for research on the helplessness-hopelessness theory.

DIRECTIONS FOR FUTURE RESEARCH

Inasmuch as the helplessness-hopelessness theory specifies the etiologic chain of events leading to anxiety and hopelessness depression in detail, and explicitly predicts many of the apparent features of comorbidity, we believe that tests of this theory may be quite fruitful in furthering our understanding of anxiety-depression comorbidity. How might we search for hopelessness depression and delineate its association with the various anxiety disorders? At the outset, we caution that a search for hopelessness depression and a determination of its relation to anxiety disorders raises some of the most basic and challenging questions facing any psychopathologist. What is a useful category of psychopathology? How can one determine whether a hypothesized psychopathologic entity exists in nature? How can one most meaningfully subdivide a group of heterogeneous disorders into their constituent types? We do not have all of the answers to these complex questions. However, we suggest that, at a conceptual level, the search for hopelessness depression and a determination of its relation to anxiety is a rather straightforward matter involving nothing more than the careful testing of the helplessness-hopelessness theory. Such a test would involve at least three components: (1) a test of the etiologic chain summarized in Figure 1 and hypothesized to culminate in the cognitions of helplessness and hopelessness; (2) an evaluation of the theory's symptom predictions summarized in Figure 2; and (3) a specific test of the theory's predictions of the four comorbidity phenomena discussed above.

In this section, we outline some possible strategies for evaluating the validity of the theory's predictions of the four features of comorbidity (for a discussion of research strategies for testing the first two components of the theory, see Alloy, Hartlage, and Abramson 1988). We emphasize that it is not our aim to provide a "cookbook" of all possible approaches and research designs one conceivably might use to evaluate the helplessness-hopelessness theory's comorbidity predictions. Instead, we suggest only a few research strategies that may be particularly appropriate for testing our theoretical perspective. More generally, in addition to providing tests of the helplessness-hopelessness theory, these strategies should also be well-suited for generating further empirical data regarding the four comorbidity phenomena themselves.

In the helplessness-hopelessness theory, the sequential relationship between anxiety and depression is explained by a change in individuals' expectations from uncertain or certain helplessness to hopelessness. When people who believe they are powerless to influence the occurrence of important personal outcomes become convinced that negative outcomes are inevitable and give up hope, the helplessness-hopelessness theory predicts that their anxiety will change to depression. This transition from helplessness to hopelessness is, in turn, dependent on the nature of the life events individuals encounter and on the attributions they make for these life events (see Figure 1). Consequently, to test the sequential prediction of the theory, longitudinal, prospective research designs would be necessary. In these studies, individuals would be assessed repeatedly for the occurrence of stressful life events, for the nature of their attributions and control perceptions for these life events, for their development of helplessness and hopelessness expectations, and for the onset of anxiety and depression symptoms (or diagnoses). Inasmuch as the transition from helplessness to hopelessness and thus from anxiety to depression may occur within relatively brief periods of time, it would be important to assess subjects' life events, cognitions, and symptoms on a frequent basis. Ideally, subjects could be asked to keep systematic diaries or to make daily ratings of their life experiences, cognitions, and symptoms. Such prospective, "follow-along" designs would be especially powerful. They would be most likely to provide an adequate test of the helplessness-hopelessness theory if they utilized a subject sample that was at high risk for developing helplessness and hopelessness over time and, therefore, anxiety and depression. According to the theory, individuals at risk for anxiety and depression would include those with dysfunctional attributional styles and perception of control styles (see Figure 1). Other at-risk individuals would be those who are likely to experience life stressors that are themselves helplessness- or hopelessness-inducing (Abramson, Alloy, and Metalsky 1988; Alloy, Clements, and Kolden 1985), such as parents or spouses of persons diagnosed with cancer or AIDS, or workers about to be laid off from their jobs.

From the perspective of the helplessness-hopelessness theory, certain anxiety disorders (e.g., panic disorder, obsessive-compulsive disorder) demonstrate greater overlap with depression than do others because they are characterized by more severe, more certain, and more pervasive helplessness. This hypothesis could be tested in a cross-sectional design in which groups of persons who meet diagnostic criteria for different anxiety disorders are compared among themselves and with a group of patients with major depression and normal controls on a variety of measures of helplessness cognitions, attributions, and perceptions of control. In conducting such a study, it would be necessary to ensure that the subjects with various anxiety disorders do not meet diagnostic criteria for any depressive disorder diagnosis and that depressed subjects do not meet diagnostic criteria for any anxiety disorder. In addition, in comparing the cognitions of the various groups, it would be important to control statistically for the effects of depressive symptoms among the anxious subjects and anxiety symptoms among the depressed subjects (K. A. Kelly and L. B. Alloy, unpublished observations).

The helplessness-hopelessness perspective also suggests that certain anxiety symptoms (e.g., panic attacks, obsessions and compulsions) that are themselves consequences of helplessness expectations may, in turn, by their own uncontrollable nature, increase the severity and certainty of the sufferer's helplessness and lead to additional symptoms of a mixed, anxiety-depression syndrome. To investigate this prediction, one could obtain a sample of panic and obsessive-compulsive disorder patients shortly after the onset of their disorders and then follow these patients longitudinally. One would hope to examine the progression of certain and generalized helplessness, hopelessness, and additional anxiety and depressive symptoms.

The relative infrequency of pure depression is explained by virtue of the logic of the helplessness-hopelessness theory: hopelessness is a subset of cases of helplessness. This hypothesis could be examined by assessing the relationships among helplessness, hopelessness, anxiety, and depression in large cross-sectional samples of normal individuals or psychiatric samples of patients with a variety of anxiety and depressive disorders. Those subjects who exhibit hopelessness should, according to the theory, also exhibit helplessness cognitions and be depressed. In contrast, only some of the subjects espousing helplessness should also exhibit hopelessness. Further, those subjects who are helpless but not hopeless should exhibit the pure, "aroused anxiety syndrome" or the mixed anxiety-depression syndrome shown in Figure 2, depending on the certainty of their beliefs in their own powerlessness.

Finally, several research strategies may be appropriate for testing the predictions regarding the development of individual affective, behavioral, cognitive, and somatic symptoms of anxiety and depression (see Figure 2). First, one could examine the onset of individual symptoms as a function of helplessness and hopelessness expectations in the context of the prospective, follow-along study described above for testing the sequential prediction of the theory. Alternatively, subjects who are experiencing anxiety and depressive symptoms could be asked to keep daily logs or records of the particular symptoms they experience, when they occur, and what they were thinking right before the symptoms were experienced (for a detailed description of such cognitive-behavioral logs, see Beck, Rush, Shaw, et al. 1979).

In conclusion, we have presented four possible features of anxiety-depression comorbidity that, if further validated, should be explained by any theory of the development and course of anxiety and depressive disorders. The helplessness-hopelessness theory is unique in directly addressing and predicting these four comorbidity phenomena and in presenting an integrated account of some types of depression and anxiety disorders. Inasmuch as the helplessness-hopelessness theory is a *process-oriented* account of anxiety and depression (see Figure 1), it makes powerful predictions about the onset, course, therapy, and prevention of anxiety and hopelessness depression (see Abramson, Alloy, and Metalsky, 1988; Abramson, Metalsky, and Alloy 1989; in press; Alloy, Abramson, Metalsky, et al. 1988; Alloy, Clements, and Kolden 1985) as well as about the intra-episode and lifetime association between these two syndromes. An application of research strategies designed to test these powerful predictions of the helplessness-hopelessness theory should greatly enhance our understanding of the psychopathology of a subset of the anxiety and depressive disorders.

Chapter 30

Psychological Defense Mechanisms and the Study of Affective and Anxiety Disorders

J. Christopher Perry, M.D., M.P.H.

PSYCHOLOGICAL DEFENSE MECHANISMS are major constructs in the description of psychodynamic psychopathology. In psychodynamic theory, defenses are construed as the individual's unconscious adaptive response to internal or external stressors as they are affected by internalized conflicts. Although defenses may not be the principal cause of symptoms per se, it is assumed that the adequacy or adaptiveness of defense responses may trigger the onset or affect the course of symptoms. This assumption suggests that it might be fruitful to study defenses as mediating variables affecting the proximate causal relationship between life stress and episodes of affective and anxiety disorders. This chapter will briefly review how defense mechanisms have been studied to date, and then discuss potential contributions to the study of anxiety and affective disorders. Examples will be taken from the author's ongoing research on personality disorders and will focus on the relationships among psychopathology, defenses, and anxiety and affective disorders. It will end with suggestions for futher exploration of whether and how particular defense mechanisms affect the susceptibility to specific affective and anxiety disorders.

Part of this work was supported by grant No. RO1-MH-34123 from the National Institute of Mental Health.

Conceptual Aspects of Psychological Defense Mechanisms

Since Freud's (1894/1960) first description of defenses in 1894, major contributions in the classification of defenses have been made by Anna Freud (1937/1966), Fenichel (1945), Vaillant (1977), Kernberg (1975), and Meissner (1985). DSM-III-R (American Psychiatric Association 1987) contains a glossary of 18 defenses that can be specified as additional features complementing Axis II psychopathology. While psychodynamic theory has at times been encumbered by specialized terms, by theoretical models, and by psychological processes that are ambiguously defined, hard to measure, and of questionable testability, defenses can be studied with fewer difficulties. This is because judging from a pattern of observable phenomena that a defense has been used requires only low levels of inference. In fact, many defenses are capable of being defined and studied from other theoretical perspectives, such as cognitive-behavioral.

Most researchers would agree with the following overall definitional assumptions. First, defenses are the individual's automatic response to internal or external stressors, which trigger what Freud (1923/1964) called the signal anxiety (i.e., anxiety that attends the perception of psychological danger). Signal anxiety occurs when internal wishes and drives conflict with internalized prohibitions or external reality. Second, defenses are generally automatic (reflexive) and function without conscious effort and often without conscious awareness. Third, individuals tend to "specialize" by characteristically employing the same defenses across different situations. The repetitive use of a defense suggests that each instance of using a defense is a manifestation of an underlying disposition or trait. Therefore, some confounding of state and trait aspects of defenses is expectable. Fourth, a defense can generally be characterized on a continuum from maladaptive to adaptive, although each defense might be very adaptive in certain unique circumstances. When least adaptive, defenses protect the subject from conflict at the expense of constricting awareness, a sense of choice, and flexibility to maximize a positive outcome. When most adaptive, defenses maximize expression, gratification of wishes and needs, and a sense of freedom to choose, while minimizing negative consequences.

Defenses appeal to clinicians because they relate to the development or maintenance of psychopathology and problems in living. Their effects are evident from the subject's report of his or her life; they also operate in the therapy situation and the transference, and they affect the ability to cooperate with treatment. Many treatment interventions are designed to counter problems of defense and resistance to treatment. Furthermore, descriptions of "the difficult patient" in any diagnostic group often describe the results of defensive operations over conflicts about being helped, getting well, facing problems, and complying with treatment.

A BRIEF REVIEW OF METHODOLOGICAL WORK AND EMPIRICAL FINDINGS

Three approaches to rating defenses have used different data sources including clinical judgment, self-report, and projective testing. Because of special problems in interpreting the results of the latter two approaches, this chapter will focus on ratings from clinical data. A review of the other approaches is available elsewhere (Perry and Cooper 1987).

Measurement Methods

Haan (1963) used written summaries of an average of 12 hours of individual interviews for rating 10 defense mechanisms and 10 coping mechanisms. The interviewer and a blind judge rated the presence of the defenses on a 1 to 5 scale based on a catalog of definitions presented in that article. All raters were clinically experienced. The mean reliability coefficients of the individual defense ratings were .66 for male subjects and .50 for female subjects.

Bellak, Hurvich, and Gediman (1973) developed the Ego Function Assessment, which uses clinical interviews to assess 12 aspects of ego functioning. Scale 8 summarizes the overall effectiveness of defensive functioning on a 13-point scale, primarily by rating evidence of symptom formation and failure to contain anxiety. It does not assess specific defenses. The original reliability of the scale was high ($r = .81$), although a Norwegian study obtained a lower estimate ($r = .13$) (Dahl 1984b). The reasons for this discrepancy are unclear.

Semrad, Grinspoon, and Fienberg (1973) developed a 45-item instrument, the Ego Profile Scale, which clinicians rate on the basis of clinical observation that yields scores for nine defenses. On a separate sample, Ablon, Carlson, and Goodwin (1974) found that the interrater reliability coefficients of the nine defense patterns ranged from .49 to .89. A factor analysis of the instrument suggested that the nine patterns could be collapsed into seven factors. The instrument was designed for inpatient settings where prolonged behavioral observation is possible; its applicability to outpatient settings has not been tested.

Vaillant (1976, 1977) devised a glossary of 18 defense mechanisms with which he rated life vignettes obtained from interviews of subjects who discussed how they dealt with important events in their lives. Vaillant selected 20 life vignettes from each subject who had been interviewed during middle age, from which blind raters determined the subject's three major defenses. The mean reliability for the defense ratings was .56 (range, −.01 to .95) for the blind raters but was somewhat higher when their combined ratings were compared to the nonblind ratings of the author (mean, .73; range, .53 to .96). Although the reliability may be somewhat lower if applied to unselected life vignettes, this method clearly captures clinically significant defensive functioning. The method does not distinguish between defenses operating at the time of describing the vignette from those operating at the time the vignette occurred. It is probably most valid when life vignettes are gathered close to the time of actual occurrence, thereby minimizing bias due to recall.

Jacobson, Beardslee, Hauser, et al. (1986a, 1986b) studied defense mechanisms among three groups of adolescents: diabetics, nonpsychotic psychiatric patients, and healthy high school students. They assessed 12 defenses and a measure of overall defense success from transcripts of open-ended interviews. Each defense had both a definition and a 5-point rating scale. In addition, they provided clinical examples of the minimal, moderate, and maximal ratings. The intraclass interrater reliability coefficients were >.60 for seven defense scales. This method uses clinical data and employs a highly specific rating scheme that measures defensive functioning in degrees. It is a promising instrument for both teaching and research.

As part of a study of the validity of borderline personality disorder, Perry and Cooper (1986a, 1986b, 1989) compared defenses used by individuals with borderline personality disorder to those used by comparison subjects with antisocial personality or bipolar type II affective disorder. They had a group of nonprofessionals rate 22 defenses after observing a videotaped dynamic interview of each subject. Their instrument, the Defense Mechanism Rating Scales, includes a definition for each defense as well as a description of its function, comments on how to discriminate it from other defenses, and an accompanying 3-point rating scale anchored with examples. The reliability of the individual defenses was acceptable when group consensus ratings were compared (median intraclass reliability, .57; range, .37 to .79). When related defenses were combined into five summary defense scales (disavowal, action, borderline, narcissistic, obsessional), reliabilities were significantly higher (median, $r = .74$). Subsequently Perry and Cooper added eight so-called mature defenses, representing the healthiest level of functioning, to the rating manual and employed all 30 defenses in rating typed summaries of prospectively gathered life vignette data on the same sample. Comparable interrater reliabilities rating defenses from the life vignette data source were obtained using professional raters. An overall maturity of defenses score can also be calculated for each subject, in which each defense rated from the life vignettes contributes an empirically derived weighting reflecting its order in a hierarchy of healthy functioning. This variable can summarize the adaptiveness of defensive responses across vignettes for comparing one time period with another or one group of subjects with another.

Diagnosis

Most of the research findings to date have focused on the relationship between defenses and diagnosis or global functioning. Studies by Vaillant and Drake (1985), Perry and Cooper (1986a), Dahl (1984a), and Goldsmith, Charles, and Feiner (1984) have demonstrated significant associations between the immature, borderline and narcissistic defenses and personality disorder diagnoses; mature defenses have been negatively associated with them. Borderline patients, in particular, have been found to have lower defensive functioning than other nonpsychotic individuals. In a study of hospitalized patients with unipolar and bipolar affective disorders, Ablon, Carlson, and Goodwin (1974) followed the course of improvement by serially rating changes in defensive functioning using the Ego Profile Scale. Two-thirds of the patients demonstrated a shift away from using distortion, denial, and projection as they clinically improved. Manic patients tended to show an increase in somatization and hypochondriasis (help-rejecting complaining) just prior to switching out of manic episodes.

Global Functioning

A consistent finding across studies is that defenses are hierarchically associated with global functioning (Battista 1982; Jacobson, Beardslee, Hauser, et al. 1986b; Vaillant 1976; Vaillant and Drake 1985). In addition, Perry and Cooper (1986b, 1989) found that defenses measured at one point in time upheld the hierarchical relationship to global functioning measured over subsequent years. Table 1 displays these findings. Psychotic-level defenses demonstrated the largest negative correlation to global functioning (range, $-.66$ to $-.48$). Immature defenses followed with these median correlations: fantasy ($-.43$), hypochondriasis ($-.35$), neurotic denial or dissociation ($-.30$), projection ($-.29$), and acting out ($-.26$). In addition, Perry and Cooper found that borderline defenses (e.g., splitting) correlated negatively with future global functioning (range, $-.35$ to $-.13$).

Table 1. Relationship of Defenses to Global Mental Health or Ego Development

	Battista (1982)	Vaillant (1976)	Vaillant and Drake (1985)	Perry and Cooper (1986b)	Jacobsen, Beardslee, Hauser et al. (1986b)
Psychotic					
Distortion	−0.48				
Psychotic denial	−0.57				
Delusional projection	−0.66				
Immature					
Neurotic denial	−0.40	−0.24[a]	−0.41[a]	−0.15	−0.30
Fantasy	−0.60	−0.28	−0.57	−0.02	
Projection	−0.22	−0.41	−0.50	−0.29	−0.26
Passive aggression	−0.07	−0.19	−0.47	−0.40	0.11
Hypochondriasis	−0.04	−0.23	−0.53	−0.46	
Acting out	−0.22	−0.37	−0.26	−0.29	−0.26
Avoidance					−0.44
Borderline-narcissistic					
Splitting self				−0.27	
Splitting other				−0.35	
Bland denial				−0.14	
Manic denial				−0.29	
Projective identification				−0.13	
Primitive idealization				0.05	
Omnipotence				0.05	
Devaluation				−0.28	

Neurotic					
Asceticism	0.29	−0.14	0.06	0.38	−0.05
Intellectualization	0.04	0.04	0.04	0.11	0.34
Repression		−0.13		0.03	−0.30
Reaction formation		−0.16		−0.17	
Displacement	−0.16		0.12	−0.01	−0.19
Dissociation[a]				0.25	
Isolation					
Rationalization				0.20	
Undoing					
Mature					
Humor	0.26	0.04	0.33		
Sublimation	0.19	0.10	0.45		
Altruism	0.25	0.57	0.46		
Suppression	0.50	0.34	0.55		
Anticipation			0.40		

[a] Vaillant's definition of dissociation includes what others define as denial.

Source. Modified, with permission, from Perry JC, Cooper SH: Empirical studies of psychological defense mechanisms, in *Psychiatry.* Edited by Michels R, Cavenar JO. Philadelphia, PA, JB Lippincott, 1987, p. 12.

Narcissistic defenses (e.g., idealization, omnipotence) were generally uncorrelated with global functioning, except for devaluation ($-.28$).

The neurotic-level defenses (e.g., repression, reaction formation) by and large demonstrated few associations with global functioning. This paucity of associations is in part because neurotic-level defenses occur in a wider range of individuals than the other defenses. The one exception is the defense of intellectualization. The median correlation with mental health in Table 1 is .29. The lowest correlations were found in Vaillant's nonpatient samples (Vaillant 1976; Vaillant and Drake 1985), which suggests that this defense is associated with higher levels of functioning in patient samples, but less so in healthier samples.

The mature defenses consistently demonstrated positive correlations with mental health. The median correlations are as follows: suppression (.43), anticipation (.40), humor (.33), altruism (.29), and sublimation (.26). These defenses enable the individual to confront emotional problems and channel conflict into avenues that exert positive effects. In the spirit of what Haan (1963) referred to as coping mechanisms, they are the most adaptive of all the defenses.

The above findings are consistent with the idea that defenses have a hierarchical relationship to the individual's general level of functioning, with certain defenses usually more maladaptive and certain ones usually more adaptive. However, it does not indicate whether there are differential relationships between specific defenses and episodes of specific Axis I disorders.

DEFENSES AND RECURRENT DEPRESSION IN PERSONALITY AND AFFECTIVE DISORDERS

The author and colleagues have been examining the relationships among stress, defense, and symptomatic episodes in a longitudinal study of personality and affective disorders. This study is comprised of a sample of subjects with borderline personality disorder originally chosen to determine its validity in comparison to two near-neighbor disorders: antisocial personality, which shares impulse pathology, and bipolar type II affective disorder, which shares affective pathology. Subsequently, the sample has been enlarged to include a schizotypal personality comparison group, which is still being collected. The overall sample is useful to study because it demonstrated a high proportion of Axis I anxiety and affective disorders by history and on follow-up, in addition to the Axis II disorders of interest. Defenses can be examined in relationship to both comorbidity of Axis I and Axis II disorders. This section will summarize some relevant findings on defenses using cross-sectional and longitudinal follow-up data.

In this sample, defenses were originally rated on 73 subjects from videotapes of unstructured initial psychiatric interviews by dynamically oriented clinicians (Perry and Cooper 1986a, 1986b, 1989). Defenses were rated according to the Defense Mechanism Rating Scales (DMRS) manual by three baccalaureate-level research assistants who together formed consensus ratings. To simplify analyses of 22 defenses, and to take advantage of the improved reliability obtained by grouping related defenses into a longer-scales, most analyses used only five summary defense scales, defined in Table 2. The sample size varied depending on the analyses employed, because some measures were introduced late into the study, because some subjects were unavailable or dropped out at the time of a given procedure, or because some more recently added subjects had insufficient data for the follow-up analyses.

Defenses and Cross-Sectional Measures

Each of the five summary defense scales demonstrated modest associations with the three major study diagnoses (Perry and Cooper 1986a). As measured by the Borderline Personality Disorder Scale (Perry and Cooper 1986a), borderline psychopathology was significantly correlated with borderline defenses (.36) and with action defenses (.26). Antisocial personality disorder was significantly corre-

Table 2. The Summary Defense Scales and Their Constituent Defenses

Action defenses: Acting out, passive-aggression, and hypochondriasis were combined because each defense releases feelings and impulses through action, often toward others.

Borderline defenses: Splitting of self and others' images, and projective identification were combined because they distort self- and object images to conform with a particular meaning or emotional state. The distinction between borderline and narcissistic defenses was supported by factor analysis (Perry and Cooper 1986a).

Disavowal defenses: Projection, neurotic (minor) denial, bland denial, and rationalization were combined because they all disavow experiences, affects, or impulses.

Narcissistic defenses: Omnipotence, primitive idealization, devaluation, and mood incongruent denial (manic or depressive denial) were combined because each serves to regulate self-esteem and mood.

Obsessional defenses: Isolation, intellectualization, and undoing, which neutralize affects without distorting external reality, were combined.

Note. The low intercorrelation of repression and other conceptually related neurotic defenses in these data did not support construction of an hysterical summary defense scale.

lated with the narcissistic defenses (.23) and with the disavowal defenses (.22). The bipolar II diagnosis was significantly correlated only with *obsessional defenses* (.37). These findings suggest that there are some relationships between defenses and Axis II disorders, but otherwise they are moderately independent. Defenses are not simply a dynamic version of Axis II.

Next the correlations were calculated between the five summary defense scales and the following self-report measures relevant to anxiety and affective symptoms: the State-Trait Anxiety Inventory (STAI) (Spielberger, Gorsuch, and Lushene 1970), the Profile of Mood States (POMS) (McNair, Lorr, and Droppleman 1971), the Eysenck Personality Questionnaire (EPQ) (Eysenck 1970) and Impulsiveness Questionnaire (Eysenck and Eysenck 1977), the Depressive Experiences Questionnaire (DEQ) (Blatt, D'Afflitti, and Quinlan 1976), and the Interpersonal Dependency Inventory (IDI) (Hirschfeld, Klerman, Gough, et al. 1977). This battery tested the overall hypothesis that the above measures would correlate with the five summary defense scales in an order congruent with the overall hierarchy of defenses in Table 1. Although a large number of correlations were obtained, the hierarchical relationship of the defenses depends on the pattern of associations with anxiety, affective, and personality scales. We examined the pattern of correlations significant at the .10 level and below. The overall hypothesis was upheld.

The action defenses summary scale demonstrated the largest number of associations with 11 correlations in the predicted direction. These defenses correlated significantly ($p < .05$) positively with STAI anxiety (generally and now), POMS total mood disturbance, anger-hostility (POMS), depression-dejection (POMS), impulsiveness (Eysenck), and lack of social self-confidence (IDI), and negatively with vigor-activity (POMS) and efficacy (DEQ). These associations suggest the hypothesis that action defenses deal poorly with the distressing affects of anger, depression, and anxiety through impulsive expression instead of more adaptive self-assertion.

The borderline defense summary scale had six correlations in the predicted direction. The most significant correlations were with emotional reliance on another (IDI) and confusion-bewilderment (POMS), followed by anger-hostility, depression-dejection, and total mood disturbance (all POMS) and lack of social self-confidence (IDI). This suggests that borderline defenses are associated with intense attachment needs and attendant feelings of subjective confusion, anger, and depression and poor ability to deal with others. This fits well with Kernberg's (1975) hypothesis that the dynamic function of borderline defenses is to protect one from intolerable contradictory feelings toward close attachment figures.

The disavowal defense summary scale had three significant correlations, those with impulsiveness (Eysenck), psychoticism (EPQ), and anxiety-now (STAI). This suggests that defenses such as projection and denial are used by impulsive individuals with some tendency to experience anxiety and distorted perceptions.

Narcissistic defenses had two correlations in the predicted direction—extraversion (EPQ) and impulsiveness (Eysenck)—but did not correlate significantly with any affective or anxiety symptom scales. These defenses appear to relate to general personality characteristics, such as being outgoing or sociable and impulsive, but not in ways that hypothetically produce or ameliorate mood symptoms.

Finally, obsessional defenses correlated negatively with four scales from the POMS and positively with the efficacy scale of the DEQ. This is consistent with the hypothesis that these defenses minimize mood symptoms while allowing some degree of effective self-assertion.

All of the above associations were in the predicted direction. Their overall pattern suggested that action and borderline defenses would be most associated with anxiety and depressive phenomena while obsessional defenses would be associated with their absence. We then began examining whether follow-up data would support this.

Defenses and Longitudinal Symptom Levels (Phase I)

During the first several years of follow-up (phase I) of the original sample, subjects were reinterviewed on average every 4 months. Of the 73 subjects who had defenses rated at intake, 67 had two or more phase 1 follow-up interviews in which the POMS was readministered and the following observer-rated scales were obtained: the Hamilton Anxiety Rating Scale (HARS) (Hamilton 1959), the Hamilton Rating Scale for Depression (HRSD) (Hamilton 1960), and the Modified Manic Rating Scale (MMRS) (Blackburn, Loudon, and Ashworth 1977). Each subject's general level of symptoms over this 1- to 2-year follow-up period was summarized by taking the median score of each scale (Perry and Cooper 1989). Spearman correlations were calculated (shown in parentheses below); values above .24 were significant at the .05 level.

The action defense summary scale was associated with higher median levels of symptoms for the HRSD (.51), MMRS (.48), and HARS (.44). It also correlated with all six of the POMS scales and the POMS total mood score (.37). This pattern of findings suggests that the action defenses, while allowing subjects to bypass awareness of internal conflicts over wishes and feelings, did not protect subjects against anxiety and affective symptoms. The association with both self-report and observer-rated symptoms suggests that subjects using these defenses subsequently suffered high levels of symptoms.

The next highest pattern of correlations was between the borderline defenses and HRSD (.29), HARS (.26), and MMRS (.25). The magnitude of the correlations was even greater for all six scales of the POMS, including the POMS total mood score (.41). This pattern suggests that borderline defenses were associated with moderate levels of observer-rated anxiety and affective symptoms, but somewhat higher levels of self-report symptoms. Thus borderline defenses are associated with a greater magnitude of subjective suffering in relation to already high levels of objectively rated symptoms.

The disavowal defenses were modestly associated with HARS (.26) and HRSD (.25). However, there were no significant correlations with the self-report POMS scales. This pattern of findings validates the overall disavowal construct: disavowal (by projection, neurotic denial, bland denial, rationalization) protects subjects from awareness of their own distress, but does not hide anxiety and affective symptoms from objective inquiry.

The narcissistic defenses demonstrated no significant correlations with affective and anxiety symptom scales, as in the cross-sectional analyses.

The obsessional defenses demonstrated a negative association with HARS ($-.39$) and HRSD ($-.32$) symptom levels. In line with the minimization of affective experience denoted by obsessional defenses, all associations with the POMS scales and POMS total mood scale ($-.41$) were in the direction of fewer symptoms. These findings also reflect that the obsessional defenses were associated with healthier individuals (with less severe diagnoses) in this sample.

Defensive Adaptation to Life Events During Phase 2 Follow-Up and Depression Recurrence

Next we examined whether there was a relationship between defensive adaptation to life events and the recurrence of depressive episodes over the follow-up period, since defenses might play a mediating role in this relationship. In the second to third year of follow-up (phase 2 follow-up), we introduced a new structured follow-up instrument, the Longitudinal Interval Follow-up Evaluation-Adapted for the Study of Personality (LIFE-ASP). This is a modification of the LIFE devised by Keller and Shapiro for the National Institute of Mental Health (NIMH) Collaborative Study of Depression (Keller and Shapiro 1982b; Keller, Lavori, Friedman, et al. 1987). Among other features, the LIFE-ASP assesses week-by-week changes in the subject's severity and course of depression. These changes were charted on a weekly calendar in relation to significant life events that occurred for each subject. Follow-up interviews were generally conducted every 3 to 6 months, with a median interval between interviews of 4½ months.

Changes in depressive symptoms were recorded on a week-by-week basis, using a 6-point scale of severity tied to the DSM-III (American Psychiatric Association 1980) criteria. Because of the interest in the recurrence of major depression or the exacerbation of depressive symptoms falling short of a major episode, increases in levels of depression were recorded using three successively more rigorous thresholds. These definitions are hierarchically arranged, with the broader definitions encompassing the narrower ones.

> D_1 (all significant increases in depressive symptoms). Low-threshold depression was the broadest definition. It was recorded whenever the subject had *any increase* in depressive symptoms.
> D_2 (full nonacute onset major depression). Medium threshold depression was recorded if (1) subject had no or minimal symptoms followed by a gradual increase in symptoms, taking 5 weeks or longer to reach full criteria for major depression; or (2) subject was partially recovered from a major depressive episode, but an exacerbation back to full criteria level occurred.
> D_3 (full acute onset major depression). High-threshold depression was recorded when a subject had at least 4 weeks of minimal symptoms or no symptoms followed by developing a full DSM-III major depressive episode within 4 weeks.

For nonacute (D_2) and acute (D_3) major depressions, the onset was coded at the time of the prodromal increase in symptoms. The rate of relapse in an individual (i.e., numbers of exacerbations or recurrences during the follow-up period) was calculated for each individual for 52 weeks of follow-up. Of the 73 subjects, 45 had a year or more of phase 2 follow-up with at least one depression recurrence by any definition.

At each follow-up interview, research assistants conducted a structured inquiry about any significant life events that occurred over the interval. A pair of raters, blind to diagnostic information, then rated a narrative of each life event for the subject's defensive responses to the event (the life vignette method). The raters followed the same DMRS manual for 30 defenses, which included the 22 defenses previously rated from the videotapes and eight mature-level defenses. Raters were allowed to score up to five defenses for each event. For most analyses, related defenses were grouped together into summary defense scales to increase the power of analyses. The score for each summary defense scale was calculated as the proportion of all defensive responses in the life vignettes over the follow-up year attributable to the respective summary group of defenses. These scores then represent a quantitative estimate of a subject's defensive functioning in response to significant life events over the follow-up period.

We calculated the correlations between the summary defense scores and the three depression recurrence rates both measured from the same phase 2 follow-up data (Perry 1988). All 52 subjects with a full year of follow-up data from phase 2 were included. The action defenses were moderately correlated with higher recurrence rates of low-threshold depression (D_1: .31, $p < .05$) and nonacute major depression (D_2: .34, $p < .05$) but not acute major depression (D_3). The borderline defenses displayed the same finding (D_1: .30; D_2: .30; both $p < .05$). This suggests that action and borderline defenses, when used in coping with life events, are associated with increased vulnerability to exacerbations in depressive symptoms and to recurrence of nonacute major depressive episodes, but not acute major depressive episodes. The narcissistic defenses were not significantly correlated with lower annualized recurrence rates of acute major depression (D_3: $-.26$, $p < .10$). This would be consistent with the defenses of omnipotence, idealization, devaluation, and mood-incongruent denial exerting a mild protective effect against the recurrence of acute major depressive episodes.

Neither obsessional nor mature defenses were associated with lower rates of depression recurrence. However, the low prevalence of mature defenses in this sample in relation to the high prevalence of less mature defenses suggests caution in interpreting this lack of a finding. Such a relationship might be demonstrated in a healthier sample with less Axis II pathology. If found, such as association would suggest that mature defenses exert a protective effect against recurrent depression.

Defenses and the Maintenance of Affective and Anxiety Disorders

We have begun to explore whether defenses and Axis II psychopathology might be differentially associated with the *total duration* of anxiety and affective disorders over follow-up. Below is a summary of findings on preliminary analyses of the bivariate relationships between defenses measured at intake and the duration of episodes of anxiety and affective disorders. For this purpose, we calculated the proportion of phase 2 follow-up weeks for which each subject was in an episode of the following Axis I disorders: major depression, dysthymia (without excluding concurrent major depression), mania (including hypomania), obsessive-compulsive disorder, agoraphobia, and panic disorder. Generalized anxiety disorder was not included on the a priori grounds that ascertainment of changes in the course of generalized anxiety disorder in this highly symptomatic population would be methodologically difficult.

These analyses were conducted on 74 subjects, which is a larger sample due to the addition of some of the new schizotypal sample. The median number of weeks of follow-up was 120 (range, 12 to 227). There were 29 males and 45 females. The principal study diagnoses included 42 subjects with definite or borderline personality disorder or significant borderline traits, 20 with antisocial personality disorder, 19 with schizotypal personality, and 18 with bipolar type 2 without the above Axis II disorders.

Nonparametric correlations between defense summary scales and the proportion of time spent in an Axis I episode demonstrated the following significant associations (all correlations are $p < .05$ unless shown).

Major depressive episodes. The proportion of follow-up spent in all episodes was negatively associated with obsessional defenses $(-.33)$. Individuals with obsessional defenses at intake tended to spend less time depressed on follow-up.

Dysthymia. The proportion of weeks dysthymic was positively associated with action defenses $(.21, p = .07)$.

Hypomania and mania. The proportion of time spent in hypomanic episodes was negatively associated with action defenses $(-.19, p = .10)$ as were manic episodes $(-.25)$. In addition, hypomania was associated with obsessional defenses $(.25)$. This may partly reflect the association between the bipolar II diagnosis and obsessional defenses.

Obsessive-compulsive disorder. The proportion of time spent with obsessive-compulsive disorder demonstrated no significant associations to defenses. However, this was the least prevalent of all the Axis I disorders.

Agoraphobia. The proportion of time spent with agoraphobia was associated with borderline defenses $(.27)$ and action defenses $(.21, p = .07)$ and negatively with obsessional defenses $(-.27)$.

Panic disorder. The proportion of follow-up weeks spent with panic disorder was associated with borderline defenses $(.30)$ and negatively with obsessional defenses $(-.27)$.

We are currently examining the relative contributions of defenses and Axis II psychopathology in predicting Axis I disorders on follow-up. Preliminary results suggest that both domains share some variance but that each domain also makes unique contributions in predicting Axis I follow-up variables.

Summary of Findings

The above findings are remarkably consistent with the empirically validated hierarchy of defenses shown in Table 1. In this largely personality-disordered sample, there is highly consistent evidence for a hierarchical relationship between the general maladaptiveness of a defense and important aspects of anxiety and affective disorders. This includes the prevalence of anxiety and affective symptoms, the recurrence rates of depressive symptoms, and overall time spent in symptomatic episodes of anxiety and affective disorders over follow-up.

The groups of defenses that are most strongly associated with anxiety and affective pathology are, in descending order, action, borderline, and disavowal defenses. The obsessional defenses were most associated with the *absence* of anxiety and affective pathology. Narcissistic defenses had the fewest associations with anxiety and affective pathology. This study did not adequately test the associations of the mature defenses because, first, they were not rated at intake, and, second, the high degree of personality pathology in the sample biased the study toward a low prevalence of mature defenses on follow-up.

FURTHER DIRECTIONS: HOW THE STUDY OF DEFENSES CAN CONTRIBUTE TO UNDERSTANDING ANXIETY AND AFFECTIVE DISORDERS

Most research to date has focused on the relationship between defenses measured at one point in time and some global characteristic of the subject, such as diagnosis or general level of functioning. While useful, such studies cannot inform about the immediate effect of defenses in the onset, maintenance, and recovery of affective and anxiety disorders. Future work could explore this in a number of ways. This chapter closes with specific suggestions for further exploration.

First, findings such as those reported in this chapter need to be replicated on both highly symptomatic and less symptomatic samples. For instance, there is a need to replicate in somewhat healthier samples whether obsessional and/or mature defenses (1) exert protective effects against recurrent depression, and (2) promote quicker recovery from any depressive episodes, and therefore (3) lead to less overall time spent in depressive episodes.

Second, the temporal relationships among stressors, the individual's defensive adaptation to the stressors, and the recurrence of symptomatic disorders need to be studied. Do defenses play a crucial role only at critical times in response to specific stressors, or do they exert their effects more by their characteristic day-to-day use? To obtain stable estimates of the mediating role of defenses will require strategies such as following a large number of subjects through multiple episodes of the affective and anxiety disorders in question.

Third, related to the above question is whether there are specific relationships among stressor, defensive adaptation and subsequent type of anxiety or affective disorder. An example is the hypothesis proposed by Freud (1917/1963) that the loss of an ambivalently held love object followed by the defensive response of turning anger inward (e.g., passive-aggression) may lead to clinical depression (melancholia). Testing hypotheses like this would require both intensive and extensive prospective follow-up studies.

Fourth, is there a relationship between characteristic defenses and whether a subject has one, or more than one, anxiety and/or affective disorder? It appears that some Axis II disorders, such as borderline personality disorder, are associated with multiple disorders on Axis I, as if the personality disorder is evidence of an underlying poly-vulnerability. It is likely that one's characteristic level of defensive adaptation bears a similar relationship to multiple Axis I disorders. Knowing this would help clinicians evaluate the probability that a patient will need multiple interventions over follow-up.

Fifth, how does the presence of an anxiety or affective disorder episode affect which defenses an individual will use, given his or her usually available repertoire? This is the state-trait issue. Studies have shown that depression affects personality variables such as neuroticism, and clinical observation suggests that the presence of depression also affects defensive functioning. Alternately, some defenses might be more likely to occur under certain affective and anxiety states (e.g., acting out, hypochondriasis), while others might be more stable despite changes in affective states (e.g., intellectualization).

Finally, some interventions can be devised to help improve defensive functioning as it affects the onset, course, and recurrence of anxiety and affective disorders. This is a very inclusive area for scientific exploration. However, it may be that existing psychological therapies exert their effects by increasing the adequacy of defensive functioning, which in turn limits the duration of symptomatic episodes or prevents future recurrences. Even if biologic vulnerability remains the same, an improvement in defensive adaptation might protect the individual from further symptomatic relapses. It may be that intervening to improve defensive functioning might not be as important for current episodes as it is for the prevention or mitigation of future episodes. Therefore, further study of defenses, response to treatment, and the problem of relapse are warranted.

Chapter 31

A Neuropsychological Perspective on Comorbid Disorders

Sheri A. Berenbaum, Ph.D.
Kimberly Kerns, B.A.
Michael A. Taylor, M.D.

PSYCHOPATHOLOGIC SYNDROMES OFTEN travel in pairs. For example, there is an association between sociopathy and Briquet's syndrome (Arkonac and Guze 1963; Cloninger and Guze 1973), affective disorder and alcoholism (Helzer and Winokur 1974; Schlesser, Winokur, and Sherman 1979), obsessive-compulsive disorder (OCD) and Tourette's syndrome (Comings and Comings 1985, 1987; Pauls, Towbin, Leckman, et al. 1986), and anxiety and affective disorders (this volume). As the chapters in this volume suggest, efforts to understand the comorbidity of anxiety disorders and depression raise important conceptual and methodological issues, including problems in diagnosis and classification, differentiation of states and traits, and variability in sampling and measurement procedures.

The use of neuropsychological constructs and techniques has proven important for understanding brain processes underlying behavior. This approach also has advantages for studying the comorbidity of anxiety disorder and depression. In this chapter, we will assess the current literature in this area and suggest strategies for future work.

One advantage of a neuropsychological approach to comorbidity is that measures can be chosen for their sensitivity to specific types of brain dysfunction; performance can be potentially informative about the neural substrate of the disorders. Second, inferences about neural involvement can suggest commonalities or differences between anxiety disorders and depression, and whether these are state- or trait-related. Third, analysis of performance on neuropsychological measures can be valuable in understanding the pathophysiology of psychopathology.

Neuropsychological studies of psychopathology rely on a variety of methods: examination of patient performance on standard neuropsychological tests; studies of perceptual asymmetries (e.g., dichotic listening), from which inferences are made about lateralization of function; electroencephalographic (EEG) recording under no stimulation or in response to stimuli that elicit characteristic EEG changes (evoked potentials or topographic EEG); and imaging studies of structural brain abnormalities (computed tomography or magnetic resonance imaging) or metabolism (regional cerebral blood flow or positron emission tomography [PET] studies of glucose use or oxygen metabolism). Sometimes data from these studies are related to clinical variables. Unfortunately, there are few studies that measure the same subjects with more than one procedure, or that measure metabolism while subjects are performing cognitive tasks. Although a few imaging studies compare anxiety disorder patients to those with affective illness, we could find no reports directly comparing these patient groups using other neuropsychological procedures. Inferences about similarities and differences between anxiety disorder and depression must derive from investigations that separately assess the two patient groups, rather than by evaluating studies that themselves make this comparison.

The typical approaches to investigating the neural substrates of anxiety disorder and depression have not been very informative, because of conceptual and methodological problems. Part of the difficulty derives from the confusion associated with neuropsychological theories of affect and psychopathology. Much of the early work on the neural basis of psychopathology attributed both normal and abnormal affect to lateralized functions of the cerebral hemispheres (e.g., Flor-Henry and Gruzelier 1983; Gur 1978). These notions about psychopathology were later fit into broader theories about the neural basis of emotion, with much of this work originating from observations of mood changes following brain trauma and stroke and from epilepsy. The result has been that some investigators have argued that the right hemisphere plays a major role in all aspects of emotional perception and expression (Levy 1983; Ley and Bryden 1982), whereas others have argued for differential hemispheric specialization by the valence of the emotion, with the right hemisphere usually associated with the perception and expression of negative emotions and the left with positive emotions (Davidson and Fox 1982; Sackheim, Greenburg, Weinman, et al. 1982). Some theorists argue for the reverse lateralization by emotional valence (Tucker and Williamson 1984). It is difficult to differentiate competing hypotheses because of speculations about inhibitory neural influences. Thus depression following left hemisphere stroke has been explained either by hypothesizing that the substrate for negative affect in the left hemisphere has been disinhibited, leading to an exaggeration in emotional tone of the damaged hemisphere (Tucker and Williamson 1984), or that the substrate for positive affect in the left hemisphere has been damaged, leading to the disinhibition of the intact right hemisphere center for negative emotion (the pathology reflecting the emotion of the undamaged side) (Davidson and Fox 1982; Sackheim, Greenburg, Weinman, et al. 1982).

Of importance for the issue of comorbidity, Tucker and Williamson (1984) differentiated among types of negative affect, suggesting that anxiety is associated with left hemisphere overactivation, and depression with right hemisphere underactivation. Euphoria, according to Tucker and Williamson, would be associated with right hemisphere overactivation. Thus some neuropsychological studies of patients with anxiety disorder have looked for evidence of intrinsic left hemisphere overactivation and/or dysfunction, whereas some studies of depressed patients have searched for intrinsic right hemisphere underactivation and/or dysfunction, and other studies have assessed disinhibition by the contralateral hemisphere.

More recent conceptualizations of the neural substrate of mood disorders have reintroduced the role of the fronto-limbic system in regulating emotional expression and experience (Gray 1982; Kolb and Taylor 1981). These concepts are supported by studies in rodents, which indicate that the limbic system and frontal connections play a part in emotion regulation (e.g., Isaacson 1982) and have recently been incorporated into neuropsychological studies of psychopathology. Damage to frontal and limbic areas have been implicated in OCD, panic disorder, affective disorders, and schizophrenia, and a variety of studies have specifically examined metabolism or behavioral indices of frontal lobe function. Unfortunately for our purposes, except for Gray's work, there have been few attempts to differentiate parts of the system for special roles in the expression of anxiety or depression.

In addition to problems raised by theoretical confusion, neuropsychological studies of anxiety and affective disorders suffer from methodological difficulties. For example, overlapping symptoms (e.g., anxiety in depressed patients) make it impossible to determine if neuropsychological similarities reflect a common neural substrate to the disorders, or to common symptoms. Because patients are rarely studied when asymptomatic, it is unclear whether we are observing neural correlates of the psychopathological state or of the trait, the latter a potential biologic marker. Diagnostic criteria vary widely across studies, and rarely are patient subgroups differentiated (e.g., melancholia versus dysthymia, unipolar versus bipolar depressed). Further, procedures for the same measure vary widely across studies, making it difficult to determine reasons for nonreplications; dependent measures are often chosen without reference to specific hypotheses about the etiology of the dysfunction or its role in depression or anxiety disorder. In addition, samples are generally small and many analyses are conducted, increasing the probabilities of both Type I and Type II error. Finally, multiple papers from a given laboratory often report data from some of the same subjects, thus making it difficult to determine true replications.

The problems with neuropsychological studies investigating anxiety disorder and depression are not merely ones of detail and refinement of constructs, measures, and methods, but also of conceptual approach—that is, adherence to the assumption that all things that look alike are alike, whether it is a syndrome (e.g., depression) or neuropsychological test performance (e.g., attention deficit). Several alternative approaches, however, might prove informative about the neural substrate of psychopathology in general, and of the comorbidity of anxiety and depression in particular. The first approach involves investigation of neural correlates of clinical features or symptoms rather than syndromes. The second approach concerns the reconceptualization of certain anxiety and depressive states as variants of personality. The last approach involves detailed specification of the behavioral or neural processes impaired in the two disorders. We will address these issues as we evaluate relevant studies, and return to them when we consider what types of studies would be informative in assessing the comorbidity of anxiety disorders and depression.

REVIEW OF THE LITERATURE

Neuropsychological Tests in Anxiety Disorders and Depression

In general, the interpretation of neuropsychological studies of psychiatric patients relies on information obtained from patients with circumscribed brain damage: poor performance implicates the damaged area in normal processing of that ability. Although the inferences from brain-damaged patients about neural representation are generally sound (as indicated by replicability and congruence with data from other sources), extrapolation to psychiatric patients is limited by the fact that these patients have a variety of problems (e.g., attentional difficulties, perceptual aberrations) that interfere with performance and limit inferences about neural substrate. In addition, studies on psychiatric patients generally rely on batteries of tasks developed for clinical purposes, or on an array of tasks developed to assess cognitive impairment in many brain regions and systems. A typical study includes measures of general intelligence, the Halstead-Reitan battery (which is sensitive to the presence of brain damage, but is not suitable for localization), and tests of fluency, motor function, simple language comprehension, and some aspects of memory. Specific assessment of hypothesized neural dysfunction in a syndrome (e.g., depression) is rarely conducted. Nevertheless, despite these problems, certain patterns of intact performance and impairment emerge in neuropsychological studies of patients with anxiety and depressive disorders. These findings are summarized in Table 1.

Many neuropsychological studies implicate the right hemisphere in depression, with depressed patients doing poorly on tests that are sensitive to right hemisphere damage, such as visuospatial abilities and attention. For example, Kronfol, Hamsher, Digre, et al. (1978) studied neuropsychological test performance in 18 depressed patients before and after electroconvulsive therapy (ECT). They concluded that right hemisphere functions were more frequently abnormal than left hemisphere functions in pre-ECT testing, and that ECT improved right hemisphere functions when the depression was ameliorated. This study is frequently cited to support the role of the right hemisphere in depression. It is important to note, however, that only one (of eight) of the increases in right hemisphere performance was significant; normative data were not reported, so there is no way to assess the abnormality of right hemispheric functions pre-ECT; and correlations between cognitive improvement and clinical improvement of depression were not reported. Nevertheless, similar impairment patterns in depressed patients have been reported by others (Abrams and Taylor 1987; Fromm-Auch 1983; Taylor and Abrams 1987; Taylor, Redfield, and Abrams 1981).

These studies are limited, however, in conclusions about the right hemisphere as the "neural locus" of depression. Many studies use tests extracted from a larger battery, and individual tests often do not have "lateralizing" or "localizing" value. Further, although right hemisphere damage affects performance on these tests, poor performance is not pathognomonic for right hemisphere damage. For example, there are some abilities (e.g., motor speed and concentration) that are more important for performance on "right hemisphere" tests than for "left hemisphere" tests. These other abilities are also impaired in depressed patients, but not lateralized to the right hemisphere, sug-

Table 1. Summary of Neuropsychological Findings in Affective and Anxiety Disorders

Method	Affective disorders	Anxiety disorders
Neuropsychological assessment	↓ performance on right hemisphere tests ↓ performance on attention and frontal lobe tests	↓ performance on right and left hemisphere tests (OCD) ↓ performance on attention and frontal lobe tests (OCD)
Perceptual asymmetries	right hemisphere dysfunction (↓ left ear advantage for nonspeech sounds)	left hemisphere overactivation (anxious normals) (right ear bias, ↓ right visual field scores)
Electroencephalography		
Visual inspection	frontal abnormalities right hemisphere abnormalities	fronto-temporal and temporal abnormalities (OCD)
Power spectral analysis	fronto-temporal deviations bilaterally parieto-occipital deviations R>L	↓ α and δ activity in temporal lobe (GAD)

Evoked potentials	↓ amplitude P300	brain-stem evoked potentials abnormal L>R (panic disorder) ↓ latencies, amplitudes N200, P300 (OCD) further ↓ latencies to complex stimuli ↑ N60 amplitudes
Blood flow		
Xenon inhalation	↑ and ↓ frontal flow right (primary motor cortex) dysfunction	
Position emission tomography		
Oxygen metabolism	↓ and ↑frontal metabolism	↑ right parahippocampal blood flow and ↑ whole brain metabolism (panic disorder)
Glucose metabolism	↓ and ↑frontal metabolism ↓ and ↑overall metabolism ↑ caudate and basil ganglia metabolism	↑ cerebral hemispheres, caudate, orbital gyri metabolism (OCD)

Note. OCD: obsessive-compulsive disorder; GAD: generalized anxiety disorder; PD: panic disorder.

gesting that the dysfunction in depressed patients is not solely in the right hemisphere.

Further evidence that depression is not just a "right hemisphere disease" comes from studies assessing frontal lobe function. For example, Taylor and Abrams (1987) reported that a large sample of melancholic patients performed poorly on tests that assess both bilateral frontal lobe function and right hemisphere function. These results are consistent with the hypofrontality found in depressed patients in brain metabolism studies.

One factor complicating interpretation of neuropsychological performance in depressed patients is the fact that performance on many tests improves (sometimes to normal levels) with clinical improvement of mood (Abrams and Taylor 1985; Brumbach, Staton, and Wilson 1980; Kronfol, Hamsher, Digre, et al. 1978; Savard, Rey, and Post 1980), suggesting that performance impairments are not trait-related but are concomitants of the depressed state. In addition, although biologic and clinical variables have been shown to differentiate subgroups of depressed patients (e.g., melancholic versus nonmelancholic patients), these subgroups exhibit similar patterns of impairment on standard neuropsychological tests (Fromm-Auch 1983), again suggesting that performance is state-related. Finally, other patient groups (e.g., schizophrenic patients) (Berman, Zec, and Weinberger 1986; Taylor and Abrams 1984, 1987) demonstrate patterns of impairment similar to those of depressed patients (poor performance on right hemisphere and frontal lobe tests), indicating that the impairment pattern in depressed patients is nonspecific and may reflect a general disruption of frontal and right hemisphere functions observed in any severe condition associated with brain damage.

Although there are many hypotheses about the neural substrate of anxiety (e.g., Gray 1982), most studies assess neurotransmitter function (Klein, Rabkin, and Gorman 1985; Redmond 1985; Stokes 1985), and few studies make use of neuropsychological methods. We could find no neuropsychological studies of generalized anxiety disorder, although there are many studies that examine "anxiety" in relation to cognitive performance in normal subjects (Eysenck 1982, 1985). These studies support the well-known Yerkes-Dodson law (Yerkes and Dodson 1908) that maximal performance is associated with intermediate levels of anxiety, while high anxiety impairs performance and low anxiety fails to enhance performance (e.g., Beck 1978; Courts 1939; Eysenck 1982, 1985). Recent findings by Gur and colleagues (Gur, Gur, Resnick, et al. 1987; Gur, Gur, Skolnick, et al. 1988) suggest a correlate to these performance differences in cerebral metabolic activity. Although these studies are interesting, they do not address the neural substrate of anxiety disorders, the relationship between normal and pathologic anxiety, or commonalities between the neural substrate for anxiety disorders and normal anxiety.

In contrast to the lack of studies on traditional anxiety disorders, there are several studies assessing neuropsychological test performance in patients with OCD. Although OCD is now included among the anxiety disorders, the validity of this classification is unknown. It is unclear whether OCD is genetically related to other anxiety disorders, although it does appear related to Tourette's syndrome (Comings and Comings 1985, 1987). Therefore, OCD may not be an appropriate model for understanding the more traditional anxiety disorders. Nevertheless, we include neuropsychological studies of OCD patients because of their possible relevance for assessing the relationship between OCD and other forms of anxiety disorder, as well as the comorbidity of OCD and depression.

The few studies that have examined neuropsychological test performance in OCD and panic patients have been used to support either left or right hemisphere dysfunction. Yeudall and colleagues (Flor-Henry, Yeudall, Koles, et al. 1979; Yeudall, Schopflocher, Sussman, et al. 1983) have found both OCD and panic patients to be impaired (relative to normals) on some tests from a large neuropsychological battery. Although these investigators interpreted their findings to implicate left hemisphere dysfunction in both patient groups, impairments were also found on tests they considered to measure right hemisphere function (e.g., nonverbal learning, rhythm). Further, findings of normal verbal and performance intelligence quotients in OCD and panic patients argue against a left hemisphere deficit (Behar, Rapoport, Berg, et al. 1984; Flor-Henry, Yeudall, Koles, et al. 1979; Insel, Donnelly, Lalakea, et al. 1983; Rapoport, Elkins, Langer, et al. 1981; Yeudall, Schopflocher, Sussman, et al. 1983). In addition, other studies have found OCD patients to do poorly on spatial (presumably right hemisphere or frontal lobe) tests (e.g., stylus maze learning, Money Road Map Test) (Behar, Rapoport, Berg, et al. 1984; Insel, Donnelly, Lalakea, et al. 1983). If anything, these data would implicate attentional disturbance or frontal lobe problems. Interpretation of these studies is confounded, however, by concurrent diagnoses of depression in the OCD patients studied, and the fact that some symptoms (e.g., fear of contamination from handling stimulus materials) may differentially affect spatial tests.

In summary, studies using neuropsychological tests reveal patients with either anxiety or depressive disorder to have some impairment. Although the results are not uniform, there is evidence of differing lateralization for anxiety disorders versus depression. Depression appears to be associated with right posterior and bilateral frontal dysfunction. OCD and panic disorder may be associated with either left or right hemisphere dysfunction, but specific assessment of attention and frontal lobe function has not been made in either disorder. There is a need for neuropsychological studies of other anxiety disorders that are likely to be comorbid with depression.

Perceptual Asymmetry Studies

Dichotic listening studies, in which competing sounds (speech or nonspeech) are simultaneously presented to both ears, support findings from studies using neuropsychological tests, in implicating the right hemisphere in depression. Most normal subjects show a right ear (i.e., a left hemisphere) advantage for speech sounds and a left ear (i.e., a right hemisphere) advantage for nonspeech sounds. Depressed patients exhibit a partial reversal or attenuation of the normal right hemisphere asymmetry for nonspeech sounds, while maintaining a normal left hemisphere advantage for language (Bruder, Sutton, and Berger-Gross 1981; Johnson and Crockett 1982; Yozawitz, Bruder, Sutton, et al. 1979). Several investigators have found this atypical asymmetry to relate inversely to severity of depressive symptomatology and to normalize with symptom remission (Johnson and Crockett 1982; Moscovitch, Strauss, and Olds 1981; Yozawitz, Bruder, Sutton, et al. 1979). Berger-Gross, Bruder, Quitkin, et al. (1985) observed the altered asymmetry to vary diurnally in association with the patient's perception of mood changes, in a pattern suggestive of altered right hemisphere activation, as Levy (1983) would suggest. These results implicate right hemisphere dysfunction in depression, but they are difficult to interpret because some studies did not use control groups; reduced or reversed asymmetries have also been reported in other neuropsychiatric disorders, including schizophrenia (Wexler and Heninger 1979), dyslexia (Bakker 1983; Bakker and Vinke 1985), and autism (Dawson, Finley, Phillips, et al. 1986) and factors other than lateralization (e.g., attention deployment) can affect asymmetries (Bryden 1982).

In one study of perceptual asymmetries in anxiety disorder, Behar, Rapoport, Berg, et al. (1984) found no significant differences between OCD and control children on dihaptic tasks (simultaneous presentation of shapes and letters that are also thought to index right- and left-hemisphere specialization, respectively). Although perceptual asymmetry has not been otherwise studied in patients with anxiety disorders, studies of normal subjects suggest that high trait and state anxiety are associated with left-hemisphere overactivation (right ear attentional bias and poor right visual field accuracy) (Tucker, Antes, Stenslie, et al. 1978). It is unclear, however, how normal variability in anxiety relates to anxiety disorders.

In sum, studies of perceptual asymmetries provide weak support for differential involvement of the left and right hemispheres in anxiety and depression, respectively. Although problems hinder interpretation of these studies, results are consistent with data derived from others methods (see Table 1).

Electrophysiologic Studies

EEG and evoked potential studies examine whether neural correlates of information processing are abnormal in psychiatric patients. Studies include visual inspection of clinical EEG tracings, power-spectral analyses, topographic EEG power-spectral analyses, and evoked response examinations (see Table 1). The last three procedures assess patients at rest and during the performance of a cognitive task. In general, these studies share several shortcomings: there is no control over the subject's cognitive activity during resting states, methodological decisions (e.g., montages, reference electrodes, and frequencies assessed) are often arbitrary and made without reference to concepts about the pathophysiology underlying the disorder being studied; and procedures for removing movement artifacts are highly variable. In studies of depression, the implications of subclassifications (unipolar and bipolar, reactive and endogenous) on EEG patterns are often ignored.

Despite these shortcomings, there appears to be a consistent association between deviant EEG activity and depression. These results are consistent with neuropsychological test data implicating the frontal lobes and right hemisphere. For example, there is an increased prevalence of nonspecific EEG abnormalities in depressed patients compared to controls (Abrams and Taylor 1979; Wegner, Struve, Kantor, et al. 1979); depressed and manic patients have similar EEG abnormalities, with differences between these groups being related to clinical severity (Abrams and Taylor 1979); and the prevalence of these abnormalities in depressed and manic patients is clearly lower than that observed in schizophrenic patients (Abrams and Taylor 1979).

It is difficult to find a specific pattern of EEG abnormality in patients with affective disorder, but several studies are suggestive. Visual inspection studies (Abrams and Taylor 1979; Abrams, Volavka, Roubicek, et al. 1970) indicate that abnormalities in melancholic patients are often diffuse, rarely circumscribed, and often frontal in location; asymmetrical patterns reveal greater abnormality in the right than in the left hemisphere. The majority of depressed patients, however, have clinically normal EEGs by this method of analysis.

Power-spectral studies (d'Elia and Perris 1973; Knot and Lapierre 1987; Monakhov, Perris, Botskarev, et al. 1979; Volavka, Abrams,

Taylor, et al. 1981) and power-spectral topographic studies (Pock-berger, Petsche, Rappelsberger, et al. 1985) also reveal consistent differences between depressed patients and normal controls, with depressed patients exhibiting fronto-temporal deviations bilaterally and parieto-occipital deviations greater on the right than on the left. There have, however, been similar findings in some schizophrenic patients (Flor-Henry and Koles 1984). Interestingly, Nystrom, Matou-sek, and Hallstrom (1986) linked EEG asymmetry to anxiety symptoms rather than to the depressive syndrome itself. Other studies apparently have not examined associations between EEG abnormalities and specific symptoms.

Evoked potential studies are less clear regarding asymmetry or other abnormalities (Blackwood, Whalley, Christie, et al. 1987; Buchsbaum, Landau, Murphy, et al. 1973; Diner, Holcomb, and Dykman 1985; Lolas and de la Para 1979; Pfefferbaum, Wenegrat, Ford, et al. 1984). These studies do indicate, however, that depressed patients have decreased P300 amplitudes but normal latencies,[1] suggesting no basic pathology in information processing, but rather disinterest in the task. Normalization of evoked response amplitude following clinical improvement supports this view (Blackwood, Whalley, Christie, et al. 1987).

EEG studies of patients with OCD have consistently found evidence for nonspecific abnormalities in the temporal and fronto-temporal areas, but not all patients display abnormalities (Flor-Henry, Yeudall, Koles, et al. 1979; Insel, Donnelly, Lalakea, et al. 1983; Jenike and Brotman 1984). Of the four studies that used visually inspected EEG in OCD patients, three reported no higher prevalence of abnormalities than would be expected in the general population, whereas the fourth reported 5 of 12 patients to exhibit fronto-temporal abnor-

---

[1]Evoked potentials are elicited in response to sensory stimulation. The different waveforms (labeled by the time since stimulus presentation) are thought to represent different levels of information processing. An early waveform, the N60, represents the registration of basic sensory stimulation and is seen with all forms of stimulation (auditory, visual, and somatosensory). The later waveforms, N200 and P300, tend to be elicited together and are considered to comprise the P3 complex, which is related to the identification and classification of relevant stimuli (Hillyard and Picton 1979). The P3 complex is influenced by a variety of emotional, motivational, and attentional factors. The amplitude of the P300 has been related to the meaningfulness of the stimulus for the subject. This includes the probability of occurrence of a stimulus and the task relevance of that stimulus (Campbell, Courchesne, Picton, et al. 1979; Johnson and Donchin 1982; Pritchard 1981); the subjective versus actual probability of stimulus occurrence (Squires, Wickens, Squires, et al. 1976); and the subject's confidence in the accuracy of his or her response (Horst, Johnson, and Donchin 1980). P300 latency appears to be determined by the time it takes the subject to recognize or classify the stimulus. The latency can be increased by degrading the stimulus, making the target more difficult to discriminate (McCarthy and Donchin 1981; Sternberg 1975).

malities. How these patients were selected for study is unclear. The one computer-analyzed EEG study of OCD (Flor-Henry, Yeudall, Koles, et al. 1979) reported patients to show reduced variability in the left temporal area and reduced variability in the right parietal area compared with a non-OCD group. The biologic implications of this are uncertain.

Among panic patients, there is no consistent evidence for EEG abnormalities. Of the three studies we could find where visually inspected clinical tracings were examined, two (Lesser, Poland, Holcomb, et al. 1985; Uhde, Roy-Byrne, Gillin, et al. 1984) reported no EEG abnormalities in patients with panic attacks, whereas the third (Edlund, Swann, and Clothier 1987) mentioned eight patients with normal EEGs and reported the cases of six others, five of whom had abnormal EEGs. In each of those five patients, however, there was evidence of seizure disorder or brain insult prior to the onset of the panic attacks. The one study examining EEG by power-spectral analysis in generalized anxiety disorder reported a decrease in slow wave and alpha activity primarily in the temporal leads (Buchsbaum, Hazlett, Sicotte, et al. 1985). Alpha activity increased frontally with successful drug treatment.

Studies of evoked potentials in patients with anxiety disorder offer little to help understand the pathophysiology of the disorder. In one study of panic disorder, brain-stem evoked potentials were reported to be more aberrant on the left than on the right (Yeudall, Schopflocher, Sussman, et al. 1983). OCD patients were reported to show abnormalities in visual and somatosensory evoked potentials, characterized by decreased latencies and amplitudes of peaks between N200 and P300, which became more deviant as the task or stimuli became more complex. In effect, OCD patients showed decreased latency to complex stimuli, whereas normal controls showed increased latency (Beech, Ciesielski, and Gordon 1983; Ciesielski, Beech, and Gordon 1981). These studies suggest that OCD patients are hyperalert, processing information too rapidly. It is unclear whether hyperalertness affects accuracy. Other studies have noted higher amplitudes in the N60 component of the evoked potential, and related this to cortical hyperexcitability (Shagass, Roemer, Straumanis, et al. 1984). Although asymmetries are rare, when they do occur, they tend to suggest left hemisphere dysfunction.

In summary, the electrophysiologic studies indicate that most patients with anxiety and depression have normal EEGs and evoked potentials. Abnormalities, when found, tend to concur with data from neuropsychological studies: right hemisphere and frontal abnormalities in depressed patients and weak evidence for left hemisphere and frontal abnormalities in patients with anxiety disorder (see Table 1).

The most interesting information is likely to come from further studies of evoked potentials, where electrical activity can be related to information-processing characteristics. These studies should include subjects with different types of anxiety and depression, and differentiate state changes from traits.

Brain Metabolism Studies

Metabolic studies (summarized in Table 1) assess the nature and extent of brain metabolic abnormalities and ask how these abnormalities are related to clinical symptomatology. Differences across studies can be attributed to differences in labeled radioactive substance (glucose or oxygen), task condition, baseline comparisons, comparison groups, or methods of assessing group differences in metabolism (e.g., absolute metabolism or relative metabolism).

Blood flow. Some reports using xenon inhalation to measure blood flow suggest that depressed patients have increased blood flow to frontal regions (Chabrol, Barrere, Guell, et al. 1986; Uytdenhoef, Portelange, Jacquy, et al. 1983), particularly when in the depressed state (Chabrol, Barrere, Guell, et al. 1986). Other studies report decreased frontal flow (Mathew, Meyer, Francis, et al. 1980). Conflicting findings may reflect differences in subject's cognitive activity during resting states and in clinical presentation (e.g., agitation or stupor). These problems are similar to those encountered with EEG studies. In the one study comparing patients to controls on task-activated blood flow (Guenther, Moser, Mueller-Spahn, et al. 1986), depressed patients showed abnormal activation during a simple motor response (squeezing a handle). In normal controls, blood flow was increased in the contralateral primary motor area, whereas depressed patients showed increased flow only in left primary motor cortex, suggesting right frontal lobe dysfunction.

PET studies. Interpretation of PET studies is complicated by difficulty in defining the best measure of metabolism: analyses include both absolute levels of metabolism and scores adjusted in various ways for whole brain or hemisphere activity. Studies typically compare small numbers of subjects in each group on a large number of measures. Occasionally, metabolism is related to treatment or clinical variables.

In two studies using overlapping samples, Buchsbaum and colleagues reported that bipolar patients (apparently in a depressed state) showed a relative decrease in frontal lobe metabolism compared to normals. It is unclear whether this result was due to increased posterior activity (Buchsbaum, DeLisi, Holcomb, et al. 1984) or decreased anterior activity (Buchsbaum, Wu, DeLisi, et al. 1986). Bipolar patients also showed higher metabolism in whole image slices than normals. Hypofrontality has also been observed in schizophrenic patients (Buchsbaum, DeLisi, Holcomb, et al. 1984; but see Gur, Resnick, Alavi, et al. 1987) and thus appears not to be specific to affective illness. Buchsbaum, Wu, DeLisi, et al. (1986) also found *hyper*frontality in a very small sample of 4 unipolar depressed patients. In subcortical regions, however, both unipolar and bipolar patients showed relative hypometabolism in caudate and basal ganglia.

Baxter, Phelps, Mazziotta, et al. (1985) also examined brain metabolism in unipolar and bipolar patients and found no abnormalities in fronto-occipital ratio. Their results do indicate, however, abnormalities in whole brain and regional metabolism, but the pattern is opposite to that reported by Buchsbaum, Wu, DeLisi, et al. (1986): bipolar depressed patients had lower metabolism than normal controls, who were lower than unipolar depressed patients, although only some comparisons were significant. They also found relative hypometabolism in the caudate in unipolar, but not in bipolar patients. In five unipolar patients who were rescanned when euthymic after drug treatment, the relative metabolism of the caudate increased nonsignificantly. Given the sample size, it is not surprising that significant effects were not obtained.

There are two studies assessing brain metabolism in anxiety: a study of oxygen metabolism in panic patients (Reiman, Raichle, Butler, et al. 1984; Reiman, Raichle, Robins, et al. 1986), and one of glucose utilization on OCD patients (Baxter, Phelps, Mazziotta, et al. 1987). Reiman and colleagues found a decreased left-right asymmetry of parahippocampal blood flow in eight panic patients vulnerable to lactate-induced panic compared to eight panic patients not vulnerable to lactate infusion and to 25 normal controls. They suggested that the abnormal asymmetry was due to increased flow to the right parahippocampus, rather than decreased left flow. Compared to normal controls and nonlactate-sensitive patients, the lactate-sensitive patients also had decreased asymmetry in parahippocampus blood volume and metabolic oxygen rate, but not in oxygen extraction. They also had increased whole brain oxygen metabolism and blood flow. Unfortunately, the fact that patients vulnerable to lactate infusion had mild uncompensated respiratory alkalosis (i.e., they hyperventilated in response to blood pH changes) makes it difficult to determine whether the observed increased brain metabolism is a trait marker or a consequence of the panic. It is possible that these changes reflect state anticipatory anxiety, and thus it would be interesting to look at parahippocampal activity in patients with other anxiety disorders under anxiety-provoking situations (e.g., in OCD patients before exposure to a contaminant, in snake phobics before exposure to a snake).

Baxter, Phelps, Mazziotta, et al. (1987) compared 14 patients with OCD to 14 patients with unipolar depression and to 14 normal controls on brain glucose metabolism during an "eyes open" resting condition. Unfortunately, there was substantial symptom overlap in the patient groups. Nevertheless, differences were observed between OCD patients and the other groups, although some differences were significant only when OCD patients were compared to depressed patients, some only when they were compared to controls, and some for both comparisons. In essence, results suggest that OCD patients have greater absolute metabolism in the cerebral hemispheres, caudate, and orbital gyri than both depressed patients and normal controls. In terms of relative glucose metabolic rates, OCD patients were higher than normals, but not depressed patients, in left-orbital-gyrus-to-hemisphere ratio. This ratio remained high after treatment with trazodone. Results were similar when depressed patients with obsessional features were excluded from analyses.

It is tempting to conclude that depression is associated with decreased metabolism in caudate and frontal areas, and OCD with increased metabolism in those areas. It is necessary to remember, however, that PET studies differ in procedure (e.g., eyes closed versus shock to forearm) and measures of metabolism (e.g., absolute versus relative to region versus relative to whole brain). Nevertheless, it will be interesting to see if these differences in metabolism between OCD and depression can be related to symptoms and other neuropsychological findings (e.g., the hypervigilance in OCD and reduced arousal in depression).

DISCUSSION

The neuropsychological test, EEG, and PET studies clearly implicate cortical and subcortical systems in both anxiety and depression. Perhaps the major conclusion to be drawn from these studies is that most types of psychopathology are associated with neural abnormalities. It is unclear whether specific disorders are associated with specific abnormalities, let alone whether these abnormalities are causal in the disorder, or whether two disorders share abnormalities because of common etiologies. It is also unclear whether it is reasonable to expect to find specific neural correlates of specific disorders. It is possible that some symptoms and some abnormalities merely represent a final common pathway of heterogeneous causes or a part of the system that is most vulnerable to breakdown.

It may be helpful to consider possible analogies from other behavioral disturbances. For example, mental retardation represents the final common pathway for hundreds of abnormalities of central nervous system function. Neuropsychological studies of mentally retarded subjects to date have not shown patterns of performance to differ for patients with retardation of differing etiologies; such studies, especially using imaging techniques, have the potential to help us understand whether observed abnormalities represent specific or general neuropathology. In terms of some functions being more vulnerable than others, studies of brain-damaged patients suggest that attentional deficits occur with a variety of types of damage (e.g., Rosvold, Mirsky, Sarason, et al. 1956), perhaps because attention is represented diffusely in the brain or because the areas involved in attention are especially vulnerable (e.g., from hypoxia). Goldberg (1988) suggested that frontal lobe pathology appears as a prominent feature in psychopathology because the frontal lobes have a low threshold for breakdown, and diffuse damage manifests itself as frontal lobe dysfunction. The clinical sign of fever is another example. Fever is common to various illnesses, but indicates little about the etiology or pathophysiology of the illness, or the "comorbidity" of diseases that are associated with fever.

This issue is harder to resolve when there are problems of diagnostic validity, as occur in neuropsychological studies of anxiety and depression. Thus subtypes of depressive disorders are rarely studied (e.g., melancholia, nonmelancholia), the relationship among the various anxiety disorders is not considered, and diagnostic groups show overlapping symptoms (e.g., depressive symptoms in OCD patients). Further, there are many studies where anxiety and depressive disorders are not differentiated from high levels of anxiety and depression in normals. We have not reviewed studies on neuropsychological and cognitive correlates of high and low state anxiety and induced mood in college students, because it is unclear whether these relate to anxiety and depressive disorders.

This does not mean that neuropsychological studies cannot be informative. We believe such studies can be uniquely valuable for understanding neural correlates—and causes—of psychopathology, and of comorbidity. Three types of studies are proposed that we believe will be useful in this regard: (1) neuropsychological studies that concentrate on symptoms rather than syndromes, (2) neuropsychological studies that relate disorders to general population variability in mood and personality, and (3) neuropsychological studies that carefully follow up on published studies, using well-defined patient groups and neuropsychological procedures that measure specific behavioral components with clear neural correlates.

With respect to the first proposal—focus on symptoms, not syndromes—neuropsychological studies of psychopathology in general and comorbidity in particular might concentrate on clinical features or symptoms rather than syndromes. Patients would be defined by the symptoms they show, rather than diagnosis. For example, it would be useful to know if depressed patients with hallucinations are more likely to show temporal lobe EEG abnormalities than depressed patients without hallucinations, or if neuropsychological commonalities between depression and anxiety disorders are associated with particular symptoms, such as changes in arousal or attention. Interestingly, in one study where such an approach was taken (Nystrom, Matousek, and Hallstrom 1986), apparent EEG correlates of depression were found to be related to anxiety symptoms rather than to the diagnosis of depression. Neuropsychological correlates of these symptoms could then be studied when patients are asymptomatic to determine whether they are state- or trait-related. Ultimately, neuropsychological factors that are found in patients with specific symptoms even when the patients are asymptomatic can be studied in relatives of these patients to determine if these neuropsychological abnormalities are part of the liability to the disorder.

Neuropsychological studies can best address issues of comorbidity by considering other work on the nature of anxiety and depression, especially diagnosis. Conflicting comorbidity data might, in part, be explained by a relationship existing between nonmelancholic depression and anxiety disorder, but not between major depression (melancholia) and anxiety disorder. Data from family studies support this idea (Noyes, Crowe, Harris, et al. 1986; Torgersen 1986; Weissman, Gershon, Kidd, et al. 1984). Further, Kendler, Heath, Martin, et al. (1986) interpret their data on comorbidity of anxiety and depressive symptoms in a normal twin sample to suggest that these symptoms may relate to personality, and that separation of such symptoms from personality may not be clear-cut or useful. Thus it might be helpful to examine in further detail comorbidity between personality dimensions related to anxiety and depression. For example, Tellegen's (1985) dimensions of positive and negative emotionality (PE and NE, respectively) encompass anxiety (high NE) and depression (both high NE and low PE). Gray's (1982) theory of personality and anxiety is tied to variability in underlying neurochemical systems. Cloninger (1987a) describes personality disorders in terms of variability on three basic personality dimensions; anxiety and depressive disorders are incorporated into his model.

Neuropsychological theories that attempt to address multiple aspects of affect can also be seen to address disorders as extremes of normal variability, and represent the second type of study we propose. For example, Tucker's hypotheses that mood disorders are associated with dysfunctions of the cerebral hemispheres (anxiety with overactivation of the left, depression with underactivation of the right) are tested with normal subjects varying in state or trait anxiety (Tucker, Antes, Stenslie, et al. 1978; Tyler and Tucker 1982) or induced into a depressed mood (Tucker, Stenslie, Roth, et al. 1981). Interestingly, constructs derived from theories of normal affect and personality are very likely to be amenable to neuropsychological study because they address the individual's characteristic ways of approaching the world. If anxiety and nonmelancholic depression represent extremes on normal continua, then these dimensions and the pathology associated with them should be amenable to description in neuropsychological terms. As such, they can also be reconciled with cognitive approaches to origins and treatment of psychopathology (e.g., Beck, Rush, Shaw, et al. 1979; Peterson and Seligman 1984). Alloy, Kelly, Mineka, et al. (Chapter 29), for example, have tried to differentiate individuals vulnerable to anxiety as opposed to depression by their cognitive approaches. It is possible that these approaches are associated both with personality as described by Tellegen (1985) and others, and with different patterns of neural organization.

The third type of informative study would be a careful extension of the current literature on neuropsychological correlates of anxiety disorders and depression. Such studies would examine carefully diagnosed patients on tests that allow inferences about underlying neuropsychological dysfunction. Measures need to be chosen for their potential ability to show *differences* between anxious and depressed patients. Most studies to date have revealed more similarities than differences between various patient groups. This may be partly due to alterations in attention and arousal that accompany most forms of behavioral disturbance and also influence task performance. Both increased arousal (as in anxiety) and decreased arousal (as in depression) will impair performance, so that examination of performance levels will be uninformative with respect to neuropsychological disturbance.

We offer two examples that we consider to represent fruitful areas for exploration in terms of the neuropsychological components that might be impaired in anxiety and depression. Oscar-Berman and colleagues (Oscar-Berman and Zola-Morgan 1980a, 1980b; Oscar-Berman, Zola-Morgan, Oberg, et al. 1982), have provided interesting demonstrations of the ways in which learning and cognition can be differentially affected by damage to different areas of the limbic and frontal systems. Their work, a comparative neuropsychological approach, consists of examination of human neuropathology in the context of experimental paradigms that are valid tests of nonhuman behavioral disruption following brain damage. Thus, although Korsakoff and Huntington patients both have deficits on visual reversal-learning, they show different patterns of poor performance. Further, Oscar-Berman and Zola-Morgan (1980b) have argued that deficits in Korsakoff patients are related to their widespread brain damage, whereas Huntington deficits are related to atrophy of frontal and temporal areas, perhaps consequent to atrophy of the caudate. As PET findings implicate the parahippocampus in panic disorder, and the caudate in OCD and depression, tasks that are differentially dependent on subcortical structures might differentiate anxious from depressed patients. For example, with respect to the role of the caudate, it might be worthwhile to compare anxious and depressed patients to Huntington patients on visual reversal-learning and other tasks used by Oscar-Berman and colleagues.

The second example would be to assess further the attention deficits reported previously in patients with anxiety disorder and in depressed patients. Mesulam (1981) suggested that directed attention is dependent on an intact, integrated network of four cerebral regions, including right parietal lobe, cingulate gyrus, frontal lobes, and reticular activating system. Each component has a unique functional role. Attention can be impaired with damage to any of these systems, but the nature of the deficit will vary with the area damaged. Lesions in only one part of the network produce partial neglect syndromes, whereas those that affect all components result in profound deficits. Thus right parietal damage will result in neglect or visuospatial attentional problems, whereas frontal damage will disturb the coordination of motor programs for exploration, scanning, reaching, and fixing. Damage to cingulate gyrus will affect the spatial distribution of motivational valence—the preferential attention to specific parts of extrapersonal space associated with specific motivational needs (e.g., a hungry animal exploring the area around the door through which the trainer is expected to enter at feeding time). Damage to the reticular-activating system will impair arousal and vigilance. It would be useful to compare patients with anxiety disorder and depressed patients on these aspects of attention, hypothesizing that depressed patients would show right parietal inattention, whereas anxious patients would show hyperarousal secondary to dysfunction in the reticular activating system.

CONCLUSION

In general, neuropsychological studies of anxiety and depressive disorders reveal that patients have abnormalities in a variety of neural systems. Because of conceptual and methodological limitations, it has been difficult either to delineate specific dysfunction in anxiety or depression, or to use existing results to understand comorbidity. Nevertheless, some tentative conclusions are warranted. States of depression appear to be associated with dysfunction or reduced activation of the right hemisphere, some frontal regions, and perhaps caudate. There is currently no indication that these abnormalities persist when subjects are well, or that they are specific to melancholia. They appear to be state phenomena. With respect to anxiety disorders, OCD is also associated with frontal and caudate abnormality, possibly overactivity. Panic attacks may be related to abnormal parahippocampal asymmetry. Some forms of anxiety may be associated with left hemisphere overactivation or dysfunction, but this is probably a state phenomenon, and it is unclear whether it is common to all forms of anxiety or just some disorders. Symptoms of anxiety and depression may co-occur as alternative manifestations of the same dysfunctional neural system; for example, both hyperactivity and hypoactivity could lead to altered arousal and impaired cognition.

Understanding of the neural substates of anxiety and depression and of their comorbidity is likely to come from studies with clear descriptions of patient's symptoms, separation of state- and trait-related correlates, description of disorders as variants of normal personality or discrete illnesses, and use of neuropsychological procedures that can be tied to underlying behavioral and brain processes.

Chapter 32

Impact of DSM-III-R Revisions on the Anxiety Disorders and on Primary Care Givers

Paula J. Clayton, M.D.

A s KARL MENNINGER et al. (1967) pointed out in his classic book, *The Vital Balance*, there are many ways to organize data, and classification is one of the basic devices for bringing order out of chaos. Physicians from the earliest times attempted to understand the mysteries of mental illnesses by developing systems of classification. Psychiatrists' most recent attempts to classify are embodied in the third edition of the *Diagnostic and Statistical Manual of Mental Disorders* (DSM-III) (American Psychiatric Association 1980) and its revision, DSM-III-R (American Psychiatric Association 1987). The chaos of such endeavors is evident in the many changes made in the 7 years from DSM-III to DSM-III-R.

The creation of a classification of morbid anxiety is newer than some of our other major mental illness categories. In the late 1800s, DaCosta (1871) described the "irritable heart syndrome" and Freud (1894/1959) "anxiety neurosis." Subsequently, many other names such as neurasthenia, neurocirculatory asthenia, nervous exhaustion, effort syndrome, and soldier's heart were used to refer to the syndrome (Breier, Charney, and Heninger 1985a). In the 1950s, Dr. Paul Dudley White, President Eisenhower's cardiologist, and collaborators in Boston conducted a study of patients seen by him in his practice whom he thought did not have organic heart disease (Wheeler,

White, Reed, et al. 1950). They chose patients for study and follow-up based on specific anxiety criteria as well as absence of organic pathology. It was a classic study of a group of patients (not psychiatric) who were separated out and labeled as anxiety neurosis. Much of what they observed and reported has been replicated and only recently extended. From their studies and review, they concluded the following: Anxiety neurosis occurs in 2% to 5% of the population, most frequently in women (two-thirds). It has its age of onset midway through the 20s, although patients may not see physicians until their early 30s. Anxiety neurosis can be provoked by numerous external stimuli (physical and psychological) and is sometimes associated with avoidance behavior. It may run in families and seldom is associated with premature death.

In the early 1960s, it was discovered that panic attacks could be precipitated with sodium lactate infusions. Moreover, panic attacks could be successfully treated with antidepressant medications, which compounds produced a remission of the panic symptoms before any remission of the other anxiety symptoms. This last discovery indicated to some that panic attacks might represent a disorder distinct from generalized anxiety, a concept adopted by the DSM-III. The more recent multicenter panic disorder trial with alprazolam (Ballenger, Burrows, DuPont, et al. 1988) indicated that drug treatment can simultaneously reduce panic, phobias, anticipatory anxiety, and more general anxiety.

Subsequently, panic attacks have been shown to be precipitated by yohimbine, caffeine, and carbon dioxide. Patients with panic disorder who develop lactate-induced panic attacks have been shown to have asymmetry in cerebral blood flow, blood volume, and oxygen metabolism, with an abnormal increase in the right parahippocampal area (Reiman, Raichle, Robins, et al. 1986) and to have strong familial transmission consistent with Mendelian inheritance. A possible linkage between panic disorder and the haptoglobin (HP) locus on chromosome 16 has been reported (Crowe, Noyes, Wilson, et al. 1987).

Table 1 displays both the DSM-III-R and the DSM-III classification of the anxiety disorders in adulthood. The old idea of anxiety neurosis was embodied in DSM-III as anxiety states, specifically as panic disorder, generalized anxiety disorder, and agoraphobia with or without panic attacks, along with social phobias and simple phobias. Obsessive-compulsive disorder was also an anxiety disorder. DSM-III-R, based on a fair amount of accumulated evidence (Ganellen, Matuzas, Uhlenhuth, et al. 1986; Thyer, Himle, Curtis, et al. 1985), returned agoraphobia to the category of panic disorder with or without agoraphobia. Those panic patients who experience agoraphobia were felt to be simply more severe or cognitively different. A third DSM-III-R

Table 1. DSM-III-R and DSM-III Classifications of the Anxiety Disorders in Adulthood

	DSM-III-R	DSM-III[a]
300.21	Panic disorder with agoraphobia	*Agoraphobia with panic attacks
300.01	Panic disorder without agoraphobia	**Panic disorder
300.22	Agoraphobia without history of panic disorder	*Agoraphobia without panic attacks
300.23	Social phobia	*Social phobia
300.29	Simple phobia	*Simple phobia
300.30	Obsessive-compulsive disorder (or obsessive-compulsive neurosis)	**Obsessive-compulsive disorder (or obsessive-compulsive neurosis)
309.89	Posttraumatic stress disorder	***Acute posttraumatic stress disorder
		***Chronic or delayed post-traumatic stress disorder
300.02	Generalized anxiety disorder	**Generalized anxiety disorder
300.00	Anxiety disorder not otherwise specified	***Atypical anxiety disorder

*phobic disorders; **anxiety states (anxiety neuroses); ***posttraumatic stress disorder.

category is agoraphobia without a history of panic disorder. Again, this concept is different than that embodied in DSM-III, which referred to it as agoraphobia without panic *attacks* (not a history of panic *disorder*). According to our recent data, there are very few patients who would qualify for this last diagnosis. The phobias are restricted to social phobia and simple phobia. Obsessive-compulsive disorder remains a separate entity. Generalized anxiety disorder and posttraumatic stress disorder are the two other disorders created in DSM-III and significantly modified in DSM-III-R. Anxiety disorders that cannot be classified are called "not otherwise specified."

RESULTS OF THE EPIDEMIOLOGIC CATCHMENT AREA (ECA) STUDY

Unfortunately, the National Institute of Mental Health (NIMH) ECA (Regier, Myers, Kramer, et al. 1984) study, which gathered data to make psychiatric diagnoses on 9,000 adults living in the community, used DSM-III criteria, so the prevalence rates do not represent our current diagnostic practices. Fortunately, in reporting the data they separated out the phobic subtypes so that revised estimates can be developed. The same cannot be said for many other same vintage studies where investigators combined all phobias to report findings and treated the less common DSM-III "panic disorder" as the prototype for the anxiety disorders (Kessler, Cleary, and Burke 1985; Von Korff, Shapiro, Burke, et al. 1987).

Table 2. Six-Month Prevalence for Three Communities of Selected Anxiety Disorders: DSM-III Disorders Regrouped According to DSM-III-R Concepts

	Men (%)	Women (%)
Panic disorder with agoraphobia and pure agoraphobia	.9 – 1.1 ⎱ 1.2 – 1.9	4.2 – 4.3 ⎱ 5.1 – 5.5
without agoraphobia	.3 – .8	.9 – 1.2
Social phobia	.9	1.5
Simple phobia	2.3 – 3.2	6.0 – 6.5
Obsessive-compulsive	.9 – 1.9	1.7 – 2.2
Total	5.3 – 7.7	12.8 – 15.7
Minus simple phobia	3.0 – 4.5	6.8 – 9.2
Alcohol abuse	8.2 – 10.4	4.5 – 5.7
Any affective disorder	2.7 – 4.6	6.0 – 8.3

Note. Generalized anxiety disorder and posttraumatic stress disorder were not included.

From the ECA study, as depicted in Table 2, the 6-month prevalence of the anxiety disorders, in collection, indicated that these disorders are extremely common (Myers, Weissman, Tischler, et al. 1984). Excluding simple phobia, the most common anxiety disorder is panic disorder with agoraphobia, which is only slightly less prevalent than the combined mood disorders. Except perhaps for simple phobia (deemed by researchers studying primary care patients as extremely common, but of questionable medical significance), the epidemiologic survey was not labeling simple distress or misery. The other categories in the anxiety disorders (i.e., generalized anxiety disorder and post-traumatic stress disorder) were not investigated in the ECA study.

The lifetime prevalences figures shown in Table 3 from the same study confirmed that the anxiety disorders are one of four important psychiatric disorders from which people suffer (Robins, Helzer, Weissman, et al. 1984). Alcohol abuse-dependence is the most prevalent, occurring in 19% to 29% of the adult male population (18 or older) and 4% of the adult female population. Depending on whether simple phobia is included or excluded, either the anxiety disorders or the affective disorders are the most common disorders of adult women. In point of fact, even with simple phobias excluded, the lifetime prevalences of these two groups of disorders are remarkably similar. If researchers believe in the diagnosis of generalized anxiety disorder and posttraumatic stress disorder, illnesses not assessed in this survey, then no doubt the anxiety disorders are adult women's most prevalent psychiatric illnesses. In adult men, drug abuse-dependence and affective disorders are similar in prevalence and would be

Table 3. Lifetime Prevalence for Three Communities of Selected Anxiety Disorders: DSM-III Disorders Regrouped According to DSM-III-R Concepts

	Men (%)		Women (%)	
Panic disorder	1.5		5.3 – 6.4	
with agoraphobia and				
pure agoraphobia		.6 – 2.7		6.9 – 8.5
without agoraphobia	.6 – 1.2		1.6 – 2.1	
Social phobia				
Simple phobia	3.8 – 4.0		8.5 – 9.4	
Obsessive-compulsive	1.1 – 2.6		2.6 – 3.3	
Total	5.5 – 9.3		18.4 – 21.2	
Minus simple phobia	1.7 – 5.3		9.9 – 11.8	
Alcohol abuse-dependence	19.1 – 28.9		4.2 – 4.3	
Drug abuse-dependence	6.5 – 7.4		3.8 – 5.1	
Major affective illness	5.3 – 7.9		8.3 – 14.6	

listed as second and third in their rankings. In adult women, drug abuse-dependence and alcohol abuse-dependence are of similar prevalence and occupy the third and fourth most frequent disorders. Except for the large sex differences, there were no other significant differences by age, race, socioeconomic status, education, or rural versus urban dwelling in this three-site comparison. The typical age of onset for all these disorders is less than 30; in some disorders it is less than 20, but they remain "cases" for years (Thyer, Parrish, Curtis, et al. 1985).

There are no similar epidemiologic data on the prevalence of generalized anxiety disorder, although it can be extrapolated from less rigorous studies. Perhaps 3% to 6% of the population qualify for such a diagnosis (Reich 1986; Uhlenhuth, Balter, Mellinger, et al. 1983). In most studies at least 50% of diagnoses of generalized anxiety disorder occur after a specific life event, and the onset is gradual compared to the sudden crescendo of a panic attack. DSM-III-R criteria for a generalized anxiety disorder are more stringent than DSM-III. The revised criteria require excessive worry in two or more life circumstances for 6 months or more, and the hierarchical rule has been retained. That is, the diagnosis cannot be made in the presence of a major depressive disorder. Most studies have shown that generalized anxiety disorder usually occurs in conjunction with many other Axis I DSM-III disorders, and a recent family study of generalized anxiety disorder (Noyes, Clarkson, Crowe, et al. 1987) showed that it is sometimes difficult to distinguish generalized anxiety disorder from adjustment disorder with anxious mood. Using the more stringent DSM-III-R criteria for generalized anxiety disorder, only 43% of the relatives diagnosed by DSM-III meet the revised criteria, leaving the authors to comment that the disturbances on a whole were relatively mild, brief, and clearly related to psychosocial stressors.

A recent epidemiologic study of posttraumatic stress disorder found it to be rare, occurring in 1% of the population (Helzer, Robins, and McEvoy 1987). In this study, the authors asked about a group of stressors, but only exposure to physical attack and being in Vietnam, particularly in combat, produced the syndrome. Of civilians exposed to physical attack, 3.5% were diagnosed as having the disorder. A similar number of Vietnam veterans who were not wounded had the disorder, whereas 20% of veterans wounded in Vietnam reported symptoms consistent with posttraumatic stress disorder.

From a different perspective we can review the disorders as they present to a specialty outpatient clinic. In a 4-month period in 1982, 133 persons contacted the phobia and anxiety clinic in Albany, New York (Di Nardo, O'Brien, Barlow, et al. 1983). Since the clinicians were undertaking a reliability study of a new structured interview, they tried to enroll all potential patients into the study. Patients were screened by telephone, and some were excluded. Sixty patients were seen twice, and given the following DSM-III diagnoses. As Table 4 indicates, 51 (85%) were given diagnoses in the anxiety disorders category. As in the ECA study, the most common diagnosis was agoraphobia with panic attack. No patient had agoraphobia without panic attack. There were 8 patients (13%) with pure panic disorder. Ten percent of the patients had generalized anxiety disorder. This percentage was actually a smaller number than those who came to the clinic and met the criteria for the affective disorders. The percentage would certainly be smaller with current criteria. There were no pa-

Table 4. Base Rates of Consensus Primary Diagnoses

Diagnosis	Patients	
	n	%
Anxiety disorders	23	38.3
Agoraphobia with panic attacks		
Agoraphobia without panic attacks	0	0
Social phobia	8	13.3
Simple phobia	2	3.3
Panic disorder	8	13.3
Generalized anxiety disorder	6	10.0
Obsessive-compulsive disorder	3	5.0
Posttraumatic stress disorder	0	0
Atypical anxiety	1	1.7
TOTAL	51	85.0
Affective disorders		
Major depression	5	8.3
Bipolar disorder, depressed	1	1.7
Dysthymic disorder	1	1.7
TOTAL	7	11.7
Other disorders		
Adjustment disorder	2	3.3
Axis III diagnoses	2	3.3
Overall total	62	103.2

Note. Percentages were computed for each diagnostic category by dividing the number of patients given the diagnosis by the total number of patients, which was 60. Since 62 diagnoses were given, the total percentage is slightly greater than 100%. (Two subjects were given two primary diagnoses). Modified from Di Nardo PA, O'Brien GT, Barlow DH, et al. (1983).

tients with posttraumatic stress disorder. How these patients relate to those seen in a general psychiatric clinic or a family practice clinic is unknown.

Even the recent Cross-National Collaborative Panic Study (Klerman 1988) decided to include in the study three groups: (1) panic disorder uncomplicated (DSM-III panic disorder); (2) panic disorder with limited phobic avoidance; and (3) panic disorder with extensive phobic avoidance (DSM-III "agoraphobia with panic disorder"). Only 5% had pure panic disorder, 16% had the limited avoidance syndrome, and 79% had the full-blown disorder (Ballenger, Burrows, DuPont, et al. 1988).

It seems fair to conclude that in psychiatry, and probably even in primary care, the major anxiety disorder is panic disorder with agoraphobia. It is this disorder that must be compared and contrasted to major depressive disorder.

DATA FROM PRIMARY CARE CLINICS

Data based on DSM-III (not DSM-III-R) from primary care clinics illustrate how these viscous, changing concepts make conclusions about the significance of anxiety disorders for the medical community (and health care providers and insurers) difficult. Patients attending a primary care group practice were screened with the Goldberg Health Questionnaire (Von Korff, Shapiro, Burke, et al. 1987). All patients who had a score of five or above (considered positive for psychiatric distress), and an equal number of those who scored four or less, were studied further. The study was designed as an intervention study. A subset of primary care physicians were given feedback about the results of the questionnaire. It was determined that the feedback had limited impact on the practitioner's assessment of mental disorder or on his or her subsequent treatment of the patient. Nevertheless, the impact of this intervention should have been referenced or factored into the analysis of this report.

Interviewers were sent to the patients' homes, where the NIMH Diagnostic Interview Schedule (DIS) (Robins, Helzer, Croughan, et al. 1981) was administered. The practitioners also completed a form that recorded whether or not they considered the patient to have had an emotional problem at the time, and their diagnostic evaluation of that problem. Of the practitioner's assessments of psychiatric distress, 83% fell into four major categories: depression not otherwise specified, anxiety not otherwise specified, adjustment reaction, and neurotic depression. The extent to which the practitioners were familiar with the diagnostic principles and criteria outlined in DSM-III is unclear.

The DIS diagnoses were limited to major depression, panic disorder, dysthymia, obsessive-compulsive disorder, and generalized anxiety disorder (added for this study). Phobias were excluded from the categories because the authors judged that the large majority of phobias were circumscribed, did not indicate significant subjective distress, and were of limited clinical significance in the context of primary care. Unfortunately, how this decision was determined is not stated, but it probably meant that a very prevalent and incapacitating anxiety disorder, panic disorder with agoraphobia, was excluded.

Von Korff, Shapiro, Burke, et al. (1987) reported that in the month preceding the interview, 1.4% of the patients qualified for panic disorder, 4.6% for generalized anxiety disorder, and 1.1% for obsessive-compulsive disorder. In a separate category, 7.8% qualified for some phobic disorder. Totally, 25% of the patients qualified for at least one of nine DIS diagnoses; 39% had elevated Goldberg Health Questionnaire scores; and 33% were assessed by the practitioners as having an emotional disorder. There was marked overlap in the diagnoses of anxiety and depressive disorders in patients assigned a diagnosis by the DIS since DSM-III diagnostic exclusion criteria were not applied. In those patients who received a diagnosis on the DIS, 82% were identified with the health questionnaire and 83% by the practitioner as cases. This high correspondence indicated that there were a group of readily identifiable cases with relatively unambiguous psychiatric symptoms among the primary care cases. These cases corresponded to what the British called "conspicuous psychiatric morbidity" (Casey, Dillon, and Tyrer 1984; Goldberg 1979).

The conclusion was that efforts should be concentrated on improving the diagnosis and treatment of these cases. Although the conclusion was probably correct, the definition of "cases" may not have been. The authors failed to identify cases classified as panic disorder with agoraphobia. In addition, by ignoring the DSM-III exclusion criteria, cases were dually classified; it is conceivable that generalized anxiety disorder was overclassified, and major depression as a single diagnosis was underclassified.

Another study (Kessler, Cleary, and Burke 1985) used the Goldberg Health Questionnaire as the screening instrument and physicians' assessment, but a different structured interview—the Schedule for Affective Disorders and Schizophrenia-Lifetime version (SADS-L) (Spitzer and Endicott 1977)—and different criteria: the Research Diagnostic Criteria (RDC) (Spitzer, Endicott, and Robins 1978a). The interview was administered twice 6 months apart. The authors found that 35% of the patients had at least one psychiatric disorder. Only 10% of the transient and episodic cases were recognized by the primary care physicians. In this study, in keeping with all other studies that classified them, "the phobias" were the most frequent remitted and continuing cases, whereas generalized anxiety disorder and panic disorder were rarer. What percentage of the phobias were agoraphobic versus simple phobia was not stated, but might be extrapolated from data displayed in Table 3, where approximately 35% of the phobias in women were agoraphobia. Agoraphobia added to panic disorder emphasizes that this combined group of patients comprise a significant number of the continuously ill for the primary care physician.

Overall, studies conclude that between 25% and 35% of patients who see primary care physicians have psychiatric disorders. The rates of the anxiety disorders vary from study to study, depending on the exclusion or inclusion of the phobias, with panic disorder with agoraphobia embedded in this category. Even in primary care, using structured interviews and strict criteria, generalized anxiety disorder does not emerge as a common disorder. This body of research exemplifies why we have difficulty communicating with each other and presenting these concepts to other physicians and mental health workers.

Only in the papers from the primary care setting has the overlap between the anxiety disorders and mood disorders been considered. From the Cross-National Collaborative Panic Study, 31% of the patients had an onset of depression occurring after the onset of the "panic" disorder (Lesser, Rubin, Pecknold, et al. 1988). My colleagues and I (Clayton, Grove, Coryell, et al. personal communication) have found that the majority of depressed patients from the collaborative study of depression had some anxiety symptoms during a depressive episode. Depressed patients with higher anxiety scores had longer times to recovery and an increased risk for primary unipolar depression among their first-degree relatives. Thus in both disorders there is an overlap of panic attacks, phobic avoidance, worry, general anxiety, and nonpsychotic depression. The family data, however, indicate that each of these disorders are distinct clinical entities. Evidence that generalized anxiety disorder is a distinct disorder is still lacking since the one family study (Noyes, Clarkson, Crowe, et al. 1987) does not present a convincing case.

DSM-IV is already being planned. One way of simplifying the anxiety disorders for psychiatry and improving our communication with primary care physicians has been proposed (Clayton 1987; Tyrer 1986a) and that is to regroup some generalized anxiety disorder with the panic disorder with agoraphobia. This regrouping would return the syndrome to the 1950 concept of anxiety neurosis and would be compatible with recent new treatment data (Ballenger, Burrows, DuPont, et al. 1988). Adjustment disorder with anxious mood could characterize some of the remaining patients now labeled as generalized anxiety disorder, whose disorder is transient (Wilson, Cadoret,

Widmer, et al. 1987); depressive disorders may absorb the rest (Clayton, Grove, Coryell, et al., personal communication). There would still be comorbidity, but perhaps its implications would be pursued with less zeal than the underlying biology of panic disorder with agoraphobia and major depressive disorder.

Chapter 33

Toward a Clinical Understanding of the Relationship of Anxiety and Depressive Disorders

Hagop S. Akiskal, M.D.

A woman at Thasos became morose as the result of a justifiable grief, and . . . she suffered from insomnia, loss of appetite . . . she complained of fears and talked too much; she showed despondency and . . . many intense and continuous pains.

Hippocrates, Aphorisms V

Patients with fear . . . of long standing are subject to melancholia.

Hippocrates, Epidemics III

HIPPOCRATES OBSERVED TWO fundamental patterns of comorbidity of anxiety and depressive disorders. The first consists of intra-episodic comorbidity when symptoms characteristic of one disorder occur during an episode of the other. The second pattern is when one disorder, followed over time, gives way to the other. Both forms of comorbidity have been observed worldwide and represent the subject of much heated current debate (this volume; Darcourt and Pringuey 1987; Racagni and Smeraldi 1987).

This chapter examines the relationship of anxiety and depressive disorders from the perspective of the medical model. Since Hippocratic times, this approach has emphasized careful bedside clinical observation consisting of description of signs and symptoms, close follow-up of cases so characterized, naturalistic explanations for the origin of the illness, and the provision of the sick role to the sufferer. For instance, Hippocrates asserted that many disturbances of behavior—he took epilepsy as a paradigm—reflected brain diseases rather than supernatural influences. This essentially biologic orientation was not meant, however, to discount sociodemographic factors, habit, seasons, and the like, which Hippocrates' disciples examined in great detail.

Although medicine is often equated with biology, systematic clinical investigation and dedication to the alleviation of suffering constitute the more fundamental foundations of the profession of medicine (Akiskal 1989). The application of this approach to psychiatry is usually credited to Kraepelin (1921). The Robins and Guze (1970) approach to validation of psychiatric disorders represents the most recent development along these lines. It lays emphasis on five perspectives: syndromal description, delimitation from other disorders, family history, laboratory investigations, and follow-up. Klein (1973) championed the perspective of treatment response, especially pharmacologic response, as an additional fundamental criterion for assessing validity.

In this chapter, I will argue that clinical comorbidity of anxiety and depressive disorders is reflected in some but not all the other perspectives. Despite the prevalence of such comorbidity, I will further argue that distinctive cross-sectional characterization of the two groups of disorders is possible. I will then discuss the therapeutic and prognostic implications of different patterns of comorbidity observed over time. Skeptics note that the differential diagnostic considerations in the interface of anxiety and depressive disorders are of theoretical rather than clinical significance. They justify such skepticism by pointing out that anxiety and depressive disorders tend to respond to antidepressants and that some benzodiazepines might also be beneficial for both conditions. In discussing these issues, I will consider critical areas of overlap of anxiety and depression that call for more complex treatment decisions.

CROSS-SECTIONAL DIFFERENTIATION

Cross-sectionally, pure anxiety states—without depressive admixtures—are more commonly observed in the clinic than the reverse (Hamilton 1983). That is to say, depressive illness seldom occurs without some anxiety component. Thus, in his description of melancholia, Hippocrates included fear along with pain, despondency, insomnia, and loss of appetite. When the two disorders are examined longitudinally, anxiety followed by depression is significantly more common than the reverse (Kendell 1974). Again, Hippocrates had insight into this aspect of the comorbidity of the two disorders, testifying to the power of the medical model in unraveling fundamental relationships in psychopathology.

The symptomatic overlap of the two disorders is documented throughout this volume. Yet those who adhere to unitarian positions do not always appreciate that key cognitive, phenomenological, psychomotor, and psychophysiologic parameters distinguish the two disorders. The pioneering studies in such differentiation were carried out by the Newcastle group (Gurney, Roth, Garside, et al. 1972; Roth, Gurney, Garside, et al. 1972) and have been followed by a more recent wave of studies highlighted in the selective review undertaken below.

The cognitive structures for the two disorders appear distinct, at least cross-sectionally (Akiskal 1985a; Beck and Emery 1985). In anxiety states the future is pregnant with dangers; the patient is tormented by uncertainty, fear of death, insecurity, and helplessness. By contrast, the central theme of clinical depression is one of loss, self-depreciation, futurelessness, hopelessness, and suicidal ideation. Phenomenologically, anxiety is experienced as heightened negative affective arousal, and depression as one of reduced positive affect (Akiskal 1986a; Tellegen 1985). At the level of psychomotor functions, increased activity is often observed in both anxiety and depressive states, whereas psychomotor retardation is unique to clinical depression (Greden and Carroll 1981; Widlöcher, Lecrubier, and Le Goc 1983). These differences in psychomotor activity are paralleled by autonomic (sympathetic) activation in anxiety states, and generally the reverse in pure depressive states (Lader 1975). This psychophysiologic distinction is particularly striking in skin conductance (Ward, Doerr, and Storrie 1983). All of these disturbances are further reflected in differential social functioning (Cassano, Perugi, Maremmani, et al. 1990); thus adjustment in sexual, interpersonal, leisure (hedonic), and work areas are all significantly more deviant in depressive patients even when compared with those with severe anxiety states, such as panic disorder with agoraphobia. These deficits in depression may arise from the fact that depression, once established, is an illness largely autonomous from the environment. The reverse is true for anxiety disorders, which show a great deal of psychophysiologic variability over time (Akiskal and Lemmi 1987). This is born out by a sleep electroencephalographic (EEG) study at our center (Akiskal, Lemmi, Dickson, et al. 1984), which showed little or no night-to-night variability of sleep measures in primary depression, but highly significant variability in those of anxiety disorders, even when contaminated by secondary depression; in addition, short rapid eye movement (REM) latency and early morning awakening characterized the primary depressions. Other differentiated vegetative signs are documented by Hamilton (1983).

The composite differentiating features of anxiety and depressive states that emerge from the foregoing considerations lead to the summary in Table 1. These clinical distinctions are also reflected in differential responses to somatic interventions (Table 2). Although some overlap occurs in response to several psychopharmacologic agents (especially those influencing noradrenergic and serotonergic systems), the differential response to somatic interventions favoring depression appears to be robust along other dimensions (e.g., those influencing the dopaminergic system, circadian rhythms, and mineral metabolism). The neurochemical aspects of the comorbidity of anxiety and depression are beyond the scope of this chapter, but it is tempting to make at least one inference from these pharmacologic response profiles. Intra-episode or symptomatic comorbidity of anxiety and depression might result in part from perturbations in neurotransmitter systems common to both conditions (e.g., the noradrenergic and the serotonergic), and unique neurochemical perturbations could be more characteristic of depression (e.g., underactivity of the dopaminergic system). This speculation finds some support in the differential neurochemistry of the "protest" and "despair" phases of primate separation (Kraemer, Ebert, Lake, et al. 1984). The hypothesized involvement of the dopaminergic system in depression might also explain the diagnostic significance of psychomotor retardation, as well as disturbed hedonic functions, in depression summarized above.

Table 1.   The Unique Cross-Sectional Profiles of Clinical Anxiety and Depression

Anxiety	Depression
Hypervigilance	Psychomotor retardation
Severe tension and panic	Severe sadness
Perceived danger	Perceived loss
Phobic avoidance	Loss of interest—anhedonia
Doubt and uncertainty	Hopelessness—suicidal
Insecurity	Self-depreciation
Performance anxiety	Loss of libido
	Early morning awakening
	Weight loss

Table 2. Response to Somatic Treatments in Anxiety and Depressive Disorders

	Anxiety	Depressive
Alprazolam[a]	+ + +	+
Phenelzine	+ + +	+ +
Imipramine	+ +	+ + +
Clomipramine	+ +	+ + +
Trazodone	+	+ +
Fluoxetine	+	+ +
Bupropion	—	+ +
Sleep deprivation	—	+
Phototherapy	?	+
Lithium	0	+
Electroconvulsive therapy	—	+ + +
Cingulotomy	+	+

Note. Summarized from Akiskal (1985b). Plus signs indicate increasing levels of clinical response, negative sign indicates clinical worsening, and zero indicates absence of any response; question mark indicates paucity of systematic data.

[a]Alprazolam is the only benzodiazepine with systematic evidence for dual action in both panic and depressive disorders; clinical evidence for anti-panic action has also been reported lately for other benzodiazepines such as clonazepam, lorazepam, and diazepam.

LONGITUDINAL OVERLAP

As pointed out by Angst, Vollrath, Merikangas, et al. (Chapter 7), once established, depressive illness is rarely followed by an anxiety disorder, whereas the reverse is true for anxiety disorders (exclusive of simple phobias). Thus, in accordance with Hippocrates' formulation, follow-up observations have shown high rates of depression in the course of anxiety disorders, especially in that of generalized anxiety, panic, and obsessive-compulsive disorders.

How should one understand this frequent association? The most parsimonious explanation lies in the biphasic primate response to separation, consisting of protest and despair stages (Akiskal and McKinney 1973; Bowlby 1960). That is, the initial response to object loss, when the finality of the loss is not fully appreciated, consists of a universal anxious-agitated search for the lost object; this is followed in 5% of adults and 25% of infants by giving up the search and retreating into a retarded-despair state. This perspective is competently reviewed by Alloy, Kelly, Mineka, et al. (Chapter 29, this volume).

What follows is how I, as a clinician, conceptualize the longitudinal relationship between anxiety and depressive disorders and how therapeutic modalities bear on them. I will make very few specific references to the literature because the existing literature in this area does not address the question of comorbidity as it is clinically conceptualized here. The relevant literature on treatment modalities is reviewed in VanValkenburg, Akiskal, Puzantian, et al. (1984) and in Akiskal (1985b).

The primate perspective might explain why equally astute observations on human bereavement can lead to "different" interpretations. Thus Parkes (1986) declares grief to be an anxiety reaction, whereas Clayton, Herjanic, Murphy, et al. (1974) consider it to be a model for reactive depression. Given that the most common life stressors consist of losses, or threats of such—and extrapolating the findings on bereavement to other forms of adversity—one can propose that much of human reaction to acute stressors consist of anxiety-depressive admixtures, what the revised version of the third edition of the *Diagnostic and Statistical Manual of Mental Disorders* (DSM-III-R) (American Psychiatric Association 1987) considers to represent adjustment disorder with "mixed-emotional" features. When such adjustment persists beyond a time frame considered adaptive, the patient will typically meet the criteria for generalized anxiety and major depressive episode simultaneously. There is no reason to believe that a specific depressive predisposition is needed for these undifferentiated emotional reactions, which are most commonly seen in such settings as community mental health, psychological counseling, and general medical practice. It is well known that somatic presentations characteristic of both anxiety and depression often dominate the clinical picture in many patients seen by the general medical practitioner (Akiskal 1983b; Goldberg and Bridges 1988). The extensive literature on acute pharmacotherapy and brief psychotherapy is generally supportive of the clinical opinion that benzodiazepines, the traditional tricyclic antidepressants (TCAs), and several among the "new generation" (especially the sedating varieties) as well as a host of brief psychotherapeutic techniques are about equally effective for such mixed emotional reactions; by contrast, they generally respond rather poorly to electroconvulsive therapy (ECT).

In another pattern, initial panic attacks are followed, several months later, by a more or less pure depressive syndrome (Uhde, Roy-Byrne, Vittone, et al. 1985), which assumes autonomy. A depressive predisposition is probably present in some, although not all, such cases. These depressions are less likely to respond to benzodiazepines (alprazolam might be an exception), and to psychotherapy alone, but would often benefit from cyclic antidepressant drugs and psychotherapy (Klerman, Weissman, Rounsaville, et al. 1984). Those unresponsive to such measures might benefit from a trial of ECT.

In a third pattern, the patient has suffered from a definable anxiety disorder (e.g., panic disorder) for many years, has had varying degrees of self-exposure to phobic situations with varying success, and, finally, succumbs to an exhausted "depressive" condition that tends to linger on a subacute or even chronic basis. This pattern can be variously interpreted as literal neurochemical "exhaustion" of relevant (e.g., noradrenergic) systems, or secondary demoralization in the sense in which Klein (1974) uses this term. There seems to be emerging consensus, although far from universal, that neither ECT nor the TCAs are particularly effective for these depressions and that monoamine oxidase inhibitors (MAOIs) might well be the drugs of choice.

Much of what is considered an "atypical depressive" syndrome (Davidson, Miller, Craig, et al. 1982) might represent a variant of the preceding pattern. Patients who have suffered from many years of low-grade neurosis consisting of varying admixtures of generalized anxiety and panic attacks—and who have received no definitive therapeutic interventions—gradually sink into insecure helplessness with brooding gloom over the uselessness of effort; insomnia in the first half of the night leads to a tendency to feel daytime fatigue and sleepiness, hence the origin of several of the key symptoms that are considered to be atypical depressive manifestations. Even in the original British reports (Sargant 1961; West and Dally 1959), these atypical depressive patients with "neurasthenic" symptoms were basically considered anxiety neurotics. In such patients studied in our sleep laboratory (Akiskal, Lemmi, Dickson, et al. 1984), polysomnographic findings have failed to reveal REM sleep findings characteristic of primary depressive illness, and instead have shown features observed in anxiety disorders (i.e., multiple awakenings in the first half of the night). Intermittent sleep deprivation in the first half of the night could hypothetically lead to many of the clinical characteristics of these patients that, depending on the presenting complaint, the sleep literature (Association of Sleep Disorders Centers 1979) classifies either as chronic psychophysiologic insomnia or chronic psychophysiologic hypersomnia. Such daytime stigmata of insufficient sleep (e.g., impaired concentration, reduced vigilance, fatigue, irritability, and gastrointestinal complaints) reproduce some of the cardinal features of so-called atypical depressions. Indirect support for this formulation comes from a study by Roy-Byrne, Uhde, and Post (1986) that found worsening of panic disorder by sleep deprivation. Hence my contention that many, if not most, atypical depressions are more appropriately subsumed under the rubric of atypical anxiety disorder and would therefore benefit from MAOIs. This is indeed the finding reported by Liebowitz, Quitkin, Stewart, et al. (1984).

Thus far I have considered anxiety-depressive admixtures where the anxiety symptoms preceded the depressive manifestations. There also exists a prevalent situation where anxiety manifestations do not precede the depression, but develop in the setting of a depressive condition. This could occur acutely (Akiskal and Lemmi 1987), or anxiety manifestations could dominate the residual phase of the depression (Cassano, Maggini, and Akiskal 1983). Both situations are most likely to occur in older individuals. The long-term use of benzodiazepines or alcohol in these individuals, often as (self-) treatment for insomnia, can lead to a state of semi-withdrawal and hence an accentuation of the anxiety features. As emphasized in DSM-III-R, an anxiety disorder rarely, if ever, begins after the age of 40. Unfortunately, this rule is often disregarded by the practitioner, and manifestations indicative of autonomic nervous system hyperactivity are automatically ascribed to a neurotic illness. What complicates differential diagnosis is the fact that some of these patients completely deny the subjective psychological symptoms of mood disorder (e.g., sadness, anhedonia, self-deprecation, and suicidal ideation). Among depressive patients presenting with medically unexplained somatic complaints (Akiskal and Lemmi 1987), about a dozen were middle-aged or elderly patients (in their 40s or older) who presented with such symptoms as sudden awakening with intense autonomic arousal and the fear of dying in their sleep. None of these patients had experienced panic attacks in their younger years or had premorbidly exhibited neurotic patterns. Elderly individuals with no psychiatric illness showed modest shortening of their REM latency. But even after taking this fact into consideration, the patients we studied with fear of dying in their sleep and other autonomic manifestations of anxiety had sleep EEG findings characteristic of primary depression. It would appear that the mere presence of anxiety attacks is not diagnostic of panic disorder in that such attacks appearing for the first time after age 40 may represent "affective equivalents." Melancholic patients presenting in this way are typically agitated and experience intense apprehension; they may even harbor delusional ideas regarding calamities to themselves and their loved ones, which confirms the diagnosis. These agitated melancholic patients should be treated like other primary depressive patients (e.g., with TCAs, other cyclic antidepressants, or ECT). The use of benzodiazepines, if ever needed, should be purely on a symptomatic basis and limited to short periods of time to supplement standard antidepressant therapy.

THE CONCEPT OF PANIC-DEPRESSIVE ILLNESS

The clinical considerations reviewed in this chapter (and throughout this volume) support the notion that some forms of anxious-depressive comorbidity might represent alternative expressions of the same diathesis (Breier, Charney, and Heninger 1985a, b; Leckman, Weissman, Merikangas, et al. 1983; Wolpe 1986). Analogous to manic-depressive illness, where manic and depressive phases occur at different points in time, and sometimes in a mixed state (Kraepelin 1921), one can postulate that existence of a triphasic "panic-depressive" disorder consisting of panic, depressive, and anxious-depressive phases (Akiskal 1986b). Furthermore, analogous to the existence of overlapping temperaments in the premorbid and inter-episodic phases of bipolar illness, one can envision the existence of overlapping personality attributes in panic-depressive illness. Indeed recent research findings suggest that the personalities of panic and nonbipolar depressive patients overlap considerably, representing variations on the theme of obsessionality, neuroticism, avoidance, and dependency (Akiskal 1988).

The hypothesized panic-depressive disorder would respond to a variety of antidepressants and to brief psychotherapeutic modalities, whether psychodynamic or cognitive-behavioral. Furthermore, beta-receptor down-regulation might represent a hypothesized final common pathway mechanism of action of both pharmacotherapy and psychotherapy (Akiskal 1985a). By contrast, cyclic depressions related to manic-depressive illness would be less responsive to such interventions and might actually get worse with TCAs (Kukopulos, Reginaldi, Floris, et al. 1980; Wehr and Goodwin 1987); therapeutic responses would occur primarily with those interventions that impact positively on circadian rhythms and mineral metabolism (e.g., sleep deprivation, phototherapy, lithium, ECT).

These considerations have important bearing on the relationship of anxiety and depressive disorders and the various dichotomies of affective illness (Kendell 1976). Some depressions seem to cluster with anxiety neuroses (Tyrer 1985), others pursue a more periodic or a cyclic course and appear to be part of a bipolar spectrum with either personal or familial history for mania (Akiskal 1983a). In other words, the various dichotomies of affective illness might be reclassified under a hypothesized dichotomy of "panic-depressive" versus "manic-depressive" illness.

OTHER CLINICAL EXPLANATIONS FOR COMORBIDITY

Much of the foregoing clinical discussion has focused on comorbidity of depression with generalized anxiety and panic disorders. Anxiety-depressive comorbidity with obsessive-compulsive, social phobic, and posttraumatic stress disorders is also common, yet more complex than what has already been presented. It is also beyond the scope of this chapter to consider mixed states of bipolar disorder where anxiety symptoms figure prominently (Akiskal and Mallya 1987; Cassano, Maggini, and Akiskal 1983). These anxious-depressive presentations of mixed bipolar states are important from the clinician's perspective as they are notoriously refractory to TCAs and MAOI drugs. Actually, TCA treatment of retarded depressions can sometimes provoke such mixed states iatrogenically (Cassano, Maggini, and Akiskal 1983); the same applies to stimulant self-treatment of retarded depressions (VanValkenburg, Akiskal, Puzantian, et al. 1984). Mixed states respond favorably to lithium carbonate (with or without neuroleptics), carbamazepine, or ECT (Akiskal 1985b). Finally, I have not discussed the varying admixtures of irritability, panic, terror, depression, and suicidal ideation (along with other pleomorphic psychopathologic manifestations) that occur in the setting of complex partial seizures or variants (Blumer, Heilbronn, and Himmelhoch 1988). The existence of this epileptiform condition lends support to Hippocrates' contention that

> from the brain, and from the brain only, arise our pleasures, joys, laughters, and jests, as well as our sorrows, pains, griefs and tears . . . It is the same thing which makes us mad or delirious, inspires us with dread and fear, whether by night or by day, brings sleeplessness, inopportune mistakes, aimless anxieties, absent-mindedness, and acts that are contrary to habit. These things that we suffer all come from the brain, when it is not healthy. [the Sacred Disease]

CONCLUDING REMARKS

The selective literature reviewed in this chapter—focusing primarily on generalized anxiety, panic, and major depressive disorders—suggest that heterogeneous clinical conditions underlie the comorbidity of anxiety and depressive disorders.

In conditions commonly encountered in primary care settings—whether mental health centers, psychological counseling, or general medical practice—such comorbidity might represent alternative expressions of the same diathesis. I have proposed the designation "panic-depressive disorder" for this entity. Whether the two affective conditions are alternative phenotypes of a common *genetic* diathesis represents an attractive possibility for which evidence is inconclusive at this time. Some evidence exists for the position that the depressions in many patients beginning with panic attacks are "secondary" to the panic disorder (i.e., without independent genetic predisposition to depression) (Crowe, Noyes, Pauls, et al. 1983; Lesser, Rubin, Pecknold, et al. 1988; Sheehan 1986). Related to this position is Torgersen's (1985b) suggestion that these depressions are due to the adverse consequences of being raised by an anxious (or panic-prone) mother.

In other cases, comorbid anxiety and depressive states might represent distinct disorders with symptomatologic overlap representing the following circumstances: (1) (atypical) depressive presentations of anxiety neurosis; (2) anxious presentations of melancholia; (3) depression plus sedative-hypnotic withdrawal; (4) depression plus stimulant (amphetamine, cocaine, or caffeine) abuse; (5) mixed (bipolar) states; and (6) pleomorphic manifestations of complex partial seizures or their variants.

Psychiatry conceived in the Hippocratic tradition has benefited greatly from naturalistic observations that support such differential outcomes for complex clinical situations as comorbid anxiety-depressive symptomatology. I have argued that the different conditions delineated in this chapter call for different—sometimes overlapping, at other times opposite—treatment approaches. As dedication to the alleviation of suffering is the most important calling of the doctor, such treatment prediction represents the most important validator of clinical phenomenology. Alternatively, although much uncertainty surrounds the biologic underpinnings of the treatments for anxiety and depressive disorders, the emerging trends in the psychopharmacologic literature tend to support the existence of overlapping as well as distinct neurobiologic substrates for anxiety and depression (Uhde, Roy-Byrne, Vittone, et al. 1985). The precise delineation of these biologic mechanisms represents one of the major challenges of the medical science of psychiatry. Cloninger, Martin, Guze, et al.'s approach (Chapter 27) to delineate selected personality attributes—with their respective hypothesized biologic substrates—in the predisposition to clinical subtypes of anxiety and dysphoric states is a promising beginning along these lines.

The medical art of psychiatry in the complex interface of anxiety and depression consists of making rational therapeutic and prognostic judgments about patients with mixed manifestations who may or may not fit into the various clinical situations discussed in this chapter. Further refinements in clinical observation, taking neurobiologic advances into consideration, are expected to shed new light into the fascinating interface of anxiety and depressive disorders.

Section VIII
Research Issues, Methodology, and Assessment

Chapter 34

Relationship Between Anxiety and Depression: Conceptual and Methodological Issues

Keith S. Dobson, Ph.D.
Elsie Cheung, M.A.

IN MANY CONTEXTS researchers attempt to eliminate experimental confounds: factors that covary with the independent or dependent variables involved in the investigation, or that add "error variance" to the results of the study. In the case of the constructs of anxiety and depression, the evidence is overwhelming that these factors covary. The current volume is a testament to the observation of confounded constructs, and the various chapters reflect the complexity of the conceptual, empirical, and methodological issues of such confounding.

This chapter will focus particularly on the methodological and statistical issues that emerge in the context of covariation of the anxiety and depression constructs. To discuss these issues adequately, some of the theoretical issues involved in construct covariation will be examined briefly, and some of the emerging patterns of observations regarding anxiety and depression covariation will be highlighted. The latter aspect of this chapter will deal with issues that derive from theoretical formulations and empirical observations, such

An earlier version of this chapter was presented at the Conference on Symptom Comorbidity in Anxiety and Depressive Disorders, Tuxedo Park, New York, September 1987.

as methods of assessment, sample characteristics, use of statistics, and research design issues. The chapter will conclude with suggestions for promising areas of future research.

MODELS OF PSYCHOPATHOLOGY

Despite the history of the observation that anxiety and depressive states tend to co-occur, it is notable that very few models of the covarying states exist (for an exception, see Costello 1976). Most of the work on these states has focused on either anxiety *or* depressive states and disorders, with only empirical or descriptive accounts of the co-variation between the two. This descriptive literature, while large and suggestive of conceptual links between the two states, has only recently been examined for potential convergence.

The importance of conceptual models cannot be understated. These models will dictate the level(s) of analysis conducted, the type(s) of data collected, the research designs employed, and the statistics used to analyze the data, all of which in turn will reflect back on the conceptual model used to drive the research investigation. For example, if the conceptual model of a particular investigator involves the definition of anxiety and depression as the results of two distinct disease or disorder processes, their research investigation is likely (1) to employ a diagnostic, categorical approach to the definition of research subjects; (2) to invoke certain a priori decision rules about the symptoms that define each disease entity; and (3) to invoke statistics that either necessitate dichotomous variables (e.g., contingency analyses) or those that employ dichotomizing procedures (e.g., analysis of variance, discriminant function analysis). By contrast, researchers who consider anxiety and depression more as dimensional constructs are (1) less likely to categorize or diagnose subjects; (2) more likely to classify subjects by assigning a dimensional score to the severity of their state; (3) likely to select subject samples from a wider range of functioning; and (4) more likely to invoke correlational statistics (e.g., Pearson product moment correlations, factor analysis) than are researchers who conceptualize anxiety and depression as distinct disorders.

The point of the above discussion is not to suggest that one or the other of the two dominant conceptual perspectives encapsulated in the two examples given is correct, or even preferred. Rather, the point is that the underlying conceptual model will be related to the methodology and statistics employed. In this context it is important for investigators to be aware of their conceptual model, to use language appropriate to their conceptual model, and to recognize that alternative perspectives exist. Within this chapter the term *comorbidity* will be used to refer to the co-variation of anxiety and depression diagnoses; the term *correlation* will be used to refer to the co-variation of dimensional anxiety and depression scores. *Co-variation* will be used as the generic term for either comorbidity or correlation. It is suggested that there are three critical aspects of conceptual models that will affect research both within each construct and in examining co-variation. These issues are those of (1) dimensional versus categorical models, (2) trait versus episodic models, and (3) the level of analysis (affect, symptom, syndrome).

Dimensional Versus Categorical Models

One of the most fundamental, and possibly the most contentious, issues facing psychopathology researchers is whether to adopt a dimensional (i.e., quantitative) or categorical (i.e., qualitative) perspective to their domain of research. Within the fields of anxiety and depression, both perspectives are evident. There are dimensional measures of anxiety (Cattell and Sheier 1961; Costello and Comrey 1967; Endler and Okada 1975; Spielberger, Gorsuch, and Luschene 1970; Zuckerman and Lubin 1965) and dimensional measures of depression (Beck, Ward, Mendelson, et al. 1961; Carroll, Feinberg, Smouse, et al. 1981; Costello and Comrey 1967; Hamilton 1960; Zuckerman and Lubin 1965; Zung 1965). There are also categorical systems for the diagnosis of both anxiety and depressive disorders such as the *Diagnostic and Statistical Manual of Mental Disorders* (DSM-III-R) (American Psychiatric Association 1987) and the Research Diagnostic Criteria (RDC) (Endicott and Spitzer 1978). The dimensional measures implicitly highlight the severity dimension of anxiety or depressive experience, while diagnostic systems highlight the judgment about the presence or absence of a clinically important anxiety or depressive experience. Clinical importance may be ascertained in a number of fashions, the chief of which have to do with the consistent clustering of symptoms, specific known psychopathologic or pathophysiologic processes that eventuate in the disorders, treatment response predicted by diagnoses, the relative purity of the diagnoses (i.e., lack of overlap with other diagnoses or discriminative validity), and the typical course or prognosis of the diagnosis.

Without reviewing each of the above areas for evidence that is supportive of either a dimensional or categorical perspective for the problems of anxiety and depression, it is a fair conclusion that the data at present are inconclusive as to whether one or the other perspective is the closest approximation of reality. Indeed, it is possible that neither model is correct and that some other, unenunciated model is the most comprehensive and accurate. It is notable that research investigations often employ both diagnostic and dimensional assessment procedures, with a view to obtaining the most possible information about research subjects. It is also notable, as one specific instance of the possible rapprochement between dimensional and categorical systems, that the diagnosis of major depressive disorder in DSM-III-R employs a dimensional model (counting the number of present symptoms) that is then converted into a categorical diagnosis (major depressive disorder or not) through the operation of a decision rule (i.e., four or more symptoms qualifies a person for the diagnosis). Such decision rules, were they to be developed and applied to other diagnostic categories, may help to make explicit the relationship between dimensional and categorical approaches to psychopathology.

Trait Versus Episodic Models

The idea that there may be a relatively stable predisposition to respond to various situations with anxiety (i.e., trait anxiety) is not a new concept (Spielberger 1975; Taylor 1953). It has also been widely accepted that state, or episodic, anxiety also exists (American Psychiatric Association 1987; Spielberger 1975). Interestingly, although the concept of state depression (i.e., episodes of depression) exists and some authors have advocated ideas about depressive personality or depressive biases (Arieti and Bemporad 1978; Beck 1976; Chodoff 1974), and even though the diagnosis of dysthymia implies a persistent depressive tendency (American Psychiatric Association 1987), there is not a well-articulated and accepted concept of trait depression (Dobson 1985c; for an exception, see Zuckerman and Lubin 1965).

Although the lack of development of a trait depression model is interesting on theoretical grounds, it is of particular relevance here due to the implications for co-variation and its assessment. Since the only shared conceptions between anxiety and depression at the state, or episodic, level have been developed, co-variation may be pursued only at this level. Current conceptual models and methodologies do not easily permit investigation of co-variation between trait (or dispositional) tendencies in anxiety and depression.

Level of Analysis

Co-variation between constructs can be approached from a number of perspectives. Dependent on the type of analysis, certain types of information may be relevant, and certain methodological and statistical conventions become possible. Within the relationship between anxiety and depression, co-variation may be examined at each of the levels of mood, symptom, and syndrome.

Examinations of mood are typically conducted through self-report scales that assess mood on a dimensional basis. For example, the Multiple Affect Adjective Check List (MAACL) (Zuckerman and Lubin 1965) assesses the degree of anxiety, depression, and hostility by examining the self-descriptiveness of affect adjectives. Such assessment tools yield dimensional scores that lend themselves readily to correlational analyses. In addition, researchers may employ affect severity scales that are uniquely created for the research setting. Examples of such methods include 1-to-7 rating scales and 100-point visual analogue scales. Although cutoff scores can be imposed to classify subjects, such procedures may artificially divide subjects who are only one or two points apart on the dimensional scale into different subject categories. Any cutoffs established for blocking subjects into groups need conceptual and empirical founding (Kendall, Hollon, Beck, et al. 1987).

Symptoms and symptom patterns have been approached from both a dimensional and categorical perspective. The severity of either specific symptoms or groups of symptoms can be examined in relation to other potential modifiers through correlational analyses. Symptom patterns have also been investigated through clinical judgment about the presence or absence of a clinically relevant amount of the symptom. These dichotomous judgments can then be examined through contingency analyses or analyses that deal with dichotomous variables (e.g., discriminant function analysis). Also, comorbidity of symptoms can be investigated through contingency analyses or other such procedures.

At the level of syndromes a priori criteria are imposed to classify subjects into diagnostic categories. These diagnoses can then be examined for evidence of comorbidity. Also, probability analyses of syndromes may be undertaken. It is important that researchers know and recognize the critical importance of the a priori criteria invoked in diagnostic categories (Frances, Widiger, and Fyer, Chapter 3). A nonexhaustive list of issues that affect subject categorization, and therefore estimates of comorbidity, includes (1) the relationship of symptoms to diagnoses; (2) inclusion and exclusion criteria for diagnostic categories; (3) implicit models of psychopathology used by diagnosticians; (4) the sensitivity and specificity of the diagnoses; and (5) the procedures used for the collection of symptom report.

In summary, the level of analyses with which the investigator approaches the issue of co-variation will be important in terms of the choice of assessment method used. The level of analysis adopted will also have direct implications for the types of statistical analyses to which the collected data can be subjected. Again, investigators need to be cognizant of their own conceptual biases and the influences that these biases have for methodological and statistical innovation.

PATTERNS OF ANXIETY-DEPRESSION CO-VARIATION

The focus of this chapter is on methodological issues involved in examining the co-variation between anxiety and depression. However, it is important to note what is emerging as the pattern of co-variation to choose optimal research strategies to investigate the phenomenon. In this section the results of both correlational and comorbidity studies will be briefly reviewed, and some suggestions about the emergent overall pattern of anxiety-depression co-variation will be offered.

It has been noted that dimensional scales of anxiety and depression are highly correlated (Dobson 1985a, 1985c; Mendels, Weinstein and Cochrane 1972). In a large review of studies that provided correlations among anxiety and depression scales, Dobson (1985c) documented that the average correlation across the constructs was approximately that within each construct. Thus he found that the average correlation was .66 among 8 anxiety scales and .69 among 30 depression scales, but that the average correlation between 34 anxiety and depression scales was .61. This pattern of results suggests a remarkable *lack* of discriminative validity between the constructs of anxiety and depression, at least in terms of dimensional systems of assessment.

It is important to keep in mind that researchers developing the scales reviewed by Dobson (1985c) were not interested in maximizing discriminative validity. Indeed, each of the researchers was most interested in providing a measure of anxiety or depression that maximized construct validity. The high intercorrelational values between anxiety and depression scales may, therefore, be a true reflection of the nature of these constructs. There are two pieces of evidence that suggest, however, that the degree of convergent validity demonstrated by existing dimensional scales is higher than perhaps it should be.

The first piece of evidence that challenges the need for high correlation between anxiety and depression scales comes from Dobson (1985b). In a series of studies he developed an interactional measure of anxiety and depression that had lower correlations than traditional measures. Beginning with a theoretical definition of anxiety and depression, Dobson collected items from existing scales of anxiety and depression and also wrote original items to reflect content not well captured in existing scales. These item pools were then administered to a large sample of subjects, and a process of item selection was begun (Jackson 1970). This selection process included the removal of items with low variance (these items are not generally able to discriminate among subjects), the comparison of item correlations within and across constructs (items with higher correlations with the opposite scale than their own scale were removed), the removal of items loading highly on social desirability, and a final confirmation of "pure" scales through factor analysis. Pure scales were then paired with potential situational determinants of anxiety and depression, and situation × person scales of anxiety and depression were formed.

These scales were then administered to large groups of male and female subjects. For 157 females, the average correlation was .68 among anxiety scales and .60 among depression scales; between anxiety and depression it was .44. Similarly, for 119 males, the average correlation was .71 among anxiety scales and .58 among depression scales; between anxiety and depression it was .41. These results suggest that construct valid scales for anxiety and depression can be developed, even while these scales show improved discriminative validity to other dimensional measures of anxiety and depression.

Another curious piece of information that suggests that current anxiety and depression scales may be able to be more "fine-tuned," to permit better discrimination of constructs, derives from studies in which subjects were classified on the basis of dimensional scales. Although the methodology of placing subjects into categories based on dimensional scales is controversial (cf., Kendall, Hollon, Beck, et al. 1987), what is relevant here is that there are several studies where attempts to establish independent two × two research groups (high versus low anxiety and depression, based on predetermined cutoff scores on dimensional scales) were thwarted by the inability to identify sufficient numbers of high depressed × low anxious subjects (Gotlib and Asarnow 1979; Kennedy and Craighead 1979; Miller, Seligman, and Kurlander 1975). Thus all of the cells to this research design were able to be filled, except the one where depression was elevated but anxiety was not. This observation again implies that anxiety and depression are correlated constructs. It also raises the idea, as yet unexplored, that the optimal line to describe the relationship between anxiety and depression is not a straight line, as is used in correlational techniques, but a curve. Figure 1 presents a hypothetical relationship between anxiety and depression that would eventuate in high correlations, but that also could account for the observation that depressed but nonanxious subjects are difficult to locate. Studies of the relationship between anxiety and depression could be conducted to locate lines of best fit in such correlational data. Such research could help to explain patterns of co-variation between these

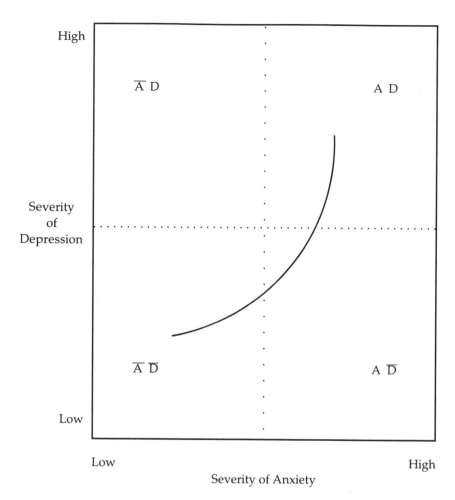

Figure 1. The hypothetical relationship between anxiety and depression dimensional scales. (A = anxiety present; D = depression present; $\overline{A}$ = anxiety not present; $\overline{D}$ = depression not present)

two constructs (Alloy, Kelly, Mineka, et al., Chapter 29).

In addition to investigations of correlational patterns between anxiety and depression scales, a growing body of literature provides estimates of the coexistence of anxiety and depressive disorders. These cross-classification studies typically examine either the presence of concomitant anxiety disorders in patients seen for affective disorders, or the converse. Another version of cross-classification studies that also bear on the issue of co-variation are those in which anxiety and depressive symptoms are examined in patients seen for affective or anxiety disorders. Although a major review of this literature is not proposed here, there is an emerging pattern of cross-classification that is noteworthy.

One of the earliest studies to examine co-variation in anxious and depressed patients was Downing and Rickels (1974). In that study patients were identified as primarily anxiety or depression cases and were assigned to a clinical trial based on this designation. Of relevance for the issue of co-variation are a set of physician ratings made on the subjects in this study. Physicians rated both anxiety and depression on a 1 to 7 scale in all subjects. Anxious patients were low on depression (mean, 3.5) but high on anxiety (mean, 4.6), whereas the depressed patients were rated high on depression (mean, 4.6) and high on anxiety (mean, 4.45). This pattern of ratings is consistent with the general conclusion from the literature reviewed above, in that it appears that while anxiety may appear as a relatively distinct condition, depression typically does not.

Further support for the hypothesis that depression in an individual predicts anxiety, but not the converse, can be gleaned from epidemiologic and clinical studies where secondary anxiety and affective diagnoses are made in patients who meet diagnostic criteria for another disorder. Although the quantity of such studies is small, the pattern that emerges from an examination of cross-classification studies is that depressed patients are also likely to be anxious, but not necessarily the reverse.

There are several studies where depressed patients have been examined for secondary disorders, including anxiety disorders (Barlow, Di Nardo, Vermilyea, et al. 1986; Leckman, Weissman, Merikangas, et al. 1983; Regier, Burke, and Burke, Chapter 6). When the comorbidity of anxiety disorders in depressed patients is examined, the rate of anxious comorbidity ranges from 42% to 100%, with an average of approximately 67%. In contrast, when rates of depression comorbidity in anxious patients are examined, the range of comorbidity is only 17% to 65%, with an average of approximately 40% (Barlow, Di Nardo, Vermilyea, et al. 1986; Clancy, Noyes, Hoenk, et al. 1978; Dealy, Ishiki, Avery, et al. 1981; Di Nardo and Barlow, Chapter 12; Regier, Burke, and Burke, Chapter 6; Roth, Gurney, Garside, et al. 1972). Although comorbidity figures of 67% and 40% must be considered approximate—due to the disparities between the above studies in diagnostic criteria, diagnostic nosologies, subject sampling methods, and the various unreliabilities associated with diagnosis in general—they tend to support the hypothesis that depressed individuals will evidence anxiety, but that anxious individuals are less likely to show diagnosable levels of depression. Obviously, even a comorbidity of 40% depression in anxiety is worth consideration, but the main point is the relative degree of comorbidity.

An extension of the above estimated rates of comorbidity between anxiety and depression would be to imagine the hypothetical joint distribution of these two disorders. Based on prevalence rates of 4% for depressive disorders and 8% for anxiety disorders, Table 1 provides a hypothesized joint distribution (the figures do not exactly correspond to cross-classification rates of 40% and 67%). One interesting line of research would be to take a large and representative community or clinical sample of subjects and to compute an actual joint distribution of diagnoses. The approximation of the hypothetical to the actual distributions could then be examined to determine if the "depression as a subset of anxiety" (Alloy, Kelly, Mineka, et al., Chapter 29) hypothesis is supported.

To conclude this section, it has been suggested that the emerging pattern of co-variation between anxiety and depression is that depression strongly predicts anxiety, but that the reverse is less likely. Alloy, Kelly, Mineka, et al. (Chapter 29) suggest that cognitive mechanisms might account for this pattern of disorders, and other authors have attempted to account for aspects of this formulation (Costello 1976; Dobson 1985c). As others also have pointed out, the field lacks an appreciable amount of longitudinal research in this area. Research on the course of these disorders could, for example, examine the future probability of developing either anxiety or depression subsequently to the other, thereby again addressing the potential pattern of depression following, or being a subset of, anxiety. There is some evidence that prior anxiety is more commonly associated with later depression than the reverse (Angst, Vollrath, Merikangas, et al., Chapter 7; Kendell 1974). This is an area deserving more research attention.

Table 1.   Hypothetical Joint Distribution of the Diagnoses of Anxiety and Depression

Anxiety condition	Depression condition		
	No diagnosis	Diagnosis given	Population %
No diagnosis	91.0	1.0	92.0
Diagnosis given	5.0	3.0	8.0
Population %	96.0	4.0	100.0

Note.   The numbers provided above are hypothetical, but are consistent with a 4% prevalence rate of depressive disorders, an 8% prevalence rate of anxiety disorders, and the emerging patterns of cross-classification.

Methodological Issues

Studies of co-variation in general, and anxiety and depression in particular, raise a number of methodological issues and problems. In this section, some of the areas where issues and problems are likely to arise will be identified, and potential methods to handle the issues and circumvent these problems will be discussed. Four major areas will be examined in turn; namely, methods of assessment, research sample characteristics, statistical methods, and research design issues.

Methods of Assessment

The areas of anxiety and depression have, by virtue of their incidence and prevalence, received considerable assessment attention. A number of distinct approaches have been pursued within the assessment literature. These approaches can be divided along the dimensions of quantitative versus qualitative, self-report versus interviewer, and trait versus state. If one reviews common exemplars of assessment instruments that are encompassed within the above categorizations, most assess self-reported state or episodic anxiety or depression (Lipman 1982; Rehm, Chapter 35; Shaw, Vallis, and McCabe 1985). Self-report diagnostic scales are a recent phenomenon, and as such are of unproven value. By contrast, there are several well-known and developed clinical interviews that are based on diagnostic systems (American Psychiatric Association 1987; Endicott and Spitzer 1978; Spitzer and Williams 1985b).

A number of issues arise in the use of self-report anxiety and depression scales. First, using these scales to assess comorbidity presupposes that respondents can adequately distinguish anxiety from depression, or at least make the discriminations demanded by the assessment scale. In global scales of anxiety and depression, such presupposition may not be valid. The overlap between anxiety and depression may be so substantial that respondents will confuse the two constructs. Alternatively, the overlap may be so substantial that respondents will view anxiety and depression as a unitary construct (Gotlib 1984; Watson and Clark 1984) and assign ratings randomly or according to whichever of the two constructs they view as the stronger exemplar of the unitary construct.

Even with self-report scales that do not employ a global assessment scheme, valid responses require the ability of the respondent to distinguish the internal signs and states being studied. In the case of the concurrent assessment of anxiety and depression, there may be a differential ability to detect these signs and states. In the domain of cognitive components, for example, it appears that depressive cognitions are reasonably amenable to assessment (Dobson and Shaw 1986; Segal and Shaw 1988; Shaw and Dobson 1979). This ease of assessment, however, is not the case for anxiety. For example, a reasonable proportion of patients with panic disorder fail to report any cognitions surrounding their anxiety states (Rachman, Levitt, and Lopatka 1987). By contrast, it may be easier to conduct valid behavioral assessments in the area of anxiety. Anxiety states involve behavioral excesses that may be easier to detect and self-report than the behavioral deficits typically associated with depressive states. For example, it may be easier to detect the presence of panic in anxiety disorders than to detect anhedonia in depression.

Just as self-report measures of anxiety and depression are open to problems of validity, interview-based methods of anxiety and depression can also be affected by the differential ease of detecting anxiety and depression symptoms. In particular, since some anxiety symptoms are more available to public observation (e.g., avoidance, withdrawal, tremulousness), these symptoms may be more easy to detect than such signs and symptoms of depression as sad affect or decreased motivation. Beyond these issues, interviewer-based assessment schemes are subject to a number of other biases (Frances, Widiger, and Fyer, Chapter 3).

Based on the above discussion, it is apparent that researchers investigating either anxiety or depression alone, or their co-variation, need to consider their assessment tools carefully. The selection of a particular dependent variable will dictate the ability of the study to demonstrate meaningful results. The informativeness and degree of ambiguity of the data are directly affected by the choice of measures.

One basic requirement for a meaningful assessment measure is that it reflects the construct of interest. One implication of this requirement in the area of co-variation is that scales should validly represent both constructs and should also be sensitive to individual differences in both areas. Another requirement for assessment measures is sensitivity to the type and magnitude of change in the construct(s). In the concurrent investigation of anxiety and depression, the measures should be sensitive to changes in both of the domains of anxiety and depression. Ideally, the measures should demonstrate (1) equal propensity for detecting change in both domains, (2) equal potential for detecting bi-directional change in both domains, and (3) freedom from the restrictions of floor and ceiling effects. These criteria become even more complicated when using multiple measures. Within the assessment of one domain, multiple measures may show discordance with each other (e.g., Prusoff, Klerman, and Paykel 1972) or show differential sensitivity to change

(Lambert, Hatch, Kingston, et al. 1986). Relatively little information exists about the differential sensitivities of assessment scales in anxiety and depression, and even less is known about the differential sensitivities of assessment scales across the two domains.

In addition to the specific problems of potential differential appropriateness and sensitivity of assessment methods in measuring the two constructs, there are some general issues that emerge. If a particular assessment method is employed and a high correlation is obtained (Dobson 1985a; Mendels, Weinstein, and Cochrane 1972), two possibilities exist. First, there may be a true relationship between the two constructs. Alternatively, the correlation may emerge as a direct result of shared method variance. To document that a correlation does not result from shared method variance, assessment methods should demonstrate both convergent validity and simultaneous discriminant validity where the measures are not conceptually related (Campbell and Fiske 1959). Such demonstrations are notably lacking in the area of the co-variation of anxiety and depression.

In summary, there are a number of ideal criteria that assessment methods will meet, whether they are assessing a single construct or are involved in the assessment of correlated constructs. A review of the domains of anxiety and depression unfortunately leads to the conclusion that the available assessment techniques may not meet the criteria very well. They are highly intercorrelated and do not demonstrate discriminant validity from each other or other domains (Gotlib 1984). Further, differential sensitivity to change has been demonstrated in depression scales. Similar research has yet to be conducted on anxiety scales. A safe conclusion is that systematic review of assessment procedures in the co-variation of anxiety and depression is timely (Rehm, Chapter 35). It is likely that some revisions of existing scales are warranted, or it may even be necessary to create new and better assessment methods.

Research Sample Characteristics

The selection of research subjects obviously has implications for the results of the individual study and their generalizability (Kazdin 1980). In this section we will focus on four subject issues that are of particular importance in the area of co-variation: (1) sociodemographic variables, (2) sex ratios, (3) psychiatric status, and (4) recruitment procedures and primary-secondary diagnoses.

Sociodemographic variables are an ever-present concern for clinical investigators, as the selection of different subject groups directly affects the investigation's generalizability. In the area of anxiety and depression, epidemiologic studies (Boyd and Weissman 1981; Reich

1986; Wing and Bebbington 1985) suggest that sociodemographic variables may be important as moderators of study results. For example, low socioeconomic status anxious patients have been demonstrated to have a qualitatively different factorial structure of their symptom patterns than those from other social classes, leading some researchers (Derogatis, Lipman, Covi, et al. 1972; Prusoff and Klerman 1974) to exclude low socioeconomic status anxious patients from their samples. This strategy improves the internal validity of the particular study, but at the expense of generalizability and external validity. To date, studies of sociodemographic variables *across* the domains of anxiety and depression are nonexistent, and constitute one area where studies are needed.

Sex ratios between anxiety and depressive disorders are generally similar (Dobson 1985c; Reich 1986; Wing and Bebbington 1985). Generalized anxiety disorder has approximately the same sex ratio as major depressive disorder. This concordance suggests that investigators must be sensitive to the sex ratio of their subject samples. Representative investigations should be sex-stratified in line with the known sex ratio (approximately two or three females to one male), or else need to identify their nonrepresentative nature explicitly. Further, to the extent that the sex ratio across diagnostic categories is disparate (Marks 1969), investigators may need samples that also reflect the sex ratios of the disorders in the population.

Subjects used to investigate co-variation between anxiety and depression will vary in their psychiatric status. Subjects used to date include college students, community volunteers, and psychiatric outpatients and inpatients. These different samples may well result in differing subject characteristics, different constellations of symptoms, and differing symptom severity. Researchers are appropriately circumspect in their desire to generalize results from one sample to others, and in qualifying their results by the psychiatric status of the sample employed. Although some phenomena appear to generalize across samples, others do not. Again, this is an area where co-variation patterns in anxiety and depression are not understood, as there is no body of literature.

A fourth area of subject selection concern has to do with the process of subject recruitment and selection. Many subjects are selected for research and treatment studies from specialty clinics whose primary focus is on either anxiety or depression. Such specialty clinics may introduce biases in research samples in at least two ways. First, the researcher may hold biases about the base rate of clinical conditions that are skewed in line with the specialty clinic's area of work. Such biases, if present, may affect diagnostic processes and decisions, subject conceptualization, and the ability to determine comorbidity.

Furthermore, specialty clinics may elicit selected responses from subjects. Patients may focus on and actually exaggerate their anxiety symptoms when presenting to an anxiety clinic, whereas patients may focus more on depressive signs and symptoms in a depression clinic.

The issue of specialty clinics and symptoms presentation dovetails with the issue of primary and secondary diagnoses. For many studies it is critical to determine if one or the other of two comorbid diagnoses is primary or predominant. Objective determination of dominant and secondary diagnoses may be made more difficult in settings where research requirements necessitate certain primary diagnoses. Researchers, to the largest extent possible, need to be aware of such potential diagnostic biases and to ensure that such biases are minimized in their practice. The convention of using standardized diagnostic instruments and decision trees (Burke, Wittchen, Regier, et al., Chapter 36) is a major development in this context.

STATISTICAL ISSUES

This section surveys the various statistical techniques that may be useful in studying the co-variation between anxiety and depression. These statistical techniques can be categorized by the various purposes that they serve (exploratory versus confirmatory). For exploratory purposes, descriptive techniques are appropriate. Descriptive techniques include correlational procedures such as simple correlations, factor analysis, cluster analysis, and multidimensional scaling. These techniques are designed to summarize the co-variation among certain items, behaviors, or symptoms. In doing so, these techniques provide descriptive information about the construct of interest. Consequently, these techniques can address such questions as what are the underlying structures or dimensions of anxiety and depression; do anxiety and depression emerge as separate constructs; and do anxiety and depression have different factorial structures?

One advantage of correlational techniques is that they can summarize a large amount of information. For example, factor analysis can determine that most of the variance of numerous self-report measures can be summarized by a few factors (Dobson 1985a; Gotlib 1984). Another advantage is that these techniques can be atheoretical; the researcher does not need specific a priori hypotheses. These techniques, however, are not entirely objective. Decisions by the researcher can affect the solution at various stages. First, the researcher decides on the pool of items (e.g., symptoms, behaviors) used in the study. The results of descriptive techniques are dependent on the pool of items because a factor cannot emerge if the relevant items that might load on that factor were not incorporated into the item pool. Second, the researcher decides on the number of dimensions (in the instance of multidimensional scaling), factors (in factor analysis), or clusters (in cluster analysis) that are interpreted in the solution to the procedure used. Although there are guidelines on such interpretations, the final decision is likely to be guided by interpretability, which is theory-driven. Even the process of labeling solutions to correlational procedures is guided by the conceptual model of the investigator and is therefore subject to subjective bias.

One example, cited by Stavrakaki and Vargo (1986), is of relevance here. They reported the similar factor analytic patterns that emerged in two studies of the relationship between anxiety and depression (Mendels, Weinstein, and Cochrane 1972; Mountjoy and Roth 1982a). Both studies found a substantial first factor of general symptom severity, which Mendels, Weinstein, and Cochrane cited as evidence of the inseparability of anxiety and depression. Mountjoy and Roth, by contrast, proceeded to interpret a second smaller "bipolar" anxiety-depression factor, which they further used in a discriminant function analysis, to emphasize the discriminability of anxiety and depression states.

In contrast to summarizing types of correlational analyses, studies may ask if and how anxiety and depression may be differentiated. In this regard, some studies have employed discriminant function analysis (e.g., Mountjoy and Roth 1982a), which attempts to determine among a set of variables which items maximally discriminate or separate categorical groups. Three points about this procedure are critical. First, as with factor analysis and other summarizing techniques, multidimensional scaling results depend on the initial pool of items in the study. Second, discriminant function analysis assumes that the categorical groups can validly be differentiated. As with any statistical methods, discriminant function analysis is "blind" to external validity and is designed to force a mathematical solution even if that solution is nonsensical or trivial. Finally, the solutions to discriminant function analyses are often specific to the subject sample. When these analyses are cross-validated with independent samples, there are often significant degrees of "shrinkage" in the groups' discriminability. Although discriminant function analyses can incorporate cross-validation (Cloninger, Sigvardsson, von Knorring, et al. 1984), the lack of cross-validation of most discriminant procedures leaves the possibility that published studies reflect inflated estimates of the discriminability of the anxiety and depression constructs.

One statistical method is that curiously absent in the anxiety-depression co-variation literature is multidimensional scaling (Torgerson 1958). Procedures such as INDSCAL (Carroll and Chang 1970) were originally designed to illustrate individual differences by taking the dimensions from a multidimensional scaling solution (similar in many respects to factor and cluster analyses), and then determining individual differences by plotting individuals on the various dimensions. This type of analysis could be applied to the study of anxiety and depression, as suggested by Blashfield (Chapter 4), in that underlying dimensions of anxiety and depression could be potentially generated from multidimensional scaling results. Individuals' anxiety and depression scores could then be entered into an INDSCAL procedure to see how individual differences in anxiety and depression are reflected in the results of the procedure. Implications for the unidimensional versus multidimensional models of anxiety and depression would be manifest in the results of such a study.

So far, this section has focused on exploratory and descriptive statistical methods. Inferential statistical methods, such as analysis of variance (ANOVA) and multivariate analysis of variance (MANOVA) try to infer whether there are significant group differences on the dependent measures used in a given study. Implicit in the use of these statistics is the validity of the independent variable. In the area of anxiety and depression, the use of ANOVA and MANOVA to assess the impact of various grouping variables (e.g., age groups, sex, ethnicity) on anxiety and depressive patterns as dependent variables is not particularly problematic.

Using anxiety and/or depression as an independent variable and assessing the impact of these categories on other dependent variables, however, may be more difficult to defend. For one, significant degrees of anxiety are also present in depression (Dobson 1985c; Downing and Rickels 1974). As such, using depression status as an independent variable means that subjects' anxiety status is also being manipulated. Although procedures such as analysis of co-variance can remove the variability in the dependent variables' scores associated with anxiety, such adjusted scores may not reflect validly the true nature of depression. Second, the potential patterns of correlation and comorbidity (see Table 1) may make the study of co-variation through the simultaneous categorization of anxiety and depression status impossible. There may simply be insufficient numbers of nonanxious but depressed subjects available for investigation.

The use of ANOVAs and MANOVAs involve certain assumptions that, when violated, may affect the validity of these procedures (Kirk 1982). Although these assumptions are likely violated in the study of anxiety and depression, they are often left untested. For example, these procedures assume that the variables studied are normally distributed. Given what is now known about the symptoms patterns of anxiety and depression, however, such an assumption is likely not valid, as the distributions of anxiety and depressive symptoms is likely positively skewed in the population. It is fortunate that ANOVA and MANOVA are quite robust with respect to violations of the assumption of normality (Pearson 1931).

A second assumption implicit in the use of ANOVAs and MANOVAs is that the variances of the experimental samples are homogeneous. Again, this assumption may not be met in studies of anxiety and depression, since diagnostic categories will vary in their degree of homogeneity versus heterogeneity (Frances, Widiger, and Fyer, Chapter 3). ANOVA and MANOVA F-tests are robust with respect to violations of the homogeneity of variance assumption only up to a certain point and only if the sample sizes are equal (Box 1954; Cochran 1947). If the samples are of unequal size, violation of this assumption can have a marked effect on tests of significance. The actual significance level will exceed the nominal level with samples drawn from more heterogeneous populations and be less than the nominal level with samples drawn from more homogeneous populations (Box 1953, 1954). These results require that researchers test the assumption of equal error variances whenever unequal sample sizes are used (Cochran 1941; Hartley 1940, 1950).

When using repeated measures analyses (also referred to as within-subjects designs, pre-post designs, or split-plot designs) (Kirk 1982), ANOVAs and MANOVAs involve another assumption, referred to as compound symmetry. The compound symmetry assumption is that all variances and co-variances among the dependent variables are homogeneous. If this assumption is tested and found to be violated, researchers should employ a more conservative F-test, perhaps downgrading the degrees of freedom. In the special case where the conservative ANOVA produces nonsignificant results but the "usual" ANOVA is statistically significant, researchers can make adjustments to the procedure using the Geisser-Greenhouse or Feldf-Huyak conservative approaches to significance testing (Kirk 1982).

To summarize this section, a wide number of statistical procedures exist that can be used productively in psychopathology and clinical research and, in particular, in the study of co-variation. We have attempted to suggest some of the uses to which these procedures may be put, and to caution researchers about considerations that must be made in using these statistics. A final caution that we would espouse is that statistical procedures are tools in aid of research. Although it is tempting to employ statistical procedures because they can be merged with a data set, our bias is that research should be theory-driven, and that statistical procedures have their place only in the service of answering theoretical questions.

RESEARCH DESIGN

In general, research designs can be categorized along a number of dimensions (Kazdin 1980; Kirk 1982). In the area of psychopathology, and the co-variation of anxiety and depression in particular, a smaller number of designs are used with regularity. In this section, we offer a few ideas related to (1) cross-sectional, (2) retrospective longitudinal, and (3) prospective longitudinal research.

Cross-sectional research designs involve descriptions within one sample of subjects, or across groups of subjects, at one point in time. These research designs are clearly the dominant type in the areas of anxiety and depression, and are useful for investigating a number of different questions. Issues of symptomatology, diagnosis, functional psychopathology, correlates of psychopathologic states, and other descriptive features of disorders can be examined using such designs. Indeed, the specific question of the concurrent comorbidity of diagnostic states can be addressed only using these methods. Cross-sectional designs are also useful in that they can suggest models of psychopathology. Unfortunately, the very cross-sectional nature of these designs is a limitation. Since most theories of psychopathology are developmental (i.e., involve changes over time), cross-sectional designs can only corroborate (or provide negative) findings from cross-sectional predictions. Dynamic processes that result in either the initiation or cessation of disorders cannot be directly examined. Most models of anxiety and depression require longitudinal research designs.

Retrospective longitudinal research is that where subjects are asked to report on past events, which can then be related to either other past events or to the present. The extensive use of life events schedules in depression is an excellent example of how retrospective events can be related to current disorder (Hammen, Mayol, de Mayo, et al. 1986; Monroe, Chapter 28; Paykel, Myers, Dienelt, et al. 1969). Retrospective designs can generally be employed to assess the adequacy of developmental models of anxiety and depression, but they are limited in a number of ways. They rely on memory for past events, which therefore makes retrospective data subject to memorial and other biases. Especially in the area of depression, where negative memory biases are known to exist (De Rubeis and Beck 1988; Dobson 1986), retrospective data must be considered suspect. Second, external validation of retrospective data is very difficult. Validation of past events is limited to those observed by others. Internal moods and psychological states are virtually impossible to validate, again rendering some of the data suspect.

Prospective longitudinal research designs hold the most promise for examining developmental models of psychopathology, or other processes over time. These designs are often employed in the context of treatment studies, where the clinical status of patients is examined over time as a function of the treatment program offered. There exist a number of powerful methodologies and statistics for conducting and analyzing the effects of such research. Beyond the use of prospective longitudinal research designs in treatment studies, however, examples of theoretical investigations of this type are virtually nonexistent (for an exception, see Lewinsohn, Steinmetz, Larson, et al. 1981). It is notable that theorists are uniform in arguing that longitudinal research is necessary to advance the fields of anxiety and depression, but such studies are rare. These studies are typically very expensive and require large samples and stable funding over a long time. Factors such as the relative infancy of developmental models of psychopathology, mixed results from retrospective longitudinal studies, and the lack of well-developed procedures for longitudinal research conspire against the funding of such studies.

SUMMARY AND CONCLUSIONS

In this chapter, we have attempted to accomplish two major tasks: (1) to review what we see as the significant patterns of co-variation between anxiety and depression that are appearing in the literature; and (2) to review the principal methodological issues that have faced, and will continue to face, researchers in this area. We have argued that investigations must maintain a clear conceptual basis and that research methodologies will, to some extent, naturally flow from these conceptual bases. In this section, we will describe four areas that have a large likelihood of making contributions to the field if they are given theoretical and experimental consideration.

We have previously noted that the concept of trait depression has not figured prominently in the field, although trait anxiety certainly has. There are only a few assessment scales that relate to trait depression (Costello and Comrey 1967; Dobson 1985b; Zuckerman and Lubin 1965), and these simply do not attract much research attention. Similarly, work on depressive personality (Chodoff 1974) has not been extensively developed. Rather, the field has focused on the parameters and correlates of episodic, or state, depression. Our argument here is not that the work to date has been misguided; indeed, the work on state depression has yielded huge gains in our understanding of depression. Rather, our concern is that more attention might be paid to the study of potential intra-individual dispositions that could be predictive of depression. Within the cognitive model of depression, considerable work has focused on the assessment of what are potentially depressogenic attitudes and beliefs (Dobson 1986; Segal and Shaw 1988; Shaw and Dobson 1979), but the available evidence does not provide strong support for such a model (Coyne and Gotlib 1983). Further research on both cognitive and other intra-individual dispositions are thus in need of both conceptual and empirical attention.

One ongoing issue in the measurement of anxiety and depression is the high correlations observed among anxiety and depression assessment scales (Dobson 1985a, 1985c; Mendels, Weinstein, and Cochrane 1972). Many of the existing scales show essentially the same magnitude of correlations within and between constructs; that is, they fail to show discriminant validity (Campbell and Fiske 1959). The lack of discriminant validity necessarily restricts the ability of researchers to identify unique anxiety or depression processes or to assess the impact of interventions on anxiety or depression differentially.

The inability of anxiety and depression assessment methods to differentiate the two constructs may be taken as evidence of (1) the fact that the constructs are truly convergent, and that the high correlations among the scales are an accurate reflection of the validity of the scales, or (2) confounded measurement, pointing to the need for the refinement of existing scales or the development of new, less confounded assessment scales. Our position is that assessment scales in this area are correlated because there is a veridical underlying co-variation between anxiety and depression (see Figure 1) (Dobson 1985c). As such, it is reasonable to have significant correlations among anxiety and depression scales. It is equally true, however, that anxiety and depression scales can be developed that show high within-construct correlations, but attenuated (although still significant) between-construct correlations (Dobson 1985b). The fact that such scales can be constructed implies that existing scales may not have the largest possible discriminative ability. Scales that are true to their to construct (anxiety or depression) but are less confounded with the other construct may be an area for future development.

A third area where we believe that insufficient work has been done is in experimental studies that use naturally occurring anxiety and depression and then examine the impact of those states on performance in various experimental tasks. Although there are some studies of this type (e.g., Beck, Brown, Steer, et al. 1987), we believe that further work of this type has the potential to explore not just the phenotypic similarity and differences between the constructs, but also the psychological and biologic processes that may distinguish these conditions. There are several areas where investigations could be initiated, and examination of differences between anxious and depressed persons could be explored (cf., Bradley and Mathews 1983;

Mogg, Mathews, and Weinman 1987). Such distinctions, if found, will have repercussions for the conceptual understanding and assessment of these states and disorders (Segal 1988).

Finally, several authors have suggested that long-term investigations of anxiety and depression are critical (Alloy, Kelly, Mineka, et. al. Chapter 29; Billings and Moos 1985; Dobson 1985c; Dobson 1986; Monroe, Chapter 28). We want to underscore this call for longitudinal investigations and to note that there exist methods and statistical procedures that can accommodate such research. There is mounting evidence that there are both psychological and biologic processes related to anxiety and depression that involve development over time. To the extent that such evidence is reflective of the actual processes involved in anxiety and depression, longitudinal research will be necessary for the field to achieve the best approximation to such processes.

Chapter 35

Extracting Comorbidity From Self-Report Instruments: A Cognitive Perspective

Lynn P. Rehm, Ph.D.

S ELF-REPORT REFERS to an assessment strategy of obtaining information with instruments to which the subject responds directly without an intervening interpretive expert. As such it defines a portion of a larger assessment matrix (Rehm 1987) that shares multiple dimensions with other perspectives. Self-report assessments may be made of overt-motor, physiologic, and cognitive behavior. The subject gives a report of various parameters of behavior (occurrence, frequency, duration, intensity, or magnitude) at various levels of abstraction (observations, estimates, opinions, attitudes, beliefs, evaluations), over various time frames, situations, and other domains of generalization.

Self-report is particularly suited as a methodology for assessing subjective components of experience. Both anxiety and depression as clinical entities or as emotional states have important subjective clinical phenomenology. Emotion per se has a subjective component, and emotional states and disorders involve many attitudes, beliefs, and evaluations. Not only the content, but the processes of cognition, such as attention, abstraction, encoding, and retrieval, may be affected by emotion. Cognitive aspects of psychopathology have been the focus of much interest in recent years, and a number of cognitive theories about the origins, maintenance, course, and treatment of anxiety and depression have been proposed.

A basic assumption of this chapter, however, is that although theory and some empirical research clearly distinguish between anxiety and depression, for the most part the instruments that are commonly used to assess these states are highly correlated and confounded. Reviews of this literature support the point clearly (Dobson and Cheung; this volume). It is surprising how little attention is given in the development of most self-report measures of anxiety or depression to discriminant validity. In most instances, new scales are validated by consensus with prior scales or rating methods, and perhaps they are demonstrated to differentiate target patients from normals or mixed control patients. When research does compare anxiety and depression measures in the same study, typically self-report measures within either construct alone may be highly intercorrelated, but correlations between anxiety and depression scales are likely to be nearly of the same magnitude (Rehm 1981). Cross-method (e.g., ratings versus self-report) correlations show the same pattern at lower magnitudes. The intent of this chapter will be to identify factors both from current theory and from relevant research that might better differentiate anxiety and depression in the cognitive self-report domain for the purposes of clinical and research assessment.

The approach of this chapter is, first, to review recent developments in cognitive theories of anxiety and depression. The aim of this review is to identify factors that may or could be contributing to the variance of self-report and subjective assessments of anxiety and depression. Factors that differentiate and factors in common will be abstracted to identify likely ways in which self-report assessments of anxiety and depression might be improved. Second, empirical studies of self-report assessment that attempt to differentiate anxiety and depression will be examined. Different methodologies and research strategies will be considered to see what they tell about the functional utility of the self-report perspective. Again, the aim is to identify ways in which current research and theory might provide improved methods for assessing the separate and overlapping components of anxiety and depression. While this distinction between theoretical and empirical approaches is at times arbitrary, it serves as a useful grouping to discuss the issues.

COGNITIVE APPROACHES TO ANXIETY

Anxiety as Conditioned Emotional Response

Many of the cognitive approaches have evolved from the more behavioral or cognitive-behavioral approaches. Two contributions to self-report assessment are worthy of note from the more behavioral approach. Behavioral approaches to anxiety have been heavily based on the assumption that anxiety can be thought of as a conditioned emotional response (Wolpe 1958). The early assumption was that classical conditioning processes could explain the pairing of previously neutral stimuli with the elicitation of an unconditioned anxiety response to produce phobic anxiety. This assumption proved to be a useful heuristic in developing treatment methods—notably systematic desensitization and its variants. The point relevant to anxiety assessment is that the assumption of anxiety as a conditioned emotional response stresses the idea of anxiety as stimulus-bound or as situational. Anxiety is seen as related to stimulus events, potentially including cognitive events. Anxiety occurs in the presence of the stimulus (internal or external) and quickly diminishes in the absence of the stimulus. For the purposes of systematic desensitization of anxiety, imaginal or actual stimuli are arranged in terms of thematic, spatial, or temporal gradients according to their power to elicit anxiety.

Assessment of anxiety from a conditioning perspective stresses that while anxiety does generalize along stimulus dimensions, the gradients of generalization are relatively steep and circumscribed. The person afraid of snakes is likely to be afraid of spiders, but not necessarily of giving a speech. This thinking was the basis for the development of the Fear Survey Schedule (Wolpe and Lang 1964). The Fear Survey Schedule consists of a long list of specific stimuli (e.g., heights, snakes, vacuum cleaners), and the subject is asked to indicate the degree of anxiety to each stimulus. A general measure of anxiety is obtained by summing the weighted ratings for each item. More recent versions of the scale have used factor analyses to identify clusters of stimuli as subscales for which scores are derived in essentially the same manner. The stimulus-response nature of anxiety is also incorporated into a multidimensional measure of trait anxiety, the S-R Inventory of General Trait Anxiousness (Endler and Okada 1975). The situationality of anxiety is clearest in the context of a discussion of phobias, but it is important to note that situationality is equally relevant to the assessment of generalized anxiety disorder. The third edition of the *Diagnostic and Statistical Manual of Mental Disorders* (DSM-III) (American Psychiatric Association 1980) and its revision, DSM-III-R (American Psychiatric Association 1987) incorporate operational criteria for depression that require that anxiety be associated with two or more domains or life circumstances and that assessment methods such as the Anxiety Disorders Interview Schedule (Di Nardo and Barlow, Chapter 12; Di Nardo, O'Brien, Barlow, et al. 1983) evaluate domains as stimulus or situation categories.

Preparedness

The assumption that phobias are conditioned does not hold up well to empirical test (cf., Rachman 1977). One of the assumptions that does not appear valid is the equipotentiality assumption; that is, that any stimulus can equally be the conditioned object of a phobia. One explanation for the lack of equipotentiality has been offered by Martin Seligman (1971), who proposed the concept of preparedness. The idea is that some stimulus-response pairings are more amenable to association because of their survival value during the evolution of our species. Evolutionary selection has left us prepared to make certain kinds of associations more readily than others. For example, children often develop fears of dogs after being frightened by them, but they seldom develop a phobia of doors after painfully pinching their fingers. Fears of threatening animals are presumed to be more prepared for conditioning. Children who did not readily fear threatening animals were less likely to contribute their genes to future gene pools. Of course, our changed modern environment may no longer favor our prepared conditionability.

An interesting extension of this concept has been developed by Öhman, Dimberg, and Öst (1985), who argue that different forms of phobias have different origins in evolution. Simple phobias are related either to situations that call for caution (e.g., heights) or to potentially dangerous types of animals (e.g., small, fast moving reptiles). These phobias are likely to be stimulus-bound and seen frequently in early childhood. Adolescence and maturity ordinarily should result in a rarer incidence of phobias, as experience and skill discriminate real danger from false. Social phobias are assumed to be based on dominance relationships. Certain kinds of situations (e.g., shared meals, dealing with authority figures, heterosexual interactions) would have special evolutionary significance. Such fears should originate in adolescence and should be more anticipatory in nature. This analysis implies that simple and social phobias have different symptoms and different courses due to different evolutionary origins. The essential point for assessment is that different types of cognition, as well as different configurations of anxiety symptoms, might be associated with different types of phobias.

Bio-Informational Theory

Peter Lang (1979, 1983, 1985) has developed a cognitive conceptualization of anxiety that he refers to as the *bio-informational theory of emotion*. From this perspective, a phobia (which, he argues, provides a useful model for considering anxiety and emotion generally) can be seen as an organized set of propositions stored in memory. When the propositional network is activated in whole or in part, the person experiences anxiety, which like any emotion has the components of valence, arousal, and dominance-control. Anxiety is characterized by negative valence, high arousal, and low dominance or control. Propositions consist of a subject, a relationship (verb), and an object. He distinguishes stimulus, response, and meaning propositions. Stimulus propositions refer to the nature of the object of the fear; response propositions refer to the qualities of the response to the object; and meaning propositions refer to inferences about and implications of the object.

The implication for self-report is that a thorough assessment of anxiety should include a survey of stimulus, response, and meaning components of fear. These measures might separate anxiety from depression or other affects not only in content but in the qualities of valence, arousal, and dominance in the propositions.

Anxiety and Coping

The work of Richard Lazarus on coping with stress has a slightly different focus than anxiety, yet a number of distinctions are made from this perspective that are useful for considering anxiety. Lazarus (1974) distinguishes between primary and secondary appraisals of situations. Primary appraisal assesses the danger in the situation in terms of what is at stake and what resources are available. The outcome of a primary appraisal is (1) acceptance of the situation, (2) a decision to act, or (3) a decision that more information is needed. Secondary appraisal concerns assessments of the ways of coping with the situation. Coping involves action coping, including attempts to change the situation, flee from it, or some other behavior. It might also involve emotional coping—that is, ways of dealing with any affect that is elicited by the situation. Emotional coping would include such tactics as denial, distortion, not thinking about it, or seeking emotional support from another person.

This model provides another outline of issues to be considered in efforts to discriminate anxiety from depression. Generalized appraisal strategies might differentiate anxiety-prone and nonanxious individuals. Self-report assessment instruments for anxiety should sample appraisal strategies that may be typical of highly anxious people. For example, anxious individuals might be more prone to want to continue seeking further information, and they might have anxious thoughts about their ability to cope and their needs for support. Lazarus and his colleagues (e.g., Coyne, Aldwin and Lazarus, 1981; Lazarus 1974) have developed various scales, such as the Hassles Scale, for assessing coping responses to specific stressors.

Anxiety and Efficacy

In his efficacy theory, Bandura (1977) makes a related distinction between outcome and efficacy expectations. Outcome expectations involve beliefs about probable outcomes in specific situations given a particular performance. These beliefs are about contingency rules that operate in the world. In contrast, efficacy expectations have to do with the conviction that one is capable of producing the particular performance. A person might know that picking up a harmless snake would not produce injury, but might not feel capable of carrying out that simple act. Efficacy expectations are influenced by prior performance accomplishments, vicarious experiences, persuasive verbal communications, and current physiologic state. Bandura argues that efficacy expectations are accurate predictors of anxious behavior. Efficacy expectations are specific to situations, but could be surveyed in general areas as part of a self-report anxiety assessment.

Of course, actual skill levels are also important determinants of efficacy expectations. A considerable literature on skill assessment in anxiety has been developed, especially for social skills, which are relevant to social interpersonal anxiety (e.g., Arkowitz 1981). Included among the assessment methods are numerous self-report instruments for assessing components of social skill.

Anxiety as Activity

Finally, mention should be made of models of anxiety that stress the activity of anxious thinking. As an example, in his work on test anxiety, Wine (1971) stressed the degree to which test-anxious persons engage in distressing anxious thoughts during tests, which interfere with effective performance. Assessments of nonassertive individuals in difficult social situations find that they engage in more negative but not positive thoughts about possible outcomes of the situation. Frequency of negative thoughts becomes the assessment parameter from this perspective. Questionnaires sometimes ask for estimates of the frequency of specific types of anxious thoughts, but other methods are also suggested. For example, self-monitoring logs of frequency of obsessive thoughts have been used (e.g., Mahoney 1971). Hurlburt and Sipprelle (1978) experimented with random sampling of cognition where subjects carry electronic devices that randomly emit a tone. At the moment of the tone, subjects are asked to write down what anxious thoughts were occurring.

Summary

In this review, a number of factors have been identified that are theoretically related to anxiety and that might provide clues for differential assessment in comparison to depression. Models of anxiety stress the reactivity of anxiety to stimulus events or situations as relevant for assessment. Various forms of cognitive activity may mediate this relationship. Thoughts can act as eliciting events or they can amplify danger and extend the meaning of a situation. Types of cognitions that could be sampled include stimulus, response, and meaning propositions. Stimuli might be assessed in clusters including those with special evolutionary significance. Appraisals of stimulus situations may involve judgments of the risks involved and resources available. Efficacy in terms of ability to perform specific acts or in terms of the range of coping skills and emotional coping strategies could be assessed. Sampling of the occurrence, type, and frequency of such thoughts may be useful for characterizing the behavior patterns that differentiate anxiety from depression.

It should be noted that many of these factors may not differentiate anxiety from depression. Factors similar to those reviewed above have also been identified by certain theories of depression. In the review of theories of depression below, comparisons and contrasts will be made to aid in these distinctions.

COGNITIVE APPROACHES TO DEPRESSION

Behavioral Theory

In contrast to anxiety, depression is not ordinarily seen as situational. While events may precipitate an episode, depression is considered to occur with relative constancy, over extended periods of time, whether or not the event is physically present. We do not usually think of "attacks" of clinical depression; that is, depression does not quickly increase and then decrease as a function of proximity to some stimulus. There is a degree to which situational factors influence normal mood and depression. Peter Lewinsohn's (1974b) original theory of depression posited that depression could be seen as analogous to an extinction phenomenon. In this view, depression could be the consequence of a loss or lack of response-contingent reinforcement. One of the implications of this model is that mood should be a function of contingent-positive and -negative events. A number of studies by Lewinsohn and others bears out the essential points of this idea (Lewinsohn and Talkington 1979; MacPhillamy and Lewinsohn 1982; Rehm 1978).

The assessment implication is that just as major life events may accrue to precipitate an episode of depression, "minor" life events accrue to influence mood on a day-to-day basis. The time-course considerations are still different from those in anxiety, but situationality is demonstrated. Lewinsohn and colleagues have used this idea to develop a therapy strategy of increasing rewarding activities (e.g., Lewinsohn 1976) and have developed assessment instruments for assessing positive and negative events: the Pleasant Events Schedule (MacPhillamy and Lewinsohn 1982) and the Unpleasant Events Schedule (Lewinsohn and Talkington 1979). Events assessed retrospectively over the last month are related to level of depression. When daily events are self-monitored, they are found to correlate with daily mood. Monitoring of the situations that are associated with poorer or better mood can provide useful information for treatment planning.

Lewinsohn's model also points to the possibility of interpersonal skill deficits in depression. Others have argued that interpersonal skill is central to depression (e.g., Coyne 1976a, 1976b; Gotlib and Asarnow 1979). Coyne (1976a) found that, in dyadic interactions, depressed persons elicited negative moods and rejection from those with whom they spoke. From the cognitive perspective of Lazarus's coping model, Coyne, Aldwin, and Lazarus (1981) found that, in appraising stressful situations, depressed subjects felt a greater need to accept a negative situation and more need for additional information. They also employed more wishful thinking, seeking help, and seeking emotional support from others. Thus both skill and strategy differences may characterize depression and differentiate it from anxiety.

Learned Helplessness

Martin Seligman's learned helplessness theory of depression has evolved from its original animal model form (Seligman 1974, 1975) to its attributional reformulation (Abramson, Seligman, and Teasdale 1978) to more recent refinements (Alloy, Clements, and Kolden 1985; Alloy, Kelly, Mineka, et al. Chapter 29). In the most recent form of the theory, a depressive attributional style acts as a contributory vulnerability factor. When an aversive event occurs, attributional style may influence the specific attribution made about the event. A helpless attribution leads to hopelessness, which is sufficient to produce certain reactive depressions.

A number of useful constructs that have potential for articulating differences between depression and anxiety are developed in this theory. The emphasis in the revised learned helplessness theory is on perceptions of control and responsibility as central to depression. The depression-prone person may have a depressive attributional style. This style is a general tendency to attribute the causes of positive events to external, unstable, and specific factors and negative events to internal, stable, and global factors. Such an attributional tendency is a contributory vulnerability factor, but it is also the case that the tendency is exaggerated among depressed individuals and may be seen as a symptom of depression. Evidence for the ability of attributional style to predict and differentiate depression from other forms of psychopathology is mixed, but generally supportive. An Attributional Styles Questionnaire (Seligman, Abramson, Semmel, et al. 1979) has been developed to assess this dimension.

Seligman made the distinction between universal and personal helplessness. Universal helplessness involves the perception that noncontingency exists as a general rule in life—that is, that no one has control over his or her life. In contrast, personal helplessness acknowledges that it may be possible for one to have some control in life, but that the particular individual feels helpless because of personal incompetence and powerlessness. The former should be related to apathy and withdrawal, the latter to guilt and low self-esteem. This distinction parallels Bandura's (1977) distinction between outcome and efficacy expectancies. The depressed person is more likely to have negative cognitions about general outcome contingencies (universal helplessness), while either an anxious or depressed person may evidence deviance in efficacy. That is, both depressed and anxious individuals may feel incapable of personally accomplishing specific tasks, but the depressed person is more likely to feel that no one can count on success at any task.

Also, as discussed earlier, the anxious person's sense of low self-efficacy is more likely to be tied to particular situations and ability to cope with those situations. The depressed person's low self-efficacy is almost, by definition, overgeneralized. It may be that as anxiety persists or generalizes, self-efficacy generalizes, and an anxiety disorder progresses to depression.

Cognitive Theory

In contrast to the learned helplessness approach, Aaron Beck's (1972) cognitive theory of depression tends to stress negativity of cognition rather than perception of control. Beck makes a useful distinction between anxiety and depression. Anxiety has to do with perceptions of danger and harm, depression with perceptions of loss. The depressed person is seen as distorting perceptions of the world, the self, and the future in a negative direction. Many studies have demonstrated the predicted negativity in a variety of self-report formats (e.g., Krantz and Hammen 1979), and a number of scales have been developed to assess negative depressive ideas—for example the Dysfunctional Attitudes Scale (Weissman and Beck 1978), the Automatic Thoughts Questionnaire (Hollon and Kendall 1980), and the Cognitive Response Test (Watkins and Rush 1983).

Self-Control Theory

My own self-control model of depression (Rehm 1977) was an attempt to integrate the factors identified by Lewinsohn, by Seligman, and by Beck into a broader self-regulatory framework. Using Kanfer's (1970) analysis of self-control, I posited that the self-management behavior of depression-prone individuals was marked by six deficits: (1) they attend selectively to negative events; (2) they attend selectively to the immediate as opposed to the delayed effects of their behavior; (3) they set stringent self-evaluative standards; (4) they make depressive attributions of causation consistent with a negative image of themselves; (5) they administer insufficient contingent self-reward effectively to motivate their behavior toward long-term goals; and (6) they administer excessive self-punishment, which interferes with effective exploration, problem solving, and persistence. The Self-Control Questionnaire (Fuchs and Rehm 1977; Rehm, Fuchs, Roth, et al. 1979) was written to assess self-control attitudes and beliefs associated with this model of depression.

The ideas of the model overlap with those of the other cognitive theorists, but add some additional points. Self-evaluation is a central concern in depression, but it is a complex and multifactored process. The self-management model suggests that standard setting or standard selection is the critical issue in self-evaluation and consequently in low self-esteem. The self-reinforcement portion of the model suggests a function effect of negative cognition in depression. Negative thoughts function as punishment, reducing initiative and persistence. Self-reinforcement tasks have been shown to differentiate depressed and normal individuals (Roth, Rehm, and Rozensky 1980; Rozensky, Rehm, Pry, et al. 1977). Finally, the theory focuses on people's attempts to obtain long-term, delayed goals. Behavior that is aimed at long-term goals is often the first to deteriorate as the person becomes depressed. Perceived loss of a long-term goal may produce depression in an otherwise unchanged environment. Although the requisite research has not been done, these self-control deficits have potential for differentiating depression from anxiety.

Memory Research

Recent cognitive theories have focused on memory processing in depression. Two major phenomena are identified by this area of research and theory. The first is mood-congruent recall (Bower 1981, 1983; Teasdale 1983a, 1983b). The concept of mood-congruent recall refers to the fact that current mood facilitates recall of information that is similar in emotional tone. The related experimental phenomenon of "emotional state-related learning" occurs when information learned during one mood is recalled better when the person is again in the same mood, and is recalled less well when the person is in a contrasting mood. If one is in a sad mood, it will be easier to recall sad events from last week (Bower 1981) or from childhood (Teasdale and Fogarty 1979). If one is asked to recall a happy childhood event, it will take longer when in a sad mood. Contrasting moods have been induced by hypnosis (Bower 1981), by recalling emotional past experiences (Leight and Ellis 1981), or by reading lists of emotional sentences (Teasdale and Fogarty 1979). Naturally occurring moods have also been used, including clinical depression, variations in clinical depression in individuals with diurnal variation in mood (Clark and Teasdale 1982), and rapid cycling manic-depressive patients who learned lists in their manic and depressed states (Weingartner, Miller, and Murphy 1977). These findings are consistent with the idea that emotion is a factor in the storage and retrieval of information. Recall bias is a potential measure of depressive information processing.

A second area of memory research in depression has investigated self-referent encoding. The idea of these studies is that an organized set of information about oneself (i.e., a self-structure) can act as a heuristic device for organizing new information for encoding and storage. In what is sometimes referred to as a depth-of-processing paradigm, subjects are asked to view a series of words and perform one of several different tasks with the words—for example, "Tell me whether the word is written in small or large letters"; "Tell me if the word means the same as X"; or "Tell me which words apply to you." Recall is better for words that were processed as self-referent (i.e., told whether they applied to you). It is assumed that under this situation, the information is more "deeply" processed because the self-structure is a powerful reference that functions to organize information as it is processed.

The relevance of this idea to depression is that a depressed person is presumed to develop a self-structure predominantly made up of negative information. It is hypothesized that depressed persons will have enhanced recall of negative self-referent adjectives and normal controls will have enhanced recall of positive self-referent adjectives. This effect has been demonstrated a number of times (e.g., Derry and Kuiper 1981; Kuiper and MacDonald 1983). The clinical relevance of this effect is that depressed persons are more aware of and selectively recall negative rather than positive feedback from others. They remember the criticism but not the praise (e.g., Gotlib 1983).

The problem is that the results do not follow from the simple hypothesis. If a depressed person has an organized self-structure, it may predominantly contain negative information, but it will still contain some positive information. Depressed subjects still indicate that *some* positive adjectives apply to them. If these positive adjectives are just as consistent with the self-structure, they should not be harder to recall. The results can be explained by saying that words are better recalled if they are self-referent *and* are consistent with current mood state. Again, emotional quality is the connection that facilitates the recall. Memory for negative self-referent adjectives is another potential measure of depressive processing.

Summary

Cognitive models of depression stress nonsituationality or lack of stimulus control. Mood is more gradually influenced by events that may sum or accumulate to produce effects. Helplessness in either a personal or a universal sense is indicated, but in either case helplessness is more generalized than in anxiety. Attributions of causality are negative for both positive and negative events. Negativity may generally characterize all inferences and judgments about the world and the future, but especially about the self. Negative self-evaluation and negative self-evaluative thoughts are frequent and may possibly be differentiated from the worried thoughts of anxious subjects. Finally, processing by depressed persons is biased toward consistency of the tone of the material to be recalled with depressed mood.

EMPIRICAL STUDIES OF SELF-REPORT OF ANXIETY AND DEPRESSION

Self-Report Instruments

There have been some attempts to develop self-report scales for the specific purpose of differentiating anxiety and depression. Mould (1975) took the straightforward tactic of choosing pairs of words from the Beck Depression Inventory (Beck, Ward, Mendelson, et al. 1961) and the State-Trait Anxiety Inventory (Spielberger, Gorsuch, and Lushene 1970) and creating forced-choice items. The idea is to indicate a differential tendency without assessing either dimension in the absolute sense. To my knowledge, the scale has not been well developed psychometrically nor used beyond the original report.

Dobson (1980) took a different approach by developing a list of 69 situations and asking subjects to rate them for their potential to elicit anxiety or depression. Using factor analyses and differential response patterns for anxiety and depression, he developed the Differential Anxiety and Depression Inventory. As an example of the structure of the scale, the depression situation factors for males, in decreasing order of magnitude, are (1) anticipation situations, (2) assertiveness-persistence situations, (3) social exits, and (4) physical danger. While the factor structures seemed to be the same for males and females, the relative importance differed. Also, situation factors that were more closely related to depression for one sex were more closely related to anxiety for the other sex; for example, anticipation situations were more related to anxiety in females. Dobson suggests that sex differences may be important in mediating situational factors in both areas. The scale is seen as a measure of specific and differential vulnerability to anxiety and depression.

Note should also be made here of the Multi-Score Depression Inventory (Berndt, Petzel, and Berndt 1980). This instrument assesses 10 dimensions of depression related to factors derived from current theory. It is an attempt to use current theory as a more differentiated way of revealing specific theory-related components of an individual's depression.

General Models of Emotion

An interesting approach to the general problem of differential emotion has been taken by Tellegen (1985) and Watson and Tellegen (1985), who argue for the relative independence of negative and positive affect in the structure of mood and personality. Within this model, anxiety is seen as being characterized by high negative affect, but not necessarily low positive affect. Depression is characterized by both high negative affect and low positive affect. As an example of this research, using DSM-III criteria, Vye (1986) assessed 16 outpatients with anxiety disorders and 16 with depressive disorders on both self-report and clinician-rating measures of anxiety, depression, negative affect, and positive affect. Both within and across assessment method, the same pattern of results occurred. Anxiety measures correlated higher with negative affect than with positive affect, and the reverse was true for depression. Positive affect but not negative affect differentiated between the two patient groups. These results are generally supportive of the model. The importance of this research is that it employed constructs that have been developed for research and theory on the basic structure of human emotion and mood, and applied them to the affective and self-report components of psychopathology.

Other theorists have suggested structural models of emotion, often employing circumplex models (e.g., Izard 1977; Plutchik 1980; Russell 1980). Russell, for example, presented evidence for a color-wheel-like array of emotions, with basic axis dimensions of pleasure-displeasure and degree of arousal. Similar to Tellegen, Russell suggests that both anxiety and depression are at the extreme on the displeasure dimension but that they differ in arousal: low for depression and high for anxiety. These dimensions are also comparable to the three dimensions cited above by Lang (1983) of valence, arousal, and control-dominance. All of these sets of dimensions are clearly parallel to the basic dimensions of connotation or affect (good-bad, active-passive, and strong-weak) suggested by the classic work on the semantic differential (Osgood, Suci, and Tannenbaum 1957).

These dimensions may underly and pervade our assessment of emotions in ways of which we are unaware. Factor-analytic studies of scales of depression and anxiety are another way that we might piece apart the components of anxiety and depression to better differentiate the two constructs. Many such analyses have been published in the self-report assessment literature. Some consistency does seem to emerge despite differences in instruments, samples, statistical models, and factor labeling. On depression scale factor analyses, typical first factors are guilty depression and motor retardation (e.g., Cropley and Weckowitz 1966). These factors appear to match valence and arousal dimensions. Control dimensions are sometimes less easy to identify, but sometimes are quite clear. It may be that factor analyses of self-report measures of depression and anxiety are not identifying independent dimensions of symptoms, but rather are identifying underlying subjective dimensions of meaning and emotion. These semantic dimensions may be basic dimensions of human affective categorization. An awareness of this possibility might lead us to be able to better use the results of factor-analytic studies for developing instruments that better differentiate anxiety and depression.

CONCLUSION

Assessment is always determined by theoretical models of the construct being measured. Assessment instruments are constructed with a model in mind of anxiety or depression as a syndrome, as a trait, or as an affective state. Instruments designed for assessment of psychopathology usually assume a syndromal constellation of interrelated symptoms in many domains. The disease model of psychopathology dominates our conceptions, and anxiety and depression are thought of as a collection of manifest symptom complaints. If the two are seen as separate (biological) entities, then self-report becomes just another method of cataloging symptoms.

In the medical model approach, symptoms are not seen as relevant functional components of the overall disorder. Emphasis in scale construction is on internal consistency and consensus with other indices of the syndrome (e.g., clinical diagnosis). Measures of severity of psychopathology assume a relatively enduring state and are often trait-like in format. Development similarly focuses on internal and external consistency with other measures of the disorder. In neither case is much attention given to the construct validity of the measure in the sense of the function or definition of depression or anxiety or to the full explication of the phenomenological state. The disease model makes discriminant validity a low priority, at best, in scale development. Scales are developed that ask about symptoms in all domains (e.g., overt-behavior and physiological), and, in the cognitive realm, they are heavily weighted with items requiring fairly high levels of abstraction that tend to measure dysphoria or negative affectivity.

If better scales are to be developed to measure the constructs of depression and anxiety, and to extract comorbidity, we must look closely at basic theory and research concerning each emotion and disorder. Until we have clear and well-supported theories of both disorders and their comorbidity, we will not have a basis for assessment. This chapter has attempted to survey a number of the possible contributions that this literature can make to this assessment problem. It has not provided a thorough critique nor an exhaustive review of the empirical literature on the problem. My intent was to open up alternative paths and ask different questions, rather than to determine the best solution.

Several themes emerge from this analysis. *Situationality* is a clear theme. Anxiety can be better assessed if it is seen as a response to external or internal stimuli. Situationality has been largely ignored in assessment of depression, but research suggests that a careful assessment of mood variations may turn up relevant situational factors that have great potential value for treatment and for the general understanding of the disorder. A second theme is that of *situation appraisal*. Both anxiety and depression are, at least in part, a function of the way in which individuals perceive and appraise situations. General dimensions of appraisal, expectancies, and self-evaluation may elucidate the nature of an individual's disorder and may also provide important avenues to understanding psychological vulnerability to depression with implications for prevention as well. Closely related is the theme of *personal control*. In the areas of both anxiety and depression, theory and research focus on constructs of efficacy, control, and helplessness. These dimensions are important aspects of the emotions themselves and are relevant to motivations and methods of treatment to be chosen. Also, the theme of *behavior or process* emerges. Symptoms are often thought of as static manifestations of some internal disorder. Theory and research suggest that we need to think of cognitive factors as ongoing behaviors and as ongoing information processing with functional significance. Assessment of these cognitive factors may have to go beyond traditional paper-and-pencil inventories to observation of problem-solving behavior, monitoring of thoughts, and evaluations of memory functions.

Extracting comorbidity from the self-report perspective will depend on using theory and research for a more detailed functional analysis of anxiety and depression (cf., Rehm 1989 and in press). That is, we need to examine how specific behaviors respond to and operate on the person's environment. Current cognitive theories of anxiety and depression should be refined to sharpen our definition of the constructs in the cognitive domain. Scales to assess specific constructs that are held to be central to depression and anxiety currently exist. These scales may offer a readily available way to study differences between the constructs. Emotion and the structure of emotion need to be viewed more broadly. Researchers must define their constructs and develop their scales cognizant of the dimensionality and interrelatedness of various emotional states and moods. We also need to look at other dimensions of cognition (e.g., thought frequency or relative accessibility of memories) to improve cognitive and self-report assessment. Finally, we need to move away from traditional conceptions of psychopathology as discrete categories of disease and look at functional behavior patterns if we are to improve assessment in ways that will be useful to diagnosis, treatment, and prevention.

Chapter 36

Extracting Information From Diagnostic Interviews on Co-Occurrence of Symptoms of Anxiety and Depression

Jack D. Burke Jr., M.D., M.P.H.
Hans-Ulrich Wittchen, Ph.D., Dipl Psych
Darrel A. Regier, M.D., M.P.H.
Norman Sartorius, M.D., Ph.D.

THIS CHAPTER REVIEWS ways that co-occurring symptoms of depression and anxiety can be assessed with well-known diagnostic interviews. To stimulate further development, we will emphasize problems that arise in trying to establish co-occurrence of anxious and depressive symptoms.

In clinical research and in clinical practice, increased recognition has been given to the importance of determining the co-occurrence of symptoms, syndromes, and disorders. For some conditions, like schizoaffective disorder, determination of co-occurring symptoms is a key part of the differential diagnosis; for conditions like bipolar disorder, the need to assess co-occurrence of syndromes over time is essential. In clinical, genetic, and epidemiologic research using a longitudinal perspective, determination of comorbidity over time has been increasingly important (Boyd, Burke, Gruenberg, et al. 1984; Carey 1987; Christie, Burke, Regier, et al. 1988; Price, Kidd, and Weissman 1987). Establishing co-occurrence usually entails gathering evidence of co-existence within the same time period, as well as identifying the pattern of onset, to determine which came first.

In general, there are three ways this assessment of overlapping conditions could be undertaken. The first is the custom-made interview. Investigators could use their own custom-made interview procedure to assess the conditions of interest in the appropriate time frame for each subject. This approach would allow each study to have a data base well suited to the question of interest, but the use of individualized interviews may limit the ability to communicate results to other investigators as well as make it more difficult for others to replicate the findings; in addition, before approving such a unique assessment method, a peer review committee may set very high expectations for demonstrations of reliability and "validity" (or at least agreement with independent clinical judgments). Perhaps because of these possible objections, this approach may not be feasible in most instances, and this review will focus on general diagnostic instruments being developed for widespread use.

The second way to assess overlapping conditions involves the use of existing interviews. Several of the best-known diagnostic interviews now in use or under development provide considerable information about the co-occurrence of depressive or anxiety disorders or syndromes in a subject's past or current experience. Their suitability for this purpose, of assessing "comorbidity" of disorders, has been demonstrated in the increasing literature about the importance of co-occurring disorders, like major depression and panic disorder, for example, as reported from the Yale family study (Price, Kidd, and Weissman 1987) and from the National Institute of Mental Health (NIMH) Epidemiologic Catchment Area (ECA) program (Boyd, Burke, Gruenberg, et al. 1984; Christie, Burke, Regier, et al. 1988). These recent publications from clinical and epidemiologic studies suggest that this problem of assessing comorbidity of disorders is being addressed adequately.

The third way involves the extension of existing interviews. It may be of interest to study the co-occurrence of *symptoms* of depression and anxiety, not just the broader question of co-occurrence of syndromes or diagnosed disorders. Rather than demonstrating some easy ways to accomplish this goal, this review may end up by suggesting that asking broad diagnostic interviews being developed for general use to provide this fine level of information may be too ambitious. Two essential problems with this request are that it demands reliability of individual interview items for each specific symptom, not just reliability for the disorder; and it introduces the challenge of documenting the time course of individual symptoms, not just episodes of illness.

In considering general diagnostic interviews that now exist or are being developed, this chapter centers on three areas: co-occurrence of disorders; co-occurrence of symptoms; and problems of dating the course of disorders and symptoms. The discussion outlines possible ways to overcome the identified problems.

BACKGROUND

This review will focus on five contemporary interviews that have won wide acceptance and are being further developed by their principal authors. Their major characteristics, including their scoring methods and linkage to classification systems, are summarized below and are abstracted in Table 1.

Present State Examination (PSE)

In the ninth edition of the PSE (Wing, Cooper, and Sartorius 1974b), 140 items are assessed by a clinical examiner who inquires about phenomena present in the month before the interview. "Cross-examination" is used to determine whether a condition is truly present and of psychiatric significance. A positive answer is probed to allow coding it on a three-point scale on the basis of severity or frequency (Table 2).

Information gathered from the interview can be entered into a computer program, CATEGO (Wing, Cooper, and Sartorius 1974b), which produces several levels of useful output: a syndrome list, including both psychotic and neurotic syndromes; a set of potential diagnostic categories; and a final unique assignment to one of 50

Table 1.　Characteristics of Major Diagnostic Interview Schedules

Diagnostic Interview	Basic time frame	Classification system	Age of onset	Determination of co-occurrence
PSE	1 month	CATEGO (ICD)	No	Implicit at symptom,
SCAN	1 month and longer	ICD-10		syndrome, category levels
SADD	1 month + current episode	ICD	Yes (affective)	Implicit
DIS	Lifetime, recency	DSM-III	Yes	Derived
CIDI	Lifetime, recency	DSM-III-R, ICD-10	Yes	Derived
SCID	Lifetime, 1 month	DSM-III-R	Yes	Implicit
SADS	Lifetime, current	RDC	Yes	Implicit

Note. PSE = Present State Examination; SCAN = Schedule for Clinical Assessment in Neuropsychiatry; SADD = Schedule for Standardized Assessment of Depressive Disorders; DIS = Diagnostic Interview Schedule; CIDI = Composite International Diagnostic Interview; SCID = Structured Clinical Interview for DSM-III-R; SADS = Schedule for Affective Disorders and Schizophrenia; ICD = International Classification of Diseases; RDC = Research Diagnostic Criteria.

Table 2. Present State Examination: Item 23

DEPRESSED MOOD

Do you keep reasonably cheerful or have you been very depressed or low-spirited recently?

Have you cried at all?
(When did you last really enjoy doing anything?)

RATE DEPRESSED MOOD

N.B. When rating clinical severity of depression remember that deeply depressed people may not necessarily cry. See definition in glossary.

☐ 23

1 = Only moderately depressed during past month, or deep depression for less than 50% of the time and tending to vary in intensity.

2 = Deeply depressed for more than 50% of the past month, and tending to be unvarying in intensity.

Note. From Wing, Cooper, and Sartorius (1974).

CATEGO classes, with a corresponding diagnostic code from the International Classification of Diseases (ICD) (Table 3). Since ICD-8 and ICD-9 (World Health Organization 1977) did not have explicit criteria, CATEGO has been produced on the basis of clinical judgment by the authors of this system. The logic of CATEGO has been set out in a monograph on the PSE and has recently been documented in flowcharts as part of the World Health Organization (WHO)-Alcohol, Drug Abuse, Mental Health Administration (ADAMHA) International Program on Classification and Diagnosis (Jablensky, Sartorius, Hirschfeld, et al. 1983).

Because the interview focuses on the previous month, it can usually be assumed that positive symptoms and syndromes occur together within that month. Exceptions to this assumption could be easily postulated; for example, it may be that one disorder is tapering off at the beginning of the month prior to interview, and another begins just 2 weeks before interview. Co-occurrence, overlap, or discontinuity of symptoms cannot be discerned for ratings of symptoms present within the 1-month period covered by the examination. Before this assumption of co-occurrence can even be used, though, information at the level of individual items or one of the early levels of CATEGO output needs to be used; if the only information used is the final stage in the output, in terms of a unique CATEGO class or a single ICD code, as commonly reported, the possibility of co-occurrence of multiple conditions may be obscured.

For instances when depressive and anxiety symptoms do coexist, one intriguing feature of the PSE-CATEGO system is the use of a differential question to determine the relative predominance of anxious or depressive symptoms. Item 26 asks the examiner, or suggests asking the subject, to rate whether the anxiety or depression is more significant (Table 4).

The PSE-CATEGO system has been perhaps the most widely used diagnostic assessment tool since the U.S.-U.K. Diagnostic Study (Cooper, Kendell, Gurland, et al. 1972), especially since it has been used in so many important crossnational studies conducted by the Division of Mental Health at the WHO. In the WHO-ADAMHA collaborative project, an effort has been made over the past 5 years to produce a new diagnostic interview with an updated version of the PSE at its core. Field testing of this instrument, the Schedule for Clinical Assessment in Neuropsychiatry (SCAN) (Wing, Babor, Brugha, et al., in press), began in early 1988 in 20 centers in different parts of the world. A major output of SCAN will be diagnostic categories assigned on the basis of the draft Diagnostic Criteria for Research being developed for the new 10th revision of the ICD. The updated PSE will be compatible with the older PSE-9, and CATEGO

Table 3. Program CATEGO Output (Sample)

SYNDROMES PRESENT INITIALLY
NS CS IS RS DD SD ON GA SA HT AF HM AH PE RE GR SF SH OH OV SL NP DE ED AG NG IR TE LE WO IT SU IC HY OD SC DI
+ +   +   + +   +   + +   + + + + +   +

NEW STAGE 3 POTENTIAL CATEGORIES
CS ECS RCS MCS PD RPD APD MPD SD ASD TSD RSD LSD MSD SA GA NS IS RS ON DD HT SS
+   +

NEW STAGE 4 POTENTIAL CATEGORIES
DS MN EMN HM DP AP OV* SL*

SYNDROMES REMAINING
NS CS IS RS DD SD ON GA SA HT AF HM AH PE RE GR SF SH OH OV SL NP DE ED AG NG IR TE LE WO IT SU IC HY OD OR SC DI
+   + +   + + + + +   +

FULL LIST OF POTENTIAL CATEGORIES
NS DS AH* DP CS ECS RCS MCS RS IS SS HM MN EMN PD RPD APD MPD SD ASD TSD RSD LSD MSD
+ +

SA GA ON HT AP OV* SL*
+

CATEGORIES PRESENT
NS CS DS DP RS SS ECS RCS MCS CNS CDS IDS MN PD AP UP XP EMN DMN RPD APD MPD MAP HM
SD SA GA ON XN ASD TSD RSD LSD MSD MAN XX NO ED HT OV* SL*
+ +

50 DESCRIPTIVE CLASSES
1 2 3 4 5 6 7 8 9 10 11 12 13 14 15 16 17 18 19 20 21 22 23 24 25
26 27 28 29 30 31 32 33 34 35 36 37 38 39 40 41 42 43 44 45 46 47 48 49 50
+

Table 4.   Present State Examination: Item 26

IF EVIDENCE OF BOTH DEPRESSION AND
ANXIETY RATE ANXIETY OR DEPRESSION PRIMARY

If subject suffers from both anxiety and depression, and both have been rated as present, try to decide which is primary.

Which seems worse, the depression or the anxiety? (Use patient's own terms).

☐ 26

0. Anxiety is primary. Depression appears to be entirely explicable in terms of the limitations placed on the subject by the symptoms of anxiety, . . .

1. Anxiety and depression both present but seem independent . . .or it is not possible to decide whether one of them is primary.

2. Depression is primary. Anxiety is either a result of the depression . . .or it takes the form of fears of catastrophe, forebodings . . .

Note.   From Wing, Cooper, and Sartorius (1974b).

output is expected to be available as well. Most likely, the key time periods assessed will be the prior month and, perhaps at the interviewer's option, the present episode of illness. Past psychiatric history will be assessed using a special module to record the temporal relationship of disorders present in past episodes (Wing, Babor, Brugha, et al., in press, Archives General Psychiatry).

WHO Schedule for Standardized Assessment of Depressive Disorders (SADD)

As part of a multi-site international Collaborative Study on the Standardized Assessment of Depressive Disorders, WHO developed the SADD (Sartorius, Davidian, Ernberg, et al. 1983), a clinical instrument for the systematic assessment of depressive symptoms and other information relevant for the assessment of depressive disorders. The WHO SADD also has a provision for recording both psychophysiologic and psychological symptoms of anxiety. In addition to ratings of symptoms, the schedule provides suggested probes for inquiring about symptoms in different cultures, a detailed glossary to define the symptoms, and examples of typical responses.

This material is assessed in detail for both the past month and for the total period of the present episode. The uncertainty of determining whether symptoms present within the past month were "co-occurring" is reduced by the expectation that the examiner will determine the dimensions of a discrete present episode of illness while conducting the interview.

One advantage of this schedule is that it has been demonstrated to be reliable for assessing subjects in different cultures. It is used in conjunction with a brief screening form used to establish whether individuals are likely to suffer from a depressive disorder.

NIMH Diagnostic Interview Schedule (DIS)

The DIS (Robins, Helzer, Croughan, et al. 1981; Robins, Helzer, Ratcliff, et al. 1982) contains a set of fully specified questions designed to meet the criteria for major diagnostic categories in DSM-III (American Psychiatric Association 1980). It is based on a lifetime framework, so questions about a symptom are characteristically asked as "Have you ever. . . ." (Table 5). Positive answers are screened, when necessary, to be sure they are of significance and are not attributable to use of drugs, alcohol, medications, or physical illness.

For each major diagnostic category, the DIS asks for age when the problem began, to determine age of onset, and for recency of the episode, to determine whether the disorder had been present in the past 2 weeks, 1 month, 6 months, or 1 year. One option that was incorporated into the DIS during the course of the NIMH ECA program was to probe each positive symptom to determine how recently it had been active as well. Another advance that Robins and Helzer have designed recently has been to ask for the age of onset of each positive symptom. Probing each positive answer for psychiatric significance, for recency, and for first onset can complicate or prolong administration of the interview, and it will be important to obtain data about the applicability of this revision outside the United States. Information from the DIS is scored by a computer program, with an emphasis on diagnoses according to DSM-III.

The WHO-ADAMHA collaborative program has also supported further development and modification of the DIS for use in international studies; this new instrument will be called the Composite International Diagnostic Interview (CIDI) (Robins, Wing, Wittchen, et al. 1988). Field tests of the interview began in 1988 in 19 centers in different countries. Additional questions to meet the draft Diagnostic

---

Table 5.   NIMH Diagnostic Interview Schedule: Depressed Mood

---

72. In your lifetime, have you ever had two weeks or more during which you felt sad, blue, depressed, or when you lost all interest and pleasure in things that you usually cared about or enjoyed?

     No . . . . [1]

     Yes . . . . [5]

Note.   From Robins, Helzer, Croughan, et al. (1981).

Criteria for Research in the tenth revision of ICD (ICD-10) are being added for major disorder categories covered in the CIDI.

Structured Clinical Interview for DSM-III-R (SCID)

The SCID (Spitzer, Williams, and Gibbon 1987) is a new interview designed specifically for administration by trained clinical examiners for DSM-III-R (American Psychiatric Association 1987). The SCID is keyed to the new set of criteria in DSM-III-R, which are printed next to the suggested questions so the examiner can see immediately what is being assessed. It is designed for administration by a clinical examiner, so cross-questioning and detailed probing by the examiner are expected, as with the PSE. Although it is possible to enter the data into a computer format for scoring and analysis, the schedule has been designed for manual scoring of diagnostic output by the examiner.

In general, the time frame covers the subject's lifetime, along with special attention to the month before the interview and to the past 5 years. The entire mood disorder section has questions to assess symptoms on both a 1-month and lifetime basis. In special cases, such as during a major depressive episode, the current and past experiences are addressed separately (Table 6). Age of onset for the disorder is also asked. One special feature is guidance for the examiner in explicitly assessing the exclusion criteria of DSM-III-R.

Schedule for Affective Disorders and Schizophrenia-Lifetime Version (SADS-L)

The SADS-L (Spitzer and Endicott 1978) has probably been the most widely used clinical diagnostic interview in the United States in the last dozen years. It provides questions keyed to the criteria in the Research Diagnostic Criteria (RDC) (Spitzer and Endicott 1978) and covers a lifetime framework as well as the current time of interview. Although computer-based scoring programs have been developed, it was designed for manual scoring by the examiner. It determines age of onset and most recent episode of illness.

A special advantage of the SADS-L is that many research teams have gained extensive experience with it. Some authorities have suggested that skilled clinical interviewers can, during the course of a SADS-L examination, determine the pattern of onset of past disorders; empirical demonstration of this use may point the way to standardizing such an achievement. Another advantage of its long use is that some research teams have developed special-purpose modifications of it, such as a SADS-L keyed to DSM-III rather than

Table 6. Structured Clinical Interview for DSM-III-R: Patient Version

CURRENT MAJOR DEPRESSIVE SYNDROME	MDS CRITERIA
Now I am going to ask you some more questions about your mood.	A. At least 5 of the following symptoms have each been present during the same two-week period (and represent a change from previous functioning); at least one of the symptoms was either [1] depressed mood or [2] loss of interest or pleasure.
In the last month . . . . . . has there been a period of time when you were feeling depressed or down most of the day nearly every day? (What was it like?) IF YES: How long did it last? (As long as two weeks?)	[1] depressed mood most of the day, nearly every day, as indicated either by subjective account or observation by others
Have you ever had a period when you were feeling depressed or down most of the day nearly every day? (What was that like?)	
(IF CURRENTLY DEPRESSED BUT FAILED TO MEET FULL CRITERIA FOR PAST MDS, SCREEN FOR PAST MDS AND MODIFY SUBSEQUENT QUESTIONS ACCORDINGLY: Has there ever been another time when you were depressed and had even more of the problems [SXS] that I just asked you about?)	
IF YES: When was that? How long did it last? (As long as two weeks?)	

Note. MDS = mood disorder section. From Spitzer, Williams, and Gibbon (1987).

just the RDC. A more extensive assessment of anxiety disorders has recently been developed (Mannuzza, Fyer, Klein, et al. 1986).

ASSESSING CO-OCCURRENCE OF ANXIETY AND DEPRESSION

These interviews can be expected to produce diagnostic assignments of reasonable usefulness according to the classification scheme they are designed to satisfy. But there are several levels to this question of how to determine co-occurrence of depression and anxiety. In this brief overview, potential problems that may seriously limit the study of co-occurrence of depression and anxiety will be emphasized.

Co-Occurrence of Disorders

Although this level, in terms of *disorders,* is the simplest of the problems facing investigators who wish to examine co-occurrence, it is not trivial. Two issues deserve consideration.

Diagnostic hierarchies. First, the diagnostic hierarchies, or "exclusion rules," have been incorporated into the interviews in some fashion and may pose problems for studies of co-occurrence. In the PSE, the unique CATEGO class is the one most commonly reported, for example, in the major epidemiologic studies from Camberwell (Bebbington, Hurry, Tennant, et al. 1981) and Canberra (Henderson, Duncan-Jones, Byrnes, et al. 1979), and the opportunity to examine co-occurrence may be lost if the prior levels of diagnostic output containing data on multiple conditions are not studied as well. In the DIS, the "exclusion rules" of DSM-III are implemented in an approximate way based on lifetime history; that is, if a subject has panic attacks without a history of major depression, the diagnostic code is 3; if there is also a history of major depression, the diagnostic code is 5, to indicate the potential of an "exclusion" based on the criteria for panic disorder in DSM-III (Table 7). In most reports of the ECA to date, the two codes have been combined to report a total rate for any reported experience with panic disorder. However, in some interviews that have used the DSM-III criteria, the exclusion rules have been used irreversibly, so it is not possible to identify subjects who may have had panic disorder at the same time as a major depressive episode, for example, the Standardized Psychiatric Examination used in Baltimore for the ECA Clinical Reappraisal study (Dr. Ernest Gruenberg, personal communication).

Reliability. Second, the reliability of these interviews on an

Table 7.   NIMH Diagnostic Interview Schedule: Example of Codes for "Excluded" Disorders

DSMPANIC

The lifetime DSM-III diagnosis of panic disorder
      No (default value) 1
      Yes (Criteria A to D fulfilled) 3
      Yes, except for Criteria C and D 5
      Missing Diagnosis . . . .

Note.   NIMH ECA Data Codebook (1986).

overall scale may be reasonably good, as shown, for example, with an early version of the SCID for major depressive disorder and generalized anxiety disorder (Riskind, Beck, Berchick, et al. 1987). However good the "overall" agreement is, it is certainly true that the reliability is variable across disorders. With the DIS, for example, the test-retest results and the agreement with a clinical examination were generally very good for major depressive episode in a range of studies (Table 8). Agreement values were much lower for panic disorder in many of the early studies (Burke 1986), but more recent papers have reported better agreement (Canino, Bird, Shrout, et al. 1987b; Semler, Wittchen, Joschke, et al. 1987). In prior discussions of these points, Dr. Ernest Gruenberg (personal communication) has emphasized the problem of comparing two interviews when each one has only moderately good reliability. The problem of studying two disorders, each of which has limited test-retest reliability, may also need to be examined carefully by statisticians (Lavori, Chapter 38).

Co-Occurrence of Symptoms

Trying to extract information about co-occurrence of depressive and anxiety *symptoms* from these general diagnostic interviews is more difficult than trying to establish co-occurrence of disorders. The interviews were each designed to provide diagnostic-level output, and the additional information about symptoms is more limited. As discussed below, studies using the DIS have given explicit attention to this problem.

     Symptom assessment.   While some information has been obtained about the test-retest reliability of depressive symptoms (Mazure, Nelson, and Price 1986), much less is known about the reliability of individual items on the interviews. Some findings from studies by Wittchen and his colleagues (Wittchen, Burke, Semler, et al. 1989) in

Table 8. Results of Studies on Diagnostic Interview Schedule Performance

	Major depression	Panic disorder
Test-retest studies		
Clinic samples		
Robins et al. 1981, 1982	0.63	0.40
Burnam et al. 1983	0.56	0.42
Community samples		
Helzer[a] et al. 1985	0.33(0.58)	0.28(0.67)
Wittchen and Semler, unpublished report	0.76	0.47
Clinical-comparison studies		
Clinic samples		
Hesselbrock et al. 1982	0.72	
Hendricks et al. 1983	1.0	
Wittchen et al. 1985	0.84	0.45
Community samples		
Anthony et al. 1985	0.25(0.71)	
Helzer et al. 1985	0.28(0.58)	0.30(0.70)
Wittchen et al. 1985	0.72	0.30

Note. Numbers are kappa values. Summarized in Burke (1986).
[a]Yule's Y in parentheses.

Germany have suggested great variability in the test-retest agreement on specific questions from interviews like the DIS, and Dr. Alan Romanosky (personal communication) and his colleagues in the Baltimore ECA demonstrated that the reliability of a DSM-III disorder is likely to be greater than for its individual symptoms. Since there are multiple ways to qualify for a diagnosis of major depression, for example, two interviews could agree that the diagnosis is present but disagree on many of the individual items contributing to the diagnosis. When individual questions are taken as the basis of data analysis, it is important to know their reliability as well. To date, not many publications report such findings, but questions have been raised about the validity of patient reports of symptoms of major depression (Bromet, Dunn, Connell, et al. 1986).

Skip-outs. Some interviews allow the examiner to skip sections once it becomes clear that a subject cannot qualify for a diagnostic rating in that category of disorder. While such skips can be suspended by investigators starting a new study, studies using skip-outs will yield an incomplete data base in terms of symptoms and cannot be used for comparison to more complete data sets.

Co-Occurrence and the Question of Timing

Discussion about the usefulness of diagnostic interviews has centered on their reliability and validity in assessing the clinical phenomena that are intended to be evaluated as criteria for a diagnostic category. However, with the advance of explicit sets of criteria that include time-related requirements, such as clustering of symptoms into an episode for major depression, or frequency of attacks for panic disorder; and with the effort to assess lifetime experience, which makes questions of onset and recency important to assess, time-related questions on diagnostic interviews have become important in establishing reliability and possibly validity, just as the clinical symptom questions themselves are. In one of the most comprehensive efforts to examine the impact of these time-related questions on diagnostic interviews, (Wittchen, Burke, Semler, et al. 1989) have recently analyzed data from their test-retest studies using the DIS and CIDI interviews. Some of their findings are relevant in this discussion as well.

Restricted focus. In assessing symptoms present in a morbid condition, the examination is often limited to the assessment of the prior 1 month of the subject's experience, as is done in the PSE and partly on the SADD and SCID (Figure 1). This period provides a fair sample of the patient's symptoms, and respondents can be expected to remember the past month's experience quite clearly. Although exceptions can be postulated, it seems fair to assume in most cases that clinical phenomena documented during this prior month have occurred at roughly the same time. But the focus on just the past month can make it difficult to understand the sequencing of symptoms and the course of illness. With focus restricted on the past month, it is also possible that the underlying nature of a disorder may be obscured. For example, some investigators would argue that it takes more than a 1-month time frame to know if the anxiety or depressive disorder is paramount, as depressive symptoms can at times "cover" the anxiety symptoms, and vice versa.

Clustering of symptoms. On interviews like the DIS or CIDI, which use a lifetime frame of reference for questioning a subject, a special difficulty arises for disorders whose symptoms must be "clustered" to determine if an episode of illness has occurred. With major depression, for example, the presence of depressed mood may be widespread in the general population, so it is important to know whether there were other concurrent symptoms that would help establish presence of an episode of major depressive illness. There has

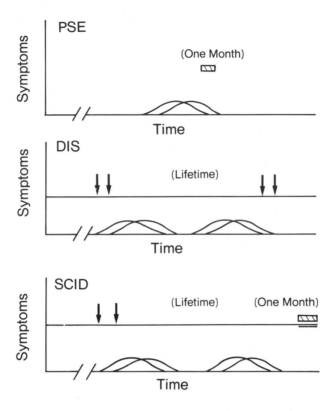

Figure 1. Assessment of Psychiatric Symptoms: Span of Time Assessed. (PSE = Present State Examination; DIS = Diagnostic Interview Schedule; SCID = Structured Clinical Interview for DSM-III-R.)

been some concern that some subjects may even report different "worst episodes" when this clustering is being assessed in a test-retest design on a lifetime interview. It seems that the definition of a "worst episode" always poses problems; it could be established as the period with most symptoms, longest duration, or greatest distress or impairment, for example, or when some unrelated life event is superimposed on the disorder.

Onset of symptoms. Another problem in timing episodes of illness is in establishing their onset. Typically interviews ask for the age of onset of a condition. It is possible to use this onset information to determine the sequence of onset of disorders, for example, in panic disorder followed by drug abuse, or alcoholism followed by depression. We have attempted to use these age of onset data in a recent analysis examining an increased risk of drug abuse following earlier onset of major depression or anxiety disorders in young adults (Christie, Burke, Regier, et al. 1988). One difficulty that arises, however, is the reliability of the age of onset reports. In Table 9, Wittchen and Teder's findings indicate that the age of onset data were acceptable for major depression and panic disorder (unpublished observations). However, for other disorders like phobias, the age of onset reports may be much worse (Wittchen, Burke, Semler, et al. 1989). In addition, a major difficulty in attempting to establish sequencing of conditions is that the age of onset in years is not a precise measure. For those subjects who report that depression and alcoholism began at the same age, for example, it is most important to know much more precisely the course of the symptoms; for these subjects, the equal ages of onset make it especially difficult to analyze co-occurrence at this overly broad level of precision.

While there are problems in timing episodes, there may be even greater problems with timing of symptoms. While Robins and her colleagues (Robins, Wing, Wittchen, et al. 1989) have found a way to get the same age of onset and recency data for individual symptoms as has been done in the DIS for episodes of illness, some investigators have expressed concern that this approach produces a very tedious interview that can increase errors by interviewers. Another problem is that the age of onset and recency data do not provide any more precise data than they do with episodes, as they record only the first and last experiences of the symptom that has been reported as present during the lifetime. What is missing is interval data, between the onset and most recent activity, to sketch the dynamic changes of symptoms over time (Figure 1).

There seem to be two difficulties in obtaining precise timing of symptoms. First, with an interview approach, which is dependent on the subject's recall, such detailed time-related information, based on the subject's memory and ability to report the information, may be a very fragile bit of evidence. Second, even if the subject had access to

Table 9. Agreement on Time-Related Questions: Diagnostic Interview Schedule Test-Retest Studies

	Major depression	Panic attack
Age of onset (kappa)	0.77	0.96
Recency questions (mean)	69.5%	62.5%[a]

Note. From Wittchen and Teder (unpublished observations).
[a]Includes generalized anxiety quesions.

this information and could report it accurately, the detailed bookkeeping required of the interviewer may detract from assessment of the clinical phenomena themselves. However, until the assessment of interval data is actually attempted, the true extent of these potential problems may not be clear. Perhaps the effort would not be so daunting in practice.

CONCLUDING REMARKS

While the general diagnostic interviews that are currently being used or are being developed are extremely helpful in providing a well-known, probably reliable basis for assessing diagnoses according to one or another classification system, one aspect of these interviews that has not been thoroughly studied is their assessment of time-related events such as the clustering of episodes, age of onset reports, and reports of recent activity of positive symptoms. The difficulty of assessing time-related activity, combined with the more tedious recording that is necessary for individual symptoms, may produce difficulties in using these general diagnostic interviews to examine the full course of overlapping symptoms of depression and anxiety, rather than the episodes of illness for which the interviews were initially designed. Despite this note of caution, however, it is possible to imagine five specific areas where progress may be within easy reach.

Full Symptom Coverage

Assessment of the full set of symptoms relevant to depression and anxiety can be accomplished easily by investigators who do not use any skip-out options for diagnostic categories that may have been provided to shorten administration of an interview.

Age of Onset Modules

While existing data about age of onset for episodes of illness, or for individual symptoms, may not be precise enough for some purposes when the sequencing of disorders or symptoms is being examined, it may be possible to write specific modules to clarify those cases whose multiple illnesses are being reported as having started at the same age, as with major depression and alcohol abuse or dependence. Such a supplementary module would not be needed very often in assessing subjects, but would provide helpful information when a subject's recall is accurate enough to permit use of the information.

Time Mapping

For those interviews that use the lifetime frame of reference to assess symptom onset and recent activity, it may be possible to elaborate the strategy used in the SCID of focusing at times on specific narrowly defined time periods, such as the past 1 month, to determine the presence of co-occurring symptoms. Events within the subject's recent memory may benefit from an increased accuracy in discriminating time-related events. A more elaborate example of this approach has been the use of a 1-year time line for graphic mapping of reported symptoms for children being assessed with the Diagnostic Interview Schedule for Children (DIS-C) in studies at Columbia University and Yale University Child Study Center (Dr. Mary Schwab-Stone, personal communication). In this approach, events such as Christmas, birthdays, and vacations are used as anchor points along the time line to illustrate the past year of the subject's experience; then positive symptoms can be graphed in relationship to these memory anchor points. A similar approach has been suggested by Wittchen and Teder (unpublished observations) based on their studies assessing time-related events.

Development of New Instruments: Children and Adolescents

The need for additional instruments can be exemplified by considering the assessment of disorders in children and adolescents. Studies examining subjects during the age of highest risk for onset of illnesses may benefit from some discussion of the most appropriate interview to use to assess these individuals in their high-risk ages. Data from the ECA and from other studies have begun to suggest that the median age of onset for drug abuse, many anxiety disorders, and major depression is in adolescence or very early adulthood (Christie, Burke, Regier, et al. 1988; Klerman, Lavori, Rice, et al. 1985). If these suggestions are correct, then the assessment of cohorts of adolescents followed into early adulthood may be of increasing importance in epidemiologic and clinical studies. However, the crossover from adolescence to adulthood raises questions about the suitability of using interviews designed for adults when the subjects are in adolescence (from puberty to age 20). An instrument like the DIS has been used as early as age 18 in the ECA, and perhaps age 15 by other investigators. The suitability of using these adult instruments in adolescents may need to be considered further, however, as more alternatives are developed, including instruments like the DIS-C, the Diagnostic Interview for Children and Adolescents (Welner, Reich,

Herjanic, et al. 1987), and similar instruments developed for this age group.

Supplementary Inventories

The need to assess co-occurring symptoms of depression and anxiety may be taken as a challenge by the interview developers and investigators interested in developing their own supplementary assessment materials. Until this challenge has been accepted and overcome, one alternative worthy of discussion is the need to use additional instruments to inventory symptoms within a focused time frame. Possible supplementary instruments include detailed symptom questionnaires; symptom checklists like those in the Association for Methodology and Documentation in Psychiatry system, which documents information from clinical interviews (Guy and Ban 1982); and structured interview-based symptom inventories like the SADD and the full version of the Schedule for Affective Disorders and Schizophrenia (Endicott and Spitzer 1978), not tied to any particular classification system but largely compatible with several of them.

In the near future, the use of more than one instrument may be required if a study has more than one focus for assessment of subjects. Greater interest in the course of illness and assessment of time-related phenomena may stimulate more refined approaches by the generally available diagnostic interviews.

Chapter 37

Treatment Trials, Comorbidity, and Syndromal Complexity

Abby J. Fyer, M.D.
Michael R. Liebowitz, M.D.
Donald F. Klein, M.D.

THE NOTION OF comorbidity has a definite meaning in internal medicine, because of a superior knowledge of etiology and pathophysiology. Comorbidity defines two separate coinciding pathologic processes (e.g., cancer and pneumonia or a compound fracture and gangrene). It is immediately comprehensible that one disease may predispose to another or interfere with its treatment.

In psychiatry, however, we rarely deal with etiologically defined diseases, but rather with polythetic syndromes. Here the notion of comorbidity becomes ambiguous at both syndromal and symptom levels. How can we distinguish syndromal complexity, both concurrent and evolving over time, from comorbid aggregation of relatively independent components?

In psychiatry, the co-occurrence of two syndromes, A and B, where at least one also occurs alone is usually referred to as comorbidity. This implies that the symptomatic similarity of the two A's (the one that stands alone and the one that co-occurs with B) reflects etiologic or at least pathophysiologic homogeneity. However, given that the etiologies of A and AB are unknown, it is also possible that the A that stands alone resembles but is not the same as the A that co-occurs with B. This is the problem of phenocopies, that is, the existence of symptoms or syndromes that are phenomenologically similar but etiologically distinct.

Internal medicine provides numerous examples where different pathologies lead to similar syndromes (e.g., hypertension, diabetes). Their symptomatic distinctions became apparent as an understanding of the underlying pathologies developed. In psychiatry it is not yet possible to peer through the veil of superficial appearance and distinguish phenocopies. Therefore, the inclusion of symptomatically similar but etiologically distinct cases within a single syndrome confounds genetic, treatment, and biologic provocation studies.

One also could argue that the more complex the syndrome, the more likely it is to be pathophysiologically homogeneous since phenocopies of simple states should be easier to generate than copies of complex ones. Therefore, syndrome ABCDE may actually be more homogeneous than syndrome A. Further, syndrome ABC may be more likely a partial expression of ABCDE than the fortuitous co-occurrence of $A + B + C$.

Comorbidity can be used to distinguish phenocopies. By a process of comparative splitting, it may be possible to bring clinical diagnoses "closer to the gene" (Carey and Gottesman 1981) or other etiologic agent. For instance, if we do not assume that the A aspect of AB is the same as an A that stands alone, then this "comorbidity" becomes a challenge to see if the two A's are not really different developmentally, symptomatically, therapeutically, genetically, and physiologically.

Longitudinal as well as cross-sectional patterns can be considered from this perspective. An example of this strategy is the finding that individuals with a lifetime history of both major depression and panic disorder (regardless of whether the two ever occur simultaneously) transmit a greater risk for major depression to their relatives than do individuals who have a lifetime history of major depression but no panic (Weissman 1985).

Can treatment trials help in understanding comorbidity or affective and anxiety disorders and symptoms? Effective treatments are now available for many of these illnesses. However, since (1) treatments have multiple physiologic effects and (2) the mechanisms by which treatments alleviate specific symptoms are not known, the leap from therapy to an understanding of pathophysiology is perilous. For example, the catecholamine theory of depression as inferred from antidepressant actions is untenable without considerably more evidence and resolution of conflicting empirical findings.

Despite these limitations, there are several situations in which pharmacologic dissection can elucidate comorbid relationships. Let us examine the example of drug response in individuals with syndrome A versus those with syndrome AB. To simplify our discussion, we will refer to the A that stands alone A_s and the A aspect of the complex AB as A_c.

Does A_s equal A_c? What is the relationship of A_c to B_c? B_c refers to the B component of the complex AB. Although it is not critical to the current discussion, B may, of course, also exist in a form that stands alone, that is, B_s.

Now assume that both syndromes are treated by the same drug and, if improvement during drug treatment is shown, that appropriate placebo-controlled trials show that this is indeed due to specific drug effect. If then, in these trials, A_s does not respond to the drug in the same fashion as A_c, this would be preliminary evidence of a real distinction between these similar syndromes.

We must distinguish the case where A_s gets better and A_c does not. Here it is possible that A_c is simply a more severe example of A_s because it is embedded in a more complex syndrome. Therefore, the difference of A_s from A_c may be due to context and severity rather than being qualitatively distinct. For instance, the fever of a mild pneumonia would more likely respond to aspirin than the fever of a severe pneumonia. This indicates that the pathophysiologic process that induces fever does differ between severe and mild pneumonia, but that the difference may be only quantitative.

It is more informative when medication benefits A_c but not A_s. Here the severity hypothesis becomes dubious; it is hard to think of a disease where the more severe case had fewer symptoms than the milder case. Therefore, A_c is probably qualitatively different from A_s. We will call this a disordinal interaction.

For example, if the panic of agoraphobia responds to imipramine but the panic of simple phobia does not, one suspects that these two panics are qualitatively different processes and may, on closer inspection, be found to differ descriptively, prognostically, genetically, and so on as well.

Other information may be gained from the effects of treatment on the respective components of a complex syndrome. For instance, if the drug causes A_c to remit while B_c remains severe over long periods of time, one would suspect that A_c did not have a maintaining role for B_c.

If, on the other hand, A_c quickly subsides and then B_c slowly subsides, one might suspect that A_c maintained B_c. By reference to the history of the illness, one might find out if A_c also regularly preceded B_c. The obvious example here is to imipramine's primary benefit on spontaneous panic (A_c) followed by secondary benefit on agoraphobic avoidance (B_c).

A converse case would be one in which B_c shows a temporary improvement but relapses on treatment cessation, while A_c remains unaffected throughout. If it had been previously shown that A_c anteceded B_c, one might hypothesize that A_c incited and maintained B_c but that the therapy had only partially helped to compensate transiently for A_c's effects. The analogy here may be the partial beneficial effects of exposure therapy on the phobic component of agoraphobia and its lack of effect on spontaneous panic.

In the sections below, we will discuss the use of clinical trials in assessment of diagnostic validity in three substantive areas: atypical depression, panic versus generalized anxiety, and social phobia. Atypical depression and panic were chosen because pharmacologic dissection has made major contributions to their nosologic development. This work provides examples of both the advantages and potential hazards of this technique. We also present recently analyzed data from an ongoing study by Liebowitz, Gorman, Fyer, et al. (1988) in which disordinal symptom comorbidity indicates possible diagnostic heterogeneity within social phobia.

ATYPICAL DEPRESSION

Atypical depression was first identified by contrasting depressions that responded to monoamine oxidase inhibitors versus those that did not. The complex syndrome of atypical depression apparently shared a common core depression with that manifested by typical depression; however, each depression showed an entirely different, and in many ways, mutually exclusive, pattern of comorbid symptoms. For instance, atypical depression was characterized by hypersomnia and hyperphagia in opposition to insomnia and anorexia.

Typical depression can be considered more severe than atypical depression because it is more commonly associated with marked social disruptions and suicide. Therefore, it would be a disordinal interaction if in the more severe illness tricyclic antidepressants were superior to monoamine oxidase inhibitors, but in the milder illness monoamine oxidase inhibitors were superior to tricyclic antidepressants. That is, if typical depression was simply a more severe variety of depression than atypical depression, then the drugs that worked the best in typical depression should surely also work the best in atypical depression.

Attempts to test the disordinal interaction hypothesis have fallen into two categories. The first approach attempts to determine statistically the relative predictors of tricyclic antidepressants (amitryptiline or imipramine) or phenelzine benefit. On the whole, this methodology has been unsatisfactory. Although several research groups have actively pursued this method, results of their studies have neither ruled out nor definitively established the existence of a subgroup of depressive patients preferentially responsive to monoamine oxidase inhibitors. Paykel and colleagues conducted a series of trials contrasting phenelzine and amitryptiline in mixed (i.e., both typical and atypical) depressive outpatients. Their initial studies demonstrated differential predictors of each drug compared to placebo, with phenelzine being superior for at least some of the features associated with atypicality (Paykel, Parker, Penrose, et al. 1979). However, a subsequent direct comparison found relatively few between-drug differences as compared to the overall number of contrasts (Paykel, Rowan, Parker, et al. 1982; Paykel, Rowan, Rao, et al. 1983; Rowan, Paykel, and Parker 1982). This research group concluded that while individuals with coexisting anxiety diagnoses in some cases responded better to phenelzine, overall the similarities between the drugs far outweighed their differences.

Robinson and Nies and colleagues (Nies 1984; Ravaris, Robinson, Ives, et al. 1980; Robinson, Kayser, Corcella, et al. 1985; Robinson, Nies, Ravaris, et al. 1973) have also used this strategy. They compared response to phenelzine and amitryptiline in outpatients who met at least one of three definitions of atypical depression: (1) mood reactivity and some evidence of reverse vegetative symptoms, (2) nonendogenous or reactive feature, or (3) preexisting or additional anxiety diagnosis or symptoms. Here also, phenelzine was significantly more effective in alleviating many symptoms associated with "atypicality" (e.g., anxiety, hypersomnia, hyperphagia, interpersonal sensitivity, and reactive depressed mood). However, a homogeneous syndromally defined subgroup of preferentially phenelzine-responsive patients could not be identified.

The Columbia group (Liebowitz, Quitkin, Stewart, et al. 1984, 1988; Quitkin, Liebowitz, and Klein 1983; Quitkin, Stewart, McGrath, et al. 1988) adopted a different approach to the problem. First, they developed a syndromal definition of atypical depression. They then attempted to demonstrate that, using this definition, the monoamine oxidase inhibitor phenelzine was superior to the tricyclic antidepressant imipramine.

Their criteria for atypical depression were: (1) presence of some type of depressive illness which meets Research Diagnostic Criteria (RDC) (Spitzer, Endicott, and Robins 1978a), (2) mood reactivity, and (3) presence of at least two of four associated symptoms (hyperphagia or weight gain, hypersomnia, rejection sensitivity, or a feeling of leaden paralysis).

In the first trial conducted by this group, 119 patients who met their atypical criteria were randomized to 6 weeks of treatment with either phenelzine (up to 90 mg/day), imipramine (up to 300 mg/day), or placebo (Liebowitz, Quitkin, Stewart, et al. 1984; Quitkin, Stewart, McGrath, et al. 1988). Responders were defined as individuals who were judged to be much or very much improved on the clinical global rating scale. At 6 weeks, 71% of patients on phenelzine, 50% of those on imipramine, and 28% of those on placebo were considered responders. Three-way comparisons indicated overall statistical significance between drug differences ($\chi^2 = 14.8$, 2df, $p = .0006$), with superiority of phenelzine ($\chi^2 = 14.8$, df, $p < .0001$) and imipramine ($\chi^2 = 4.5$, df, $p = .03$) over placebo. There was a trend for phenelzine to be superior to imipramine ($\chi^2 = 3.2$, df, $p = .08$).

Phenelzine was significantly superior to placebo on scales and items that encompass the definition of atypical depression: mood reactivity ($p < .02$), oversleeping ($p < .02$), overeating ($p < .03$), self-pity ($p < .00001$), and the Hopkins Symptom Check List (Derogatis, Lipman, Rickels, et al. 1974) interpersonal sensitivity, paranoia, and psychoticism subscales. Imipramine was not superior to placebo for any of the specific atypical items (reactivity, overeating, oversleeping, self-pity), nor was it superior to phenelzine for any measure at week 6. These findings have recently been replicated in a second group of 120 outpatients who met these specific criteria for atypical depression (Quitkin, personal communication).

Quitkin, Stewart, McGrath, et al. (1988) have also found phenelzine to be superior to imipramine and placebo in a slightly more broadly defined group of "probable" atypical depressive patients. Probable atypical depression as defined in this study was identical to atypical depression, except that individuals were required to have only one rather than two associated "atypical" features (i.e., either hyperphagia, hypersomnia, rejection sensitivity, or leaden paralysis) in addition to reactive mood and RDC depressive illness.

Sixty patients with probable atypical depression were randomized to 6 weeks of treatment with either phenelzine, imipramine, or placebo. Dosage ranges and assessments and definition of response were identical to those in the first trial described above. Response rates in the sample as a whole were 71% for phenelzine, 47% for imipramine, and 29% for placebo. There was a significant overall between-drug effect ($p = .03$). Phenelzine was significantly superior to placebo ($p < .01$) and showed a nonsignificant trend toward superiority to imipramine ($p = .08$). Imipramine was not significantly superior to placebo. Since it has been assumed that imipramine is superior to phenelzine in typical depression, the finding that the monoamine oxidase inhibitors are superior to tricyclics in patients with atypical depression is a type of disordinal interaction. Therefore, the atypical pattern seems qualitatively distinct from the endogenomorphic pattern. In other words, these data suggest that we have two distinct complex syndromes rather than syndromes that differ only quantitatively.

Unfortunately, it has become less clear that the monoamine oxidase inhibitors are inferior to the tricyclics in non-atypical endogenous depression. More recent studies (e.g., McGrath, Stewart, Harrison, et al. 1986) indicate that, in many non-typical depressions, the monoamine oxidase inhibitors have at least an equivalent effect to the tricyclic antidepressants. Probably this equivalence reflects an unrecognized heterogeneity within the non-atypical depressions. However, the fact that imipramine is inferior to monoamine oxidase inhibitors within the less severe class of depressions, but at least equal to monoamine oxidase inhibitor within the more severe class, still argues for a qualitative discontinuity.

PANIC ATTACKS AND GENERALIZED ANXIETY

Klein (1964) observed that, within the complex syndrome of agoraphobia, imipramine alleviated spontaneous panic attacks within a matter of several weeks, but that both high levels of chronic anxiety and phobic avoidance were maintained for a much longer period, although they too eventually disappeared. This observation led him to postulate that spontaneous panic attacks incited the development of secondary, chronic, anticipatory anxiety and tertiary avoidant behaviors, which then developed substantial functional autonomy. Klein (1967, 1981) postulated that spontaneous panics could not simply be the quantitative extreme of chronic generalized anxiety, since it would be strange that the same drug that eliminated the most severe form had little immediate effect on the more minor form.

It followed that if the generalized, chronic anxiety of agoraphobia was like the generalized, chronic anxieties of other panic-free anxious states, then imipramine may be useless in the treatment of those states.

This prediction was followed by Klein and colleagues' studies on simple phobia, in which it was shown that these chronically anxious patients did not respond to imipramine (Klein, Zitrin, Woerner, et al. 1983; Zitrin, Klein, Woerner, et al. 1983). Therefore, the observation of the disjunction of effects within agoraphobia led to a comparison of agoraphobia with simple phobia, which showed a disordinal interaction. Both the panics and eventually the generalized anxiety of the severe agoraphobic patients showed specific drug effects, whereas the chronic anxiety of the mildly impaired simple phobic patients did not.

Klein (1981) further substantiated his belief that panic was different than generalized anxiety by pointing to the fact that benzodiazepines were effective on generalized anxiety, but not on spontaneous panic. This differential treatment outcome, however, is not a disordinal interaction, but could be simply a severity effect. In fact, it has been shown that alprazolam and clonazepam, which are high-potency benzodiazepines, have an antipanic effect (Ballenger 1986;

Chouinard, Annable, Fontaine, et al. 1982; Dunner, Ishiki, Avery, et al. 1986; Liebowitz, Fyer, Gorman, et al. 1986a; Spier, Tesar, Rosenbaum, et al. 1986). One possibility is that alprazolam and clonazepam have other specific effects that are distinct from the ordinary benzodiazepines. Another possibility is that there are indeed some aspects of the spontaneous panic that are benzodiazepine-sensitive. This possibility remains to be elucidated. A more telling attack on the qualitative distinction between panic and generalized anxiety would be if it were shown that imipramine was effective as an anti-generalized-anxiety agent.

Almost all studies that have attempted to assess possible antianxiety effects of imipramine or to contrast them with those of the benzodiazepines have included a mixture of anxious, depressed, and phobic patients. This fact makes the imipramine benefit impossible to specify because its antidepressant and antipanic effects could well account for any observed advantage over the benzodiazepines.

The most convincing evidence for a distinct anxiolytic effect of imipramine, unrelated to its antipanic effect, comes from the study by Kahn, McNair, Lipman, et al. (1986) in which the anti-generalized-anxiety effects of imipramine, chlordiazepoxide, and placebo were compared in nondepressed anxious outpatients. Unfortunately, patients with panic disorder and with agoraphobia with panic attack were not prospectively excluded. Therefore, although a significant imipramine antianxiety effect was found, it is not possible to assess to what extent this was due to the drug's antipanic action.

Kahn, McNair, Lipman, et al. (1986) attempted to address this issue by retrospectively excluding 35 panic-phobic-type patients from their 242 patient sample. The criteria for this exclusion process are not given in their report. However, the proportion (14%) of panic patients seems small (Barlow 1985; Boyd 1986). Further, severe cases of panic disorder, in which panic is masked by chronic high levels of anticipatory anxiety, or mild ones in which infrequent panic attacks did not warrant a diagnosis of panic disorder, might have been missed using these retrospective methods.

Kahn, McNair, Lipman, et al. (1986) also undertook a multiple regression analysis in an attempt to show that the imipramine antianxiety effects demonstrated by their study are independent of antipanic effects. However, the reliability of this analysis is dependent on the reliability of the assessments of panic and generalized anxiety. Since the panic assessments were retrospective, their reliability must be considered questionable. This flaw significantly compromises the overall result. Kahn, McNair, Lipman, et al. (1986) agree that replication is necessary.

To sum up, the qualitative distinction between panic and generalized anxiety is still supported by the differential effects of comorbidity of agoraphobia by imipramine and by the lack of imipramine effects in simple phobia. The efficacy of imipramine in treating generalized anxiety disorder awaits an appropriately designed prospective study.

SOCIAL PHOBIA

Social phobia is a common disorder whose course is associated with considerable comorbidity (Aimes, Gelder, and Shaw 1983; Liebowitz, Gorman, Fyer, et al. 1983; Marks 1969). Until recently, effective treatments were not available for most patients.

The DSM-III (American Psychiatric Association 1980) defined the central feature of social phobia as persistent and irrational fear of humiliation while being observed by others in the course of certain activities. Common social phobic fears include public speaking, eating in public, writing in public, talking to strangers, attending social occasions such as parties, or speaking with authority figures. Either avoidance or endurance with dread of one or more of this type of situation was required for a diagnosis. However, the DSM-III definition described most sufferers as having only one or two fears.

In the course of two open medication trials with social phobic patients, Liebowitz, Fyer, Gorman, et al. (1986b) and Gorman, Liebowitz, Fyer, et al. (1985) observed two types of socially anxious patients. The first type were individuals who conformed closely to the DSM-III description. Each had discrete fears of one to several situations in which they were convinced that they would be humiliated or shamed if observed by others. Typical fears in this group were of speaking, writing, or eating in public. However, despite their phobias, these discrete social phobic patients usually had normal interpersonal relationships. Most were married and/or had active social lives. They enjoyed and were relaxed in contact with others, provided they were not faced with their specific phobic situations.

In contrast, a second group of patients presented with pervasive avoidance of or severe anxiety during most or all activities involving social interaction. This subgroup, labeled generalized social anxiety, also feared humiliation through observation by others. However, their fears included a wide range of interpersonal encounters. Most had few friends and severely restricted or nonexistent romantic lives. Some had no contact with individuals outside of their immediate family.

The discrete social phobic patients may be considered to have a simple form (A_s). The generalized social phobic patients are the complex comorbid form (A_cB_c).

To investigate the treatment response characteristics of these subcategories, patients with DSM-III social phobia participating in a double-blind trial of phenelzine, atenolol, and placebo were prospectively classified as either generalized or discrete social phobic patients (Liebowitz, Gorman, Fyer, et al. 1988). Preliminary results are described here.

Atenolol was chosen instead of propanolol for two reasons. Propanolol is thought to be both centrally and peripherally active. In contrast, since atenolol's activity is confined to peripheral β-receptors, use of this drug enables more specific hypothesis testing. Atenolol's longer half-life also allows for a simpler once-daily dosage.

To date, 56 patients have completed the acute 8-week treatment trial. Twenty of the completers had been randomized to placebo, 18 to atenolol, and 18 to phenelzine. At week 8, 5 (25%) of the 20 patients on placebo, 5 (28%) of 18 on atenolol, and 13 (72%) of 18 on phenelzine were considered responders. The overall difference between rates was significant ($p = .02$). Phenelzine was significantly more effective than placebo and atenolol. Placebo and atenolol responses were not significantly different.

Of the 56, 41 (73%) completers were classified as having generalized social anxiety. The remaining 15 (27%) met criteria for the discrete subtype. Response rates among the generalized social phobics were 79% (11/14) for phenelzine, 15% (2/13) for atenolol, and 21% (3/14) for placebo ($p < .001$). Phenelzine remained significantly more effective than both atenolol and placebo. Placebo and atenolol again did not differ significantly.

In contrast, among the 15 discrete social phobic patients, only 1 of 4 on phenelzine, of 5 (60%) 3 on atenolol, and 2 (33%) of 6 on placebo were judged responders. The current sample size is clearly too small to allow conclusions.

However, these preliminary results do suggest a disordinal pattern of phenelzine response, in that it showed superiority in the more severe group. Phenelzine effectively treated 79% (11/14) of the generalized social anxiety patients (the complex A_cB_c form) as compared to only 25% (1/4) of the discrete subgroup (the simple A_s alone form). Despite small numbers, this difference showed a trend toward significance. Within the atenolol group, 15% (2/13) of those with generalized social anxiety responded versus 60% (3/5) for discrete social phobia (Fisher exact test, two-tailed, $p = .10$). The response to the peripheral β-blocker atenolol (if eventually definitive) is compatible with either a quantitative or qualitative distinction.

CONCLUSION

Comorbidity and syndromal complexity are widely prevalent among individuals with anxiety and affective disorder diagnoses. Although complicated, these phenomena may also present a valuable setting for further work in the continued effort to bring nosologic systems into closer proximity with underlying genetic, environmental, and/or pathophysiologic causative processes. The presence of comorbid syndromes can be used as a guideline for comparative splitting of existing diagnostic groups. Family, genetic, developmental, biologic challenge, and therapeutic studies can then be used to test the validity of these subdivisions.

Therapeutic trials are of limited use until methods are developed for determination of mechanism of drug action in specific situations. In most instances, pharmacologic dissection serves only an initial function of suggestion and hypothesis generation. However, in one special case, where a disordinal interaction is observed between severity of subtype and drug response, therapeutic outcome may definitively establish the existence of qualitative distinctions between syndromes.

The examples described above illustrate the potential power of pharmacologic dissection in this specific setting and highlight the importance of the concept of phenocopies in understanding psychiatric nosology. Future clinical trials will benefit from consideration of the possibilities of this design.

Chapter 38

Double Diagnosis: The Role of the Prior Odds on Each Disorder

Philip W. Lavori, Ph.D.

COMORBIDITY OF PSYCHIATRIC illness involves complex philosophical issues, such as the nature of disease entities; measurement issues, such as the appropriate nosologic classification schemes; and data handling and analysis issues, such as the decision of how much detail to retain in data bases. The philosophical or clinical-nosologic issues will not be discussed at length here because they can be found in other chapters. A brief excursion into this area will serve to set the stage for a pragmatic consideration of statistical issues. Thereafter the discussion will proceed on the premise that two diseases have been identified for study, and that it is possible, in principle, to imagine them co-occurring. This chapter will deal only with the problem of current diagnosis, rather than of continued follow-up or past diagnosis. The resulting narrow area of discussion is central and basic to any consideration of comorbidity.

Assume, therefore, that each individual may or may not have either or both of two disorders and that the diagnostic process for each disorder is independent of the knowledge of the presence or absence of the other disorder. To fix ideas, suppose that the two disorders are depression and panic disorder, and the diagnosis is to be made by a structured clinical interview such as the Structured Clinical Interview for DSM-III-R (SCID) (Spitzer, Williams, and Gibbon 1987) or Schedule for Affective Disorders and Schizophrenia (SADS) (Endicott and Spitzer 1978), using standard criteria, such as DSM-III-R (American Psychiatric Association 1987) or the Research

Diagnostic Criteria (RDC) (Spitzer, Endicott, and Robins 1978a). Now suppose that an individual has been diagnosed with both disorders. How valuable is this information? It will help first to consider some issues involved in a single diagnosis and then generalize to two or more diagnoses.

A standard measure of the information contained in a positive diagnosis is the "positive predictive value (PV +)," defined as the probability that the disease is truly present given the positive diagnosis:

$$PV + = P \text{ (Disease } | \text{ Diagnosis } +)$$

This quantity can be thought of in Bayesian terms as the posterior probability of disease given the "data," (i.e., the interview results). To keep these distinctions clear, one must distinguish between the presence of the disorder (i.e., the true state of nature) and the presence of the diagnosis (i.e., the data). The relationship between the true state of disease and the categories of diagnosis is expressed by certain relations of conditional probability:

$$\text{Sensitivity} = P(\text{Diagnosis} + | \text{ Disease}) = \frac{P(\text{Diagnosis} + \text{ \& Disease})}{P(\text{Disease})}$$

$$\text{Specificity} = P(\text{Diagnosis} - | \text{ No Disease}) = \frac{P(\text{Diagnosis} - \text{ \& No Disease})}{P(\text{No Disease})}$$

Sensitivity and specificity (which are conditional probabilities) are collectively called the "operating characteristics" of the diagnostic process. They may vary from disease to disease, so that there are separate operating characteristics for both the affective disorder and panic disorder. In addition, these conditional probabilities may vary from patient to patient since some patients may have more informative and definite presentations than others.

The term *operating characteristics* originated in signal-detection methodology, in an engineering context. Kraemer (1988) reviewed the generalizations of these methods to the biobehavioral context. Her analysis concerns the important case that there is both a "test" and a "gold-standard" diagnosis, as well as the unknown true state of the patient (referred to as the "signal," for historical reasons). In that context, the sensitivity and specificity are analysed as properties of the test, relative to the gold-standard diagnosis, which itself imperfectly represents the signal. The focus of that presentation is the performance of the test as a representation of the diagnosis, as in the common situation that an inexpensive screening procedure or short diagnostic interview is used as a surrogate for the gold-standard diagnostic procedure. Thus, although Kraemer's generalization to the biobehavioral model permits the diagnosis to have less than perfect reliability and correlation with the signal, the analysis of cost in her model depends only on the relationship between the test and diagnosis.

For example, Kraemer's cost analysis assigns a loss to discrepant test and diagnosis, regardless of the true state of the patient (the signal). This formulation would not be appropriate if the actual loss is a function of the discrepancy between the true state and the "decision" about the state (referred to here as the "diagnosis," most closely related to Kraemer's "test"). A concrete example serves to clarify this issue.

Suppose that the purpose of the diagnostic decision is to assign a subject to either the affected or unaffected category in an analysis of genetic linkage to some marker, and that the analysis will proceed by the affected relatives strategy (Lander and Botstein 1986). In this situation, the null hypothesis is that the hypothetical locus associated with the disease has recombination frequency 0.5 with the marker, and thus is distant in the sense of the recombination probability metric. The alternative hypothesis is that the disease locus is close to the marker, in terms of recombination frequency. These hypotheses are framed by the context that there is a genetic locus associated uniquely with the disease, and it is important to note that a nongenetic disease or a genetic lesion at a different locus tends to produce data that support the null hypothesis and reduce the lod scores. For the purposes of the linkage analysis, the true disease state of the subject is well-defined: the subject has the disease if the subject has a particular (unknown) genetic quality. If there is no such locus or it is not close to the marker, then "recombinations" (real or apparent) will tend to occur at random, and the lod score will reflect this tendency. If there is such a locus, close to the marker, then the null hypothesis is false, and the investigator will be interested in minimizing the probability of failing to reject the (false) null hypothesis (Type II error). A major component of the risk of Type II error comes from misclassification of subjects as affected when they do not have the specific lesion. This may occur as a result of nongenetic forms of the clinical syndrome masquerading as genetic, or there may be another genetic locus associated with a similar clinical picture.

A false positive in this context is the assignment of a positive diagnosis (T+ in Kraemer's notation, or D+ if the investigator uses the gold-standard diagnostic procedure) to a subject who does not have the specific lesion at the linked locus and thus does not have the signal in Kraemer's sense, or the disease in the sense used in this chapter. The "cost" to the investigator of such an error comes from the effect that these errors have on the linkage analysis: such subjects tend to add evidence apparently in favor of the null hypothesis; thus the Type II error is increased. The investigator might have some (a priori) decisions to make about whether to include all "diagnosis +" family members as affected cases in a linkage analysis, or to restrict the affected group to a more certainly positive set of diagnoses—perhaps the most severe or "clear-cut" cases, or those diagnosed by an experienced clinician. If the investigator decides to weigh the consequences of such a selective inclusion (sample size versus specificity), the appropriate measure of the certainty of a positive diagnosis is the posterior probability of disease, given a positive diagnosis (PV +).

There are circumstances when the investigator might be concerned with the relationship of a test result to the hypothetical result that would have been obtained by a particular gold-standard diagnostic procedure. In such cases, Kraemer's approach may be helpful. The diagnostic value of sleep characteristics (rapid eye movement latency), biologic measures (dexamethasone suppression test), and symptom scales (Hamilton 1960) have been assessed in this way. In particular, the test specificity and sensitivity could be considered relative to the diagnosis, rather than the "true" disease state, which may be unobservable or even undefined. (If the investigator does not postulate a unitary disease model, such as the linkage analysis requires, but rather an operational model based on the available diagnostic procedures, then it may be fruitless to pursue the "disease." To paraphrase Gertrude Stein, "there may be no there there.") For example, in the family-genetics substudy of the Collaborative Depression Study—National Institute of Mental Health Clinical Research Branch Collaborative Study of the Psychobiology of Depression-Clinical (Katz, Secunda, Hirschfeld, et al. 1979)—one object of study was the distribution of diagnoses in a set of families of affectively ill individuals. About half of the first-degree relatives and spouses of the probands (affectively ill individuals who were the index cases on which the families were ascertained) were available for direct interview by study raters, using the Schedule for Affective Disorders and Schizophrenia-Lifetime version (SADS-L) (Spitzer and Endicott 1977). All family members were diagnosed by the family history (FH) method using the RDC (Andreasen, Rice, Endicott, et al. 1986), based on interviews of the proband and at least one other "informant" in the family. The interview and FH-RDC data were combined into a consensus diagnosis when both were available, otherwise the consensus diagnosis was based on the two-informant FH-RDC. The consensus based on interview and FH might be thought of as a gold standard, and the FH alone might be thought of as a test. A question posed by Lavori and Keller (1988) was: "What would the rate of major affective disorder be in the uninterviewed relatives if they had been interviewed?" In this context, the PV+ and PV−refer to the posterior probabilities of diagnosis by consensus of FH-RDC and (hypothetical) interview, given the results (+ or −) of the FH-RDC. Thus the consensus diagnosis takes on the role of disease since it is the principal object of inquiry, and the FH-RDC diagnosis takes on the role of diagnosis since it is the observable result. Some information on operating characteristics (OC) were available from the "overlap" group of relatives who received both a direct interview and FH-RDC.

The interpretation of results may depend considerably on whether the "state of nature" is taken to be a hypothetical unitary disease (as in linkage) or an operational gold standard (as in consensus diagnosis), but the same theoretical development serves for both situations. To preserve the link to usual clinical usage, the state of nature will be referred to in this chapter as the disease (absent or present), and the results of the test will be referred to as a diagnosis. The value of a positive or negative diagnosis will then be analyzed using the Bayesian method.

The conditional probabilities of disease given the diagnostic results sum up the *value* of the diagnostic procedure. They express the state of certainty (or uncertainty) about the presence or absence of disease after the diagnosis is made (+ or −). They are called "posterior" probabilities, to reflect the fact that they are "updated" estimates of the uncertainty about the true state *after* ("posterior" to) the results of the diagnostic procedure. Posterior probabilities are related to the "prior" probabilities (sometimes called the base rates) of disease by Bayes' rule:

$$PV+ \; = \; P(\text{Disease} \mid \text{Diagnosis} +) \; = \; \frac{P(\text{Disease \& Diagnosis} +)}{P(\text{Diagnosis} +)}$$

$$= \; \frac{P(\text{Diagnosis} + \mid \text{Disease}) \, P(\text{Disease})}{P(\text{Diagnosis} + \mid \text{Disease}) P(\text{Disease}) \; + \; P(\text{Diagnosis} + \mid \text{No Disease}) P(\text{No Disease})}$$

$$= \; \frac{S_e P_D}{S_e P_D \; + \; (1-S_p)(1-P_D)}$$

where S_e = sensitivity, S_p = specificity, and P_D = P(Disease).

The relationship of these posterior probabilities to cost of decisions can be seen by imagining that a cost accounting is made of the consequences of decisions based on the results of the diagnosis, such as "if diagnosis is +, treat with antidepressants, otherwise place under observation," or "if diagnosis is +, use this individual as affected in a linkage analysis." In the treatment-decision context, there are several possible "identifications" of the state of nature (disease), while in the linkage context the state of nature has a unique identification. In both contexts, the "losses" or "gains" are contingent on the "fit" between the true state of nature and the decision, so that if the disease has an operational definition, the validity of the cost analysis will depend on the aptness of that definition. With that caveat, the overall costs will be weighted averages of posterior probabilities.

It is convenient to calculate the posterior odds on disease given a positive diagnosis, since the denominators cancel:

$$\frac{P(\text{Disease} \mid \text{Diagnosis} +)}{P(\text{No Disease} \mid \text{Diagnosis} +)} = \frac{\dfrac{P(\text{Disease \& Diagnosis} +)}{P(\text{Diagnosis} +)}}{\dfrac{P(\text{No Disease \& Diagnosis} +)}{P(\text{Diagnosis} +)}} = \frac{P(\text{Disease \& Diagnosis} +)}{P(\text{No Disease \& Diagnosis} +)}$$

$$= \frac{S_e P_D}{(1 - S_p)(1 - P_D)} = \frac{S_e}{(1 - S_p)} \frac{P_D}{(1 - P_D)}$$

Thus the occurrence of a positive diagnosis multiplies the prior odds on disease by a factor, $S_e/(1\text{-}S_p)$, sometimes called the Bayes factor. A similar result obtains in the case of a negative diagnosis. Thus if the sensitivity is .90 and the specificity is .80, the multiplier for a " + " diagnosis is $.90/.20 = 4.5$. The remaining uncertainty also depends on the prior odds. In a group of individuals with an overall 50% rate of disease (odds = 1:1), the rate of illness in those with a positive diagnosis would be $4.5/5.5 = 81\%$ (odds of 4.5:1). If the overall rate were only 5% (odds of 1:19), then the posterior odds would be 4.5:19, corresponding to a probability of $4.5/23.5 = 19\%$.

What does this have to do with comorbidity? In a clinical setting, patients may arrive from two intake streams (e.g., an anxiety clinic and an depression clinic). In both kinds of patients, we may make the dual diagnosis of depression and panic. However, the base rates of panic disorder may be less than 5% in the patients who arrive through the depression clinic and more than 50% in the anxiety clinic patients. Suppose for a moment that the two diagnostic processes (corresponding to the two diseases) have the same (excellent) OC of, say, 95% sensitivity and 90% specificity, and that these OC do not vary from clinic to clinic. The resulting Bayes factor is $.95/.10 = 9.5$. Then the diagnosis of panic disorder will be very valuable in the group of anxiety clinic patients (posterior probability over 90%) and nearly worthless in the depression clinic patients (posterior probability less than 40%).

If the specificity and sensitivity were so near perfect that the odds multiplier always overwhelmed the prior odds, we could ignore this problem. However, as long as we are interested in diagnosis when the prior odds are 1:20 or less, we need odds multipliers of over 20 to have confidence in a positive diagnosis, requiring sensitivities and specificities in the .95 range. To get truly accurate diagnosis, we might want a sensitivity of 1 and a specificity of .98. If two clinicians had these OC, their kappa (in the 50:50 situation) would be at least .95 (much higher than likely with current methods). Thus at current operating characteristics of diagnostic methods, the prior odds of disease (and therefore the intake stream) must be taken into account in evaluating the uncertainty of diagnosis.

The investigator may have limited confidence in estimates of the OC of the diagnostic methods and the prior odds (base rates) of the diseases in the population being sampled, but may have some idea about the relative sizes of these quantities, even if that idea is expressed as a range of plausible values. For example, the investigator may believe strongly that the prevalence of depression is at least 5 times but no more than 20 times the prevalence of panic disorder (in the particular intake stream) and that the sensitivities of the diagnoses are at least .9, while the specificities are each between .7 and .9.

To get an idea of the relative value of the positive diagnoses of depression and panic disorder, it is instructive to contrast the PV+ of each disorder. By taking the ratio of the posterior odds on each disease given a positive diagnosis of each, one obtains a measure of the relative certainty of each diagnosis. From the equation above, one obtains a ratio of posterior odds for, say, depression and panic, that is the product of two terms: the ratio of Bayes factors for the two disorders and the ratio of prior odds of the two disorders. The Bayes factor reflects the amount by which the positive diagnosis changes the prior odds and is a function of the OC of the diagnosis. If the diagnoses of panic and depression have equal OC, then the ratio of posterior odds will be just the ratio of prior odds. Thus if the one disease is much less prevalent than another, the posterior odds after a positive diagnosis will be much lower for the less prevalent disorder, unless the Bayes factor for the less prevalent diagnosis is correspondingly higher (greater sensitivity and specificity).

In the example above, the most favorable ratio of Bayes factors for the panic disorder diagnosis that is consistent with the beliefs of the investigator occurs when the sensitivity of panic disorder diagnosis is 1.0 and depression diagnosis is .9, while the corresponding specificities are .9 and .7, so that the Bayes factor for panic diagnosis is $1/(1 - .9) = 10$ and the Bayes factor for depression diagnosis is $.9/(1 - .7) = 3$. The ratio of these factors is $10/3 = 3.3$, so that even under the extreme assumption that the prior odds of depression are only five times those of panic, the posterior odds on depression exceed the posterior odds on panic, after both are diagnosed as "present." Thus the investigator will be less sure of the panic disorder diagnosis under any circumstance that is consistent with the range of possibilities set out above. This analysis is "quick and dirty" because it does not take into account the possible associations between the diseases, or the possibly complex relationship between the diagnostic procedures for the two disorders, but it provides outer limits for the relative values of the diagnoses. A more realistic analysis is developed below.

Since the source of patients for a study heavily influences the prior odds of each disease, and thus the posterior odds, it would be desirable to have some discussion of the determinants of the prior odds, such as "presenting complaint" or "catchment area" or "referral pattern" in presentations of the results of diagnostic studies. In this way, the reader could make informed guesses about the true value of the diagnoses. The investigator could go further by providing estimates (or ranges) of the prior odds and the Bayes factors. This may seem a lot to require, and the investigator might wonder how to find estimates of these quantities, but in the light of the above discussion it is fair to turn the question around and ask how the investigator values diagnostic rates presented in isolation, without a calibrating framework of OC and prior odds. At the very least, the investigator ought to discuss any asymmetry in sampling that might be relevant to the PV +. For example, the "found" diagnosis of panic disorder in patients whose presenting complaint is depression may carry much less value than the same diagnosis in patients presenting with phobic avoidance to a specialist in anxiety, after referral by a primary care provider. It is hard to see how the "consumer" of diagnoses can make sensible use of the results without making assumptions about this auxiliary information. Since variance in implicit assumptions can lead to explicit disagreements about content, it would be preferable to expose the necessary assumptions to scrutiny.

It is clear from the mathematics that if subgroups of patients (defined by intake stream as well as other characteristics) differ widely in prior odds of disease, then this should be reflected by providing separate prior estimates for these groups. Similarly, the OC of a given diagnostic method might vary considerably, due to measurable features of the patient (such as how close to the threshold of diagnosis the symptom pattern or number was). Different patients might have received diagnoses based on different methods (FH versus family study, SCID versus SADS, clinical interview versus lay person or computer interview). Thus the Bayes factors might be estimated separately for subgroups of patients. More appropriate prior odds and Bayes factors for subgroups of patients will lead to better estimates of the PV +. The resulting empirical distribution of PV + across the sample would make it possible to estimate the net content of the positive diagnoses in the sample. The average (or modal) posterior probability of disease given a positive diagnosis could be used as a "weight" to adjust the usually reported figure (percentage of positive diagnosis) to reflect more closely the amount of true diagnosis in the sample.

These methods would also provide a framework for incorporating the estimates of "reliability" that are sometimes available at the time of interview, by using them to adjust the multipliers. Much more work of a methodological nature needs to be done in this area, but a good start has been made by Rice, Endicott, Knesevich, et al. (1987). These investigators have developed models for predicting the stability of diagnosis over time. It would be a logical step to build such models into an overall assessment of the multipliers for prior odds.

THE PREDICTIVE VALUE OF DOUBLE DIAGNOSIS

So far this discussion has treated the problem of "double diagnosis" as if the diagnoses were made independently and in isolation from each other. But it is more realistic to consider the entire diagnostic process as a single measurement process, with four outcomes (both diagnoses positive, both negative, or the two cases of single diagnosis). If both diagnoses are made in the same individual, one may ask what is the conditional probability of actually having both diseases, given a double diagnosis, since this is obviously the minimal case of comorbidity. Suppose we consider the comorbidity of an anxiety disorder and depression. Let A denote the true presence of anxiety, and a its absence, similarly, D and d shall denote the presence and absence (respectively) of depression. If the event of a simultaneous positive diagnosis on each disorder is denoted by $++$, it is possible to inquire into the PV $++$:

$$P(AD \mid ++) = \frac{P(++ \mid AD)P(AD)}{P(++)}$$

$$= \frac{P(++ \mid AD)P(AD)}{P(++ \mid AD)P(AD) + P(++ \mid Ad)P(Ad) + P(++ \mid aD)P(aD) + P(++ \mid ad)P(ad)}$$

$$= \frac{S_e P(AD)}{S_e P(AD) + X_{Ad}P(Ad) + X_{aD}P(aD) + X_{ad}P(ad)}$$

where X_{Ad}, etc. are the various conditional probabilities of mistakenly giving a diagnosis of $++$ given the true states Ad, etc. and S_e is the "sensitivity" of the double diagnosis.

In the double diagnosis situation, there are three "nonspecificities" that affect the performance of the diagnosis; these are X's in the denominator of the equation above. The weight of each nonspecificity is determined by the corresponding probability of the joint occurrence of the states Ad (anxiety without depression), Da (depression without anxiety), and ad (neither disorder).

To see how this might work out in a simple situation, suppose that the two disorders have a joint distribution described by the following two-way table of probabilities:

	D	d
A	.3	.2
a	.2	.3

This is the situation that would reflect 50:50 marginal distributions for each disorder and a 9/4 odds ratio, indicating modest association of the disorders. It is not necessarily realistic, but will suffice to give the flavor. Suppose that the sensitivity is as high as 90%; that is, given that both disorders are present, a + + diagnosis will be made 90% of the time. Suppose also that the probability of a + + diagnosis is very small if neither disorder is present (ad), say 10%. Suppose further that the probabilities of a + + diagnosis if only one of the diagnoses is present (aD and Ad) are both equal to 20%. Then the posterior probability is

$$(.3 \times .9)/(.3 \times .9 + .2 \times .2 + .2 \times .2 + .3 \times .1) = .71$$

so that prior probability of comorbidity (30%) has been "updated" to only 71% after the joint positive finding.

In disorders (such as anxiety and depression) that have many common presenting features, it is likely that the presence of one of the disorders will substantially increase the likelihood that the other will be diagnosed, even if it is not present. This nonspecificity may be greater than 20%, in which case the denominator will increase and further erode the value of the double diagnosis. When the comorbid state is less likely a priori (perhaps because the association is less strong), there will be a similar decline in the numerator, and the denominator may rise because the nonspecificities will have greater play. The moral of this story may be that avoiding the "carryover" of one disorder's symptoms to the other disorder's diagnosis is the best way to ensure a high value for the double diagnosis of comorbidity.

Another simplified case occurs when the disorders are independent of each other, the sensitivity is perfect, and the last nonspecificity is zero (diagnosis + + is never made when neither disorder is present). If either disorder (for the sake of argument, anxiety) occurs half the time, then the PV + + simplifies to $p(D)/(P(D) + X)$ where X is the remaining inspecificity (the probability of a + + if only one disorder is present) and P(D) is the probability of depression. This illlustrates the fact that the posterior probability of comorbidity may be considerably less than 100% if the "carryover nonspecificity" is at all substantial. If the carryover nonspecificity exceeds the prior probability of the depressive disorder, under these simplified conditions, then the PV + + will be less than 50%. This would easily occur if the depressive disorder were truly uncommon, but the anxiety disorder had symptoms that made it easy to get a false-positive diagnosis of depression when only anxiety was present. Again, the thrust of this argument is the need to avoid carryover nonspecificity.

This issue takes on great importance in the analysis of genetic data, in particular in linkage analysis, where the avoidance of false positives is a critical need. Heterogeneity and lack of penetrance may be overcome by the newest methods of analysis based on multiple marker maps, but only if the rate of false positives is kept near zero. When the diagnostic systems and the state of nature are such as to make it easy for one disorder to masquerade as another, then the phenocopy problem becomes acute, even if one restricts positive diagnosis to the apparently comorbid cases.

The Comorbid Versus "Other" Diagnosis

When the investigator is interested in all four combinations of diagnostic status, such as in an investigation of the association between the disorders in individuals, it is necessary to consider an analysis of the type considered above, based on the cross-classification of the disorders and the corresponding cross-classification of the diagnoses. When the investigator is interested in the comorbid cases per se, as in a linkage study, or a subtype analysis where the typology is determined by comorbidity, then one may consider the true state as binary —comorbid or not—and similarly categorize the diagnosis as + + or not. In this case, the problem is formally equivalent to the single diagnosis situation, although it must be emphasized that the definitions of sensitivity, specificity, and prior odds all change to reflect the collapsing of three states into one. The investigator may try to estimate the PV + by using estimates of the sensitivity and specificity provided by other studies, and an internal estimate of the prior base rate. The probability of positive diagnosis is related to the prevalence, sensitivity, and specificity by the following equation:

$$P(\text{Diagnosis}+) = P_D S_e + (1 - P_D)(1 - S_p)$$

where P_D is the prior probability of disease.

Using the observed rate of diagnosis P_{Dx} as the estimator of the left-hand term, and solving for P_D, one obtains the estimate of prevalence (Rogan and Gladen 1978):

$$P_D = (P_{Dx} - (1 - S_p))/(S_e + S_p - 1)$$

Substituting this estimate of the prevalence into the equation for the PV+ yields an estimate for the PV+:

$$est(PV+) = [S_e/(S_e + S_p - 1)][1 - (1 - S_p)/P_{Dx}]$$

Suppose that the sensitivity is perfect; then the estimate simplifies to:

$$(1/S_p)\{1 - (1 - S_p)/P_{Dx}\}$$

Since the true rate must be positive, P_{Dx} must be greater than $1 - S_p$, so that implicit in the use of such a diagnosis is the assumption that the specificity is at least as great as the observed rate of "negative diagnosis." If the specificity is at all close to the rate of "negative diagnosis," the PV+ will be close to zero; thus, for observed comorbidity of 20% or less, one needs specificities of 90% or more to obtain PV+ over 50%.

The sampling variability of the PV+ can be estimated from the formula above. Gastwirth (1987) provides a formula for the variance of the PV+ that takes account of the extra variability inherent in the fact that estimates of the sensitivity and specificity are based on finite samples. That article contains important results applied to the enzyme-linked immunosorbent assay (ELISA) test for acquired immune deficiency syndrome (AIDS) that have direct relevance to the comorbidity problem.

CONCLUSION

Comorbidity of psychiatric disorders is an important topic that is currently under intense investigation by many clinical researchers. Reports of high levels of "other" disorders appear in the literature of each disease specialty: anxiety on depression, depression on alcoholism, and personality disorders everywhere. These findings may be real, but some comorbidity owes more to nonspecificity than to disease. Disentangling the false clues from the true cases will require punctilious attention to the goals of nosologic classification as well as the technology of diagnosis. In the meantime, the investigator who masters the consequences of the imperfections of the current diagnostic techniques will avoid false starts on fruitless paths and take the reports of comorbidity with the appropriate amount of salt.

Chapter 39

Relationships Between Anxiety and Depression Affecting Development of Antidepressant and Antianxiety Drugs

Donald S. Robinson, M.D.
Neil M. Kurtz, M.D.

THE COMORBIDITY OF anxiety and depressive disorders must be considered in the development of new treatments for anxiety and depressive disorders. The pharmaceutical industry is quite sensitive, in general, to issues of diagnostic specificity because a firm is obligated by regulatory agencies, as a prerequisite of approval, to demonstrate efficacy of its agent in carefully defined nosologic categories. Issues that obfuscate diagnostic precision affect both regulatory agencies and investigators, perhaps contributing to inconsistent research results and problems in interpretation of findings. Methodological imprecision serves to retard the discovery process for novel psychoactive drugs.

Before discussing specific concerns about comorbidity of anxiety and depression and their effects on drug discovery, it may be useful to gain some insight into the developmental process. We will briefly review the three phases of clinical development required to achieve critical decision points by a drug sponsor and to satisfy the requirements of the Food and Drug Administration (FDA).

DRUG DEVELOPMENT PROCESS

Phase I

The aim here is to determine in normal subjects whether a drug is safe and well tolerated. Experimental designs involve single-dose and multiple-dose safety and tolerability studies with careful laboratory and medical surveillance to establish the safety of the compound. Pharmacokinetic data also are obtained to provide preliminary information about absorption, distribution, metabolism, and excretion of the drug in humans. This information will be important in designing definitive Phase II and Phase III efficacy trials.

Phase II

This stage includes studies involving relatively small numbers of patients to gain preliminary evidence of efficacy for the targeted indication. A major objective of Phase II is to allow an internal decision to be made as to the therapeutic potential of a compound. Additional goals are to determine whether a compound is safe and well tolerated by patients and to secure further insight about effective dosage range and dosing strategy for designing the definitive (pivotal) Phase III efficacy trials.

Generally, a drug regulatory agency will not accept symptom amelioration alone as evidence of therapeutic effect. The FDA requires that diagnostic entities show change, not simply symptoms in ill-defined populations. For example, if one wants to develop a drug effective in depression, it is not acceptable merely to show that the agent ameliorates the symptoms of dysphoria, motor retardation, suicidal ideation, and appetite disturbance. One must establish that patients meeting diagnostic criteria for depression benefit from drug therapy. The third edition of the *Diagnostic and Statistical Manual of Mental Disorders* (DSM-III) (American Psychiatric Association 1980) defines nosologic criteria regarded by the FDA as essential to the development process. Other diagnostic criteria, such as the Feighner criteria (Feighner, Robins, Guze, et al. 1972) or the Research Diagnostic Criteria (RDC) (Spitzer, Endicott, and Robins 1978a, b), have been used previously, but a preference is evolving for DSM-III, and now DSM-III-R (American Psychiatric Association 1987).

Phase III

In this later development phase, a sponsor conducts large-scale, so-called pivotal, efficacy trials to establish efficacy conclusively for regulatory purposes. To obtain approval for a putative anxiolytic or antidepressant drug in the United States, the preferred design for efficacy studies is either two-arm or three-arm, placebo-controlled trials using parallel treatment groups. A pivotal study is defined as one that a group of qualified experts would regard as providing unequivocal evidence of efficacy in the target patient population.

The sample size must be large enough to ensure adequate statistical power to distinguish active treatment and placebo. This decision is based on the inherent variability of the sample and the therapeutic activity of the drug estimated from Phase II studies and from the literature. It is also based on the Type I and Type II error risks one is willing to accept. Symptom co-occurrence and nosologic uncertainty contribute to increased variance and tend to obscure drug effects. These factors dictate larger samples to counter the greater variability. Increasing sample size mandates studies that have greater cost, are more time consuming, and may necessitate a multicenter rather than a single-site design.

Recently, increased emphasis has been placed on obtaining long-term safety data to ensure that a compound is safe and well tolerated over a prolonged period of administration. Although the FDA does not specify patient numbers to be used in such investigations, in general at least 100 patients with an anxiety or depressive disorder treated continuously for at least 6 months is acceptable. Issues relating to drug approval in European countries are beyond the scope of this chapter, but requirements vary considerably. As a result, placebo-controlled trials play a less central role in psychopharmacologic drug development in the majority of nations outside of the United States.

COMORBIDITY, NOSOLOGY, AND DRUG DEVELOPMENT STRATEGY

The comorbidity of anxiety and depressive disorders, by affecting diagnostic precision, influences the developmental strategy of anxiolytic or antidepressant compounds. This issue is particularly relevant if the experimental agent has both putative and antianxiety and antidepressant properties.

The comorbidity issue is complicated by the fact that there are no symptoms absolutely pathognomonic of either anxiety or depressive disorders. Highlighting this fact is the Bristol-Myers experience from two recently conducted studies (data on file, Bristol-Myers Co.), one with gepirone, a putative anxiolytic-antidepressant, and the other with nefazodone, a putative antidepressant agent. The gepirone study involved 140 patients meeting the inclusion criterion of manifest anxiety symptoms present for at least 4 weeks, which in the investigator's judgment required drug treatment. Existence of a DSM-III Axis I diagnosis other than generalized anxiety disorder (GAD) was an exclusion factor. In the nefazodone study, 100 patients were enrolled meeting DSM-III criteria for major depressive disorder with the proviso that they could have no other Axis I diagnosis. In both studies, at baseline, patients completed the Symptom Checklist-90 (SCL-90) (Derogatis 1977), a self-rated symptom checklist consisting of an anxiety factor, a depression factor, and other symptom dimensions relevant to mood disorders.

When the authors examined specific symptom items reported by patients in each study, an interesting pattern emerged. In general, neither depressed nor anxious patients reported symptoms unique to that particular sample. This lack of specificity may not be particularly surprising for the depressed group, as it is well-known that depressed patients experience considerable anxiety. Given the hierarchical nature of DSM-III, many depressed patients could, in fact, also meet symptom criteria for GAD. What is less easily explained is why patients with anxiety disorder shared many symptoms with the depressed patients. All of the SCL-90 depression items were also reported by patients in the anxiety trial with gepirone. The principal difference in symptom profile between the two samples was a severity dimension. This difference is consistent with Leff's (1978) study, which concludes that patients cannot discriminate accurately between the experiences of anxiety and depression.

Consistent with these SCL-90 findings were observer-rated Hamilton Rating Scale for Depression (HRSD)(Hamilton 1960) scores. There were no real qualitative differences in HRSD symptom profiles (except for severity) between the anxiety and depressed samples, as rated by the physician. However, physicians tended to rate the severity of depressive symptoms in the anxiety study population lower than did the patients with GAD themselves. One explanation is that physicians may be more sensitive to the predominant mood disorder, while discounting symptoms relating to a secondary diagnosis or syndrome. Another possibility is bias on the part of the screening physician in rating symptoms specified as inclusion criteria for the study. A possible consequence of such bias could be poor concurrence in patient selection and diagnosis from center to center.

Findings of coexistent depressive and anxiety symptoms in these populations are consistent with a unitary hypothesis postulating that most individuals lie somewhere along a continuum between pure anxiety disorder and pure depressive disorder. The symptom mix may shift back and forth as a function of time, and with advancing age there appears to be a trend to progress from anxiety to depressive disorder (Kendell 1974). This progression is supported by the observation that, in elderly patients, a GAD diagnosis is relatively uncommon, whereas major depressive disorder is much more prevalent. While this fact has implications for the pathogenesis of anxiety and depression, it holds particular relevance for the field of drug development. Many patients during an index depressive episode have been previously diagnosed as suffering an anxiety disorder and have been treated with an anxiolytic drug. Subsequent inclusion of such patients in an antidepressant drug trial could be questioned during an audit performed by a regulatory agency. Of possible theoretic importance, although not well studied, is the likelihood that history of anxiety disorder affects treatment response to antidepressants. By and large, the pharmaceutical industry is committed to a simple cross-sectional approach to nosology, with the index episode determining entry into a study. The complexities of longitudinal clinical data have not been addressed in drug development, nor have they been addressed by the field at large.

CLINICAL TRIAL METHODOLOGIES FOR NOVEL ANXIOLYTIC-ANTIDEPRESSANT DRUGS

In studies to develop an anxiolytic drug, a principal criterion for patient entry is that the subject manifest significant anxiety symptoms for a sustained period. To obviate questions about whether the condition represents merely an adjustment reaction, it is generally wise to specify a minimum duration of continuously present symptoms. DSM-III requires a 4-week duration for GAD; DSM-III-R specifies 6 months (American Psychiatric Association 1987). In the aforementioned gepirone study, the entry criterion was simply manifest anxiety symptoms of 4 weeks duration rather than requiring that patients meet GAD criteria. However, physicians were asked to complete a "DSM-III symptom checklist" to allow the sponsor to make a DSM-III diagnosis retrospectively, if necessary. It was found that 100% of patients, in fact, met GAD criteria, and 36% had a history of major depression and/or dysthmia. Even though the cross-sectional diagnosis at entry to the gepirone trial was GAD (and by definition not major depressive disorder or dysthymia), this requirement does not infer absence of any depressive symptoms. In fact, as shown above, depressive symptoms were common in the patients with GAD, and, as stated above, patients rated themselves as more depressed than did the ratings of their physicians.

A standard study design for an anxiolytic drug is to administer it for 4 to 6 weeks, comparing drug to placebo response. Major outcome measures are subjective rating scales completed either by the investigator and/or the patient. A commonly employed rating scale is the

Hamilton Anxiety Rating Scale (HARS) (Hamilton 1959). While the HARS has established utility, its positive features, not the least of which are published data validating its use, do not meet all needs. One limitation is that the anxiety scale includes nonspecific symptoms common to several mood disorders. It was never intended to be a diagnostic instrument, but rather was to be used to detect changes in symptom severity among patients undergoing treatment. Complicating interpretation, the HARS has largely been validated in treatment studies of anxiety disorders involving benzodiazepines. Its popularity and continued use by sponsors in anxiolytic drug development may be attributed, in part, to the fact that it is a good benzodiazepine rating scale. The HARS actually gives "credit" to prominent benzodiazepine side effects (e.g., sedation and sleep induction). Amelioration of these symptoms does not necessarily infer clinically significant antianxiety activity, but rather nonspecific central nervous system depressant activity.

In trying to develop a nonbenzodiazepine anxiolytic that does not share these properties, a drug developer may be penalized by use of the HARS and overlook important antianxiety properties of a novel compound. Such was the case when comparing the anxiolytic profile of buspirone to diazepam in placebo-controlled trials in anxiety disorders. Diazepam treatment produces prompt decreases in HARS scores of many patients, principally due to immediate sedative effects. On the other hand, buspirone therapy produces a gradual reduction in scores on the HARS, reflecting its anxioselective effects. The HARS data have been interpreted as showing that benzodiazepines have a more rapid anxiolytic effect than the so-called anxioselective agents. When the individual scale items were analyzed in the buspirone and gepirone studies, however, a different interpretation emerged. It appeared that items relating to muscle relaxation and sedation showed the greatest early changes. However, representative core anxiety items—that is, tension, nervousness, restlessness, dread, anticipatory concerns, and autonomic symptoms (e.g., heart pounding, sweating, gastrointestinal discomfort)—show gradual improvement over 7 to 14 days with both buspirone and diazepam. If buspirone were compared to diazepam on only these items, significant differences in therapeutic effects between the two drugs were not evident. In responders, buspirone treatment ameliorated muscle tension and insomnia, but this was presumably a secondary, or indirect, rather than a direct pharmacologic effect. Therefore, because of its nonspecificity, the HARS has significant limitations in developing new anxiolytic agents, particularly those described as being anxioselective.

Additional problems become apparent when dealing with an anxiolytic compound that has putative antidepressant properties. The choice of rating instruments for depression can be particularly complex. As cited above, many patients meeting DSM-III criteria for major depressive disorder not only have a past history of anxiety episodes, but are currently experiencing anxiety symptoms resembling GAD. In these patients, the physician must weigh the preponderance and severity of the anxiety and depressive symptoms based purely on his or her judgment. In some instances, the accuracy of the diagnosis could be questioned by auditors based on the historical information. A potential problem is that amelioration of anxiety in a patient with a comorbid diagnosis of major depressive disorder might infer that the agent lacks intrinsic antidepressant activity and is merely treating the anxiety component. This problem is confounded by the use of the HRSD and HARS because of overlapping items and the nonspecificity issue. It is quite likely that a purely anxiolytic drug given to a depressed patient will decrease the total HRSD score.

A critical issue is whether core depressive symptoms can be identified that do not occur to any significant degree in anxiety disorders and are responsive to antidepressant treatments. No consensus exists about core depression symptoms; agreement and validation are badly needed. Since there are no known symptoms truly pathognomonic of depression at the present time, one is left to decide which symptoms are more likely to be prominent in depression rather than in anxiety.

The impact of symptom comorbidity on the drug-development process of a putative anxiolytic-antidepressant is perhaps best illustrated by The Upjohn Company's recent experience with an antidepressant claim for alprazolam. Upjohn conducted prospective double-blind, placebo-controlled trials in patients who met DSM-III criteria for major depressive disorder and was able to show significant differences in HRSD scores between drug- and placebo-treated patients (Rickels, Feighner, and Smith 1985). One rationale given by the FDA for rejecting the evidence for alprazolam in depression was a failure to show an advantage for alprazolam on the so-called core symptoms of depression. It was contended that the Hamilton ratings could be significantly influenced by a "purely" anxiolytic drug as well as by "true" antidepressants. However, there is no unanimity as to what constitutes core depressive symptoms, and groups of experts may not concur on depression-specific symptoms. This issue is difficult and complex and deserves careful study with a goal of reaching consensus. Efforts are underway to attempt to develop improved scales with greater specificity (Rehm, Chapter 35; Rehm and O'Hara 1985).

Due to the present ambiguity, a pharmaceutical sponsor of a putative broad-spectrum anxiolytic-antidepressant faces a difficult task in gaining acceptance and approval of a novel agent with both anxiolytic and antidepressant effects. An overreliance on nosology has further complicated this issue. Present evidence suggests that prototypic antidepressants, especially the tricyclics and monoamine oxidase inhibitors, possess anxiolytic efficacy under certain conditions (Mountjoy, Roth, Garside, et al. 1977; Robertson and Trimble 1982; Tyrer, Gardner, Lambourn, et al. 1980). On the other hand, the evidence that anxiolytic drugs also may be effective antidepressants is less robust and still controversial (Fyer, Liebowitz, and Klein, Chapter 37; Johnstone, Cunningham, Owens, et al. 1980; Klein 1964; Lipman 1982).

Given the current degree of diagnostic imprecision, particularly in patients with both significant anxiety and depressive symptoms, it is possible that an appreciable number of patients currently diagnosed as having GAD would be categorized as depressed under different circumstances by other experienced clinicians and investigators. Likewise, a significant percentage of patients diagnosed as having major depressive disorder also meet criteria for GAD. For clinicians whose threshold for accepting depressive symptoms is set high, a greater number of patients would be diagnosed as having an anxiety disorder. This is underscored by the study of Riskind, Beck, Berchick, et al. (1987), in which there was considerable diagnostic disagreement among clinicians for patients with GAD and depressive symptoms. It is likely, therefore, that many patients currently being treated successfully with benzodiazepines for anxiety would, by some clinicians, be diagnosed as being depressed. Similarly, patients who are being treated for depression with antidepressants would probably be diagnosed as having an anxiety disorder by certain clinicians. Given these diagnostic uncertainties relating to symptom co-occurrence, the implications for development of a new drug are formidable.

CLINICAL EXPRESSION OF ANXIETY AND DEPRESSION RATING SCALES

Despite the problem of poor diagnostic precision, studies have found distinctions between patients diagnosed as anxious or depressed. Differing phenomenology and symptoms have been described based on clinical ratings (Lipman 1982; Mountjoy, Roth, Garside, et al. 1977; Prusoff and Klerman 1974) and physiologic measures, such as electrocortical (Shagass 1955) and electrogalvanic (Lader and Wing 1969) responses. Nevertheless, one cannot escape the fact that patients with heterogeneous diagnoses who seek treatment have similar complaints. The diagnostic label applied often depends on the bias and interests of the screening personnel. Given the current status of clinical assessment, the value of lumping patients into categorical entities is purely heuristic. Of greater significance is understanding which symptoms respond preferentially to a particular drug class, rather than overdefining poorly validated disease categories. Addressing such questions may provide insight into the underlying mechanism and pathogenesis of mood disorders. The question is not whether a 5-HT uptake inhibitor is an effective antidepressant, but rather which symptoms respond preferentially as compared to a noradrenergic uptake inhibitor or a 5-HT$_{1A}$ agonist. This information would be extremely valuable to the practicing clinician who is faced with selecting the preferred agent. Drugs with specific actions are likely to prove uniquely effective in a limited patient population. It is important to try to better define patient samples so that clinicians can select the most appropriate treatment. Such information could be obscured by requiring patients in clinical trials to be categorized primarily with a nosologic label and by ignoring other symptomatology.

In comparing anxiety and depressive disorders, it appears that items relating to (1) depressed mood, (2) work and interest, and (3) psychomotor retardation may best discriminate depression and anxiety (Rehm and O'Hara 1985). At Bristol-Myers, we have chosen to select these three HRSD items as representing the core symptoms of depression. By requiring patients to have significant ratings on these three items for entry in a study, and by examining change in these items relative to placebo, it is our contention that one could distinguish an antidepressant from an anxiolytic effect. Further efforts are required to modify and adapt the HRSD to make it a more sensitive instrument for purposes of drug development. Emphasis should be placed on constructing more specific scales capable of detecting and differentiating anxiolytic and antidepressant effects. Utilizing scales merely to detect change is very limiting in clinical research.

The HRSD was validated largely in the era of tricyclic antidepressant drug trials. Its 17 items can be thought of as a useful assay of treatment response in patients meeting criteria for major depression with melancholia, since it gives weight to endogenous symptoms. However, the majority of patients warranting treatment for depressive disorders do not meet melancholic criteria, suffering instead nonendogenous or atypical depressions. Many of these patients could benefit from pharmacologic intervention. However, most psychopharmacologic studies tend to target endogenous depression, which was thought to respond preferentially to somatic treatments. It is questionable how useful the 17-item HRSD is in assessing treatment effects in nonendogenous and atypical depressions, or in patients with dysthymic disorder. Many symptoms experienced by nonmelancholic patients are not addressed or rated in this scale. In developing novel antidepressants for targeted depression subgroups other than melancholia, improved rating instruments will be necessary. Again, scale development work is sorely needed. Furthermore, regulatory agencies must become receptive to new scales with appropriate validation. Despite its limitations, the tradition of the HRSD persists.

SPECIFICITY OF THERAPEUTIC EFFECTS OF DRUGS

Pharmacologic response of patients to psychotherapeutic agents has been used in psychobiology to elucidate mechanisms of action and to differentiate nosologic categories. Patients responding to antidepressants are regarded as being "depressed" while patients are "anxious" because they respond to an anxiolytic drug. The validity of this approach is subject to question because the therapeutic specificity of existing agents has not been thoroughly and systematically studied.

There is a paucity of studies assessing the anxiolytic properties of antidepressants, including the prototype tricyclics: imipramine and amitriptyline. The anxiolytic effects of these drugs need to be assessed in patients with GAD. The literature suggests that imipramine is, in fact, a useful anxiolytic drug (Kahn, McNair, Lipman, et al. 1986). However, to our knowledge, there has been only a single study with imipramine in a carefully selected GAD patient sample, as defined by DSM-III criteria; the results showed imipramine to be efficacious in GAD (Fyer, Liebowitz, and Klein, Chapter 37; Kahn, McNair, and Frankenthaler 1987).

When treating an anxiety disorder with a tricyclic, significant numbers of patients can be predicted to drop out because of side effects. In addition, the onset of therapeutic activity (as defined by the HARS) may lag behind the standard drug control, usually a benzodiazepine. However, for patients who remain in treatment, it might be expected that significant drug-placebo differences would be seen. If this proved to be the case, what interpretations would be possible? One would be that the patients were misdiagnosed and were really depressed. However, an alternative explanation is that no one should place undue reliance on arbitrary nosologic categories, but rather should focus on core symptom profiles.

A similar issue arises if one attempts to assess the antidepressant effects of anxiolytics. The response of depression to benzodiazepines has been widely studied (Johnson 1985; Schatzberg and Cole 1987a, 1987b). In general, it does not appear that the benzodiazepines are classic antidepressants. Although the benzodiazepines do improve overall HRSD scores in depressed patients, they have less consistently shown a benefit for core symptoms, especially in the endogenous depression symptom profile. It is possible that the triazolobenzodia-zepine, alprazolam, is unique for this clinical application (Rickels, Feighner, and Smith 1985). However, this compound's antidepres-sant efficacy is still controversial. Severely depressed inpatients with DSM-III major depressive disorder with melancholia and exhibiting shortened rapid eye movement latency did not respond to alprazolam (Dawson, Jue, and Brogden 1984). This negative outcome might infer that the drug is not effective in treating classic depression. It appears to be the accepted opinion that the benzodiazepines have limited, if any, utility in the treatment of patients with endogenous or severe depression. That the tricyclics are beneficial in treating anxiety, while benzodiazepines are marginally effective in severe depression, is con-sistent with the interpretation that anxiety and depressive disorders lie along a continuum, with the greater severity toward the depressive pole of the spectrum.

Pharmacologic Specificity of Panic Disorder

Panic disorder is the area where response to pharmacologic treatment has been utilized extensively as evidence of a distinct nosologic group. It has been reported that panic disorder responds preferen-tially to antidepressant drugs, such as the monoamine oxidase inhibi-tors (Sheehan, Ballenger, and Jacobsen 1980) and the tricyclic antide-pressants (Pecknold, McClure, and Appeltauer 1982). Recently, other studies show that potent, short-acting benzodiazepines such as alpra-zolam (Chouinard, Annable, Fontaine, et al. 1982; Tyrer 1984; Uhde, Siever, and Post 1984) and clonazepam (Beaudry, Fontaine, Mercier, et al. 1985) reduce spontaneous panic attacks. Higher doses of the less-potent benzodiazepines such as chlordiazepoxide (McNair and Kahn 1981) and diazepam (Noyes, Anderson, Clancy, et al. 1984) also improve spontaneous panic attacks, but the doses needed to treat patients with panic disorder would be more impairing, if not prohibi-tive. If benzodiazepines are found to be equieffective to antidepres-sant drugs in treating panic disorder, then one criterion used to differentiate panic disorder from other anxiety disorders would have to be rethought.

Categorization of Anxiety and Depressive Disorders: Is It Possible?

A lesson to be drawn from this discussion is that caution should be exercised before reification of current nosologic classifications. A case in point would be the history of DSM-III and DSM-III-R with regard to GAD. Because the DSM-III GAD diagnosis lacked construct validity and reliability, the diagnostic criteria were revised in DSM-III-R, again without validation studies to justify the changes that were adopted. It may be that similar problems will arise with diagnostic categories other than panic disorder, and subsequent versions of DSM may be extensively revised.

Unvalidated DSM-III-R syndromes create problems in new drug development. In the regulatory process there is a tendency to treat nosologic categories as valid clinical entities. For a variety of reasons, regulatory agencies place undue emphasis on, or at least tacitly accept as valid, these nosologic criteria for mood disorders. While this acceptance is understandable, it contributes to premature codification of DSM criteria, with resulting far-reaching, and often unappreciated, implications on the conduct of clinical research.

Drug sponsors are placed in an awkward situation. When it is required that a drug be tested by treating a diagnosis rather than a cluster of symptoms, some patients in the trial may receive a somewhat arbitrary diagnosis, and the precise clinical disorder may thereby be obscured. An interpretation is made that if a compound is effective in depression, it may not be effective in GAD or in panic disorder. However, the weight of evidence appears to be that these nosologic distinctions are blurred and do not hold up under pharmacologic scrutiny (e.g., imipramine's broad effectiveness in depression and anxiety disorders). There is little evidence suggesting antidepressant agents would not be effective antipanic or antianxiety agents, while most anxiolytics appear effective in panic disorder. The lack of psychopharmacologic specificity calls into question assumptions about drugs prescribed for mood disorders. Included among such questions are those demands made by the FDA that require separate preliminary evidence of efficacy for the same agent in depression, GAD, and panic disorder before fecund females may be entered into clinical trials. This requirement places an unnecessary burden of added cost on the drug sponsor.

The issue of comorbidity has academic interest. It is of primary interest to clinical investigators hoping to identify more homogeneous populations in an attempt to understand pathophysiology better. Practitioners, on the other hand, may not be particularly troubled by problems of symptom comorbidity. The clinician listens to patients' complaints and interprets the symptoms in terms of their preponderance and severity before choosing a therapy. In essence, the strategy is not to treat the nosology, but rather the symptoms. For the patient complaining of both anxiety and depressive symptoms, a preponderance involving the depressive spectrum would indicate the choice of an antidepressant, whereas if it were predominantly anxiety, an anxiolytic drug would be selected.

In the final analysis, all pharmacologic agents prescribed for the mood disorders predominately treat symptoms. Admittedly, some drugs are more effective in certain symptom clusters than others. Characteristic symptoms clusters often overlap nosologic categories. This situation is not unique to anxiety and depression. Rather, it is the case for all of psychopathology, as evidenced by the fact that antipsychotic drugs are not specifically antischizophrenic; symptoms of mania, psychotic depression, and drug-induced psychosis respond nicely to them.

Psychiatry is faced with an interesting problem. The benzodiazepines, the most widely prescribed class of drugs worldwide, are not indicated, as defined in the approved labeling, for a specific DSM-III diagnosis. For whom are these drugs being prescribed? Benzodiazepines represent the best example of the fact that clinicians treat symptoms and not nosologic categories. In none of the diagnoses selected for the Epidemiologic Catchment Area study (Regier, Myers, Kramer, et al. 1984) were benzodiazepines considered the drug of first choice, despite their widespread use. What is clear is that patients are being prescribed benzodiazepines to treat those symptoms that, in the clinician's judgment, respond to benzodiazepines.

In this regard, regulatory agencies are out of step, since they tend to adhere to nosologic criteria in making decisions about drug development. By pressuring pharmaceutical companies to "pigeonhole" patients into diagnostic entities, useful information is almost certainly lost and considerable time is added to the drug development process. For example, it is the policy of the FDA that before a compound can be used in fecund females, it must be shown to have efficacy. The ability to show efficacy in one anxiety disorder does not extend to another anxiety disorder for this purpose, even though a relationship might be inferred and the target symptoms of anxiety are the same.

For the sponsor developing a broad-spectrum antianxiety drug, this limitation means that for each separate anxiety classification, costly controlled trials must be done to show preliminary evidence of efficacy in nonfecund females for each separate DSM-III anxiety disorder. In essence, drug firms are expected to treat patient populations that are not necessarily the most typical for a disorder, in the effort to obtain preliminary evidence of efficacy. Because of the sample being studied, treatment studies may yield confusing results, especially since the patient sample of preliminary interest (i.e., younger women) is precluded from the study. This omission clearly adds to the development time of a new agent, especially the more novel compounds.

By requiring pharmaceutical companies to undergo a lengthy and somewhat arbitrary development process, the FDA contributes to the growing development costs of new psychopharmacologic agents.

These costs are ultimately passed on to consumers and detract from research support in other sectors.

If such FDA decisions were based on scientific merit, there could be little argument. Lack of consensus about the comorbidity of anxiety and depressive disorders and confusion about current nosologic distinctions should be reassessed as they apply to drug development. Experts in the field clearly disagree over the validity of certain diagnostic entities and the notion of drug specificity for many of the agents currently used to treat mood disorders.

The comorbidity issue calls for flexible regulatory policies regarding anxiolytic and antidepressant drug development. Emphasis should be placed on the measurement of specific symptomatic improvement with a particular therapeutic agent, in keeping with how drugs are used clinically. Reporting in a clinical trial that a patient has an anxiety or depressive disorder may result in overlooking important information about intrinsic drug activity.

Nosologic categories should infer meaningful clinical distinctions regarding heritability, clinical course, and treatment response. Present knowledge does not allow such conclusions regarding DSM-III or DSM-III-R. While categorical definition of diseases is a goal for which psychiatry should aim, this state of knowledge has not yet been attained. With our limited knowledge of how the central nervous system functions, we are left with an ability only to identify symptom patterns that respond preferentially to a given psychopharmacologic treatment.

The use of DSM-III should be primarily etiologic and descriptive and should not reify diagnostic categories. However, there is considerable concern that to some extent reification has occurred, with resultant adverse effects on clinical research and drug development. "Patients with major depressive disorders are different than patients with GAD who, in turn, differ from those with panic," argue many people, "because, after all, DSM-III says they're different."

Chapter 40

The Sampling of Experience: A Method of Measuring the Co-Occurrence of Anxiety and Depression in Daily Life

Marten W. de Vries, M.D.
Chantal I.M. Dijkman-Caes, Dr.S.
Philippe A.E.G. Delespaul, Dr.S.

A NXIETY AND DEPRESSION are today recognized as the most frequently occurring mental disorders in the general population, especially in women (American Psychiatric Association 1980; Pitts 1971; Robins, Helzer, Weissman, et al. 1984; Wittchen 1986). Moreover, symptoms of anxiety and depression commonly coexist in both clinical and normal populations (Dobson 1985a; Hamilton and Alagna 1985; Roth and Mountjoy 1982). These data suggest that anxiety and depression are comorbid conditions. Although not an entirely new observation, comorbidity has created a conundrum for researchers

This chapter is partly derived from data presented elsewhere for which permission for republication has been granted: de Vries MW, Delespaul Ph, Dijkman-Caes CIM: Affect and anxiety in daily life, in Anxious Depression: Assessment and Treatment. Edited by Racagni G, Smeraldi E. New York, Raven Press, 1987, pp 21–32; de Vries MW: Introduction: investigating mental disorders in their natural settings (special issue). J Nerv Ment Dis 175:503–509, 1987.

The research was supported by the University of Limburg and by the Dutch Science Foundation (Medigon; grant 900.556.046).

Individuals seeking startup consultation, training, or apparatus should contact: M. W. de Vries, IPSER Institute, Box 214, 6200 AE Maastricht, The Netherlands.

who have worked largely in separate camps on each disorder. It is unclear whether the phenomenon of comorbidity is related to methodological shortcomings, artifacts or classification procedures, or new discoveries.

In this chapter, we will focus on methods that offer a supplementary research strategy for investigating the co-occurrence of anxiety and depression symptoms in daily life. With this method, we first propose a decreased reliance on cross-sectional, one-time assessments of traits that require retrospective recall by the patient. There is now ample evidence that historical and retrospective data of this kind provide only one fragment of reality about pathologic processes. Since this fragment is of indeterminant size, it may be misleading (Lamiell 1981). Moreover, cross-sectional measures of depression and anxiety have such an extensive overlap that they may contribute directly to the problem of discriminating anxiety and depression (Dobson 1985a).

We advocate the repeated measures of clinical phenomena by means of interrupting the flow of a person's experience. Information is thereby acquired with greater frequency and ecological detail. Second, we suggest that the phenomena should be examined by means of self-reports within the real-time and natural environment of daily life. This method would partly solve the problem of unreliable, retrospective reporting and increase the ecological validity of the findings. Research that adequately describes the person in context, however, has proved difficult, in part due to the lack of readily available and replicable assessment methods with which to describe the places and social contexts of interest to psychiatry. Researchers have paid insufficient attention to the variability and patterning of conscious experience over time and may have overlooked important features of psychopathology.

In this chapter, we explore the daily interplay of anxiety and depression in a group of individuals diagnosed with primary anxiety disorders. A new time-sampling method, the experience sampling method (ESM), is used; it provides data on time allocation and mental state gathered in real-life situations by signaling subjects to complete self-report forms at random intervals (de Vries 1987; Larson and Csikszentmihalyi 1984). The method is quantitative and replicable. ESM produces a high level of situational and temporal detail, made possible by advances in ambulatory signaling devices, computer science, and statistical methods that enable investigators to acquire, store, and analyze vast amounts of useful information about individual subjects. Such advances have allowed time-sampling techniques to move to the forefront of behavioral science research over the last 10 years (Gross 1984; Pervin 1985).

A key problem is that the foundation of the third edition of the *Diagnostic and Statistical Manual of Mental Disorders* (DSM-III) (American Psychiatric Association 1980) rests on the criteria of exclusivity. The notion of exclusivity has obviously been useful for classification and research purposes, but little evidence for symptom exclusivity can be found in the accounts of illness experience of individual patients. The individual experience of psychopathologic symptoms is more complex, dynamic, and interrelated (de Vries 1987). Our approach to the problem is to seek quantifiable phenomenological descriptions of the co-occurrence of different symptoms on a moment-to-moment basis in individuals, in this case, with presumed comorbid anxiety and affective disorders. Clinically, this group deserves our attention, regardless of the outcome of the nosologic debate concerning depression and anxiety because they tend to be sicker. Whether they are anxiety patients with concurrent depressive symptoms or depressive patients with concurrent symptoms of anxiety, these individuals suffer greater morbidity and poorer psychosocial outcome than patients with depression alone or with anxiety alone (Stavrakaki and Vargo 1986; Van Valkenburg, Akiskal, Puzantian, et al. 1984). In exploring anxiety and depression, a key problem remains that we have discovered an important clinical entity but lack a means of defining it adequately. To this end we offer a supplementary research strategy that takes time, situations, and subjective experience more fully into account.

TIME-SAMPLING TECHNIQUES IN PSYCHIATRY

Historically, psychiatry has not been blind to the influence of temporal and situational factors on mental disorders. They were recognized in the late 19th century by Kahlbaum, Kraepelin, and Bleuler in their detailed descriptions of schizophrenia. Today they are the focus of study in life history and life event research. The research reported here extends this interest and borrows further from a variety of time-sampling approaches that date back at least to the ethnographies of Malinowski (1935). Further contributions have been made by the more systematic application of time-observation techniques in naturalistic field studies (Barker 1978; Chapple 1970; Munroe and Munroe 1971a, 1971b), by ethological research strategies applied in psychiatry (McGuire and Polsky 1979; Reynolds 1965), and by behavior-monitoring techniques (Nelson 1977).

Another important influence has come from research on circadian rhythms, which has evolved from the early work of Wada (1922), who described rhythmicity in gastric motility, to the discovery and detailed exploration of cyclical rapid eye movements in different stages of sleep (Kleitman 1963; Kripke 1983). Several investigators have sought a comparable rhythmicity affecting cycles of arousal and behavioral activity in the waking person. Although this line of research has not yet been successful, it has highlighted the profound influence of "zeitgebers," daily environmental time setters (Minors and Waterhouse 1981; Reynolds 1965). Temporal and setting effects in daily life have also been shown to influence a variety of biologic and behavioral measures (Dimsdale 1985; Palmer and Harrison 1983).

One of the key ancestors of the studies presented here has been the time-budget survey. Although scientific study of time budgets goes back many generations, there has been a recent surge of activity focused on a variety of social problems (Michelson 1978; Robinson 1977). A good example is the International Time-Budget Study (Robinson 1977; Stone and Nicolson 1987; Szalai 1972). This massive undertaking obtained 25,000, 24-hour diaries in 12 countries and represented more than 640,000 events. Information was gathered on what people did, when they did it, for how long they did it, where it took place, and in what social context. Information was provided about the frequency, duration, and sequence of circumstances and events. The International Time Budget Study ascertained that time-use variations differentiated populations on the basis of cultural-political, class, occupational, and personal factors (Szalai 1972). Extention of this approach to clinical groups could serve a number of psychiatric purposes by broadening the mental status examination, supplementing intake procedures, clarifying points for therapeutic interventions, and improving clinical reasoning and psychosocial formulations.

ESM, a time-based ambulatory monitoring, data-gathering strategy enabling the study of mental disorders in the natural context has been introduced to psychiatry (de Vries 1987). ESM provides a representative sample of moments in a person's daily life. It uses an electronic signaling device that directs subjects to fill out self-reports at preselected but randomized time points, thus providing information about an individual's mental status or symptoms within the context and flow of experience. The method avoids the problem of global and retrospective recall that haunts the one-time sampling procedures of psychiatric research (Fiske 1971; Lamiell 1981; Mischel 1968; Willems 1969; Yarmey 1979).

The self-report forms request a range of information about the subject's objective and subjective state 4 to 20 times per day for 1 week. Information such as where subjects are, what they are doing, and who they are with, as well as information about their thoughts, moods, activities, select somatic as well as psychological symptoms and specific aspects of their social and environmental context, are reported. Responses are noted in small booklets of self-report forms (see Figure 1).

what were you thinking at the moment of the beep? ....

was this thought:

	not	a little	rather	very much
pleasant?	1 2	3 4	5 6	7
clear?	1 2	3 4	5 6	7
normal?	1 2	3 4	5 6	7
distorted?	1 2	3 4	5 6	7

at the moment of the beep, did you feel:

	not	a little	rather	very much
relaxed?	1 2	3 4	5 6	7
sad?	1 2	3 4	5 6	7
lonely?	1 2	3 4	5 6	7
satisfied?	1 2	3 4	5 6	7
anxious?	1 2	3 4	5 6	7
listless?	1 2	3 4	5 6	7
angry?	1 2	3 4	5 6	7
self-assured?	1 2	3 4	5 6	7

at the moment of the beep, were your complaints present?

	not	a little	rather	very much
1st complaint?	1 2	3 4	5 6	7
2nd complaint?	1 2	3 4	5 6	7

at the moment of the beep, did you:

	not	a little	rather	very much
feel short of breath, chocking?	1 2	3 4	5 6	7
have palpitations, pain on the chest?	1 2	3 4	5 6	7
feel weak, dizzy, unsteady?	1 2	3 4	5 6	7
feel unreal?	1 2	3 4	5 6	7
afraid to die, go crazy, to lose control?	1 2	3 4	5 6	7

what were you doing at the moment of the beep? ....

	not	a little	rather	very much
were you concentrated?	1 2	3 4	5 6	7
were you active?	1 2	3 4	5 6	7
did you want to do it?	1 2	3 4	5 6	7
was it difficult?	1 2	3 4	5 6	7
was the environment stimulating?	1 2	3 4	5 6	7
did you feel obliged to do it?	1 2	3 4	5 6	7

where were you at the moment of the beep? ....
were you alone? no yes
if not: with how many people? ....

name	what did you do together?

	not	a little	rather	very much
a pleasant company?	1 2	3 4	5 6	7

at the moment of the beep:

	not	a little	rather	very much
were you hungry?	1 2	3 4	5 6	7
were you tired?	1 2	3 4	5 6	7
did you feel sick?	1 2	3 4	5 6	7

since the last beep:

did you use? tobacco coffee alcohol drugs ....

did something important happened? no yes
what? ....
did your complaints troubled you? no yes
how? ....

what time is it now? ...... hour .... minutes

notes: ....

Figure 1. Experience sampling format for anxiety.

One of the earliest lines of investigation was begun at the University of Chicago by Csikszentmihalyi and associates, who obtained general data on daily activities and experience of adolescents (Csikszentmihalyi and Larson 1987; Hormuth 1986). Similar techniques were developed by de Vries and associates for the study of psychopathology (de Vries 1983; de Vries, Delespaul, and Dijkman-Caes 1987; de Vries, Delespaul, Theunissen, et al. 1986); by Hurlburt (1979, 1980) and Hurlburt and Melancon (1987) for the study of thought content; by Klinger, Barta, and Maxeimer (1980), for the study of stream-of-conscious thought in daily life; by Massimini, Csikszentmihalyi, and Carli (1987) for the study of high school students; and by Hormuth (1986) for the study of urban uprooting. In these studies, self-report questionnaires, instructional procedures, coding, and data analysis were developed and validated with a population of more than 600 subjects. Early research focused on critical aspects of ESM, such as reactivity effects, subjects' self-selection biases, missing data, validity of self-reports, and comparisons across subjects.

These studies have relied on self-reports because of the methodological limitation of observing psychiatric phenomena outside the clinic or laboratory. This shortcoming of observational methods (Harré and Secord 1972) and the apparent strength of verbal self-reports (Ericsson and Simon 1985; Simon 1969) support the shift to such methods with human subjects. Of course, subject compliance is the key element that can make or break an ESM study. Procedures that ensure a research alliance with subjects have been of paramount importance in the investigation reported here.

ESM has been used to investigate the following issues:

1. Time allocation characteristics of disordered and nondisordered subjects. Variations in the use of time and the selection of places and activities discriminate many diagnostic disorders and developmental stages (Csikszentmihalyi and Larson 1984; Delespaul and de Vries 1987; de Vries, Delespaul, Theunissen, et al. 1986).

2. Clinically significant within-day variations in experience and symptoms. The occurrence of symptoms in many disorders is overestimated in global, retrospective reports when compared with actual measures in daily life. (Freedman, Janni, Ettedgui, et al. 1985; Margraf, Ehlers, and Roth 1986; Taylor, Sheikh, Agras, et al. 1986), and variability of mental states is the rule. For example, rapid fluctuations in state perception of "alternates" is found in multiple personality disorder (Loewenstein, Hamilton, Alagna, et al. 1987).

3. Patterning of experiences; contributions of context and setting to illness or well-being. Mood fluctuates across the menstrual cycle

(Hamilton and Alagna 1985); both binge eating and anxiety have a dynamic relationship with affect (de Vries, Delespaul, and Dijkman-Caes 1987; Johnson and Larson 1982); social contexts have a different impact on symptoms of acutely ill schizophrenic patients (Delespaul and de Vries 1987); and recovery from alcoholism demonstrates a temporal pattern (Filstead, Reich, Parella, et al. 1985).

4. Refinement of current diagnostic categories with time-sampling data. Avoidant behavior appears to be a general characteristic of anxiety disorders and not a behavior that discriminates one class of anxiety from another (Dijkman and de Vries 1987), and experienced autonomic panic symptoms do not provide a basis for classifying panic disorder (Margraf, Taylor, Ehlers, et al. 1987).

5. The influence of positive psychological experience on well-being and illness states. It is important whether or not there is balance between challenges and skills when a subject is engaged in an activity that is related to self-assessment of general well-being (Massimini, Csikszentmihalyi, and Carli 1987).

The above studies illustrate that methods assessing variability and context relatedness of behavior and mental state over time can provide supplementary information as important to psychiatry as the genealogical chart has been to kinship studies and family risk factor research.

Measuring mental state and concurrent context frequently, as these studies have done, creates a large data set. Such studies may seem excessive and potentially overwhelming at the data level. Making sense of data collected from different individuals, or from the same individual at different times, with self-reports that are often randomly sampled across contexts, requires care with regard both to the coding of data into meaningful categories of experience and the choice of appropriate statistical procedures. Statistical analyses that have been developed ensure that the data are not falsely inflated. Conversely, these analyses must safeguard the very information these methods are meant to uncover by not letting them be inadvertently obscured by an overly conservative approach (Delespaul and de Vries 1987; Margraf, Taylor, Ehlers, et al. 1987). Further, the application of time-series statistics (e.g., Markov chain models and event history analysis) are already producing interesting results (Allison 1984). New strategies using ascending cross-classification analysis may also empirically test "daily-life" variables against other diagnostic criteria (Fink 1986; Van Meter 1986; Van Meter, de Vries, Kaplan 1987).

METHODOLOGICAL CONSIDERATIONS

The theoretical objective of ESM is to obtain a representative sample of a person's or a population's daily experiences. The method's usefulness as a research technique depends on how much it measures up to this ideal. Four issues generally arise about potential shortcomings: (1) the adequacy of the sampling of ill persons; (2) the adequacy of the sampling of experiences; (3) experimental effects of the method; and (4) construct validity of the self-reports. In the following section each of these is considered in light of previous studies on daily life and mental disorders.

The Sampling of Ill Persons

Although one is generally skeptical of the potential applicability of the method for clinical research, ESM studies demonstrate that it can be used with a broad range of persons. Thus far, ESM has gathered useful data from respondents as old as 65 years and as young as 10 years, and with individuals who exhibit a wide range of mental disorders. From schizophrenic and depressive patients to the elderly and drug abusers, compliance was generally high and dropout rates are remarkably low given the intensive involvement that the research requires of the subject.

The Sampling of Experience With Normal and Ill Participants

Missing signals are caused by a variety of factors. Across samples, individuals responded to 80% of the signals sent. Apparently, most missed signals either occurred early in the morning or late in the evening, when subjects were asleep, or were due to problems with the apparatus. Less frequent sources of missing data were respondents forgetting the beeper, leaving the booklet at home, or the nature of the activity at the time the signal was transmitted (e.g., taking a shower).

The delay in responding to the beeper is typically quite short. In a study of adolescents, 64% of the subjects responded immediately, and 87% responded within 10 minutes (Csikszentmihalyi and Larson 1987). In Hormuth's (1985) study of 101 German adults, 50% of the signals were responded to immediately, 80% within 5 minutes after the signal, and 90% within 18 minutes. Similar results were obtained in other studies. Delays are usually due to being engaged in activities that cannot be interrupted. In the studies reported here, forms filled out more than 10 minutes after the signal are discarded.

Analyses of posttest interview responses suggest that the method is not felt to be excessively intrusive. Among U.S. adults, 32% said that the beeper was getting disruptive or annoying by the end of the week; 22% of German adults complained that it did disrupt daily routine (Hormuth 1985). In the current study, complaints of disruption have been reduced to near 10%. Among U.S. and Dutch adults, 90% felt that the reports captured their week's experiences well; 80% of the German adults felt the same. When asked whether they would participate again in such a study, 75% of the German subjects said they would.

How adequately daily life is sampled may be demonstrated by matching ESM self-reported activities with the profiles of time use gathered in time-diary research. For the Chicago adult sample, the percentages of ESM reports in 18 standard daily activity categories (e.g., working at a job, eating meals, socializing, grooming, watching television, driving a car) were found to be nearly identical with adult time distribution found in major time-budget studies (Robinson 1977; Szalai 1972). A Spearman rank-order correlation between diary reports and ESM frequencies for the 18 categories was .96 (Csikszentmihalyi and Larson, 1987).

The method might be suspected of systematically missing or underrepresenting aspects of people's experience, although current information suggests that this is not a major source of error. One might not expect to get a complete reporting of certain types of activities (e.g., sex and criminal behavior). Nonetheless, studies have obtained numerous reports of sex, drug abuse, aggression, and fantasies as well as numerous other private reports. Studies with such likely noncompliers as schizophrenic patients and heroin addicts have also obtained a wide range of candid reports about psychopathologic and criminal experiences. When observations are used as a means of checking accuracy, observer-patient correlations on observable measures ranged from .70 to .90 (de Vries 1983).

Experimental Effects

A subsample of 34 high school students was asked whether carrying the beeper and participating in the study had any influence on their activities, mood, and thoughts during the week (Larson 1983). Eight reported effects on activities, mood, or thoughts or that carrying the beeper made them more self-conscious and self-aware than they would have been otherwise. Other studies have investigated if the ESM raised the level of self-consciousness in subjects. Fenigstein, Scheier, and Buse (1975) expected such a finding, but no significant differences in test scores on a self-consciousness scale before and after the test period were found, suggesting that whatever the change in consciousness produced by the method, it seems not to alter report validity detectably. Indeed subjects have spontaneously mentioned that they learned important insights about their lives and activities. A more subtle and quantitative assessment of effects of the procedure on people's experience can be obtained by looking at changes in their response patterns over the reporting period. That is, if there are experimental effects, they should be evident in shifts from the beginning to the end of the sampling period to more stereotyped responses; in fact the variability of responses remained remarkably stable from the first to the second half of the study week (Csikszentmihalyi and Larson 1987).

Self-Reports and Construct Validity

While we tacitly assume that respondents can and will accurately describe relevant experiences and behaviors, we know from experience that this is not always the case. One practical method to minimize inaccuracy in self-reports is the building of a research alliance and offering pretest instructions, during which the items and their meanings are clarified and agreed on (Nelson 1977). To minimize bias further and to increase validity, the self-report forms are constructed using the psychometric techniques of Likert-type scales and specific descriptions of events and persons. While the validity of self-reports may vary across types of subjects, items, and situations, the method itself is likely to increase subject sensitivity to behavioral dispositions and, therefore, to increase reporting accuracy (Wegner and Vallacher 1980), as has been the case with behavioral self-monitoring (Hayes and Cavoir 1977; Nelson, Lipinski, and Boykin 1978).

Although self-reports may claim many positive attributes, such as cost efficiency, sensitivity in a broad range of environments, and most of all the ability to test the respondents themselves, they also introduce a number of potential liabilities, which include the effects of personal defenses and the insertion of acquiesence and social desirability into the reports. A strong effort has been made to track these effects using patient interviews and statistical techniques, but response biases remain complex and difficult to determine (Fiske 1971; Norman 1967; Rorer 1965; Wiggins 1964). Methods can be employed to ensure reporting accuracy further: discarding first-day data, using split-half or daily comparisons, and evaluating and rating compliance during the debriefing procedure at the end of the test period. In addition, validity checks are made through correlations with other measures of clinical state (Chapman and Chapman 1980; Docherty, van Kammen, Siris, et al. 1980; Marks and Matthews 1979; Spielberger, Gorsuch, and Lushene 1970). This self-report format, then, does not present insurmountable problems and compares favorably to other research procedures that depend on reconstruction and recollection.

The validity of thought-sampling methods is being addressed. Thought-sampling approaches have relied heavily on retrospective reports (Singer 1975, 1978). The momentary random sampling of thoughts is a rather new approach, and validity is currently being investigated (Hurlburt 1980). For mood sampling, however, there is a substantial literature demonstrating the validity of self-reports. Researchers have shown associations between reports of emotional states and ratings of facial expression, voice print analysis, bodily cues, and physiologic measures. Significant correlations have also been reported between mood self-ratings and work productivity, social withdrawal, school performance, and psychiatric status (Izard 1972). It should be noted, however, that most analyses with ESM data do not employ single reports, but composite measures based on many self-reports (e.g., all of a person's self-reports or all of the person's reports when alone). The validity of a questionnaire does not depend on a single item; it is the validity of the aggregate scores that is critical.

Common sense findings substantiate the construct validity of the ESM measures. People report being more sociable when they are with friends, constrained when they are working, relaxed when watching television, and lonely when alone. Workers dissatisfied with their jobs report worse mood when they are at work than do satisfied workers. Good students report better moods in class that do poor students. Agoraphobic patients are more anxious out of the house than are other general anxiety patients.

For the purposes of psychiatric research, ESM is capable of sensitively capturing mental state fluctuations over time and in different contexts. For our purposes in this study, the interplay of affect and anxiety in daily life could be successfully measured using ESM.

ESM WITH ANXIETY AND DEPRESSION

In this study, we aim to illustrate variations in time allocation, self-reports of mental states, and temporal properties of anxious subjects with different degrees of depression. We are thus investigating the effect of the co-occurrence of anxiety and affect in daily life in individuals with varying degrees of comorbidity. To do this we need to obtain self-reports about a representative sample of mental reactions to moments in a subject's life. Subjects carry a wristwatch (Seiko 1000 wrist terminal) that signals them on a programmed quasi-random schedule, with 10 beeps a day between 7:30 A.M. and 11:00 P.M. The mean interval between two signals is 90 minutes; the minimal interval is 15 minutes in this study. Because the set of signals is to be representative and unpredictable, randomization is essential to prevent the person anticipating the signals. When signaled, the person completes a self-report form that includes a range of questions about his or her objective and subjective states. Reports also include information about where they are, what they are doing, and who they are with, as well as their thoughts, mood, activities, and (individualized) somatic and psychological complaints (see Tables 1 and 2).

An anxiety module, based primarily on the DSM-III criteria for panic attacks, was included (see Table 3). The repeated administration

Table 1. ESM 7-Point Likert-Type Scales Within Previously Defined Subsets of Thoughts, Mood, Motivation, and Physical Concerns

About the *thoughts*	About activity *motivation*
Pleasant	Like to do this
Clear	Active
Excited	In control
Normal	Can concentrate on this
About *mood*	About *physical concerns*
Cheerful	Hungry
Secure	Tired
Social	Not feeling well
Relaxed	
Calm	
Friendly	

Note. 1 = not at all; 7 = totally true.

Table 2. ESF Open-Ended Questions With Coding Information

About *context* (with coding categories)
Where are you (home *vs.* family—network—health care—public spaces)
What are you doing (nothing—self-care—household—work—leisure—travel)
Who are you with (alone *vs.* being with family—friends—colleagues—strangers)

Additional *thought* variables
Congruence of thought and activity
Thought pathology (focused thinking—daydreaming—worrying—preoccupation—circular thoughts—psychotic—derealized)
Thought content (nothing—leisure—travel—self-care—friends—sex—aggression—money—religion—work—past—environment—ESM—future—abstract thoughts—miscellaneous)

Note. Codebook available.

Table 3. The 7-Point Likert-Type Scales Related to Anxiety

At the moment of the beep:	Not	A Little		Rather		Very Much	
did you feel short of breath, choking?	1	2	3	4	5	6	7
did you have palpitations, pain on the chest?	1	2	3	4	5	6	7
did you feel weak, dizzy, unsteady?	1	2	3	4	5	6	7
did you feel unreal?	1	2	3	4	5	6	7
were you afraid to die, to go crazy, to loose control?	1	2	3	4	5	6	7

of this module may be regarded as an attempt to capture repeated diagnosis of anxiety.

In a briefing phase, the method was introduced using standardized instructions to the patient. Two individualized complaints (a psychological one and a physical one) to be assessed during the research period were selected. In addition, subjects completed the State-Trait Anxiety Inventory (STAI) (Spielberger, Gorsuch, and Lushene 1970), as well as the Fear Questionnaire (Marks and Matthews 1979), and were instructed to fill out the checklist every time a beep was heard on the random-signal watch. ESM data were collected during the next 6 days. After the sixth day, another meeting with the subject was arranged. In this debriefing phase, information about possible missing data and the impact of the beeper on the patient's daily life was gathered. In a separate interview, the therapist provided information about the patient's life history.

Subjects complaining about anxiety and depression were recruited from three mental health care settings: a behaviorally oriented phobia treatment ward, a psychotherapeutic unit, and several ambulatory mental health care teams in Maastricht, the Netherlands. They were usually referred to the research group by the mental health clinicians. They represent a convenience sample gathered from sequential admissions, equally derived from a hospital and community outpatient clinic during the spring and summer of 1986. The subjects selected had scored one standard deviation above the mean on the STAI as well as scoring one standard deviation below the mean on the Zung Scale for Depression (Zung 1965).

Diagnostically, the group demonstrated both significant depression as well as anxiety. The group is similar to the patients defined by Van Valkenburg, Akiskal, Puzantian, et al. (1984) as the anxious depression group (Overall 1974; Paykel, Prusoff, Klerman, et al. 1973).

Our goal was to report data on anxiety patients with low and high depression scores, but of the 15 clients sampled, all clustered in the moderate-high or high-high categories for both depression and anxiety (Table 4). Although there is some overlap in the STAI and Zung measures, which may contribute to the co-occurrence (Dobson 1985a), the clustering of individuals in this way is in itself an interesting finding. We thus restricted our research to two groups: 6 patients in a high anxiety-moderate depression group and 5 in a high anxiety-high depression group. The findings reported thus compare two high anxiety groups that differ from one another by one standard deviation on reports of depression measured on the Zung.

RESULTS

The two groups are compared using three types of data. First, we present variations in ecological descriptions and time allocation; second, we present differences in the self-rating of mental state; and third, we describe temporal properties of depression and anxiety. In Table 5 the differences in frequency distributions of the ESM variables between the two groups can be seen. For all coded ESM categories, except thought-activity congruence, strong differences were found. The groups differed in thought-content, reported psychopathology, where they were, what they were doing, and with whom they were.

A more detailed breakdown of these differences in global categories is instructive. For example, thought content differentiated the groups. In this cluster, thoughts about leisure were found 10% of the time in the moderately depressed group and 21% in the highly depressed group; "thinking about nothing" was found 1% in the moder-

Table 4. Sample Overview: Anxiety × Depression

	Zung (with standard scoring)		
STAI state	Low (-1 SD)	Medium (-1 SD$><+1$ SD)	High ($+1$ SD)
Low (-1 SD)			1
Medium (-1 SD$><+1$ SD)		2	1
High ($+1$ SD)		6	5

Note. Zung = Zung Scale for Depression; STAI = State-Trait Anxiety Inventory.

ate group and 8% in the high group, and thoughts about work were found 11% in the moderate group and 25% in the high group. Excessive worrying and rumination occurred 2% of the time in the moderate group and 11% in the high group. In terms of activities, the moderate group was found to be involved in self-care 7% of the time and the high group 14% of the time; inversely the moderate group was caring for another 18% of the time, but the high group did so only 7% of the time. The moderately depressed group was also found significantly more in public places than the high group. The variable "whom they were with" also differentiated the groups. Although both the moderately and highly depressed groups were alone about equal amounts of time (21% and 26%, respectively), the moderately depressed group spent 47% of their time with family and the highly depressed only 33%. This relationship switched for friends and colleagues, and the moderately depressed group was with friends 13% of the time and the high group 23% of the time.

In summary, the highly depressed group had more idle thoughts, ruminated more, experienced less focused thoughts in public, and registered most self-care and less care and involvement with others. Socially, the highly depressed group was at home more and with the family less. They also tended to report more diffuse and vague somatic and psychological complaints than the moderately depressed group. These findings are in accordance with clinical characteristics of this group as having a higher degree of morbidity than individuals with only anxiety or only depression alone.

In Figure 2, these relationships are plotted using the likelihood that an individual will be found in the same place on two sequential signals, indicated as percentages, for the variable "where." Here we observe a subtle and dynamically different picture for each group. The

Table 5: Difference in Frequency Distribution of Nominal Variables Between Groups: High Anxiety-Moderately Depressed Versus High Anxiety-Highly Depressed

	χ^2 of frequency distributions	df	p
Thought-activity congruence	4.111	2	NS
Thought content	57.787	16	.001
Psychopathology	31.475	5	.001
Where	13.063	6	.05
What	31.840	6	.001
Who	54.425	6	.001

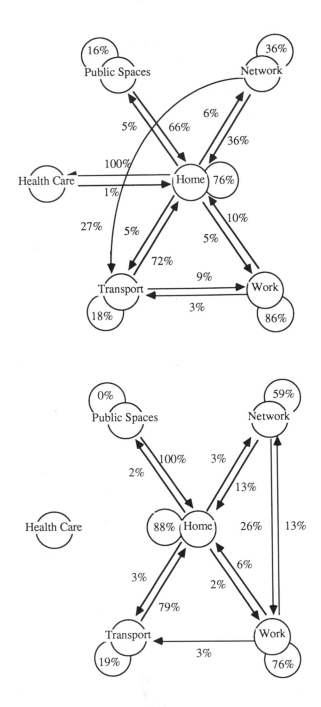

Figure 2. Setting changes from time t to time t + 1. *Top*: Moderately depressed anxious subjects. *Bottom*: Highly depressed anxious subjects.

moderate group demonstrated a more diverse and dynamic network, with quantitatively more social contexts and transitions from place to place. The figure also demonstrates one way that ESM data may be used to provide a quantitatively derived picture of the social network of patients with different disorders or degree of severity.

SELF-RATINGS OF MENTAL STATE

While frequency distributions clearly differentiated the two groups on ecological and time-allocation variables, the psychological reactions to similar situations, such as being alone or being at home, did not differentiate the groups significantly. A difference was found for the entire group, however, on the congruence between the self-rating of thoughts and the activity being carried out (i.e., thinking about what you are doing). This measure differentiated both groups from other ESM samples of mental disorders. For example, in contrast with schizophrenic patients, who showed marked more incongruence of thought and activity when alone at home (de Vries, Delespaul, and Dijkman-Caes 1987), both anxiety groups were less congruent when they were away from home. The anxiety groups report more disorganization when they are with people, whereas the schizophrenic patients report more unfocused thoughts when they are alone than when they are with company. In summary, self-ratings of mental state, measures of affect, motivation, and reactions to situations did not differentiate the moderate and high groups.

TEMPORAL PATTERNS

Diurnal patterns in anxiety and depression scores in the highly and moderately depressed groups were explored by applying a linear regression technique to the entire sequence of beeps per subject and collapsed over subjects per group. For the moderately depressed group, no daily pattern was found for anxiety or depression symptoms, but for the highly depressed group, a within-day significant fluctuation was found for depression ($t = -2.06$, $p < .04$). This significant effect was produced by one subject who demonstrated a strong late-in-the-day mood upswing ($t = -3.93$, $p < .001$), which was, in addition, supported by a trend in the other four subjects. Inter-day differences per subject were also detected, but this effect disappeared at the group level.

We next asked if we could separate the two groups on other temporal dimensions such as the recovery rate or decay time from high anxiety states. To demonstrate this, we tracked the recovery of anxiety within a day from a high anxiety or panic experience point at

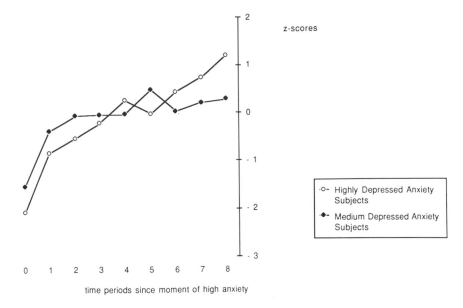

Figure 3. Recovery from anxious episodes in moderately depressed and highly depressed anxiety subjects.

least one standard deviation below the individual's mean mental state on anxiety. The anxiety was tracked over subsequent signals that day to manufacture a recovery or decay curve for each group. Figure 3 shows the temporal recovery curve in the course of the day from anxiety states in moderately and highly depressed subjects.

The highly depressed group recovered from anxiety more slowly. At the end of the day, a rebound or a diurnal decrease in anxiety is reported by the highly depressed group. This finding is greater than may be expected from the expected regression to the mean shown by the moderately depressed group.

In Figure 4, we replicate the above analysis for 10 normal controls and graph the recovery from the high anxiety as well as depressed moments reported by this group. Rather than the gradual decrease in anxiety observed in the clinical group, we see a precipitous return to the mean for anxiety symptoms. Depressive feelings returned to the mean at an expected slower rate.

This result suggests that the recovery from anxiety states occurs at different rates with varying degree and perhaps type of psychopathology. The rate of recovery is clearly affected by comorbidity and severity, an interesting finding for planning treatment. These data illustrate the utility of examining the temporal properties of mental states. Subsequent samples will employ larger numbers of subjects to

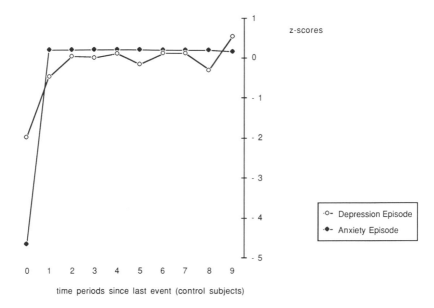

Figure 4. Recovery from anxious episodes and depressive episodes in normal subjects.

describe these processes more fully and reliably.

We further sought to determine if mood states or anxiety states predicted one another. To do this we carried out a cross-lag analysis to determine whether low mood or high anxiety scores had a temporal relationship. At lag-0, anxiety and depression are significantly correlated with each other for the highly depressed group ($r = .42$, $SE = .131$, $p < .001$). The analysis of further lags in the highly depressed group demonstrated a nonsignificant trend of depression predicting anxiety.

DISCUSSION

Between these subtly defined groups of high anxiety with moderate depression and high anxiety with high depression, characteristic differences in daily activities and temporal aspects of anxiety and depression were found using ESM. These differences were particularly strong for data at the behavioral level representing activities selected by the subjects in each group, and at the temporal level in terms of each group's differential capacity to recover and rebound from high anxiety episodes.

ESM separated the groups on self-report scores of thought content and psychopathology as well as the situation and activities selected. Mean self-report scores of moment-to-moment mental states did not separate the groups nor did the situations in which they occurred. Behavioral indices in this case measured by means of time-allocation frequencies appear a stronger indicator of differences in mental state and psychopathology than averaged or cross-sectional scale scores based on reports of the self-perception of state. Future assessments of anxiety and depression should therefore include these seemingly more robust behavior measures.

The data on temporal relationships, while exploratory, also lead to some tentative conclusions and suggestive mechanisms. The two findings, the slow decay of anxiety in the highly depressed group and the trend of mood predicting anxiety, suggest that depression in a day-to-day sense renders an individual more sensitive to the experience of anxiety. The co-occurrence of the two pathologic processes clearly increase experienced severity. The temporal recovery curves of symptoms and the behavioral time-allocation data, when taken together, suggest a mechanism for why the addition of depression to anxiety should result in greater morbidity. This process of anxiety evolving to increased morbidity and depression is currently considered the natural course of the disorder over the life span and is also discernible diurnally in the delayed recovery curves. The greater delay in recovery from anxiety observed with increasing severity of comorbid depression could be a result of the behavioral inhibition, evident on the time-allocation data, when increasing levels of depression are present. Depression could thus worsen the anxiety disorder by inhibiting the behavioral adjustments that could potentially lead to a more rapid restitution of the anxiety symptom. The data on normal subjects further suggest this since they utilize a broad range of activities and recover rapidly. The findings and suggested mechanisms reported here will be pursued further to safeguard against ecologically fallacious and tautological arguments. Larger samples analyzed in different and divergent ways should accomplish this and generate a more comprehensive description of phenomena of depression and anxiety in temporal and contextual terms. The data base gathered using time-based techniques may not only be useful in solving current diagnostic controversies, but may also be useful in providing new avenues for treatment based on the frequency and dynamic nature of actual illness phenomenon, its context, and its temporal recovery properties.

References and Author Index

Aagesen CA. 295

Abbott PJ. 243, 246

Abelman E. 388

Ablon SL, Carlson GA, Goodwin FK: Ego defense patterns in manic-depressive illness. American Journal of Psychiatry 131:803–807, 1974. 547, 549

Abraham A: Selected Papers of Karl Abraham. London, Hogarth Press, 1927. 24, 35

Abrams R. 567, 570, 573

Abrams R, Taylor MA: Differential EEG patterns in affective disorder and schizophrenia. Archives of General Psychiatry 36:1355–1358, 1979. 573

Abrams R, Taylor MA: A prospective follow-up study of cognitive functions after electroconvulsive therapy. Convulsive Therapy 1:4–9, 1985. 570

Abrams R, Taylor MA: Cognitive dysfunction in melancholia. Psychological Medicine 17:359–362, 1987. 567

Abrams R, Volavka J, Roubicek J, Dornbush R, Fink M: Lateralized EEG changes after unilateral and bilateral electroconvulsive therapy. Diseases of the Nervous System (GWAN Suppl) 31:28–33, 1970. 573

Abramson LY. 499, 500, 506–509, 510, 511, 513, 515, 516–518, 519, 528–530, 543, 641

Abramson LY, Alloy LB, Metalsky GL: The cognitive diathesis-stress theories of depression: toward an adequate evaluation of the theories' validities, in Cognitive Processes in Depression. Edited by Alloy LB. New York, Guilford, 1988. 510, 512, 541, 543

Abramson LY, Metalsky GL, Alloy LB: The hopelessness theory of depression: does the research test the theory? in Social Cognition and Clinical Psychology: A Synthesis. Edited by Abramson LY. New York, Guilford, 1988.

Abramson LY, Metalsky GL, Alloy LB: Hopelessness depression: a theory-based subtype of depression. Psychological Review 96:358–372, 1989. 510, 511, 512, 513, 515, 518, 527, 528

Abramson LY, Seligman MEP, Teasdale JD: Learned helplessness in humans: critique and reformulation. Journal of Abnormal Psychology 87:49–74, 1978. 509, 516, 517, 527, 528, 640

Ádám G: Interception and Behaviour: An Experimental Study. Budapest, Akademiai Kiado, 1967. 246

Adcock S. 120, 659

Adrian C. 354–358

Aggarwal AK. 505

Aghajanian GK. 425

Agras WS. 392, 712, 713

Agras WS: Stress, panic, and the cardiovascular system, in Anxiety and the Anxiety Disorders. Edited by Tuma AH, Maser JD. Hillsdale, NJ, Lawrence Erlbaum Associates, 1985. 509

Ahles TA. 251

Aimes P, Gelder M, Shaw P: Social phobia: a comparative clinical study. British Journal of Psychiatry 142:174–179, 1983. 677

Akil H. 433

Akiskal HS. 52, 53, 306, 341, 346, 378, 478, 602, 606, 599, 604, 606, 709, 719

Akiskal HS: The bipolar spectrum: new concepts in classification and diagnosis, in Psychiatry Update: American Psychiatric Association Annual Review, Vol 2. Edited by Grinspoon L. Washington, DC, American Psychiatric Press, 1983a. 605

Akiskal HS: Diagnosis and classification of affective disorders: new insights from clinical and laboratory approaches. Psychiatric Developments 2:123–160, 1983b. 602

Akiskal HS: Dysthymic disorder: psychopathology of proposed chronic depressive subtypes. American Journal of Psychiatry 140:11–20, 1983c. 320

Akiskal HS: Anxiety: definition, relationship to depression, and proposal for an integrative model, in Anxiety and the Anxiety Disorders. Edited by Tuma AH, Maser JD. Hillsdale, NJ, Lawrence Erlbaum Associates, 1985a. 51, 508, 509, 599, 605

Akiskal HS: The clinical management of affective disorders, in Psychiatry, Vol 1. Edited by Michels R, Cavenar JO, Brodie HKH, et al. Philadelphia, JB Lippincott, 1985b. 601, 602, 606

Akiskal HS: Mood disturbances, in The Medical Basis of Psychiatry. Edited by Winokur G, Clayton P. Philadelphia, WB Saunders, 1986a. 599

Akiskal HS: A multifactorial approach to depression: the inadequacy of pharmacologic inference and psychosocial hypotheses. Psychiatrie et Psychobiologie 1:49–59, 1986b. 605

Akiskal HS: Personality in anxiety disorders. Psychiatrie et Psychobiologie 3 (special B): 161s–166s, 1988. 605

Akiskal HS: Classification of mental disorders, in Comprehensive Textbook of Psychiatry, 5th Edition. Edited by Kaplan HI, Sadock BJ. Baltimore, Williams & Wilkins, 1989, pp 583–598. 598

Akiskal HS, King D, Rosenthal TL, Robinson D, Scott-Strauss A: Chronic depressions, part I. Journal of Affective Disorders 3:297–315, 1981. 322

Akiskal HS, Lemmi H: Sleep EEG findings bearing on the relationship of anxiety and depressive disorders, in Anxious Depressions: Assessment and Treatment. Edited by Racagni G, Smeraldi E. New York, Raven, 1987. 599, 604

Akiskal HS, Lemmi H, Dickson H, King D, Yerevanian B, Van Valkenburg C: Chronic depressions, part 2: sleep EEG differentiation of primary dysthymic disorders from anxious depressions. Journal of Affective Disorders 6:287–295, 1984. 599, 603

Akiskal HS, Mallya G: Criteria for the "soft" bipolar spectrum: treatment implications. Psychopharmacological Bulletin 23:68–73, 1987. 606

Akiskal HS, McKinney WT Jr: Depressive disorders: toward a unified hypothesis. Science 182:20–29, 1973. 601

Akiskal HS, Rosenthal TL, Haykal RF, Lemmi H, Rosenthal RH, Scott-Strauss A: Characterologic depressives: clinical and sleep EEG findings separating "subaffective dysthymias" from "character spectrum disorders." Archives of General Psychiatry 37:777–783, 1980. 317, 325, 327

Akiskal HS, Yeravanian BI, Davis GC, King D, Lemmi H: The nosologic status of borderline personality: clinical and polysomnographic study. American Journal of Psychiatry 142:192–198, 1985. 47

Alagna SW. 707, 712, 713

Alavi A. 570

Albala AA. 387, 403, 427, 613

Aldenhoff JB, Gruol DL, Rivier J, Vale W, Siggins GR: Corticotropin releasing factor decreases postburst hyperpolarizations and excites hippocampal neurons. Science 221:875–877, 1983. 419

Alderson LM. 289

Aldwin C. 637, 640

Alessi NE, Robbins DR, Dilsaver SC. Panic and depressive disorders among psychiatrically hospitalized adolescents. Psychiatry Research 20:275–283, 1987. 277, 280

Alexander J. 472

Allison PD: Event-history analyses. Sage University, paper series on quantitative applications in the social sciences. Beverly Hills, LA, Sage, 1984. 713

Alloy LB. 500, 505, 506, 509, 510, 511, 512, 513, 515, 516–518, 527, 528, 530, 541, 543

Alloy LB: The role of perceptions and attributions for response-outcome noncontingency in learned helplessness: a commentary and discussion. Journal of Personality 50:443–479, 1982. 527

Alloy LB, Abramson LY: Depressive realism: four theoretical perspectives, in Cognitive Processes in Depression. Edited by Alloy LB. New York, Guilford, 1988. 530

Alloy LB, Abramson LY, Metalsky GL, Hartlage S: The hopelessness theory of depression: attributional aspects. British Journal of Clinical Psychology 27:5–21, 1988. 510, 511, 512, 513, 515, 518, 528, 543

Alloy LB, Clements C, Kolden G: The cognitive diathesis-stress theories of depression: therapeutic implications, in Theoretical Issues in Behavior Therapy. Edited by Reiss S, Bootzin R. New York, Academic, 1985. 513, 518, 530, 541, 543, 640

Alloy LB, Hartlage S, Abramson LY: Testing the cognitive diathesis-stress theories of depression: issues of research design, conceptualization and assessment, in Cognitive Processes in Depression. Edited by Alloy LB. New York, Guilford, 1988. 510, 513, 517, 518

Alloy LB, Kayne NT, Romer D, Crocker J: Predicting increases and decreases in depression in the classroom: a test of the diathesis-stress and causal mediation components of the hopelessness theory. Manuscript under editorial review. 517

Alloy LB, Koenig LJ: Hopelessness: on some of the antecedents and consequences of pessimism. Manuscript in preparation, Northwestern University, Evanston, IL. 518

Alloy LB, Tabachnik N: Assessment of covariation by humans and animals: the joint influence of prior expectations and current situational information. Psychological Review 91:112–149, 1984. 516, 517

Alterman IS. 308, 571, 574

Altmann MW. 248

Altschuler KZ, Weiner MF: Anorexia nervosa and depression: a dissenting view. American Journal of Psychiatry 142:328–332, 1985. 255

Amado H. 666, 667

Amalric M. 420

Ambrose MJ. 419, 425, 496

Ambrosini P. 273

American Psychiatric Association: Diagnostic and Statistical Manual of Mental Disorders, 1st Edition. Washington, DC, American Psychiatric Association, 1952. 18, 88, 155, 283, 499

American Psychiatric Association: Diagnostic and Statistical Manual of Mental Disorders, 2nd Edition. Washington, DC, American Psychiatric Association, 1968. 18, 43, 91, 283, 318, 499

American Psychiatric Association: Diagnostic and Statistical Manual of Mental Disorders, 3rd Edition. Washington, DC, American Psychiatric Association, 1980. 8, 14, 41, 61, 83, 93, 114, 123, 155, 190, 205, 264, 273, 283, 310, 317, 331, 350, 372, 392, 447, 473,499, 557, 585, 635, 677, 694, 707, 709

American Psychiatric Association: Diagnostic and Statistical Manual of Mental Disorders, 3rd Edition, Revised. Washington, DC, American Psychiatric Association, 1987. 4, 25, 41, 44, 61, 85, 120, 140, 200, 206, 240, 264, 284, 313, 319, 332, 351, 524, 546, 585, 613, 614, 621, 635, 681, 694, 697

American Psychiatric Association Task Force on the Use of Laboratory Tests in Psychiatry: The dexamethasone suppression test: an overview of its current status in psychiatry. American Journal of Psychiatry 144:1253–1262, 1987. 36, 404, 500, 602

Amsterdam JD. 390

Amsterdam JD, Kaplan M, Potter L, Bloom L, Rickels K: Adinazolam, a new triazolobenzodiazepine, and imipramine in the treatment of major depressive disorder. Psychopharmacology 88:484–488, 1986. 414

Amsterdam JD, Maislin G, Winokur A, Kling M, Gold P: Pituitary and adrenocortical responses to the ovine corticotropin releasing hormone in depressed patients and healthy volunteers. Archives of General Psychiatry 44:775–781, 1987. 388

Amsterdam JD, Winokur A, Abelman E, Lucki I, Rickels K: Cosyntropin (ACTH alpha-1-24) stimulation test in depressed patients and healthy subjects. American Journal of Psychiatry 140:907–909, 1983. 389

Andersen A. 254

Anderson C. 418, 424–426, 431

Anderson CA, Arnoult LH: Attributional style and everyday problems in living: depression, loneliness, and shyness. Social Cognition 3:16–35, 1985. 518

Anderson CD: Expression of affect and physiological response in psychosomatic patients. Journal of Psychosomatic Research 25:143–149, 1981. 244

Anderson DJ. 703

Anderson JC. 279

Anderson K. 49, 51, 476, 480

Andorn AC. 428

Andrasik F. 251

Andreasen NC. 84, 294, 295, 296, 297, 301, 346, 347, 378, 556, 666

Andreasen N: Concepts, diagnosis and classification, in Handbook of Affective Disorders. Edited by Paykel E. New York, Guilford, 1982. 52, 55

Andreasen NC, Rice J, Endicott J, Reich T, Coryell W: The family history approach to diagnosis. Archives of General Psychiatry 43:421–429, 1986. 684

Andreasen NC, Winokur G: Secondary depression: familial, clinical and research perspectives. American Journal of Psychiatry 136:62–66, 1979. 294, 296

Andrews D. 513

Andrews G. 371

Angst J: Recurrent brief depression: a new concept of mild depression. Psychopharmacology, XIVth CINP Congress, Munich, August 15–19, 1988, p. 123. 125

Angst J: The kaleidoscope of anxiety states. International Symposium of the International Prevention and Treatment of Depression Committee (Kielholz P, Chairman; Adams C, Coordinator), working session on February 1–2, 1988, Suvretta House, St. Moritz, in press. 125

Angst J, Dobler-Mikola A: The Zurich study, VI: a continuum from depression to anxiety disorders? European Archives of Psychiatry and Neurological Sciences 235:179–186, 1985. 124, 125

Angst J, Dobler-Mikola A, Binder J: The Zurich study: a prospective epidemiological study of depressive, neurotic and psychosomatic syndromes, I: problem, methodology. European Archives of Psychiatry and Neurological Science, 234:13–20, 1984. 124, 125

Angst J, Vollrath M, Koch R: New aspects on epidemiology of depression. Presented at the International Symposium on Lofepramine in the Treatment of Depressive Disorders: Review of the Past 10 Years and Future Prospects, Lugano, Switzerland, October 22–24, 1987. 125

Annable L. 676, 703

Antes JR. 572, 581

Anthony JC. 115, 165, 168, 171, 589

Anthony JC, Folstein M, Romanoski AJ, Von Korff MR, Nestadt GN, Chahal R, Merchant A, Brown CH, Shapiro S, Kramer M, Gruenberg EM: Comparison of Lay DIS and a standardized psychiatric diagnosis: experience in eastern Baltimore. Archives of General Psychiatry 42:667–675, 1985. 661

Antoni FA, Palkovits M, Makara GB, Linton EA, Lowry PJ, Kiss JZ: Immunoreactive corticotropin-releasing hormone in the hypothalamo-infundibular tract. Neuroendocrinology 36:415–423, 1983. 418

Antram MC. 79, 90

Apley J, Keith RM, Meadow R: The Child and His Symptoms: A Comprehensive Approach. Oxford, Blackwell Scientific Publications, 1978. 245

Appeltauer L. 703

Arana GW, Baldessarini RJ, Ornsteen M: The dexamethasone suppression test for diagnosis and prognosis in psychiatry. Archives of General Psychiatry 42:1193–1204, 1985. 388

Arato M. 404, 427

Arato M, Banki CM, Nemeroff CB, Bissette G: Hypothalamic-pituitary-adrenal axis and suicide. Annals of the New York Academy of Sciences 487:263–270, 1986. 428

Arieti S: Manic-depressive psychosis, in American Handbook of Psychiatry, Vol 1, 1st Edition. Edited by Arieti S. New York, Basic Books, 1959. 519

Arieti S, Bemporad J: Severe and Mild Depression. New York, Basic Books, 1978. 614

Arkonac O, Guze SB: A family study of hysteria. New England Journal of Medicine 268:239–242, 1963. 240, 563

Arkowitz H: Assessment of Social Skills: Behavioral Assessment: A Practical

Handbook, 2nd Edition. Edited by Hersen M, Bellack AS. Elmsford, NY, Pergamon, 1981. 638

Arnoult LH. 517

Aronoff MS. 279

Asarnow RF. 505, 617, 640

Asberg M. 256

Ashworth CM. 554

Askenasy AR. 466

Association of Sleep Disorders Centers and the Association for the Psycho-physiological Study of Sleep: Diagnostic classification of sleep and arousal disorders. Sleep 2:5–129, 1979. 603

Aston-Jones G. 419, 420, 425, 426, 431

Astrachan D. 423

Atkinson RM. 189

Augerinos P. 430, 433

Avegerinos PC. 255

Averill JR. 519

Avery DH. 337, 338, 394, 472, 502, 505, 619, 676

Avery DH, Osgood TB, Ishiki DM, Wilson LG, Kenny M, Dunner D: The DST in psychiatry outpatients with generalized anxiety disorder, panic disorder or primary affective disorder. American Journal of Psychiatry 142:844–848, 1985. 386, 387

Babor TF. 235, 285, 286, 288, 300, 302, 653, 655, 656, 664

Baer L. 314, 387

Bagshaw VE. 79, 90

Bagshaw VE, McPherson FM: The applicability of the Foulds and Bedford hierarchy model to mania and hypomania. British Journal of Psychiatry 132:293–295, 1978. 90

Bailey WH. 425

Bakker DJ: Hemispheric specialization and specific reading retardation, in Developmental Neuropsychiatry. Edited by Rutter M. New York, Guilford, 1983. 572

Bakker DJ, Vinke J: Effects of hemisphere-specific stimulation on brain activity and reading in dyslexics. Journal of Clinical and Experimental Neuropsychology 7:505–525, 1985. 572

Baldessarini RJ. 388

Balla JI, Moraitis S: Knights in armour: a follow-up of injuries after legal settlement. Medical Journal of Australia 2:355–361, 1970. 247

Ballenger JC. 387, 703

Ballenger JC: Pharmacotherapy of the panic disorders. Journal of Clinical Psychiatry 47 (6 Suppl): 27–31, 1986. 675

Ballenger JC, Burrows GD, DuPont RL Jr, Lesser IM, Noyes R Jr, Pecknold JC, Rifkin A, Swinson RP: Alprazolam in panic disorder and agoraphobia: results from a multicenter trial, I: efficacy in short-term treatment, Archives of General Psychiatry 45:413–422, 1988. 586, 592, 594

Balon R. 392

Balter MB. 477, 590

Ban TA. 667

Bandura A: Self-efficacy: toward a unifying theory of behavior change. Psychological Review 84:191–215, 1977. 509, 522, 523, 527, 637, 641

Banerjee SP, Kung LS, Riggi SJ, Chanda SK: Development of β-adrenergic receptor subsensitivity by antidepressants. Nature 286:455–456, 1977. 431

Banki CM. 428

Banki CM, Bissette G, Arato M, O'Connor L, Nemeroff CB: CSF corticotropin-releasing factor-like immunoreactivity in depression and schizophrenia. American Journal of Psychiatry 144:873–877, 1987. 404, 427, 429, 430

Barabash W. 571, 575

Barker RG: Habitats, Environments and Human Behavior: Studies in the Ecological Psychology and Eco-Behavioral Science of the Midwest. Psychological Field Station: 1947–1972. San Francisco, Jossey-Bass, 1978. 709

Barlow DH. 207, 208, 209, 219, 223, 224, 225, 226, 228, 230, 523, 590, 591, 635

Barlow DH: The classification of anxiety disorders. Paper presented at the conference on DSM-III: An Interim Appraisal, sponsored by the American Psychiatric Association, Washington, DC, October 1983. 218

Barlow D: The dimensions of anxiety disorders, in Anxiety and the Anxiety Disorders. Edited by Tuma A, Maser J. Hillsdale, NJ, Lawrence Erlbaum Associates, 1985. 46, 54, 208, 221, 509, 676

Barlow DH: Anxiety and Its Disorders: The Nature and Treatment of Anxiety and Panic. New York, Guilford, 1988. 229, 230

Barlow DH, Blanchard EB, Vermilyea JA, Vermilyea BB, Di Nardo PA: Generalized anxiety and generalized anxiety disorder: description and reconceptualization. American Journal of Psychiatry 143:40–44, 1986. 43, 46, 51, 223

Barlow DH, Cohen AS, Waddell MT, Vermilyea BB, Klosko JS, Blanchard EB, Di Nardo PA: Panic and generalized anxiety disorders: nature and treatment. Behavior Therapy 15:431–449, 1984. 227

Barlow DH, Di Nardo PA, Vermilyea BB, Vermilyea J, Blanchard EB: Co-morbidity and depression among the anxiety disorders: issues in diagnosis and classification. Journal of Nervous and Mental Disease 174:63–72, 1986. 44, 45, 49, 51, 55, 62, 63, 64, 67, 69, 70, 71, 76, 190, 200, 207, 209, 213, 472, 619

Barlow DH, Vermilyea J, Blanchard EB, Vermilyea BB, Di Nardo PA, Cerny JA: The phenomenon of panic. Journal of Abnormal Psychology 94:320–328, 1985. 221

Barlow SM, Knight AF, Sullivan FM: Plasma corticosterone response to stress following chronic oral administration of diazepam in the rat. Journal of Pharmacy and Pharmacology 31:23–26, 1979. 422

Barnhardt TM. 572, 581

Barouche F. 388

Barrabee EL. 242

Barrere M. 576

Barrett J. 554

Barrett JE: The relationship of life events to the onset of neurotic disorders, in Stress and Mental Disorder. Edited by Barrett JE. New York, Raven, 1979. 482, 483

Barsky AJ: Patients who amplify bodily symptoms. Annals of Internal Medicine 91:63–70, 1979. 239, 246

Barsky AJ, Klerman GL: Overview: hypochondriasis, bodily complaints, and somatic styles. American Journal of Psychiatry 140:273–283, 1983. 249

Barsuhn C. 422

Barta S. 712

Bartett D. 673

Barton WE. 22

Basoglu M. 310

Bateman DE. 244

Bates WM. 285, 290

Battista JR: Empirical test of Vaillant's hierarchy of ego functions. American Journal of Psychiatry 139:356–357, 1982. 549, 550

Baumgartner A, Graf KJ, Kurthen I: Serial dexamethasone suppression tests in psychiatric illness, part II: a study in major depressive disorder. Psychiatry Research 18:25–43, 1986. 388

Baxter LR, Phelps ME, Mazziotta JC, Schwartz JM, Gerner RH, Selin CE, Sumida RM: Cerebral metabolic rates for glucose in mood disorders. Archives of General Psychiatry 42:441–447, 1985. 577

Baxter LR, Phelps ME, Mazziotta JC, Guze BH, Schwartz JM, Selin CE: Local cerebral glucose metabolic rates in obsessive-compulsive disorder. Archives of General Psychiatry 44:211–218, 1987. 577, 578

Baxter N. 388

Bayton JA. 661

Beardslee WR. 354–357, 548, 549, 550

Beardslee WR, Bemporad J, Keller MB, Klerman GL: Children of parents with major affective disorder: a review. American Journal of Psychiatry 140:825–832, 1983. 354

Beaudry P, Fontaine R, Mercier P, Annable L, Chouinard G: Clonazepam in the treatment of patients with recurrent panic attacks. Abstract, Society of Biological Psychiatry 40th Annual Convention and Scientific Program, Dallas, 1985. 703

Beaumont VJP. 311

Bebbington P. 468, 471, 478, 487, 490, 624

Bebbington P: Depression distress or disease? British Journal of Psychiatry 149:479, 1986. 468, 477, 486, 487

Bebbington P, Hurry J, Tennant C, Sturt E, Wing J: Epidemiology of mental disorders in Camberwell. Psychological Medicine 11:561–579, 1981. 120, 659

Beck AT. 219, 506, 528, 615, 617, 629, 641, 700

Beck AT: Depression: Clinical, Experimental, and Theoretical Aspects. New York, Harper & Row, 1967. 23, 508, 509, 511, 513, 517, 519, 527, 528, 530, 531, 533

Beck AT: Depression: Causes and Treatment. Philadelphia, University of Pennsylvania Press, 1972. 641

Beck AT: Cognitive Therapy and the Emotional Disorders. New York, International Universities Press, 1976. 225, 500, 508, 509, 525, 527, 530, 533, 614

Beck AT: Depression Inventory. Philadelphia, Center for Cognitive Therapy, 1978. 256, 570

Beck AT, Brown G, Steer RA, Eidelson JI, Riskind JH: Differentiating anxiety and depression: a test of the cognitive content-specificity hypothesis. Journal of Abnormal Psychology 96:179–183, 1987. 218, 496, 509, 528, 631

Beck AT, Emery G: Cognitive therapy of anxiety and phobic disorders. Philadelphia, Center for Cognitive Therapy, 1979. 225

Beck AT, Emery G: Anxiety Disorders and Phobias: A Cognitive Perspective. New York, Basic Books, 1985. 500, 508, 509, 519, 523, 525, 527, 528, 530–533, 599

Beck AT, Kovacs M, Weissman A: Hopelessness and suicidal behavior: an overview. Journal of the American Medical Association 234:1146–1149, 1975. 528

Beck AT, Laude R, Bonhert M: Ideational components of anxiety neurosis. Archives of General Psychiatry 31:319–325, 1974. 225

Beck AT, Riskind JH, Brown G, Sherrod A: A comparison of likelihood estimates for imagined positive and negative outcomes in anxiety and depression. Paper presented at Eastern Psychological Association, New York, 1986. 225

Beck AT, Riskind JH, Brown G, Steer RA: Levels of hopelessness in DSM-III disorders: a partial test of content-specificity in depression. Cognitive Therapy and Research 12:459–470, 1988. 528, 529

Beck AT, Rush AJ, Shaw BF, Emery G: Cognitive Therapy of Depression. New York, Guilford, 1979. 513, 543, 581

Beck AT, Steer RA, Kovacs M, Garrison B: Hopelessness and eventual suicide: a 10-year prospective study of patients hospitalized with suicide ideation. American Journal of Psychiatry 142:559–563, 1985. 528

Beck AT, Ward CH, Mendelson M, Mock J, Erbaugh J: An inventory for measuring depression. Archives of General Psychiatry 4:561–571, 1961. 213, 226, 613, 644

Beck LH. 579

Beck NC. 275, 279, 317, 322, 360, 361

Beck RC. 528

Beck RC: Motivation: Theories and Principles. Englewood Cliffs, NJ, Prentice-Hall, 1978.

Becker JT. 290

Becker JT, Kaplan RF: Neurophysiological and neuropsychological concomitants of brain dysfunction in alcoholics, in Psychopathology and Addictive Disorders. Edited by Meyer RE. New York, Guilford, 1986. 289

Becker RE. 225, 226

Beck-Friis J. 394

Bedford A. 79, 80

Bedford A, Foulds GA: Validation of the Delusions-Signs-Symptoms Inventory. British Journal of Medical Psychology 50:163–171, 1977. 79

Bedford A, Presly AS: Symptom patterns among chronic schizophrenic inpatients. British Journal of Psychiatry 133:176–178, 1978. 90

Beech HR. 575

Beech HR, Ciesielski KT, Gordon PK: Further observations of evoked potentials in obsessional patients. British Journal of Psychiatry 142:605–609, 1983. 575

Begleiter H. 290

Begleiter H, DeNoble V, Porjesz B: Protracted brain dysfunction after alcohol withdrawal in monkeys, in Biological Effects of Alcohol. Edited by Begleiter H. New York, Plenum, 1980. 290

Begleiter H, Porjesz B: Persistence of brain hyperexcitability following chronic alcoholic exposure to rats. Advances in Experimental Medicine and Biology 85b:209–222, 1977. 290

Behar D. 24

Behar D, Rapoport JL, Berg CJ, Denckla MB, Mann L, Cox C, Fedio P, Zahn T, Wolfman MG: Computerized tomography and neuropsychological test measures in adolescents with obsessive-compulsive disorder. American Journal of Psychiatry 141:363–369, 1984. 571, 572

Beidel DC. 53, 228, 230

Beis A. 120

Beiser M. 154, 157, 159

Beiser M: A psychiatric follow-up of 'normal' adults. American Journal of Psychiatry 21:56–78, 1971. 154

Beiser M, Benfari RC, Collomb H, Ravel JL: Measuring psychoneurotic behavior in cross-cultural surveys. Journal of Nervous and Mental Disease 163:10–23, 1976. 154, 157

Bell DA. 251

Bell J. 395

Bell SE. 305

Bellack AS. 476

Bellak L, Hurvich M, Gediman H: Ego Functions in Schizophrenics, Neurotics and Normals. New York, John Wiley, 1973. 547

Belluzzi JD. 415

Bembinski A. 420

Bemporad J. 354, 614

Benfari RC. 154, 157

Benfari RC, Beiser M, Leighton AH, Mertens CJ: Some dimensions of psychoneurotic behavior in an urban sample. Journal of Nervous and Mental Disease 155:77–90, 1972. 154, 157

Benfari RC, Beiser M, Leighton AH, Murphy JM, Mertens CJ: The manifestation of types of psychological states in an urban sample. Journal of Clinical Psychology 30:471–483, 1974. 154, 159

Benham L. 116

Benkert O. 45

Bennet EA: The Neuroses in Modern Practice in Psychological Medicine. Edited by Rees JR. London, Butterworth, 1949. 314

Benshoof B: A comparison of anxiety and depressive symptomatology in the anxiety and affective disorders. Poster presented at the Annual Meeting of the Association for the Advancement of Behavior Therapy, Boston, November 1987. 508, 509

Benson DF. 310

Benson H, Herd J, Morse W, Kelleher R: Hypotensive effects of chlordiazepoxide, amobarbital and chlorpromazine on behaviorally induced elevated blood pressure in the squirrel monkey. Journal of Pharmacology and Experimental Therapeutics 173:399–406, 1970. 422

Berchick RJ. 700

Berchou R. 392

Berg CJ. 571, 572

Berger-Gross P. 572

Berger-Gross P, Bruder GE, Quitkin F, Goetz R: Auditory laterality in depression: relation to circadian patterns and EEG sleep.Biological Psychiatry 20:611–622, 1985. 572

Berglund M: Suicide in alcoholism. Archives of General Psychiatry 41:888–891, 1984. 302

Bergman E. 528

Berkson J: Limitations of the application of fourfold table analysis to hospital data. Biometric Bulletin 2:47–53, 1946. 116, 333

Berman KF, Zec RF, Weinberger DR: Physiologic dysfunction of dorsolateral prefrontal cortex in schizophrenia. Archives of General Psychiatry 43:126–135, 1986. 570

Bernadt M. 287, 289

Berndt DJ, Petzel TP, Berndt, SM: Development and initial evaluation of a Multiscore Depression Inventory. Journal of Personality Assessment 44:396–403, 1980. 645

Berndt SM. 645

Berney TP. 274

Bernstein GA, Garfinkel BD: School phobia: the overlap of affective and anxiety disorders. Journal of the American Academy of Child Psychiatry 25:235–241, 1986. 277, 360, 361

Berrettini WH. 393, 415

Berridge CW. 421, 431

Berridge CW, Dunn AJ: Corticotropin-releasing factor elicits naloxone sensitive stress-like alterations in exploratory behavior in mice. Regulatory Peptides 16:83–93, 1986. 421, 426

Berridge CW, Dunn AJ: A corticotropin-releasing factor antagonist reverses the stress-induced changes of exploratory behavior in mice. Hormones and Behavior 21:393–401, 1987a. 423

Berridge CW, Dunn AJ: Corticotropin-releasing factor (CRF) and norepinephrine involvement in the regulation of exploratory behavior. Social Neuroscience Abstracts 13:427, 1987b. 421

Berwick DM. 161

Bes A. 576

Better SR, Fine PR, Simison D, Doss GH, Wells RT, McLaughlin DE: Disability benefits as disincentives to rehabilitation. Health and Society 57:412–427, 1979. 247

Bhat A. 673

Bhate SR. 274

Bibb JL, Chambless DL: Alcohol use and abuse among diagnosed agoraphobics. Behavior Research and Therapy 24:49–58, 1986. 291

Biddle N. 388, 406

Biederman J. 254

Biederman J, Rivinus T, Kemper K, Hamilton D, MacFadyen J, Harmatz J: Depressive disorders in relatives of anorexia nervosa patients with and without a current episode of nonbipolar major depression. American Journal of Psychiatry 142:1495–1496, 1985. 254

Bierer LM. 387

Bifulco A. 469, 478, 494

Billings AG, Moos RM: Psychosocial stressors, coping and depression, in Handbook of Depression: Treatment, Assessment and Research. Edited by Beckham E, Leber W. Homewood, Ill, Dorsey Press, 1985. 632

Bilski J. 420

Binder J. 124, 125

Bingham SF. 284, 285

Birbaumer N. 244

Bird HR. 317, 321, 660

Birley JLT. 475

Bishop YMM, Fienberg SE, Holland PW: Discrete Multivariate Analysis: Theory and Practice. Cambridge, MA, MIT Press, 1975. 130, 165

Bissette G. 404, 415, 418, 424–426, 427, 428, 430, 431–433

Bissette G, Reynolds GP, Kilts CD, Nemeroff CB: Corticotropin-releasing factor-like immunoreactivity in senile dementia of the Alzheimer type: reduced cortical and striatal concentrations. Journal of the American Medical Association 254:3067–3069, 1985. 430

Bixler EO. 327

Black A: The natural history of obsessional neurosis, in Obsessional States. Edited by Beech HR. London, Methuen, 1974. 306, 314

Black DW. 294, 296, 302

Black DW, Winokur G, Bell SE, Nasrallah A, Hulbert J: Complicated mania: comorbidity and immediate outcome in mania. Archives of General Psychiatry 45:232–240, 1988. 305

Black DW, Winokur G, Nasrallah A: Mortality in patients with primary unipolar depression, secondary unipolar depression, and bipolar affective disorder: a comparison with general population mortality. International Journal of Psychiatry in Medicine 17:351–360, 1987a. 296

Black DW, Winokur G, Nasrallah A: Treatment and outcome in secondary depression: a naturalistic study of 1087 patients. Journal of Clinical Psychiatry 48:438–441, 1987b. 296, 301

Blackburn IM. 574

Blackburn IM, Loudon JB, Ashworth CM: A new scale for measuring mania. Psychological Medicine 7:453–458, 1977. 555

Blackwell D. 248

Blackwood DHR, Whalley LJ, Christie JE, Blackburn IM, St Clair DM, McInnes A: Changes in auditory P3 event-related potentials in schizophrenia and depression. British Journal of Psychiatry 150:154–160, 1987. 574

Blanchard EB. 43, 44, 45, 46, 49, 51, 55, 62, 63, 64, 67, 69, 70, 71, 76, 190, 200, 207, 208, 209, 213, 221, 223, 227, 228, 472, 590, 591, 619, 635

Blanchard EB, Andrasik F, Ahles TA, Teders SJ, O'Keefe D: Migraine and tension headache: a meta-analytic review. Behavior Therapy 11:613–631, 1980. 251

Blashfield RK. 80

Blashfield RK: The Classification of Psychopathology. New York, Plenum, 1984. 42, 49, 477

Blatt SJ, D'Afflitti FP, Quinlan DM: Experience of depression in normal young adults. Journal of Abnormal Psychology 85:383–389, 1976. 554

Blazer DG. 115, 159, 321, 415, 588, 705

Blazer D, Hughes D, George LK: Stressful life events and the onset of a generalized anxiety syndrome. American Journal of Psychiatry 144:1178–1183, 1987. 433

Blodgett AN. 387

Bloom FE. 419, 420, 421, 425, 431

Bloom L. 414

Blowers GH. 392

Blumberg SH. 54, 508

Blumer D, Heilbronn M, Himmelhoch J: Indications for carbamazepine in mental illness: atypical psychiatric disorder or temporal lobe syndrome? Comprehensive Psychiatry 29:108–122, 1988. 606

Bohman M. 245, 285, 440, 447, 448, 453, 461, 626

Bohman M, Cloninger CR, von Knorring AL: An adoption study of somatoform disorders, III: cross-fostering analysis and genetic relationship to alcoholism and criminality. Archives of General Psychiatry 41:872–878, 1984. 245

Bolles RC: Reinforcement, expectancy, and learning. Psychological Review 79: 394–409, 1972. 527

Bolton J. 417

Bonhert M. 225

Bonner RT. 581

Boodoosingh L. 273, 274

Booth JD. 431

Bootzin R, Engle-Friedman M: Sleep disturbances, in Handbook of Clinical Gerontology. Edited by Carstensen LL, Edelstein BA. Elmsford, NY, Pergamon, 1987. 528

Bootzin RR, Max D: Learning and behavioral theories, in Handbook on Stress and Anxiety. Edited by Kutash, IL, Schlesinger LB, et al. San Francisco, Jossey-Bass, 1980. 508

Bootzin R, Nicassio P: Behavioral treatment in insomnia, in Progress in Behavior Modification, Vol 6. Edited by Hersen M, Eisler R, Miller P. New York, Academic, 1978. 528

Borenstein M. 387

Borg S. 288, 290

Borkovec TD: The role of cognitive and somatic cues in anxiety and anxiety disorders: worry and relaxation-induced anxiety, in Anxiety and the Anxiety Disorders. Edited by Tuma AH, Maser JD. Hillsdale, NJ, Lawrence Erlbaum, 1985, pp 463–478. 509

Borrell J. 422

Borus JF. 161

Botskarev VK. 572

Botstein D. 683

Boulenger JP. 393, 415, 523, 575, 602, 607

Bowen RC, Cipywnyk D, D'Arcy C, Keegan D: Alcoholism, anxiety disorders, and agoraphobia. Alcoholism: Clinical and Experimental Research 8:48–50, 1984. 290

Bowen RC, Kohout J: The relationship between agoraphobia and primary affective disorders. Canadian Journal of Psychiatry 24:317–322, 1979. 503

Bower GH: Mood and memory. American Psychologist 36:129–147, 1981. 642, 643

Bower GH: Affect and cognition. Philosophic Transactions of the Royal Society of London B302:387–402, 1983. 642

Bowlby J. 503, 509, 511, 519

Bowlby J: Separation anxiety. International Journal of Psycho-analysis 41:89–113, 1960. 503, 601

Bowlby J: Attachment and Loss, Vol 1: Attachment. New York, Basic Books, 1969. 533

Bowlby J: Attachment and Loss, Vol 2: Separation: Anxiety and Anger. New York, Basic Books, 1973. 272, 281, 500, 533, 534, 536

Bowlby J: Attachment and Loss, Vol 3: Loss: Sadness and Depression. New York, Basic Books, 1980. 272, 281, 500, 503, 504, 533–536

Box GEP: Nonnormality and tests of variances. Biometrika 40:318–335, 1953. 628

Box GEP: Some theorems on quadratic forms applied in the study of analysis of variance problems; I: effects of inequality of variance in the one-way classification. Annals of Mathematical Statistics 25:290–302, 1954. 628

Boyd JH. 115, 116, 165, 168, 171, 317, 322, 589, 649, 650, 664, 666

Boyd JH: Use of mental health services for the treatment of panic disorder. American Journal of Psychiatry 143:1569–1574, 1986. 676

Boyd JH, Burke JD, Gruenberg E, Holzer CE III, Rae DS, George LK, Karno M, Stoltzman R, McEvoy L, Nestadt G: Exclusion criteria of DSM-III: a study of co-occurrence of hierarchy-free syndromes. Archives of General Psychiatry 41:983–989, 1984. 6, 44, 45, 61, 63, 118, 120, 137, 190, 204, 206, 221, 305, 307, 308, 311, 332, 367, 439, 455, 649, 650

Boyd JH, Burke JD, Gruenberg E, Holzer CE III, Rae DS, George LK, Karno M, Stoltzman R, McEvoy L, Nestadt G: The exclusion criteria of DSM-III: a study of the co-occurrence of hierarchy-free syndromes, in Diagnosis and Classification in Psychiatry: A Critical Appraisal of DSM-III. Edited by Tischler GL. New York, Cambridge University Press, 1987. 93, 95, 97, 109

Boyd JH, Regier DA, Burke JD: The contribution of epidemiology to the advancement of nosology. Presented at the World Psychiatric Association Conference on International Classification in Psychiatry: Unity and Diversity, Montreal, Canada, June 27, 1985. 116

Boyd JH, Weissman MM: Epidemiology of affective disorders: a reexamination and future directions. Archives of General Psychiatry 38:1039–1046, 1981. 168, 623

Boyer RM, Hellman LD, Roffwarg H, Katz J, Zumoff B, O'Connor J, Bradlow HL, Fukushima D: Cortisol secretion and metabolism in anorexia nervosa. New England Journal of Medicine 296:190–193, 1977. 255

Boykin RA. 716

Bradley B, Mathews A: Negative self-schemata in clinical depression. British Journal of Clinical Psychology 22:173–181, 1983. 631

Bradlow HL. 255

Brambilla F, Cavagnini F, Invitti C, Poterzio F, Lampertico M, Sali L, Maggioni M, Candolfi C, Panerai AE, Muller EE: Neuroendocrine and psychopathological measures in anorexia nervosa: resemblances to primary affective disorders. Psychiatry Research 16:165–176, 1985. 255

Brannon WS. 512

Bransome ED. 579

Brantley T, Sutker TP: Antisocial behavior disorders, in Comprehensive Handbook of Psychopathology. Edited by Adams AG, Sutker T. New York, Plenum, 1984. 285

Bravo M. 317, 321, 660

Brehm JW. 504, 521, 527

Breier A. 390

Breier A, Charney DS, Heninger GR: Major depression in patients with agoraphobia and panic disorder. Archives of General Psychiatry 41:1129–1135, 1984. 94, 109, 472, 473, 487, 489, 495, 496, 502

Breier A, Charney DS, Heninger GR: The diagnostic validity of anxiety disorders and their relationship to depressive illness. American Journal of Psychiatry 142:787–797, 1985a. 54, 271, 472, 487, 489, 495, 496, 585, 605

Breier A, Charney DS, Heninger GR: Agoraphobia with panic attacks: development, diagnostic stability, and course of illness.Archives of General Psychiatry 142:787–797, 1985b. 271, 472, 487, 489, 495, 496, 605

Breier A, Charney DS, Heninger MD: Agoraphobia with panic attacks: development, diagnostic stability, and course of illness. Archives of General Psychiatry 43:1029–1036, 1986. 217

Brenner R. 387

Breslau N, Davis G: Refining DSM-III criteria in major depression: an assessment of the descriptive validity of criterion symptoms. Journal of Affective Disorders 9:199–206, 1985. 48

Breslau N, Davis GC, Prabucki K: Searching for evidence on the validity of generalized anxiety disorder: psychopathology in children of anxious mothers. Psychiatry Research 20:285–297, 1987. 354, 355, 356, 357

Brezinova V. 431

Bridge L. 494

Bridges A. 255

Bridges KW. 602

Bridges KW, Goldberg DP: Somatic presentation of DSM-III psychiatric disorders in primary care. Journal of Psychosomatic Research 29:563–569, 1985. 248

Bridges M. 524

Bridges M, Yeragani VK, Rainey JM, Phol R: Dexamethasone suppression test in patients with panic attacks. Social and Biological Psychiatry 21:849–853, 1986. 387

Briley MS, Langer SZ, Raisman R, Sechter D, Zerifian E: Tritiated imipramine binding sites are decreased in platelets of untreated depressed patients. Science 209:303–305, 1980. 414

Britton DR, Britton KT: A sensitive open field measure of anxiolytic drug activity. Pharmacology, Biochemistry and Behavior 15:577–582, 1981. 422

Britton DR, Koob GF, Rivier J, Vale W: Intraventricular corticotropin-releasing factor enhances behavioral effects of novelty. Life Sciences 31:363–367, 1982. 421, 422

Britton DR, Varela M, Garcia A, Rosenthal M: Dexamethasone suppresses pituitary-adrenal but not behavioral effects of centrally administered CRF. Life Sciences 38:211–216, 1986. 420, 421

Britton KT. 409, 410, 422

Britton KT, Koob GF: Alcohol reverses the proconflict effect of corticotropin-releasing factor. Regulatory Peptides 16:315–320, 1986. 422

Britton KT, Lee G, Dana R, Risch SC, Koob GF: Activating and 'anxiogenic' effects of corticotropin releasing factor are not inhibited by blockade of the pituitary-adrenal system with dexamethasone. Life Sciences 39:1281–1286, 1986. 420

Britton KT, Morgan J, Rivier J, Vale W, Koob GF: Chlordiazepoxide attenuates response suppression induced by corticotropin-releasing factor in the conflict test. Psychopharmacology 86:170–174, 1985. 422

Brocco KJ. 453

Brockington IF. 661

Brogden SRN. 703

Bromet EJ, Dunn LO, Connell MM, Dew MA, Schulberg HC: Long-term reliability of diagnosing lifetime major depression in a community sample. Archives of General Psychiatry 43:435–440, 1986. 178, 489, 661

Brophy C. 274

Brotman AW. 574

Brotman AW, Jenike MA: Monosymptomatic hypochondriasis treated with tricyclic antidepressants. American Journal of Psychiatry 141:1608–1609, 1984. 315

Brown AC. 247

Brown CH. 661

Brown FW: Heredity in the psychoneuroses. Proceedings of the Royal Society of London: Medicine 35:785–788, 1942. 306

Brown G. 218, 225, 528, 529, 631, 700

Brown GB. 219

Brown GM. 424

Brown GW. 45, 470, 474, 486–488, 490, 493–497, 509, 520

Brown GW: Meaning, measurement, and stress of life events, in Stressful Life Events: Their Nature and Effects. Edited by Dohrenwend BS, Dohrenwend BP. New York, John Wiley, 1974. 466, 471

Brown GW: Life events, psychiatric disorder and physical illness. Journal of Psychosomatic Research 25:461–473, 1981. 466, 467

Brown GW, Bifulco A, Harris T, Bridge L: Life stress, chronic subclinical symptoms and vulnerability to clinical depression. Journal of Affective Disorders 11:1–19, 1986. 494

Brown GW, Bifulco A, Harris TO: Life events, vulnerability and onset of depression: some refinements. British Journal of Psychiatry 150:30–42, 1987. 469

Brown GW, Birley JLT: Crises and life changes and the onset of schizophrenia. Journal of Health and Social Behavior 9:203–214, 1968. 475

Brown GW, Harris T: Social Origins of Depression. New York, Free Press, 1978a. 467, 470, 475, 479, 484, 487, 511, 519, 536

Brown GW, Harris T: Social origins of depression: a reply. Psychological Medicine 8:577–588, 1978b. 468

Brown GW, Harris T: Fall-off in the reporting of life events. Social Psychiatry 17:23–28, 1982. 468

Brown GW, Harris T: Establishing causal links: the Bedford College studies of depression, in Life Events and Psychiatric Disorders: Controversial Issues. Edited by Katschnig H. Cambridge, England, Cambridge University Press, 1986. 467, 468, 469, 470, 471, 475, 476, 478, 479, 481, 488, 492

Brown GW, Harris TO, Bifulco A: Long-term effect of early loss of parent, in Depression in Childhood: Developmental Perspective. Edited by Rutter M, Izard C, Read P. New York, Guilford, 1985. 478

Brown MR. 420

Brown M: Corticotropin releasing factor: central nervous system sites of action. Brain Research 399:10–14, 1986. 420

Brown MR, Fisher LA: Central nervous system effects of corticotropin releasing factor in the dog. Brain Research 280:75–79, 1983. 420

Brown MR, Fisher LA, Spiess J, Rivier C, Rivier J, Vale W: Corticotropin-releasing factor: actions on the sympathetic nervous system and metabolism. Endocrinology 111:928–931, 1982. 420

Brown MR, Fisher LA, Webb V, Vale WW, Rivier JE: Corticotropin-releasing factor: a physiologic regulator of adrenal epinephrine secretion. Brain Research 328:355–357, 1985. 423

Brown MR, Gray TS, Fisher LA: Corticotropin-releasing factor receptor antagonist: effects on the autonomic nervous system and cardiovascular function. Regulatory Peptides 16:321–329, 1986. 423

Brown N. 151

Brown R, Kocsis J, Caroff S, Amsterdam J, Winokur A, Stokes P, Frazer A: Differences in nocturnal melatonin secretion beween melancholic depressed patients and control subjects. American Journal of Psychiatry 143:811–816, 1985. 390

Brown WA, Haier RJ, Qualls CB: Dexamethasone suppression test identifies subtypes of depression which respond to different antidepressants. Lancet 1:928–929, 1980. 404

Bruce ML. 317, 321, 323, 327

Bruder GE. 572

Bruder G, Sutton S, Berger-Gross P: Lateralized auditory processing in depression: dichotic click detection. Psychiatry Research 4:253–266, 1981. 572

Brugha T. 653, 655

Brumbach RA, Staton RD, Wilson H: Neuropsychological study of children during and after remission of endogenous depressive episodes. Perceptual and Motor Skills 50:1163–1167, 1980. 570

Brus I. 151

Bryden MP. 564

Bryden MP: Laterality: Functional Asymmetry in the Intact Brain. New York, Academic, 1982. 572

Buchsbaum MS. 276, 571

Buchsbaum MS, DeLisi LE, Holcomb HH, Cappelletti J, King AC, Johnson J, Hazlett E, Dowling-Zimmerman S, Post RM, Morihisa J, Carpenter W, Cohen R, Pickar D, Weinberger DR, Margolin R, Kessler RM: Anteroposterior gradients in cerebral glucose use in schizophrenia and affective disorders. Archives of General Psychiatry 41:1159–1166, 1984. 577

Buchsbaum MS, Hazlett E, Sicotte N, Stein M, Wu J, Zetin M: Topographic EEG changes with benzodiazepine administration in generalized anxiety disorder. Biological Psychiatry 20:832–842, 1985. 575

Buchsbaum MS, Landau S, Murphy DL, Goodwin FK: Average evoked response in unipolar affective disorders: relationship to sex, age of onset, and monoamine oxidase. Biological Psychiatry 7:199–212, 1973. 574

Buchsbaum MS, Wu J, DeLisi LE, Holcomb H, Kessler R, Johnson J, King AC, Hazlett E, Langston K, Post RM: Frontal cortex and basal ganglia metabolic rates assessed by positron emission tomography with [18F]2-deoxyglucose in affective illness. Journal of Affective Disorders 10:137–152, 1986. 577

Buck RC, Hull DL: The logical structure of the Linnean hierarchy. Syst Zool 15:97–111, 1966. 64

Budman SH. 161

Buell U. 576

Bueno JA, Sabanes F, Gascon J, Gasto C, Salamero M: Dexamethasone suppression test in patients with panic disorder and secondary depression. Archives of General Psychiatry 41:723–724, 1984. 387

Bugnon C. 418

Buller R. 339, 340, 346, 347

Buller R, Maier W, Benkert O: Clinical subtypes in panic disorder: their descriptive and prospective validity. Journal of Affective Disorders 11:105–114, 1986. 45

Bunney WE Jr, Davis JM: Norepinephrine in depressive reactions: a review. Archives of General Psychiatry 13:483–494, 1965. 431

Burdick CA. 512

Burge D. 354, 355, 356, 357, 358

Burke JD. 6, 44, 45, 61, 63, 93, 95, 97, 109, 115, 116, 118, 120, 137, 165, 168, 171, 190, 204, 206, 221, 305, 307, 308, 311, 317, 321, 332, 333, 364, 439, 455, 588, 589, 592, 593, 649, 650, 653, 655, 656, 660, 662, 664, 666, 707

Burke JD: Diagnostic categorization by the Diagnostic Interview Schedule: a comparison with other methods of assessment, in Mental Disorders in the Community: Findings From Psychiatric Epidemiology. Edited by Barrett JE, Rose RM. New York, Guilford, 1986. 660, 661

Burnam A. 115, 246, 322

Burnam MA. 247, 317, 322

Burnam MA, Karno M, Hough RL, Escobar JI, Forsythe AB: The Spanish Diagnostic Interview Schedule: reliability and comparison with clinical diagnoses. Archives of General Psychiatry 40:1189–1196, 1983. 661

Burns BH. 588, 592, 593

Burns BH, Nichols MA: Factors related to the localization of symptoms to the chest in depression. British Journal of Psychiatry 121:405–409, 1972. 247

Burroughs J. 254, 311

Burrows GD. 387, 390, 393, 586, 592, 594, 607

Buse AH. 715

Bushing JA. 409

Butler FK. 396, 577

Butler MC, Jones AP: The Health Opinion Survey reconsidered: dimensionality, reliability, and validity. Journal of Clinical Psychology 35:554–559, 1979. 157

Byrne DG. 120, 659

Byrne E: Idiopathic chronic fatigue and myalgia syndrome (myalgic encephalomyelitis): some thoughts on nomenclature and aetiology. Medical Journal of Australia 2:80–82, 1988. 151

Cadoret RJ. 9, 594

Cadoret RJ: Psychopathology in adopted-away offspring of biologic parents with antisocial behavior. Archives of General Psychiatry 35:176–184, 1978. 240

Cadoret R, Troughton E, Widmer R: Clinical differences between antisocial and primary alcoholics. Comprehensive Psychiatry 25: 1–8, 1984. 285

Cadoret RJ, Widmer RB, Troughton EP: Somatic complaints: harbinger of depression in primary care. Journal of Affective Disorders 2:61–70, 1980. 242

Callies AL. 327

Calloway SP. 488

Camarri F. 420

Cameron OG. 43, 53, 387, 586, 590

Cameron V. 417

Campbell DT, Fiske D: Convergent and discriminant validation by the multi-trait-multimethod matrix. Psychological Bulletin 56:81–105, 1959. 623, 631

Campbell KB, Courchesne E, Picton TW, Squires KC: Evoked potential correlates of human information processing. Biological Psychology 8:45–68, 1979. 574

Campeas R. 672, 676–678

Candolfi C. 255

Canino GJ, Bird HR, Shrout PE, Rubio-Stipec M, Bravo M, Martinez R, Sessman M, Guevara LM: The prevalence of specific psychiatric disorders in Puerto Rico. Archives of General Psychiatry 44:727–735, 1987a. 317, 321

Canino GJ, Bird HR, Shrout PE, Rubio-Stipec M, Bravo M, Martinez R, Sessman M, Guzman A, Guevara LM, Costas H: The Spanish Diagnostic Interview Schedule. Archives of General Psychiatry 44:720–726, 1987b. 660

Canter S. 291

Cantor N, Genero N: Psychiatric diagnosis and natural categorization: a close analogy, in Contemporary Issues in Psychopathology. Edited by Millon T, Klerman G. New York, Guilford, 1986. 52

Cantwell DP. 273, 279

Cantwell DP, Sturzenberger RS, Burroughs J, Salkin B, Green JK: Anorexia nervosa: an affective disorder? Archives of General Psychiatry 34:1087–1095, 1977. 254, 311

Cappell H, Herman CP: Alcohol and tension reduction: a review. Journal of Studies on Alcohol, 33:33–64, 1972. 290

Cappelletti J. 577

Carcangiu P. 420

Carette S, McCain GA, Bell DA, Fam AG: Evaluation of amitriptyline in primary fibrositis. Arthritis and Rheumatism 29:655–659, 1986. 251

Carey G: Big genes, little genes, affective disorder, and anxiety: a commentary. Archives of General Psychiatry 44:486–491, 1987. 371, 649

Carey G, Gottesman II: Defining cases of genetic criteria, in What Is a Case? Edited by Wing JK, Bebbington P, Robins LH. London, Grant McIntyre, Medical & Scientific, 1981. 670

Carey RJ. 314

Carli M. 712, 713

Carlson GA. 273, 275, 279, 317, 322, 360, 361, 547, 549

Carlson GA, Cantwell DP: A survey of depressive symptoms in a child and adolescent psychiatric population. Journal of the American Academy of Child Psychiatry 18:587–599, 1979. 279

Carmichael SK. 79, 90

Caroff S. 390, 570

Carpenter WT Jr. 179, 577

Carr DB, Sheehan DV, Surman OS, Coleman JH, Greenblatt DJ, Heninger GR, Jones KJ, Levine PH, Watkins WD: Neuroendocrine correlates of lactate-induced anxiety and their response to chronic alprazolam therapy.

American Journal of Psychiatry 143:483–494, 1986. 392

Carroll B: Letter to the editor: from the researcher's perspective. American Journal of Psychiatry 138:705–707, 1981. 36

Carroll BJ. 424, 599

Carroll BJ: The dexamethasone suppression test for melancholia. British Journal of Psychiatry 140:292–304, 1982. 387

Carroll BJ, Curtis GC, Davis BM, Mendels J, Sugerman AA: Urinary free cortisol excretion in depression. Psychological Medicine 6:43–50, 1976. 427

Carroll BJ, Feinberg M, Greden JF, Tarika J, Albala AA, Haskett RF, James NM, Kronfol Z, Lohr N, Steiner M, de Vigne JP, Young E: A specific laboratory test for the diagnosis of melancholia: standardization, validation, and clinical utility. Archives of General Psychiatry 38:15–22, 1981. 387, 403, 427

Carroll BJ, Feinberg M, Smouse PE, Lawson SG, Greden JF: The Carroll Rating Scale for Depression: I. Development, reliability, and validation. British Journal of Psychiatry 138:194–200, 1981. 261, 613

Carroll JD, Chang JJ: Analysis of individual differences in multidimensional scaling via an N-way generalization of the "Eckart-Young" decomposition. Psychometrika 35:283–319, 1970. 626

Carsia RV, Weber H, Perez FM Jr: Corticotropin-releasing factor stimulates the release of adrenocorticotropin from domestic fowl pituitary cells. Endocrinology 118:143–148, 1986. 417

Carson SW, Halbreich U, Yeh C-M, Goldstein S: Altered plasma dexamethasone and cortisol suppressibility in patients with panic disorders. Biological Psychology 24:56–62, 1988. 406

Caruso KA. 350

Carver CS, Gaines JG: Optimism, pessimism, and postpartum depression. Cognitive Therapy and Research 11:449–462, 1987. 512

Carver CS, Scheier MF: Control theory: a useful conceptual framework for personality-social, clinical, and health psychology. Psychological Bulletin 92:111–135, 1982. 509

Casey PR, Dillon S, and Tyrer PJ: The diagnostic status of patients with conspicuous psychiatric morbidity in primary care. Psychological Medicine 14:673–681, 1984. 593

Casper RC. 256, 263, 266

Casper RC, Eckert ED, Halmi KA, Goldberg SC, Davis JM: Bulimia: its incidence and clinical importance in patients with anorexia nervosa. Archives of General Psychiatry 37:1030–1035, 1980. 258

Casper RC, Jabine LN: Psychological functioning in anorexia nervosa: a comparison between anorexia nervosa patients on follow-up and their sisters, in Proceedings of the 15th European Conference on Psychosomatic Research. Edited by Lacey JH, Sturgeon DA, John Libbey & Co, 1986, pp 172–178. 254, 255

Casper RC, Redmond DE, Katz MM, Schaffer CB, Davis JM, Koslow SH: Somatic symptoms in primary affective disorder: presence and relationship to the classification of depression. Archives of General Psychiatry 42:1098–1104, 1985. 256, 260, 264, 265

Casper RC, Schlemmer RF, Javaid JI: A placebo-controlled crossover study of oral clonidine in acute anorexia nervosa. Psychiatry Research 20:249–260, 1987. 260

Cassano GB, Maggini C, Akiskal HS: Short-term, subchronic and chronic sequelae of affective disorders. Psychiatric Clinics of North America 6:55–67, 1983. 604, 606

Cassano GB, Perugi G, Maremmani I, Akiskal HS: Social adjustment in dysthymia, in Dysthymic Disorder. Edited by Burton S, Akiskal HS. London, Gaskell, Royal College of Psychiatrists, 1990, pp 78–85. 599

Cassem NH: Depression, in Massachusetts General Hospital Handbook of General Hospital Psychiatry, 2nd Edition. Edited by Hackett TP, Cassem NJ. Littleton, MA, PSG Publishing, 1987. 327

Cassidy WL, Flanagan NB, Spellman M, Cohen ME: Clinical observations in manic-depressive disease: a quantitative study of 100 manic-depressive patients and 50 medically sick controls. Journal of the American Medical Association 164:1535–1546, 1957. 260

Cattell RB: The Scientific Analysis of Personality. Chicago, Aldine, 1966. 71

Cattell RB, Sheier I: The meaning and measurement of neuroticism and anxiety. New York, Ronald Press, 1961. 613

Cavagnini F. 255

Cavoir N. 716

Cerny JA. 221

Chabrol H, Barrere M, Guell A, Bes A, Moron P: Hyperfrontality of cerebral blood flow in depressed adolescents. American Journal of Psychiatry 143:263–264, 1986. 576

Chahal R. 661

Chamberlain K. 528

Chambers WJ, Puig-Antich J, Hirsch M, Paez P, Ambrosini PJ, Tabrizi MA, Davies M: The assessment of affective disorders in children and adolescents by semistructured interview. Archives of General Psychiatry 42:696–702, 1985. 273

Chambless DL. 291

Chanda SK. 431

Chang JJ. 626

Chapman JP. 716

Chapman LJ, Chapman JP: Scales for rating psychotic and psychotic-like experiences as continua. Schizophrenia Bulletin 6:476–489, 1980. 716

Chappell P. 430

Chappell PB, Smith MA, Kilts CD, Bissette G, Ritchie J, Anderson C, Nemeroff CB: Alterations in corticotropin-releasing factor-like immunoreactivity in discrete rat brain regions after acute and chronic stress. Journal of Neuroscience 6:2908–2914, 1986. 418, 424–426, 431

Chapple ED: Culture and Biological Man: Explanations in behavioral anthropology. New York, Holt Rinehart & Winston, 1970. 709

Chapron DJ. 289

Charles E. 549

Charney DS. 54, 94, 109, 217, 271, 389, 390, 391–393, 407, 472, 473, 487, 489, 495, 496, 502, 585, 605

Charney DS, Heninger GR: Abnormal regulation of noradrenergic function in panic disorders: effects of clonidine in healthy subjects and patients with agoraphobia and panic disorder. Archives of General Psychiatry 43:1042–1054, 1986a. 389, 390

Charney DS, Heninger GR: Serotonin function in panic disorders: the effect of intravenous tryptophan in healthy subjects and panic disorder patients before and during alprazolam treatment. Archives of General Psychiatry 43:1059–1065, 1986b. 393

Charney DS, Heninger GR, Breier A: Noradrenergic function in panic anxiety: effects of yohimbine in healthy subjects and patients with agoraphobia and panic disorder. Archives of General Psychiatry 41:751–763, 1984. 390

Charney DS, Heninger GR, Jatlow PI: Increased anxiogenic effects of caffeine in panic disorders. Archives of General Psychiatry 42:233–243, 1985. 392

Charney DS, Heninger GR, Sternberg DE: Failure of chronic antidepressant treatment to alter growth hormone response to clonidine. Psychiatry Research 7:135–138, 1982. 390

Charney DS, Menkes DB, Phil M, Heninger GR: Receptor sensitivity and the mechanism of action of antidepressant treatment. Archives of General Psychiatry 38:1160–1180, 1981. 419, 432

Charney DS, Nelson JC, Quinlan DM: Personality traits and disorder in depression. American Journal of Psychiatry 138:1601–1604, 1981. 327

Charney DS, Woods SW, Goodman WK, Heninger GR: Neurobiological mechanisms of panic anxiety: biochemical and behavioral correlates of yohimbine-induced panic attacks. American Journal of Psychiatry 144:1030–1036, 1987. 389, 390, 391, 392

Charry JM. 425

Chaudhry DR. 364, 386, 387, 478, 580

Chen JJ. 503

Cheslow DL. 315

Chestnut EC. 273

Chewluk J. 570

Chodoff P. 554

Chodoff P: The depressive personality: a critical review, in The Psychology of Depression: Contemporary Theory and Research. Edited by Friedman RJ, Katz MM. Washington, DC, V.H. Winston & Sons, 1974. 614, 630

Chouinard G. 703

Chouinard G, Annable L, Fontaine R, Solyom L: Alprazolam in the treatment of generalized anxiety and panic disorders: a double-blind placebo-controlled study. Psychopharmacology 77:229–233, 1982. 676, 703

Christie JE. 574

Christie KA, Burke JD, Regier DA, Rae DS, Boyd JH, Locke BZ: Epidemiologic evidence for early onset of mental disorders and increased risk of drug abuse in young adults. American Journal of Psychiatry 145:971–975, 1988. 649, 650, 664, 666

Chrousos GP. 255, 404, 417, 427, 429–433

Ciesielski KT. 575

Ciesielski KT, Beech HR, Gordon PK: Some electrophysiological observations in obsessional states. British Journal of Psychiatry 138:479–484, 1981. 575

Cipywnyk D. 290

Ciraulo DA. 286, 290

Ciraulo DA, Alderson LM, Chapron DJ, Jaffe JH, Subbarao B, Kramer PA: Imipramine disposition in alcoholics. Journal of Clinical Psychopharmacology 2:2–7, 1982. 289

Ciraulo DA, Jaffe JH: Tricyclic antidepressants in the treatment of depression associated with alcoholism. Journal of Clinical Psychopharmacology 1:146–150, 1981. 289

Cisin IH. 477, 590

Clancy J. 334, 335, 337, 344, 338, 386, 387, 703

Clancy J, Noyes R, Hoenk PR, Slymen DJ: Secondary depression in anxiety neurosis. Journal of Nervous and Mental Disease 166:846–850, 1978. 217, 472, 619

Clark DC, Gibbons RD, Fawcett J, Aagesen CA, Sellers D: Unbiased criteria for severity of depression in alcoholic inpatients. Journal of Nervous and Mental Disease 173:482–487, 1985. 295

Clark DM, Teasdale JD: Diurnal variation in clinical depression and accessibility of memories of positive and negative experiences. Journal of Abnormal Psychology 91:87–95, 1982. 643

Clark LA. 55, 508, 621

Clark WB: Loss of control, heavy drinking and drinking problems in a longitudinal study. Journal of Studies on Alcohol 37:1256–1290, 1976. 302

Clarkin JF. 48, 62, 279

Clarkson C. 343, 590, 594

Clarkson SE. 279

Claycomb B. 387

Clayton PJ. 10, 84, 180, 286, 287, 291, 294, 295, 296, 310, 337, 338, 346, 347, 378, 439, 440, 449, 453, 455–457, 500

Clayton P: Anxious depression: a reemerging subtype of depression, in Anxious Depression: Assessment and Treatment. Edited by Racagne G, Smeraldi E. New York, Raven, 1987. 594

Clayton PJ, Herjanic M, Murphy GE, Woodruff R: Mourning and depression; their similarities and differences. Canadian Journal of Psychiatry 19:309–312, 1974. 602

Cleary PA. 158

Cleary PD. 588, 593

Clements C. 513, 518, 530, 541, 543, 640

Clements CM, Alloy LB: Affective and behavioral consequences of perception of control styles. Northwestern University, Evanston, Ill (in press). 515

Clements CM, Alloy LB, Greenberg MS, Kolden G: Depression, anxiety, and self-schemata: a test of Beck's theory. Northwestern University, Evanston, Ill. (in press). 505, 517

Clifford CA. 287, 289

Clifford CA, Hopper JL, Fulker DW, Murray RM: A genetic and environmental analysis of a twin family study of alcohol use, anxiety, and depression. Genetic Epidemiology 1:63–79, 1984. 344, 345

Clinthorne J. 477, 590

Cloninger CR. 10, 180, 245, 439, 440, 447–449, 453, 455–457, 461

Cloninger CR: Somatoform and dissociative disorders, in The Medical Basis of Psychiatry. Edited by Winokur G, Clayton P. Philadelphia, WB Saunders, 1986a, pp 123–131. 239, 243, 246

Cloninger CR: A unified biosocial theory of personality and its role in the development of anxiety states. Psychiatric Developments 3:167–226, 1986b. 449, 455, 458, 459, 461, 462, 500

Cloninger CR: Neurogenetic adaptive mechanisms in alcoholism. Science 236: 410–416, 1987a. 285, 453, 459, 461, 462, 580

Cloninger CR: A systematic method for clinical description and classification of personality variants: a proposal. Archives of General Psychiatry 44:573–588, 1987b. 459, 462

Cloninger CR: A unified biosocial theory of personality and its role in the development of anxiety states: a reply to commentaries. Psychiatric Developments 2:83–120, 1988. 459, 461

Cloninger CR, Bohman M, Sigvardsson S: Inheritance of alcohol abuse: cross fostering analysis of adopted men. Archives of General Psychiatry 38:861–868, 1981. 285

Cloninger CR, Guze SB: Psychiatric illness in the families of female criminals: a study of 288 first degree relatives. British Journal of Psychiatry 122:697–703, 1973. 563

Cloninger CR, Martin RL, Guze SB, Clayton P: A blind follow-up and family study of anxiety neuroses: preliminary analysis of St. Louis 500, in Anxiety: New Research and Changing Concepts. Edited by Klein DF, Rabkin J. New York, Raven, 1981, pp 137–150. 337, 338, 378, 455, 456, 457, 500

Cloninger CR, Martin RL, Guze SB, Clayton PJ: Diagnosis and prognosis in schizophrenia. Archives of General Psychiatry 41:58–70, 1985. 84, 447

Cloninger CR, Reich T, Sigvardsson S, von Knorring A-L, Bohman M: Effects of changes in alcohol use between generations on inheritance of alcohol abuse, in Alcoholism: Origins and Outcome. Edited by Rose RM, Barrett J. New York, Raven, 1988. 285

Cloninger CR, Reich T, Wetzel R. Alcoholism and the affective disorders: familial association and genetic models, in Alcoholism and the Affective Disorders. Edited by Goodwin D, Erickson C. New York, Spectrum Press, 1979. 453

Cloninger CR, Sigvardsson S, Bohman M: Childhood personality predicts alcohol abuse in young adults. Alcoholism: Clinical and Experimental Research 12:494–505, 1988. 453, 461

Cloninger CR, Sigvardsson S, von Knorring A-L, Bohman M: An adoption study of somatoform disorders, II: identification of two discrete somatoform disorders. Archives of General Psychiatry 41:863–871, 1984. 440, 447, 626

Cloninger CR, von Knorring A-L, Sigvardsson S, Bohman M: Symptom patterns and causes of somatization in men, II: genetic and environmental independence from somatization in women. Genetic Epidemiology 3:171–185, 1986. 453

Clothier J. 575

Clouse RE, Lustman PJ: Psychiatric illness and contraction abnormalities of the esophagus. New England Journal of Medicine 309:1337, 1983. 249

Coccaro E. 387

Cochran WG: The distribution of the largest of a set of estimated variances as a fraction of their total. Annuals of Ergonomics 11:47–52, 1941. 628

Cochran WG: Some consequences when the assumptions for the analysis of variance are not satisfied. Biometrics 3:22–38, 1947. 628

Cochrane C. 51, 54, 499, 505, 616, 623, 626, 631

Coe C, Wiener S, Rosenberg L, Levine S: Endocrine and immune responses to separation and maternal loss in nonhuman primates, in The Psychobiology of Attachment and Separation. Edited by Reite M, Fiedl T. New York, Academic, 1985. 503, 521

Coffman GA. 52, 192

Cohen AS. 227

Cohen DJ. 24, 32, 299, 310, 563

Cohen ME. 242, 260, 585

Cohen ME, Robins E, Purtell JJ, Altmann MW, Reid DE: Excessive surgery in hysteria. Journal of the American Medical Association 151:977–986, 1953. 248

Cohen R. 577

Cohen S, Wills TA: Stress, social support, and the buffering hypothesis. Psychological Bulletin 98:310–357, 1985. 470, 471

Cole BJ, Koob GF: Propranolol antagonises the enhanced conditioned fear produced by corticotropin releasing factor but not FG 7142, an anxiogenic beta-carboline, in press. 423, 426

Cole HW. 227

Cole JO. 22, 702

Coleman LL. 288

Costello AJ. 191

Costello CG: Depression: loss of reinforcers or loss of reinforcer effectiveness? Behavior Therapy 3:240–247, 1972. 508

Costello CG: Anxiety and Depression: The Adaptive Emotions. Montreal, McGill-Queen's University Press, 1976. 612, 620

Costello CG, Comrey AL: Scales for measuring depression and anxiety. Journal of Psychology 66:303–313, 1967. 506, 613, 630

Costello RM: Alcoholism and the "alcoholic" personality, in Evaluation of the Alcoholic: Implications for Research Theory, and Treatment. Edited by Meyer RE, Glueck BC, O'Brien JE, Babor TF, Jaffe JH, Stabenau Jr. (NIAAA Research Monograph, No 5, DHHS Publ No ADM-81-1033). Washington, DC, U.S. Government Printing Office, 1981.

Cottler L. 116

Courchesne E. 574

Courts FA: Relation between experimentally induced muscular tension and memorization. Journal of Experimental Psychology 25:235–256, 1939. 570

Covi L. 54, 158, 234, 240, 256, 261, 508, 509, 624, 674, 676, 702

Cowley DS. 392

Cowley DS, Dager SR, Dunner DL: Lactate-induced panic in primary affective disorder. American Journal of Psychiatry 143:646–648, 1986. 392

Cowley DS, Dager SR, Dunner DL: Lactate infusions in major depression without panic attacks. Journal of Psychiatric Research 21:243–248, 1987. 392

Cowley DS, Dager SR, Foster SI, Dunner DL: Clinical characteristics and response to sodium lactate of patients with infrequent panic attacks. American Journal of Psychiatry 144:795–797, 1987. 392

Cox C. 571, 572

Cox DP. 387

Cox DJ, Freundlich A, Meyer BG: Differential effectiveness of electromyographic feedback, verbal relaxation instructions, and medication placebo with tension headache. Journal of Consulting and Clinical Psychology 43:892–898, 1975. 213

Cox DR: Analysis of binary data. London, Methuen, 1970. 130

Coyle PK, Sterman AB: Focal neurologic symptoms in panic attacks. American Journal of Psychiatry 143:648–649, 1986. 396

Coyne JC: Depression and the response of others. Journal of Abnormal Psychology 85:186–193, 1976a. 640

Coyne JC: Toward an interaction description of depression. Psychiatry 39:14–27, 1976b. 640

Coyne JC, Aldwin C, Lazarus RS: Depression and coping in stressful episodes. Journal of Abnormal Psychology 90:439–447, 1981. 637, 640

Coyne JC, Gotlib IH: The role of cognition in depression: a critical appraisal. Psychological Bulletin 94:472–505, 1983. 631

Craig DT. 260, 603

Craig TKJ, Brown GW, Harris TO: Depression in the general population: comparability of survey results. British Journal of Psychiatry 150:707–708, 1987. 487

Craighead WE. 505, 617

Crisp AH. 254, 255

Crocetti GM. 157

Crocker J. 517, 530

Crocker J, Alloy LB, Kayne NT: Self-esteem, depression, and attributional style (in press). 516

Crockett D. 572

Cropley AJ, Weckowitz TE: The dimensionality of clinical depression. Australian Journal of Psychology 18:18–25, 1966. 646

Croughan JL. 93, 159, 592, 656, 661

Croughan JL, Miller P, Matar A, Whitman BY: Psychiatric diagnosis and prediction of drug and alcohol dependence. Journal of Clinical Psychiatry 43:353–356, 1982. 302

Crouse-Novak MA. 276, 322, 360, 362

Crowe RR. 335, 337, 338, 341, 342, 343, 344, 364, 386, 387, 478, 580, 590, 594, 703

Crowe RR, Noyes R, Pauls DL, Slymen DS: A family study of panic disorder. Archives of General Psychiatry 40:1065–1069, 1983. 340, 364, 607

Crowe RR, Noyes R, Wilson AF, Elston RC, Ward LJ: A linkage study of panic disorder. Archives of General Psychiatry 44:933–937, 1987. 586

Crowe RR, Pauls DL, Slymen DJ, Noyes R: A family study of anxiety neurosis: morbidity risk in families of patients with and without mitral valve prolapse. Archives of General Psychiatry 37:77–79, 1980. 335, 338

Csikszentmihalyi MR. 708, 712, 713

Csikszentmihalyi MR, Larson R: Being Adolescent: The Daily Experience of American Teenagers. New York, Praeger, 1984. 712

Csikszentmihalyi MR, Larson R: Validity and reliability of the experience sampling method. Journal of Nervous and Mental Disease 175:526–537, 1987. 712, 714, 715, 716

Cummings JL. 310

Cummings S, Elde R, Ellis J, Lindall A: Corticotropin-releasing factor immunoreactivity is widely distributed within the central nervous system of the rat: an immunohistochemical study. Journal of Neuroscience 3:1355–1368, 1983. 425

Cunningham O. 700

Cunningham-Rundles C. 151

Curtis GC. 43, 53, 427, 586, 590

Curtis GC, Cameron OG, Nesse RM: The dexamethasone suppression test in panic disorder and agoraphobia. American Journal of Psychiatry 139:1043, 1982. 387

Cutler GB Jr. 430, 431

Cytryn L. 279

DaCosta JM: On irritable heart: a clinical study of a form of functional cardiac disorders and its consequences. American Journal of the Medical Sciences 61:17, 1871. 585

D'Afflitti FP. 554

Dager SR. 392, 394

Dager SR, Cowley DS, Dunner DL: Biological markers in panic states: lactate-induced panic and mitral valve prolapse. Biological Psychiatry 22:339-359, 1987. 392

Dahl AA: Ego function assessment of hospitalized adult psychiatric patients with special reference to borderline patients, in The Broad Scope of Ego Function Assessment. Edited by Bellak L, Goldsmith LA. New York, John Wiley, 1984a. 549

Dahl AA: A study of agreement among raters of Bellak's Ego Function Assessment test, in The Broad Scope of Ego Function Assessment. Edited by Bellak L, Goldsmith LA. New York, John Wiley, 1984b.

Dahl AA: Some aspects of the DSM-III personality disorders illustrated by a consecutive sample of hospitalized patients. Acta Psychiatrica Scandinavica Supplementum 328:61–67, 1986. 190

Dally PJ. 603

Dana R. 420

Dancu CY. 228

Dann R. 570

Dantzer R. 421, 423

Darcourt G, Pringuey D (eds): Anxiété, Dépression—Rupture ou Continuité? Paris, Grandes Escoles Medecine, 1987. 597

D'Arcy C. 290

Darwin C: The Expression of the Emotions in Man and Animals. New York, Philosophical Library, 1872/1955. 519

Dasgupta S, Mukherjee B: Effect of chlordiazepoxide on stomach ulcers in rabbits induced by stress. Nature 215:1183, 1967. 422

Dave M, Wanck B: Depression in alcoholics: implications for treatment. Journal of the American Medical Association 254:231, 1985. 295

Davidian H. 655

Davidson JRT, Miller RD, Craig DT, Sullivan JL: Atypical depression. Archives of General Psychiatry 39:527–534, 1982. 260, 603

Davidson RJ. 213

Davidson RJ, Fox NA: Asymmetrical brain activity discriminates between positive and negative affective stimuli in human infants. Science 218:1235–1237, 1982. 565

Davies A. 395

Davies BM. 388, 406, 427

Davies M. 260, 273, 362

Davies RK. 288

Davies SO. 676

Davis B. 429

Davis GC. 47, 48, 354–357

Davis JM. 256, 258, 260, 264, 265, 266, 431

Davis K, Davis B, Mohs R, Mathe A, Vale W, Krieger D: CSF corticotropin releasing factor in neuropsychiatric diseases, in New Research Abstracts, 137th Annual Meeting of the American Psychiatric Association. Washington, DC, American Psychiatric Press, 1984. 429, 432

Davis M: Diazepam and fluorazepam: effects on conditioned fear as measured with the potentiated startle paradigm. Psychopharmacology 62:1–7, 1979a. 423

Davis M: Morphine and naloxone: effects on conditioned fear measured with the potentiated startle paradigm. European Journal of Pharmacology 54:341–347, 1979b. 423

Davis M, Astrachan D: Spinal modulation of acoustic startle: opposite effects of clonidine and d-amphetamine. Psychopharmacology 75: 219–225, 1981. 423

Davis Y. 263

Dawson G, Finley C, Phillips S, Galpert L: Hemispheric specialization and the language abilities of autistic children. Child Development 57:1440–1453, 1986. 572

Dawson GW, Jue SG, Brogden SRN: Alprazolam—A review of its pharmacodynamic properties and efficacy in the treatment of anxiety and depression. Drugs 27:132–147, 1984. 703

Dawson ME. 244, 246

Dealy RS, Ishiki DM, Avery DH, Wilson LG, Dunner DL: Secondary depression in anxiety disorders. Comprehensive Psychiatry 22:612–618, 1981. 337, 338, 414, 472, 502, 505, 619

Dean C, Surtees P, Sashidharian SP: Comparison of Research Diagnostic Systems in an Edinburgh Community Sample. British Journal of Psychiatry 142:247–256, 1983. 120

de la Para G. 574

de la Vega E. 407

Delespaul PhAEG. 712, 713, 723

Delespaul PhAEG, de Vries MW: The daily life of ambulatory chronic mental patients. Journal of Nervous and Mental Disease 175:537–545, 1987. 712, 713

d'Elia G, Perris C: Cerebral functional dominance and depression. Acta Psychiatrica Scandinavica 49:191–197, 1973. 573

DeLisi LE. 577

Delizio R. 504, 522

de Mayo R. 518, 629

Demura H. 420, 426, 430

Denckla MB. 571

De Noble V. 290

Depue RA, Monroe SM: Conceptualization and measurement of human disorder in life stress research: the problem of chronic disturbance. Psychological Bulletin 99:36–51, 1986. 477, 475, 481, 490, 491, 493, 494

Depue RA, Slater JF, Wolfstetter-Kausch H, Klein D, Goplerud E, Farr D: A behavioral paradigm for identifying persons at risk for bipolar depressive disorder: a conceptual framework and five validation studies. Journal of Abnormal Psychology 90:381–437, 1981. 323

Derogatis LR. 158

Derogatis LR: SCL-90: Administration, Scoring and Procedures Manual-I for the R (Revised) Version and Other Instruments of the Psychopathology Rating Scale Series. Chicago, Johns Hopkins University School of Medicine, 1977. 696

Derogatis LR, Cleary PA: Factorial invariance across gender for the primary symptom dimensions of the SCL-90. The British Journal of Social and Clinical Psychology 16:347–356, 1977. 158

Derogatis LR, Covi L, Lipman RS, Rickels K: Dimensions of outpatient neurotic pathology: comparison of a clinical vs. an empirical assessment. Journal of Consulting and Clinical Psychology 34:164–171, 1970. 158

Derogatis LR, Lipman RS, Covi L: The SCL-90: an outpatient psychiatric rating scale. Psychopharmacology Bulletin 9:13–28, 1973. 234, 261

Derogatis LR, Lipman RS, Covi L, Rickels K: Factorial invariance of neurotic symptom dimensions in anxious and depressive neuroses. Archives of General Psychiatry 27:659–665, 1972. 54, 158, 508, 509, 624

Derogatis LR, Lipman RS, Rickels K, Uhlenhuth EH, Covi L: The Hopkins Symptom Check List (HSCL): a self-report symptom inventory. Behavioral Science 19:1–15, 1974. 158, 240, 256, 674

Derry PA, Kuiper K: Schematic processing and self-reference in clinical depression. Journal of Abnormal Psychology 90:286–297, 1981. 509, 643

DeRubeis R, Beck AT: Cognitive therapy, in Handbook of Cognitive-Behavioral Therapies. Edited by Dobson K. New York, Guilford, 1988. 629

De Souza FVA. 488

Devereux R. 395

de Vigne JP. 387, 403, 427, 613

de Vries MW. 712, 713

de Vries MW: Temporal patterning of psychiatric symptoms (abstract). Vienna, WPA Congress, 1983. 712, 715

de Vries MW: Investigating mental disorders in their natural settings: introduction, special issue: mental disorders in their natural settings: the application of time allocation and experience sampling techniques in psychiatry. Journal of Nervous and Mental Disease 175:509–514, 1987. 708, 709, 710

de Vries MW, Delespaul Ph, Dijkman-Caes CIM: Affect and anxiety in daily life, in Anxious Depression: Assessment and Treatment. Edited by Racagni G, Smeraldi E. New York, Raven, 1987, pp 21–32. 712, 713, 723

de Vries MW, Delespaul PhAEG, Theunissen J, Dijkman CIM: Temporal and situational aspects of severe mental disorders, in L'Esperienze Quotidiana. Edited by Massimini F, Inghilleri PI. Milano, Franco Angeli, 1986, pp 21–33. 712

Dew MA. 178, 489, 661

Dewald L. 504

Deykin EY, Levy JC, Wells V: Adolescent depression, alcohol and drug abuse. American Journal of Public Health 77:178–182, 1987. 287

Dibble ED. 254, 580

Dickman W. 502

Dickson H. 599, 603

Dickstein S. 322, 323

Dienelt MN. 483, 629

Digre K. 567, 570

Dijkman CIM. 712

Dijkman CIM, de Vries MW: The social ecology of anxiety: theoretical and quantitative perspectives. Journal of Nervous and Mental Disease 175:550–558, 1987. 713

Dijkman-Caes CIM. 712, 713, 723

Dillon S. 593

Dilsaver SC. 277, 280

Di Mascio A. 719

Dimberg U. 636

Dimsdale JE: A psychosomatic perspective on anxiety, in Anxiety and the Anxiety Disorders. Edited by Tuma AH, Maser J. Hillsdale, NJ, Lawrence Erlbaum Associates, 1985. 710

Di Nardo PA. 43, 44, 45, 46, 49, 51, 55, 62, 63, 64, 67, 69, 70, 71, 76, 190, 200, 207, 209, 213, 219, 221, 223, 227, 230, 472, 619

Di Nardo PA, O'Brien GT, Barlow DH, Waddell MT, Blanchard EB: Reliability of DSM-III anxiety disorder categories using a new structured interview. Archives of General Psychiatry 40:1070–1075, 1983. 207, 208, 209, 228, 590, 591, 635

Diner BC, Holcomb PJ, Dykman RA: P300 in major depressive disorder. Psychiatry Research 15:175–184, 1985. 574

Dinerman H. 251

Dintzer L. 516

Discipio WJ. 309

Dixon KN. 254

Dobler-Mikola A. 124, 125

Dobson KS. 622, 631

Dobson KS: Assessing anxiety and depression: development and application of the differential anxiety and depression inventory. Unpublished doctoral dissertation, University of Western Ontario, London, Canada, 1980. 644

Dobson KS: An analysis of anxiety and depression scales. Journal of Personality Assessment 49:522–527, 1985a. 616, 623, 625, 631, 707, 708, 720

Dobson KS: Defining an interactional approach to anxiety and depression. Psychological Record 35:471–489, 1985b. 616, 630, 631

Dobson KS: The relationship between anxiety and depression. Clinical Psychology Review 5:307–324, 1985c. 52, 54, 504, 505, 614, 616, 620, 624, 627, 631, 632

Dobson KS: The self-schema in depression, in Perception of Self in Emotional Disorders and Psychotherapy. Edited by Hartman LM, Blankstein K. New York, Plenum, 1986. 629, 632

Dobson KS, Shaw BF: Cognitive assessment with major depressive disorders. Cognitive Therapy Research 10:13–29, 1986. 622, 631

Docherty JP, van Kammen DP, Siris SG, Marder SR: Stages of onset of schizophrenic psychosis. American Journal of Psychiatry 135:420–426, 1980. 716

Dodge CS. 225, 226

Dodson JD. 570

Doerr H. 599

Dohrenwend BP. 178, 180, 181, 182, 466, 475, 477

Dohrenwend BP: Problems in defining and sampling the relevant populations of stressful life events, in Stressful Life Events: Their Nature and Effects. Edited by Dohrenwend BS, Dohrenwend BP. New York, John Wiley, 1974. 466

Dohrenwend BP: The epidemiology of mental disorders, in Handbook of Health, Health Care, and the Health Professions. Edited by Mechanic D. New York, Free Press, 1983, pp 157–194. 178

Dohrenwend BP, Dohrenwend BS: Social Status and Psychological Disorder. New York, John Wiley, 1969. 475

Dohrenwend BP, Krasnoff L, Askenasy AR, Dohrenwend BS: Exemplification of a method for scaling life events: The PERI Life Events Scale. Journal of Health and Social Behavior 19:205–229, 1978. 466

Dohrenwend BP, Levav I, Shrout PE: Screening scales from the Psychiatric Epidemiology Research Interview (PERI), in Community Surveys of Psychiatric Disorders. Edited by Weissman MM, Myers JK, Ross C. New Brunswick, NJ, Rutgers University Press, 1986. 180

Dohrenwend BP, Levav I, Shrout P, Link BG, Skodol AE, Martin JL: Life stress and psychopathology. American Journal of Community Psychology 15:677–715, 1987. 180, 181

Dohrenwend BP, Link BG, Kern R, Shrout PE, Markowitz J: Measuring life events: the problem of variability within categories, in Psychiatric Epidemiology. Edited by Cooper B. London, Croom Helm, 1987. 466

Dohrenwend BP, Shrout PE, Egri G, Mendelsohn S: Measures of nonspecific psychological distress and other dimensions of psychopathology in the general population. Archives of General Psychiatry 37:1229–1236, 1980. 178

Dolan RJ, Calloway SP, Fonagy P, De Souza FVA, Wakeling A: Life events, depression and hypothalamic-pituitary-adrenal axis function. British Journal of Psychiatry 147:429–433, 1985. 488

Dolce JJ, Raczynski JM: Neuromuscular activity and electromyography in painful backs: psychological and biomechanical models in assessment and treatment. Psychological Bulletin 97:502–520, 1985. 244

Dolinisky ZS. 235, 285, 286, 288, 300, 302

Donald RA, Redekopp C, Cameron V, Nicholls MG, Bolton J, Livesey J, Espiner EA, Rivier J, Vale W: The hormonal actions of corticotropin-releasing factor in sheep: effect of intravenous and intracerebroventricular injection. Endocrinology 113:866–870, 1983. 417

Donchin E. 574

Donnelly EF. 308, 571, 574

Dopplet HG. 229

Doran AR. 429, 430, 432, 488

Dorer DJ.354–357

Dornbush R. 573

Dorus W, Kennedy J, Gibbins RD, Ravi SD: Symptoms and diagnosis of depression in alcoholics. Alcoholism: Clinical and Experimental Research 11:150–154, 1987. 288

Doss GH. 247

Doterall G. 250

Dow JT. 191, 192

Dowie C. 700

Dowling-Zimmerman S. 577

Downing R. 676, 702

Downing RW, Rickels K: Mixed anxiety-depression—fact or myth? Archives of General Psychiatry 30:312–317, 1974. 506, 619, 627

Downs NS, Britton KT, Gibbs DM, Koob GF, Swerdlow NR: Supersensitive endocrine response to physostigmine in dopamine-depleted rats: a model of depression? Biological Psychology 21:775–786, 1987. 409, 410

Drake ME: Panic attacks and excessive aspartame ingestion. Lancet 1:61, 1986.

Drake RE. 549, 550, 552

Draspa LJ: Psychological factors in muscular pain. British Journal of Medical Psychology 32:106, 1959. 250

Droler K. 292

Droppleman LF. 554

Dube S. 411

Dube S, Jones DA, Bell J, Davies A, Ross E, Sitaram N: Interface of panic and depression: clinical and sleep EEG correlates. Psychiatry Research 19:119–133, 1986. 395

DuBois FS: Compulsion neurosis with cachexia. American Journal of Psychiatry 106:107–115, 1949. 310

Dubois, RE. 151

Duffy P. 420

Dugger D. 11

Duncan C. 52

Duncan-Jones P. 120, 659

Dunleavy DLF. 431

Dunn AJ. 421, 423

Dunn AJ, Berridge CW: Corticotropin-releasing factor administration elicits a stress-like activation of cerebral catecholaminergic systems. Pharmacology, Biochemistry and Behavior 27:685–691, 1987. 421, 426, 431

Dunn AJ, File SE: Corticotropin-releasing factor has an anxiogenic action in the social interaction test. Hormones and Behavior 21:193–202, 1987. 423

Dunn LO. 178, 489, 661

Dunner DL. 337, 338, 386, 387, 392, 394, 414, 472, 502, 505, 619

Dunner DL, Ishiki D, Avery DH, Wilson LG, Hyde TS: Effect of alprazolam and diazepam on anxiety and panic attacks in panic disorder: a controlled study. Journal of Clinical Psychiatry 47:458–460, 1986. 676

Dunner D, Myers J, Khan A, Avery D, Ishiki D, Pyke R: Adinazolam—a new antidepressant: findings of a placebo-controlled, double-blind study in outpatients with major depression. Journal of Clinical Psychopharmacology 7:170–172, 1987. 414

Du Pont RL Jr. 586, 592, 594, 607

Dykman RA. 574

Easton CR. 586

Eaton WW. 115, 159, 321, 588, 705

Eaton WW, Holzer CE, VonKorff M, Anthony JC, Helzer JE, George L, Burnam A, Boyd JH, Kessler LG, Locke BZ: The design of the Epidemiologic Catchment Area surveys: the control and measurement of error. Archives of General Psychiatry 41:942–948, 1984. 115

Eaton WW, Kessler L (eds): Epidemiologic Field Methods in Psychiatry: The NIMH Epidemiologic Catchment Area Program. New York, Academic, 1985. 115

Eaves LJ. 120, 344, 370, 478, 487, 490, 497, 580

Eaves M. 420

Eaves M, Thatcher-Britton K, Rivier J, Vale W, Koob GF: Effects of corticotropin-releasing factor on locomotor activity in hypophysectomized rats. Peptides 6:923–926, 1985. 420

Ebert MH. 254, 255, 310, 430, 600

Eckert ED. 258, 263

Eckert ED, Goldberg SC, Halmi KA, Casper RC, Davis JM: Depression in anorexia nervosa. Psychological Medicine 12:115–122, 1982. 256, 266

Edlund MJ, Swann AC, Clothier J: Patients with panic attacks and abnormal EEG results. American Journal of Psychiatry 144:508-509, 1987. 575

Edwards BC. 623

Edwards G: The alcohol dependence syndrome: a concept as stimulus to enquiry. British Journal of Addiction 81:171–183, 1986. 300

Edwards G, Gross MM: Alcohol dependence: provisional description of a clinical syndrome. British Medical Journal 1:1058–1061, 1976. 300

Egeland JA: Affective disorders among the Amish, 1976–1980. Unpublished paper presented at the annual meeting of the American College of Neuropsychopharmacology, Puerto Rico, December 1980. 36

Egri G. 178

Ehlers A. 227, 712, 713

Ehlers CL. 409

Ehlers A, Margraf J, Roth WT, Taylor CB, Maddock RJ, Sheikh J, Kopell ML, McClenahan KL, Gossard D, Blowers GH, Agras WS, Kopell BS: Lactate infusions and panic attacks? Do patients and controls respond differently? Psychiatry Research 17:295–308, 1985. 392

Ehlers CL, Henriksen SJ, Wang M, Rivier J, Vale W, Bloom FE: Corticotropin releasing factor produces increases in brain excitability and convulsive seizures in rats. Brain Research 278:332–336, 1983. 420

Eidelson JI. 218, 496, 509, 631

Eklund K. 427, 428, 430

Elde R. 425

Elkins R. 276, 571

Ellis HC. 643

Ellis J. 425

Elston RC. 586

Emery G. 225, 500, 508, 509, 513, 519, 523, 525, 527, 528, 530–533, 581, 599

Emken RL. 414

Endicott J. 22, 24, 42, 84, 92, 93, 114, 181, 205, 232, 236, 256, 273, 286, 294, 295, 296, 297, 298, 300, 301, 318, 322, 325, 339, 346, 347, 378, 405, 427, 483, 494, 502, 556, 593, 657, 659, 666, 673, 682, 684, 689, 694

Endicott J, Spitzer RL: A diagnostic interview: the Schedule for Affective Disorders and Schizophrenia. Archives of General Psychiatry 35:837–844, 1978. 22, 115, 181, 256, 297, 488, 613, 621, 667

Endicott J, Spitzer RL: Use of the Research Diagnostic Criteria and the Schedule for Affective Disorders and Schizophrenia to study affective disorders. American Journal of Psychiatry 136:52–56, 1979. 256

Endicott J, Spitzer RL, Fleiss JL, Cohen J: The Global Assessment Scale: a procedure for measuring overall severity of psychiatric disturbance. Archives of General Psychiatry 33:766–771, 1976. 32, 299

Endler NS, Okada M: A multidimensional measure of trait anxiety: the S-R Inventory of General Trait Anxiousness. Journal of Consulting and Clinical Psychology 43:319–329, 1975. 613, 635

Engle-Friedman M. 528

Erbaugh J. 213, 226, 613, 644

Ericsson AK, Simon HA: Protocol analysis; verbal reports as data. Cambridge, MA, MIT Press, 1985. 712

Ernberg G. 655

Escobar JI. 317, 322, 661

Escobar JI, Burnam A, Karno M, Forsythe A, Golding JM: Somatization in the community. Archives of General Psychiatry 44:713–720, 1987. 246

Espiner EA. 417

Essen-Möller E, Larsson H, Uddenberg CE, White G: Individual traits and morbidity in a Swedish rural population. Acta Psychiatrica et Neurologica Scandinavica Supplement 100:1–160, 1956. 140

Essen-Möller E, Wohlfahrt S: Suggestions for the amendment of the official Swedish classification of mental disorders: report on the 8th Congress of Scandinavian Psychiatrists. Acta Psychiatrica et Neurologica Scandinavica Supplement 47:551–555, 1949. 140

Esveldt-Dawson K. 528

Ettedgui E. 392, 712

Ettedgui E, Bridges M: Post traumatic stress disorder. Psychiatric Clinics of North America 8:89–103, 1985. 524

Evans DL, Nemeroff CB: The clinical use of the dexamethasone suppression test in DSM-III affective disorders: correlation with the severe depressive subtypes of melancholia and psychosis. Journal of Psychiatric Research 21:185–194, 1987. 427

Evans L. 387

Ewusi-Mensah I. 287, 289

Extein I, Pottash ALC, Gold MS, Sweeney DR, Martin DM, Goodwin FK: Deficient prolactin response to morphine in depressed patients. American Journal of Psychiatry 137:845–846, 1980. 407

Eysenck HJ. 554

Eysenck HJ: Dimenson of Personality. London, Routledge & Kegan Paul, 1947. 157

Eysenck HJ: Behavior Therapy and the Neuroses. London, Pergamon, 1960. 499

Eysenck HJ: A dimensional system of psychodiagnostics, in New Approaches to Personality Classification. Edited by Mahrer AR. New York, Columbia University Press, 1970. 71, 554

Eysenck HJ: The definition of personality disorders and the criteria appropriate for their description. Journal of Personality Disorders 1:211–219, 1987. 80

Eysenck M. 532

Eysenck MW: Attention and Arousal: Cognition and Performance. Berlin, Springer, 1982. 570

Eysenck MW: Anxiety and cognitive-task performance. Personality and Individual Differences 6:579–586, 1985. 570

Eysenck SBG, Eysenck HJ: The place of impulsiveness in a dimensional system of personality. British Journal of Social Psychology 16:57–68, 1977. 554

Fabrega H, Mezzich J, Mezzich A, Coffman G: Descriptive validity of DSM-III depressions. Journal of Nervous and Mental Disease 174:573–584, 1986. 52

Fairburn CG. 256, 257

Fallahi C. 275, 279, 317, 322, 360, 361

Fam AG. 251

Famularo R, Stone K, Popper C: Preadolescent alcohol abuse and dependence. American Journal of Psychiatry 142:1187–1189, 1985. 200

Fanelli C. 386

Farmer A. 656, 661, 664

Farr D. 323

Farr RK. 322

Fawcett J. 295

Fawcett J, Kravitz HM: Anxiety syndromes and their relationship to depressive illness. Journal of Clinical Psychiatry 44:8–11,1983. 281, 472

Fedio P. 571, 572

Feighner J. 699, 703

Feighner JP, Robins E, Guze SB, Woodruff RA, Winokur G, Munoz R: Diagnostic criteria for use in psychiatric research. Archives of General Psychiatry 26:57–63, 1972. 8, 10, 24, 91, 114, 205, 254, 294, 337, 439, 449, 455, 457, 694

Feinberg M. 261, 387, 403, 427, 613

Feinberg TL. 276, 322, 360, 362

Feinberg T, Goodman B: Affective illness, dementia and pseudodementia. Journal of Clinical Psychiatry 45:99–103, 1984. 190

Feiner K. 549

Feinstein AR. 6, 7, 331

Feinstein AR: The pre-therapeutic classification of co-morbidity in chronic disease. Journal of Chronic Diseases 23:455–468, 1970. 5, 11, 331

Feinstein AR: Clinical Epidemiology. New Haven, CT, Yale University Press, 1984. 26

Fellman D, Bugnon C, Gouger A: Immunocytochemical demonstration of corticoliberin-like immunoreactivity (CLI) in neurons of the rat amygdala central nucleus (ACN). Neuroscience Letters 34:253–258, 1982. 418

Felson DT. 251

Fenichel O: The Psychoanalytic Theory of Neurosis. New York, WW Norton, 1945. 546

Fenigstein A, Scheier MF, Buse AH: Public and private self-consciousness: assessment and theory. Journal of Consulting and Clinical Psychology 43:522–527, 1975. 715

Fenton FR. 474, 655

Fenton WS, McGlashan TH: The prognostic significance of obsessive compulsive symptoms in schizophrenia. American Journal of Psychiatry 143:437–441, 1986. 307

Fichter M. 311

Fielding U. 416

Fienberg SE. 130, 165, 547

Fierko B. 418

Fieve RR. 388

File SE. 423

Filstead W, Reich W, Parella D, Rossi J: Using electronic pagers to monitor the process of recovery in alcoholics and drug abusers. Paper presented at the 34th International Congress on Alcohol, Drug Abuse and Tobacco, Calgary, 1985. 713

Finch AJ. 274

Finder E. 488

Fine PR. 247

Finesinger JE. 242

Fink M. 433, 573

Fink WL. Microcomputers and phylogenetic analysis. Science 734:1133–1139, 1986. 713

Finkelstein R. 276, 277, 322, 360, 362

Finlay-Jones R: Showing that life events are a cause of depression: a review. Australian and New Zealand Journal of Psychiatry 15:229–238, 1981. 467, 468, 479, 492

Finlay-Jones R, Brown GW: Types of stressful life events and the onset of anxiety and depressive disorders. Psychological Medicine 11:803–815, 1981. 45, 484, 486, 487, 488, 490, 495, 497, 520

Finley C. 572

First MB. 100

First MB, Williams JBW, Spitzer RL: Decision trees for differential diagnosis, in Diagnostic and Statistical Manual of Mental Disorders, 3rd Edition, Revised. Washington, DC, American Psychiatric Association, 1987. 101

Fisher AK. 22, 168

Fisher LA. 420, 423

Fisher LA, Jessen G, Brown MR: Corticotropin-releasing factor (CRF): mechanism to elevate mean arterial pressure and heart rate. Regulatory Peptides 5:153–161, 1983. 420

Fisher LA, Rivier J, Rivier C, Spiess J, Vale W, Brown MR: Corticotropin-releasing factor (CRF): central effects on mean arterial pressure and heart rate in rats. Endocrinology 110:2222–2224, 1982. 420

Fisher S. 676, 702

Fishman R. 308

Fiske D. 623, 631

Fiske D: Measuring the concept of personality. Chicago, Aldine, 1971. 710, 716

Flanagan NB. 260

Fleiss J. 32, 208, 299, 572

Fleiss JL, Spitzer RL, Endicott J, Cohen J: Quantification of agreement in multiple psychiatric diagnosis. Archives of General Psychiatry 26:168–171, 1972. 24

Flor-Henry P, Gruzelier J (eds): Laterality and Psychopathology. Amsterdam, Elsevier Science Publishers, 1983. 564

Flor-Henry P, Koles ZJ: Statistical quantitative EEG studies of depression, mania, schizophrenia and normals. Biological Psychiatry 19:257–279, 1984. 574

Flor-Henry P, Turk DC, Birbaumer N: Assessment of stress-related psychophysiological reactions in chronic back pain patients. Journal of Consulting and Clinical Psychology 53:354–364, 1985. 244

Flor-Henry P, Yeudall LT, Koles ZJ, Howarth BG: Neuropsychological and power spectral EEG investigations of the obsessive-compulsive syndrome. Biological Psychiatry 14:119–130, 1979. 571, 574, 575

Florio L. 317, 321, 323, 327

Floris G. 605

Foa EB: Failure in treating obsessive compulsives. Behaviour Research and Therapy 17:169–176, 1979. 309

Foa E, Foa U: Differentiating depression and anxiety: is it possible? is it useful? Psychopharmacological Bulletin 18:62–68, 1982. 48, 508, 509

Foa EB, Grayson JB, Steketee GS, Dopplet HG, Turner RM, Latimer PL: Success and failure in the behavioral treatments of obsessive-compulsives. Journal of Consulting and Clinical Psychology 51:287–297, 1983. 229

Foa EB, Steketee G, Kozak MJ, Dugger D: Effects of imipramine on depression and obsessive-compulsive symptoms. Psychiatry Research 21:123–136, 1987. 11

Foa UG. 48, 508, 509

Fogarty SJ. 643

Folstein M. 661

Fonagy P. 488

Fontaine R. 676, 703

Foote SL. 419, 420, 425, 426, 431

Foote SL, Bloom FE, Aston-Jones G: Nucleus locus coeruleus: new evidence of anatomical and physiological specificity. Physiological Reviews 63:844–914, 1983. 419, 425, 431

Ford CV. 246

Ford CV: The Somatizing Disorders: Illness as a Way of Life. New York, Elsevier, 1983. 239, 246, 249

Ford JM. 574

Forgus R, Shulman BH: Personality: A Cognitive View. Englewood Cliffs, NJ, Prentice-Hall, 1979. 525

Forster B. 488

Forsythe A. 246, 661

Foster SI. 392

Foulds GA. 79

Foulds GA: Personal continuity and psychopathological disruption. British Journal of Psychology 55:269–276, 1964. 78, 79

Foulds GA: Personality and Personal Illness. London, Tavistock, 1965. 78, 79, 90

Foulds GA: The Hierarchical Nature of Personal Illness. New York, Academic, 1976. 88, 90, 164, 201

Foulds GA, Bedford A: Hierarchy of classes of personal illness. Psychological Medicine 5:181–192, 1975. 79, 90

Fowles DC. 477, 480, 487, 493, 494, 499, 505, 506

Fowles DC, Gersh FS: Neurotic depression: the endogenous-neurotic distinction, in The Psychobiology of the Depressive Disorders: Implications for the Effects of Stress. Edited by Depue RA. New York, Academic 1979. 475

Fox NA. 565

Fox P. 396, 577, 586

Frances AJ. 44, 47, 48, 50, 51, 62, 317, 318, 325, 326

Frances A: The DSM-III personality disorders section: a commentary. American Journal of Psychiatry 137:1050–1054, 1980. 52, 190, 318

Frances A: Categorical and dimensional systems of personality diagnosis: a comparison. Comprehensive Psychiatry 23:516–527, 1982. 52

Frances A, Widiger T: The classification of personality disorders: an overview of problems and solutions, in Psychiatry Update: American Psychiatric Association Annual Review, Vol 5. Edited by Frances AJ, Hales RE. Washington, DC, American Psychiatric Press, 1986a. 52

Frances A, Widiger TA: Methodological issues in personality disorder diagnoses, in Contemporary Directions in Psychopathology. Edited by Millon T, Klerman GL. New York, Guilford, 1986b. 72

Francis DJ. 576

Francis G. 277, 359, 360

Frank E, Jarrett DB, Kupfer DJ, Grochocinski VJ: Biological and clinical predictors of response in recurrent depression: a preliminary report. Psychiatry Research 13:315–324, 1984. 235

Frank E, Kupfer DJ, Jacob M, Jarrett D: Personality features and response to acute treatment in recurrent depression. Journal of Personality Disorders 1:14–26, 1987. 233

Frank JD. 250

Frank JD: Persuasion and Healing. Baltimore, Johns Hopkins University Press, 1973. 178

Frankel M, Cummings JL, Robertson MM, Trimble M, Hill MA, Benson DF: Obsessions and compulsions in Gilles de la Tourette's syndrome. Neurology 36:378–382, 1986. 310

Frankenburg FR. 326

Frankenthaler LM. 676, 702

Franklin J. 630

Fraser S. 394

Fratta W. 420

Frazer A. 390

Freedman DX. 237

Freedman R, Janni P, Ettedgui E, Puthezhath N: Ambulatory monitoring of panic disorders. Archives of General Psychiatry 42:244–248, 1985. 712

Freis ED: Mental depression in hypertensive patients treated for long periods with large doses of reserpine. New England Journal of Medicine 251:1006–1008, 1954. 431

French NH. 528

Freud A: The Ego and the Mechanisms of Defense, Revised Edition. New York, International Universities Press, 1937/1966. 546

Freud S: The justification for detaching from neurasthenia a particular syndrome: the anxiety-neurosis, in Collected Papers, Vol 1. Edited by Jones E. New York, Basic Books, 1894/1959. 585

Freud S: The neuro-psychoses of defense, in The Standard Edition of the Complete Psychological Works of Sigmund Freud, Vol 8. Translated and edited by Strachey J. London, Hogarth Press, 1894/1960. 546

Freud S: The Standard Edition of the Complete Psychological Works of Sigmund Freud, Vol 3. Translated and edited by Strachey J. London, Hogarth Press, 1895, p 112. 332, 333, 347

Freud S: Mourning and melancholia, in The Standard Edition of the Complete Psychological Works of Sigmund Freud, Vol 14. Translated and edited by Strachey J. London, Hogarth Press, 1917/1963. 561

Freud S: New Introductory Lectures. New York, WW Norton, 1917/1945. 24

Freud S: The ego and the id, in The Standard Edition of the Complete Psychological Works of Sigmund Freud, Vol 19. Translated and edited by Strachey J. London, Hogarth Press, 1923/1964. 546

Freud S: Inhibitions, symptoms, and anxiety, in The Standard Edition of the Complete Psychological Works of Sigmund Freud, Vol 20. Translated and edited by Strachey J. London, Hogarth Press, 1926/1959. 501, 534

Freud S: Character and anal eroticism, in The Standard Edition of the Complete Psychological Works of Sigmund Freud, Vol 2. Translated and edited by Strachey J. London, Hogarth Press, 1948. 314

Freud S: The Origins of Psychoanalysis: Letter to Wilhelm Fliess, Drafts and Notes: 1887–1902. Edited by Bonaparte M, Freud A, Kris E; translated by Mosbacher E, Strachey J. New York, Basic Books, 1954. 254

Freundlich A. 213

Friedhof AJ. 310

Friedman B. 297, 556

Friedman CTH. 246

Friedman RC, Clarkin JF, Corn R, Aronoff MS, Hurt SW, Murphy MC: DSM-III and affective pathology in hospitalized adolescents. Journal of Nervous and Mental Disease 170:511–521, 1982. 279

Frith CD. 700

Fromm-Auch D: Neuropsychological assessment of depressed patients before and after drug therapy: clinical profile interpretations, in Laterality and Psychopathology. Edited by Flor-Henry P, Gruzelier J. Amsterdam, Elsevier Science Publishers, 1983. 567, 570

Frommer EA: Depressive illness in childhood (special pub): British Journal of Psychiatry 2:117–136, 1968. 272

Fuchs CZ. 642

Fuchs CZ, Rehm LP: A self-control behavior therapy program for depression. Journal of Consulting and Clinical Psychology 45:206–215, 1977. 642

Fuiji I. 655

Fuiji S, Kachi T, Sobue I: Chronic headache: its psychosomatic aspect. Japanese Journal of Psychosomatic Medicine 21:411–419, 1981. 244

Fukushima D. 255

Fulker DW. 344, 345

Fulop G, Strain JJ, Vita J, Lyons JS, Hammer JS: Impact of psychiatric comorbidity on length of hospital stay for medical/surgical patients: a preliminary report. American Journal of Psychiatry 144:878–882, 1987. 11, 305

Fyer AJ. 391, 392, 415, 432, 659, 672, 676–678

Gabbard GO: The role of compulsiveness in the normal physician. Journal of the American Medical Association 254:2926–2930, 1985. 313

Gaines JG. 512

Gallager DW. 415

Gallucci W. 255

Galpert L. 572

Gammon GD. 45, 275, 350, 354–358, 360, 361, 363, 364, 377, 499

Ganellen RJ, Matuzas W, Uhlenhuth EH, Glass R, Easton CR: Panic disorder, agoraphobia, and anxiety-relevant cognitive style. Journal of Affective Disorders 11:219–225, 1986. 586

Ganguli R. 192

Gantz NM. 151

Garber J, Miller SM, Abramson LY: On the distinction between anxiety states and depression: perceived control, certainty, and probability of goal attainment, in Human Helplessness: Theory and Applications. Edited by Garber J, Seligman MEP. New York, Academic, 1980. 499, 500, 506–509, 511, 518, 519, 528–530

Garbutt JC. 394

Garcia A. 420, 421

Gardner M. 700

Gardos G: Is agoraphobia a psychosomatic form of depression? in Anxiety: New Research and Changing Concepts. Edited by Klein DF, Raskin J. New York, Raven, 1981. 502

Garfinkel BD. 277, 360, 361

Garfinkel PE. 256, 261

Garfinkel PE, Moldofsky H, Garner DM: The heterogeneity of anorexia nervosa: bulimia as a distinct subgroup. Archives of General Psychiatry 37:1036–1040, 1980. 258

Garmezy N, Streitman S: Children at risk: the search for the antecedents of schizophrenia, I: conceptual models and research methods. Schizophrenia Bulletin 8:14–90, 1974. 353

Garner DL, Garfinkel PE: The Eating Attitudes Test: an index of the symptoms of anorexia nervosa. Psychological Medicine 9:273–279, 1979. 261

Garner DM. 258

Garner DM, Olmstead MP, Polivy J: Development and validation of a multidimensional eating disorders inventory for anorexia nervosa and bulimia. International Journal of Eating Disorders 2:15–35, 1983. 261

Garside RF. 54, 331, 506, 508, 509, 599, 619, 700

Garside RF, Roth M: Multivariate statistical methods and problems of classification in psychiatry. British Journal of Psychiatry 133:53–67, 1978. 71

Garvey M, Tuason V: The relationship of panic disorder to agoraphobia. Comprehensive Psychiatry 25:529–531, 1984. 53

Gascon J. 387

Gaspar M. 655

Gasto C. 387

Gastwirth JL: The statistical precision of medical screening procedures: application to polygraph and AIDS antibody test data. Statistical Science 2:213–238, 1987. 692

Gatchel RJ, Paulus PB, Maples CW: Learned helplessness and self-reported affect. Journal of Abnormal Psychology 84:732–734, 1975. 528

Gatchel RJ, Proctor JD: Physiological correlates of learned helplessness in man. Journal of Abnormal Psychology 85:27–34, 1976. 528

Gatsonis C. 276, 279, 280, 281

Gediman H. 547

Geertz C: Local Knowledge. New York, Basic Books, 1983. 474

Gelder M. 677

Geller B, Chestnut EC, Miller MD, Price DT, Yates E: Preliminary data on DSM-III associated features of major depressive disorder in children and adolescents. American Journal of Psychiatry 142:643–644, 1985. 273

Gelles L. 387

Genero N. 52

George DT. 430

George LK. 6, 44, 45, 61, 63, 93, 95, 97, 109, 115, 118, 120, 137, 159, 190, 204, 206, 221, 305, 307, 308, 311, 332, 333, 364, 433, 439, 455, 649, 650

George WCG. 311

Georgotas A, McCue RE, Kim M, Hapworth WE, Reisberg B, Stoll PM, Sinaiko E, Fanelli C, Stokes PE: Dexamethasone suppression in dementia, depression and normal aging. American Journal of Psychiatry 143:452–456, 1986. 386

Gerken A. 430

German PS. 116, 588, 592, 593

Gerner RH. 255, 577

Gerner RH, Wilkins JN: CSF cortisol in patients with depression, mania, or anorexia nervosa and in normal subjects. American Journal of Psychiatry 140:92–94, 1983. 255

Gersh FS. 475

Gersh FS, Fowles DC: Neurotic depression: the concept of anxious depression, in The Psychobiology of the Depressive Disorders: Implications for the Effects of Stress. Edited by Depue RA. New York, Academic, 1979. 477, 480, 487, 493, 494, 499, 505, 506

Gershon ES. 393, 394, 580

Gershon E: The genetics of affective disorders, in Psychiatry Update: The American Psychiatric Association Annual Review, Vol 2. Edited by Grinspoon L. Washington, DC, American Psychiatric Press, 1983, pp 434–457. 346

Gershon ES, Liebowitz JH: Social-cultural and demographic correlates of affective disorders in Jerusalem. Journal of Psychiatric Research 12:37–50, 1975. 36

Gershon ES, Schreiber JL, Hamovit JR, Dibble ED, Kaye WH, Nurnberger JI, Andersen A, Ebert MH: Clinical findings in patients with anorexia nervosa and affective illness in their relatives. American Journal of Psychiatry 141:1419–1422, 1984. 254

Gershon S. 411

Geschwind N. 565

Gessa GL. 420

Geyer MA. 423

Ghoneim MM. 703

Gibbins RD. 288

Gibbon M. 323, 657, 658, 681

Gibbons JE. 431

Gibbons RD. 237, 295

Gibbs DM. 409, 410

Gibson JG. 244

Giel R. 653, 655

Gildea EF. 248

Giles DE. 256

Gill D. 571, 575

Gillespie RD: The clinical differentiation of types of depression. Guy's Hospital Reports 79:306–344, 1929. 475

Gillin JC. 276, 308, 411, 571, 575

Gilmore MM. 48, 62, 190, 201, 325

Gittelman R: Childhood anxiety disorders: correlates and outcome, in Anxiety Disorders of Childhood. Edited by Gittelman R. New York, Guilford, 1986. 279

Gittelman R, Klein DF: Relationship between separation anxiety and panic and agoraphobic disorders. Psychopathology 17:56–65, 1984. 272

Gittelman R, Klein DF: Childhood separation anxiety and adult agoraphobia, in Anxiety and the Anxiety Disorders. Edited by Tuma AH, Maser J. Hillsdale, NJ, Lawrence Erlbaum Associates, 1985. 272

Gittleson NL: The fate of obsessions in depressive psychosis. British Journal of Psychiatry 112:705–708, 1966. 309

Gladen B. 692

Gladis MA. 255, 256

Glanville K. 311

Glaser K. Masked depresson in children and adolescents. American Journal of Psychotherapy 1:565–574, 1968. 272, 280

Glass R. 586

Glassman AH. 255, 256

Glavin GB: Stress and brain noradrenaline: a review. Neuroscience and

Biobehavioral Reviews 9:233–243, 1985. 425

Glover E: On the Development of Mind, Vol 1. New York, International Universities Press, 1956. 24, 35

Glowinski J. 425

Goetz DM. 672, 673, 678

Goetz R. 260, 572

Gold A. 700

Gold MS. 407

Gold PW. 388, 417, 429–432

Gold PW, Chrousos GP: Clinical studies with corticotropin-releasing factor: implications for the diagnosis and pathophysiology of depression, Cushing's disease, and adrenal insufficiency. Psychoneuroendocrinology 10:401–419, 1985. 404, 427, 430

Gold PW, Chrousos G, Kellner C, Post R, Roy A, Augerinos P, Schulte H, Oldfield E, Loriaux DL: Psychiatric implications of basic and clinical studies with corticotropin-releasing factor. American Journal of Psychiatry 141:619–627, 1984. 430, 433

Gold PW, Gwirtsman H, Avegerinos PC, Nieman L, Galluci WT, Kaye W, Jimerson D, Ebert M, Rittmaster R, Loriaux DL, Chrousos GP: Abnormal hypothalamic-pituitary-adrenal function in anorexia nervosa. New England Journal of Medicine 314:1335–1342, 1986. 255

Gold P, Loriaux DL, Roy A, Kellner C, Post RM, Pickar D, Avgerinos P, Paul SM, Schulte H, Oldfield E, Cutler G, Chrousos G: The corticotropin releasing factor stimulation test: implications for the diagnosis and pathophysiology of hypercortisolism in primary affective disorders and Cushing's disease. New England Journal of Medicine 314:1329–1335, 1986. 430

Goldberg DP. 248

Goldberg DP: Detection and assessment of emotional disorders in primary care. International Journal of Mental Health 8:30–48, 1979. 593

Goldberg D, Blackwell D: Psychiatric illness in general practice. British Medical Journal 3:439–443, 1970. 248

Goldberg D, Bridges K: Somatic presentation of psychiatric illness in primary care settings. Journal of Psychosomatic Research 32:137–144, 1988. 602

Goldberg E: The nonspecificity of frontal-lobe dysfunction. Paper presented in Symposium on Frontal-lobe Dysfunction and the Schizophrenia Syndrome at the 16th annual meeting of the International Neuropsychological Society, New Orleans, LA, January 1988. 579

Goldberg SC. 256, 258, 263, 266

Goldberger EL. 315

Goldenberg DL: Psychologic studies in fibrositis. American Journal of Medicine 81:67–70, 1986. 249

Goldenberg DL, Felson DT, Dinerman H: A randomized, controlled trial of amitriptyline and naproxen in the treatment of patients with fibromyalgia. Arthritis and Rheumatism 29:1371–1377, 1986. 251

Golding JM. 246

Goldsmith LA, Charles E, Feiner K: The use of EFA in the assessment of borderline pathology, in The Broad Scope of Ego Function Assessment. Edited by Bellak L, Goldsmith LA. New York, John Wiley, 1984. 549

Goldstein S. 406

Goleman DJ. 213

Gomez J. 480

Good BJ, Kleinman AM: Culture and anxiety: cross-cultural evidence for the patterning of anxiety disorders, in Anxiety and the Anxiety Disorders.

Edited by Tuma AH, Maser JD. Hillsdale, NJ, Lawrence Erlbaum Associates, 1985. 15

Goodman B. 190

Goodman PA. 425, 496

Goodman WK. 389, 390–392

Goodwin DW, Guze SB, Robins E: Follow-up studies in obsessional neurosis. Archives of General Psychiatry 20:182–187, 1969. 306, 307

Goodwin FK. 407, 547, 549, 574, 605

Goplerud E. 323

Gordon D. 354–358

Gordon PK. 575

Gorman JM. 391, 392, 570, 672, 676–678

Gorman J, Liebowitz M, Fyer A, Klein DF: Treatment of social phobia with atenolol. Journal of Clinical Psychopharmacology 5:298–301, 1985. 677

Gorsuch RL. 213, 554, 613, 644, 716, 719

Gosnell BA. 421, 423

Gosnell BA, Morley JE, Levine AS: A comparison of the effects of corticotropin releasing factor and sauvagine on food intake. Pharmacology, Biochemistry and Behavior 19:771–775, 1983. 421

Gossard D. 392, 712

Gotlib IH. 631

Gotlib IH: Perception and recall of interpersonal feedback: negative bias in depression. Cognitive Therapy Research 7:399–412, 1983. 643

Gotlib IH: Depression and general psychopathology in university students. Journal of Abnormal Psychology 93:19–30, 1984. 621, 623, 625

Gotlib IH, Asarnow RF: Interpersonal and impersonal problem-solving skills in mildly and clinically depressed university students. Journal of Consulting and Clinical Psychology 47:86–95, 1979. 505, 617, 640

Gottesman I. 670

Gouger A. 418

Gough HG. 554

Grace MC. 421, 423, 503

Graf KJ. 388

Grande TP. 453

Gray JA: The Neuropsychology of Anxiety: An Enquiry into the Functions of the Septo-hippocampal System. New York, Oxford University Press, 1982. 496, 565, 570, 580

Gray TS. 418, 423

Grayson JB. 229

Greden JF. 261, 386, 387, 403, 427, 613

Greden JF, Carroll BJ: Psychomotor function in affective disorders: an overview of new monitoring techniques. American Journal of Psychiatry 138:1441–1448, 1981. 599

Green AR. 415

Green BL, Lindy JD, Grace MC: Post traumatic stress disorder: toward DSM-IV. Journal of Nervous and Mental Disease 173:406–411, 1985. 503

Green HS, Kane JM: Review: The dexamethasone suppression test in depression. Clinical Neuropharmacology 6:7–24, 1983. 387

Green JK. 254, 311

Green RC. 310, 312

Greenberg J. 509, 527

Greenberg MS. 505, 565

Greenberg MS, Alloy LB: Depression versus anxiety: processing of self- and other-referent information (in press). 505, 506, 509

Greenberg MS, Beck AT: Depression versus anxiety: schematic processing of self, world, and future referent information. Journal of Abnormal Psychology 98:9–13, 1989. 506

Greenberg MS, Vazquez CV, Alloy LB: Depression versus anxiety: differences in self and other schemata, in Cognitive Processes in Depression. Edited by Alloy LB. New York, Guilford, 1988. 500, 505, 509, 530

Greenblatt DJ. 392

Greenhouse JB. 237

Gregg JR: The Language of Taxonomy. New York, Columbia University Press, 1954. 64

Gregory M. 393

Greten H. 420

Grings WW, Dawson ME: Emotions and Bodily Responses: A Psychophysiological Approach. New York, Academic, 1978. 244, 246

Grinker RR: Anxiety and psychopathology, in Anxiety and Behavior. Edited by Spielberger CD. New York, Academic, 1966. 499, 505

Grinker RR, Nunnally JC: The phenomena of depressions, in The Role and Methodology of Classification in Psychiatry and Psychopathology. Edited by Katz MM, Cole JO, Barton WF. Chevy Chase, MD, U.S. Public Health Service, 1968. 505

Grinspoon L. 547

Grochocinski VJ. 235, 237

Gross DR: Time allocation: a tool for the study of cultural behavior. American Review of Anthropology 13:519–558, 1984. 708

Gross MM. 300

Grove WM, Andreasen NC, Clayton PJ, Winokur G, Coryell WH: Primary and secondary affective disorders: baseline characteristics of unipolar patients. Journal of Affective Disorders 13:249–257, 1987. 295, 296

Grove WM, Andreasen NC, Winokur G, Clayton PJ, Endicott J, Coryell WH: Primary and secondary affective disorders: unipolar patients compared on familial aggregation. Comprehensive Psychiatry 28:113–126, 1987. 294, 296

Gruenberg E. 6, 44, 45, 61, 63, 93, 95, 97, 109, 118, 120, 137, 165, 168, 190, 204,206, 221, 305, 307, 308, 311, 317, 321, 332, 333, 364, 439, 455, 589, 649, 650, 661, 707

Grunhaus L, Flegel P, Haskett RF, Greden JF: Serial dexamethasone suppression tests in simultaneous panic and depressive disorders. Biological Psychiatry 22:332–338, 1987. 386, 387

Grunhaus L, Tiongco D, Haskett RF, Greden JF: The dexamethasone suppression test in inpatients with panic attacks. Biological Psychiatry 22:513–517, 1987. 386, 387

Gruol DL. 419

Gruzelier J. 564

Guaza C. 422

Guell A. 576

Guenther W, Moser E, Mueller-Spahn F, von Oefele K, Buell U, Hippius H: Pathological cerebral blood flow during motor function in schizophrenic and endogenous depressed patients. Biological Psychiatry 21:889–899, 1986. 576

Guevera LM. 317, 321, 660

Guidano VF, Liotti G: Cognitive Processes and Emotional Disorders. New York, Guilford, 1983. 525

Guillemin R: Hypothalamic hormones: releasing and inhibiting factors, in

Neuroendocrinology. Edited by Krieger DT, Hughes JC. Sunderland, MA, Sinauer Associates, 1980, pp 23–32. 416

Gulbinat W. 655

Gull WW: The address in medicine delivered before the annual meeting of the B.M.A. at Oxford. Lancet 2:171–176, 1873. 254

Gunderson JG. 326

Gunderson JG: DSM-III diagnoses of personality disorders, in Current Perspectives of Personality Disorders. Edited by Frosch JP. Washington, DC, American Psychiatric Press, 1983. 285

Gunderson J: Borderline Personality Disorder. Washington, DC, American Psychiatric Press, 1984. 53

Gur RC. 565, 577

Gur RC, Gur RE, Resnick SM, Skolnick BE, Alavi A, Reivich M: The effect of anxiety on cortical cerebral blood flow and metabolism. Journal of Cerebral Blood Flow and Metabolism 7:173–177, 1987. 570

Gur RC, Gur RE, Skolnick BE, Resnick SM, Silver FL, Chewluk J, Muenz L, Obrist WD, Reivich M: Effects of task difficulty on regional cerebral blood flow: relationships with anxiety and performance. Psychophysiology 1988. 570

Gur RE. 570

Gur RE: Left hemisphere dysfunction and left hemisphere overactivation in schizophrenia. Journal of Abnormal Psychology 87:226–238, 1978. 564

Gur RE, Resnick SM, Alavi A, Gur RC, Caroff S, Dann R, Silver FL, Saykin AJ, Chewluk JB, Kushner M, Reivich M: Regional brain function in schizophrenia, I: a positron emission tomography study. Archives of General Psychiatry 44:119–125, 1987. 577

Gurland B. 572, 653

Gurling HMD. 287, 289

Gurney C. 54, 331, 506, 508, 509, 599, 619

Gurney C, Roth M, Garside RF, Kerr TA, Schapira K: Studies in the classification of affective disorders: the relationship between anxiety states and depressive illness, Part 2. British Journal of Psychiatry 121:162–166, 1972. 599

Guroff JJ. 580

Gursky DM. 223

Guttman L: The Cornell technique for scale and intensity analysis. Educational and Psychological Measurement 7:247–280, 1947. 156

Guttman L: The basis for scalogram analysis, in Measurement and Prediction. Edited by Stouffer SA, Guttman L, Suchman EA, Lazersfeld P, Star SA, Clausen JA. Princeton, NJ, Princeton University Press, 1950, pp 60–90. 156

Guy W, Ban TA (eds and translators): The AMDP-System: Manual for the Assessment and Documentation of Psychopathology. Berlin, Springer-Verlag, 1982. 667

Guze SB. 8, 10, 24, 52, 84, 91, 113, 114, 163, 180, 205, 240, 254, 287, 291, 294, 306, 307, 337, 338, 378, 439, 440, 447, 449, 456–457, 500, 563, 577, 598, 694

Guze SB, Cloninger CR, Martin RL, Clayton PJ: A follow-up and family study of schizophrenia. Archives of General Psychiatry 40:1273–1276, 1983. 453, 456

Guze SB, Cloninger CR, Martin RL, Clayton PJ: Alcoholism as a medical disorder. Comprehensive Psychiatry 27:501–510, 1986a. 456

Guze SB, Cloninger CR, Martin RL, Clayton PJ: A follow-up and family study of Briquet's syndrome. British Journal of Psychiatry 149:17–23, 1986b. 455, 456

Guze S, Roth M (eds): Psychiatric Developments 4:3, 1986. 24

Guze SB, Woodruff RA, Clayton PJ: Secondary affective disorders: a study of 95 cases. Psychological Medicine 1:426–428, 1972. 286, 294, 295, 296

Gwirtsman HE. 255, 430

Gwirtsman HE, Roy-Byrne P, Yager J, Gerner RH: Neuroendocrine abnormalities in bulimia. American Journal of Psychiatry 140:559–563, 1983. 255

Haan N: Proposed model of ego functioning: coping and defense mechanisms in relationship to IQ change. Psychological Monographs 77:1–23, 1963. 547, 552

Haefely W: Actions and Interactions of GABA and Benzodiazepines. Edited by Bowery NG. New York, Raven, 1984, p 263. 415

Hagnell O. 140, 144, 147

Hagnell O: A Prospective Study of the Incidence of Mental Disorder: A Study Based on 24,000 Person Years of the Incidence of Mental Disorders in a Swedish Population Together with an Evaluation of the Aetiological Significance of Medical, Social, and Personality Factors. Lund, Svenska Bokförlaget, 1966. 140, 141, 142, 143, 144, 149, 151

Hagnell O: The 25-year follow-up of the Lundby Study: incidence and risk of alcoholism, depression, and disorders of the senium, in Mental Disorders in the Community. Edited by Barrett JE, Rose RM. New York, Guilford, 1986a, pp 89–110. 140

Hagnell O: Mental disorder in the welfare state—Sweden: a prospective, longitudinal, psychiatric-epidemiologic study of a total population over 25 years, 1947–1972. The Lundby Study. American Journal of Social Psychiatry 6:230–248, 1986b. 140

Hagnell O: The psychiatric fatigue syndrome: incidence and course in the longitudinal Lundby Study. Unpublished paper presented at the WPA Symposium on Psychiatric Epidemiology and Primary Health Care, Toronto, Canada, May 31–June 2, 1989. 149

Hagnell O, Lanke J, Rorsman B, Öjesjö L: Are we entering an age of melancholy? Depressive illness in a prospective epidemiologic study over 25 years: the Lundby Study, Sweden. Psychological Medicine 12:279–289, 1982. 144, 168

Hagnell O, Lanke J, Rorsman B, Öjesjö L: The incidence of mental illness over a quarter of a century: a longitudinal study of mental illnesses in a total Swedish population during 1947 to 1972 based on 50,000 observation years. Almquist & Wiksell (in press). 144

Hagnell O, Tunving K: Prevalence and nature of alcoholism in a total population. Social Psychiatry 7:190–201, 1972. 147

Haier RJ. 404

Halberstadt LJ. 517

Halberstadt LJ, Andrews D, Metalsky GI, Abramson LY: Helplessness, hopelessness, and depression: a review of progress and future directions, in Personality and Behavior Disorders. Edited by Endler NS, Hunt J. New York, John Wiley, 1984. 513

Halbreich U. 406

Hallmayer J. 339, 340, 346, 347

Hallstrom T. 574, 580

Halmi KA. 256, 258, 266

Halmi KA: Relationship of eating disorders to depression: biological similarities and differences. International Journal of Eating Disorders 4:667–680, 1985. 255

Halmi KA, Goldberg SC, Casper RC, Eckert E, Davis Y: Pretreatment predic-

report of a pilot study. Archives of General Psychiatry 40:1061–1064, 1983. 341, 342, 364

Harris GW: Neural control of the pituitary gland. Physiological Reviews 28:139–179, 1948. 416

Harris TO. 467, 468, 469, 470, 471, 474, 475, 478, 479, 481, 484, 486–488, 492–494, 511, 518, 536

Harrison B. 223

Harrison GA. 710

Harrison WM. 260, 604, 673, 674, 675

Hart PJ. 405, 406

Hartlage S. 510, 512, 513, 515, 517, 518, 528, 543

Hartley HO: Testing the homogeneity of a set of variances. Biometrika 31:249–255, 1940. 628

Hartley HO: The maximum F-ratio as a short-cut for hetereogeneity of variances. Biometrika 37:308–312, 1950. 628

Harvey JH, Ickes WJ, Kidd RF: New Directions in Attribution Research, Vol 1. Hillsdale, NJ, Lawrence Erlbaum Associates, 1976. 516

Harvey JH, Ickes WJ, Kidd RF: New Directions in Attribution Research, Vol 2. Hillsdale, NJ, Lawrence Erlbaum Associates, 1978. 516

Harvey JH, Ickes WJ, Kidd RF: New Directions in Attribution Research, Vol 3. Hillsdale, NJ, Lawrence Erlbaum Associates, 1981. 516

Hasin D, Endicott J, Keller MB: RDC alcoholism in patients with major affective syndromes: 2-year course. American Journal of Psychiatry 146:318–323, 1989. 300

Haskett RF. 386, 387, 403, 427, 613

Hatch DR. 623

Hathaway SR, McKinley JC: Minnesota Multiphasic Personality Inventory: Manual for Administration and Scoring. Minneapolis, MN, University of Minnesota Press, 1951. 256, 283

Hauch J. 223

Hauser ST. 548, 549, 550

Hayes SC, Cavoir N: Multiple tracking and the reactivity of self-monitoring. Behavior Therapy 8:819–731, 1977. 716

Haykal RF. 318, 325, 327

Hays LR. 386

Hays P. 30

Hazlett E. 575, 577

Heath AC. 344, 370, 371, 478, 487, 490, 497, 580

Heather N, Rollnick S, Winston M: A comparison of objective and subjective measures of alcohol dependence as predictions of relapse following treatment. British Journal of Clinical Psychology 22:11–17, 1983. 300

Hecht HM, Fichter M, Postpischil F: Obsessive compulsive neurosis and anorexia nervosa. International Journal of Eating Disorders 2:69–77, 1983. 311

Hecker E: Uber Iarvirte und abortive angstzustande bei neurasthenie zentralbl. Nervenheilk 133:565–572, 1893. 332

Heilbronn M. 606

Heimberg RG, Klosko JS, Dodge CS, Shadick R, Becker RE, Barlow DH: Anxiety disorders, depression, and attributional style: a further test of the specificity of depressive attributions. Cognitive Therapy and Research 13:21–36, 1989. 226

Heimberg RG, Vermilyea JA, Dodge CS, Becker R, Barlow DH: Attributional style, depression, and anxiety: an evaluation of the specificity of depressive attributions. Cognitive Therapy and Research 11:537–550, 1987. 225

Heitz PU. 424

Hellman LD. 255, 427

Helzer JE. 93, 115, 159, 165, 168, 286, 313, 317, 321, 589, 592, 656, 661, 664, 707

Helzer JE, McEvoy LT, Robins LN, Spitznagel E, Stoltzman RK, Farmer A, Brockington IF: Results of the St. Louis ECA Physician Reexamination Study of the DIS Interview. Archives of General Psychiatry 42:657–666, 1985. 661

Helzer JE, Robins LN, McEvoy L: Post-traumatic stress disorder in the general population. New England Journal of Medicine 317:1630–1634, 1987. 315, 321, 590

Helzer JE, Winokur G: A family interview study of male manic depressives. Archives of General Psychiatry 31:73–77, 1974. 563

Henderson AS. 344, 345, 370

Henderson S, Duncan-Jones P, Byrne DG, Scott R, Adcock S: Psychiatric disorder in Canberra: a standardized study of prevalence. Acta Psychiatrica Scandinavica 60:355–374, 1979. 120, 659

Hendricks LE, Bayton JA, Collins JL, Mathura CB, Macmillen SR, Montgomery TA: The NIMH Diagnostic Interview Schedule: a test of its validity in a population of black adults. Journal of the American Medical Association 75:667–671, 1983. 661

Heninger GR. 54, 94, 109, 217, 271, 392, 389, 390–393, 419, 432, 472, 473, 487, 489, 495, 496, 502, 572, 585, 605

Heninger GR, Charney DS, Price LH: Alpha-2 adrenergic receptor sensitivity in depression: the plasma MHPG, behavioral, and cardiovascular responses to yohimbine. Archives of General Psychiatry 1988. 390

Heninger GR, Charney DS, Sternberg DE: Serotonergic function in depression: prolactin responses to intravenous tryptophan in depressed patients and healthy subjects. Archives of General Psychiatry 41:398–402, 1984. 393, 407

Henriksen SJ. 420

Henry BW, Market JR, Emken RL, Overall JE: Drug treatment of anxious depression in psychiatric outpatients. Diseases of the Nervous System 31:684–691, 1970. 414

Herd J. 422

Herjanic B. 332, 666, 667

Herjanic M. 602

Herman CP. 290

Herscovitch P. 396, 577, 586

Hersen M. 277, 359, 360, 476

Hershberg SA, Carlson GA, Cantwell DP, Strober M: Anxiety and depressive disorders in psychiatrically disturbed children. Journal of Clinical Psychiatry 43:358–361, 1982. 273

Herzberger S. 516

Herzog DB. 254, 255

Hesbacher PT, Rickels K, Morris RJ, Newman H, Rosenfeld H: Psychiatric illness in family practice. Journal of Clinical Psychology 41:6–10, 1980. 158, 159

Hesselbrock MN. 302, 661

Hesselbrock MN, Babor TF, Hesselbrock V, Meyer RE, Workman K: "Never believe an alcoholic?" On the validity of self-report measures of alcohol dependence and related constructs. International Journal of the Addictions 18:593–609, 1983. 300

Hesselbrock MN, Meyer RE, Keener JJ: Psychopathology in hospitalized alcoholics. Archives of General Psychiatry 42:1050–1055, 1985. 284, 285, 288, 290

Hesselbrock V. 300

Hesselbrock VM, Hesselbrock MN, Workman-Daniels KL: Effect of major depression and antisocial personality on alcoholism: course and motivational patterns. Journal of Studies on Alcohol 47:207–212, 1986. 302

Hesselbrock V, Stabenau J, Hesselbrock M, Mirkin P, Meyer R: A comparison of two interview schedules: the Schedule for Affective Disorders and Schizophrenia-Lifetime and the National Institute for Mental Health Diagnostic Interview Schedule. Archives of General Psychiatry 39:674–677, 1982. 661

Higgins ET: Self-discrepancy: a theory relating self and affect. Psychological Review 94:319–340, 1987. 500, 537, 538

Hill MA. 310

Hillyard SA, Picton TW: Event-related brain potentials and selective information processing in man, in Progress in Clinical Neurophysiology, Vol 6: Cognitive Components in Cerebral Event-related Potentials and Selective Attention. Edited by Desmedt JE. Basel, Karger, 1979. 574

Himle J. 43, 53, 586

Himmelhoch JM. 191, 288, 476, 606

Himmelhoch JM: Cerebral dysrhythmia, substance abuse, and the nature of secondary affective illness. Psychiatric Annals 17:710–727, 1987. 323

Hinde RA: Animal Behavior. New York, McGraw-Hill, 1970. 421

Hinrichs JV. 703

Hippius H. 576

Hippocrates: Hypocratic Writings. Translated and edited by Lloyd GER. Hammondsworth, England, Penguin, 1983.

Hiroto D. 354–358

Hirsch M. 273

Hirschfeld RMA. 296, 297, 346, 347, 378, 653, 666, 684

Hirschfeld RMA: Situational depression: validity of the concept. Archives of General Psychiatry 139:297–305, 1981. 488

Hirschfeld RMA, Klerman GL, Gough HG, Barrett J, Korchin SJ, Chodoff P: A measure of interpersonal dependency. Journal of Personality Assessment 41:610–618, 1977. 554

Hirschfeld RMA, Kosier T, Keller MB, Lavori PW, Endicott J: The influence of alcoholism on the course of depression. Journal of Affective Disorders 16:151–158, 1989. 298

Hodgson RJ. 291, 308, 503

Hoehn-Saric R. 227

Hoehn-Saric R: Characteristics of chronic anxiety patients, in Anxiety: New Research and Changing Concepts. Edited by Klein DR, Rabkin J. New York, Raven, 1981. 227

Hoehn-Saric R, Maisami M, Wiegand D. Measurement of anxiety in children and adolescents using semistructured interviews. Journal of the American Academy of Child and Adolescent Psychiatry 26:541–545, 1987. 272

Hoenk PR. 217, 334, 335, 337, 344, 338, 472, 619

Hoeper EW. 275, 279, 317, 322, 360, 361

Hoffman H. 283, 284

Hoffman LJ. 419, 425, 496

Holcomb C. 575

Holcomb HH. 577

Holcomb PJ. 574

Hole DJ. 479, 492

Holland PW. 130, 165

Hollander E. 672, 678

Hollister LE. 505

Hollon SD. 615, 617

Hollon SD, Kendall PC: Cognitive self-statements in depression: development of an automatic thoughts questionnaire. Cognitive Therapy and Research 4:383–397, 1980. 641

Holmes GP, Kaplan JE, Gantz NM, Komaroff AL, Schonberger LB, Straus SE,
Jones JF, Dubois RE, Cunningham-Rundles C, Pahwa S, Tosato G, Zegans
LS, Purtillo DT, Brown N, Schooley RT, Brus I: Chronic fatigue syndrome: a
working case definition. Annals of Internal Medicine 108:387–389, 1988. 151

Holmes TH, Rahe RH: The Social Readjustment Rating Scale. Journal of
Psychosomatic Research 11:213–218, 1967. 465, 466

Holsboer F: The dexamethasone suppression test in depressed patients: clinical and biochemical aspects. Journal of Steroid Biochemistry 19:251–257,
1983. 387

Holsboer F, von Bardeleben U, Gerken A, Stalla GK, Müller OA: Blunted
corticotropin and normal cortisol response to human corticotropin-releasing factor in depression (letter). New England Journal of Medicine 311:1127,
1985. 430

Holsboer F, Gerken A, Stalla GK, Muller OA: Blunted aldosterone and ACTH
release after human CRF administration in depressed patients. American
Journal of Psychiatry 144:229–231, 1987. 430

Holzer CE III. 6, 44, 45, 61, 63, 93, 95, 97, 109, 115, 118, 120, 137, 165, 168, 171,
190, 204, 206, 221, 305, 307, 308, 311, 332, 333, 364, 439, 455, 589, 649, 650

Hong B. 453

Hong B, Smith MD, Robson AM, Wetzel RD: Depressive symptomatology
and treatment in patients with end-stage renal disease. Psychological Medicine 17:185–190, 1987. 456

Hopper JL. 344, 345

Hormuth SE: Methoden für Psychologische Forschung im Feld (Diskussion-
spapier nr. 43). Heidelberg, Psychologischen Institut der Universität Heidelberg, 1985. 714, 715

Hormuth SE: The random sampling of cognitions and behavior. Journal of
Personality 54:262–293, 1986. 712

Horst RL, Johnson R, Donchin E: Event-related brain potential and subjective
probability in a learning task. Memory and Cognition 8:476–488, 1980. 574

Hough RL. 115, 159, 317, 321, 322, 588, 661, 705

Houlihan J. 548–550

Houseworth S. 254

Howard D. 673

Howarth BG. 571, 574, 575

Hsu LKG, Crisp AH, Harding B: Outcome of anorexia nervosa. Lancet
1:61–65, 1979. 254, 255

Huang Y. 415, 419, 425, 432

Hucek A. 387

Hudson JI, Hudson MS, Pliner LF: Fibromyalgia and major affective disorder:
a controlled phenomenology and family history study. American Journal of
Psychiatry 142:441–446, 1985. 249

Hudson JI, Hudson MS, Rothschild AJ, Vignati L, Schatzberg AF, Melby JC: Abnormal results of dexamethasone suppression tests in nondepressed patients with diabetes mellitus. Archives of General Psychiatry 41:1086–1089, 1984. 386

Hudson JI, Pope HG, Jonas JM, Laffer PS, Hudson MS, Melby JM: Hypothalamic-pituitary-adrenal axis hyperactivity in bulimia. Psychiatry Research 8:111–118, 1983a. 255

Hudson JI, Pope HG, Jonas JM, Yorgelun-Todd D: Phenomenologic relationship of eating disorders to major affective disorder. Psychiatry Research 9:345–354, 1983b. 255

Hudson MS. 249, 255, 386

Huey LY. 407

Hughes CC. 154, 171

Hughes CC, Tremblay MA, Rapoport RN, Leighton AH: People of Cove and Woodlot: The Stirling County Study. New York, Basic Books, 1960. 154

Hughes D. 433

Hulbert J. 305

Hull DL. 64

Hungerbuhler JP. 565

Hurlburt RT: Random sampling of cognitions and behavior. Journal of Research in Personality 13:103–111, 1979. 712

Hurlburt RT. Validation and correlation of thought sampling with retrospective measures. Cognitive Therapy and Research 4:235–238, 1980. 712, 717

Hurlburt RT, Melancon SM: Single case study: "goofed-up" images: thought-sampling with a schizophrenic woman. Journal of Nervous and Mental Disease 175:575–578, 1987. 712

Hurlburt RT, Sipprelle CN: Random sampling of cognitions in alleviating anxiety attacks. Cognitive Therapy and Research 2:165–170, 1978. 638

Hurry J. 120, 468, 471, 478, 487, 659

Hurst MW. 465

Hurt SW. 48, 62, 279

Hurvich M. 547

Hyde TS. 354–358, 394, 676

Ickes WJ. 516

Ickes WJ, Layden MA: Attributional styles, in New Directions in Attribution Research, Vol 2. Edited by Harvey J, Ickes W, Kidd R. Hillsdale, NJ, Lawrence Erlbaum Associates, 1978. 517

Illich I: Medical Nemesis: The Expropriation of Health. London, Pantheon Books, 1976. 21

Imaki T, Shibasaki T, Masuda A, Demura H, Shizume K, Ling N: Effects of adrenergic blockers on corticotropin-releasing factor-induced behavioral changes in rats. Regulatory Peptides 19:243–252, 1987. 420, 426

Imber SD. 250

Ingram IM: Obsessional illness in mental hospital patients. Journal of Mental Science 107:382–402, 1961. 306, 311

Ingram RE. 615, 617

Ingram RE: Information Processing Approaches to Clinical Psychology. New York, Academic, 1986. 525

Innes G, Millar WM: Mortality among psychiatric patients. Scottish Medical Journal 15:143–148, 1970. 173

Innis RB, Charney DS, Heninger GR: Differential 3H-imipramine platelet binding in patients with panic disorder and depression. Psychiatry Research 21:33–41, 1986. 393

Insel TR, Akiskal HS: Obsessive compulsive disorder with psychotic features: a phenomenologic analysis. American Journal of Psychiatry 143:1527–1533, 1986. 306

Insel TR, Donnelly EF, Lalakea ML, Alterman IS, Murphy DL: Neurological and neuropsychological studies of patients with obsessive-compulsive disorder. Biological Psychiatry 18:741–751, 1983. 308, 571, 574

Insel TR, Mueller EA, Gillin JC, Siever LJ, Murphy DL: Biologic markers in obsessive-compulsive and affective disorders. Journal of Psychiatric Research 18:407–423, 1984. 308

Invitti C. 255

Isaacson RL: The Limbic System, 2nd Edition. New York, Plenum, 1982. 565

Ishiki DM. 337, 338, 386, 387, 414, 472, 502, 505, 619, 676

Itil TM. 264

Iverson LL, Mackay AVP: Pharmacodynamics of anti-depressants and anti-manic drugs, in Psychopharmacology of Affective Disorders. Edited by Paykel ES, Coppen A. New York, Oxford University Press, 1979, pp 60–90. 431

Iverson SD. 415

Ives A. 673

Izard CE: The Face of Emotion. Meredith, NY, Appleton-Century-Crofts, 1971. 506

Izard CE: Patterns of Emotions. New York, Academic, 1972. 717

Izard CE: Human Emotions. New York, Plenum, 1977. 506, 645

Izard C, Blumberg S: Emotion theory and the role of emotions in anxiety in children and adults, in Anxiety and the Anxiety Disorders. Edited by Tuma AH, Maser JD. Hillsdale, NJ, Lawrence Erlbaum Associates, 1985. 54, 508

Jabine LN. 254, 255

Jablensky A. 474, 653, 655, 656, 664

Jablensky A: Approaches to the definition and classification of anxiety and related disorders in European psychiatry, in Anxiety and the Anxiety Disorders. Edited by Tuma AH, Maser JD. Hillsdale, NJ, Lawrence Erlbaum Associates, 1985. 505, 508

Jablensky A, Sartorius N, Hirschfeld R, Pardes H: Diagnosis and classification of mental disorders and alcohol- and drug-related problems: a research agenda for the 1980s. Psychological Medicine 13:907–921, 1983. 653

Jackman H. 408

Jackson DN: A sequential system for personality scale development, in Current Topics in Clinical and Community Psychology, Vol 2. Edited by Spielberger CD. New York, Academic, 1970. 617

Jackson DN, Messick S: Response styles on the MMPI: comparison of clinical and normal samples. Journal of Abnormal and Social Psychology 5:285–299, 1962. 80

Jackson SW: Melancholia and Depression. New Haven, CT, Yale University Press, 1986. 473, 475

Jacob M. 233

Jacob RG, Moller MB, Turner SM, Wall C: Otoneurological examination in panic disorder and agoraphobia with panic attacks: a pilot study. American Journal of Psychiatry 142:715–720, 1985. 396

Jacobs C. 254

Jacobson AM, Beardslee W, Hauser ST, Noam GG, Powers SI: An approach to evaluating ego defense mechanisms using clinical interviews, in Empirical Studies of the Ego Mechanisms of Defense. Edited by Vaillant GE. Washington, DC, American Psychiatric Press, 1986a. 548

Jacobson AM, Beardslee W, Hauser ST, Noam GG, Powers SI, Houlihan J, Rider E: Evaluating ego defense mechanisms using clinical interviews: an empirical study of adolescent diabetic and psychiatric patients. Journal of Adolescence 9:303–319, 1986b. 548, 549, 550

Jacobson G. 703

Jaeckle RS, Kathol RG, Lopez JF, Meller WH, Krummel SJ: Enchanced adrenal sensitivity to exogenous cosyntropin (ACTH alpha-1-24) stimulation in major depression. 44:233–240, 1987. 389

Jaenicke C. 354–358

Jaffe JH. 289, 290

Jaffe JH, Ciraulo DA: Alcoholism and depression, in Psychopathology and Addictive Disorders. Edited by Meyer RE. New York, Guilford, 1986. 286

James N McI. 387, 403, 427, 613

James RH. 393

Janet P: Les Obsessions et la Psycasthenie, 2nd Edition. Paris, Balliere, 1908. 313

Janni P. 712

Janowski AJ. 432

Janowsky DS. 407, 411

Jardine R. 371

Jardine R, Martin NG, Henderson AS: Genetic covariation between neuroticism and the symptoms of anxiety and depression. Genetic Epidemiology 1:89–107, 1984. 344, 345, 370

Jarrett DB. 233, 235

Jaspers K: General Psychopathology, 7th Edition. Translated by Hoenig J, Hamilton MW. Manchester, Manchester University Press, 1962. 89, 90, 164

Jatlow PI. 391, 392

Javaid JI. 260

Javoy F. 425

Jenike MA. 310, 312, 315

Jenike MA, Baer L, Minichiello WE, Schwartz CE, Carey RJ: Concomitant obsessive compulsive disorder and schizotypal personality disorder. American Journal of Psychiatry 143:530–532, 1986. 314

Jenike MA, Brotman AW: The EEG in obsessive-compulsive disorder. Journal of Clinial Psychiatry 45:122–124, 1984. 574

Jenkins CD, Hurst MW, Rose RM: Life changes: do people really remember? Archives of General Psychiatry 36:379–384, 1979. 465

Jesberger JA, Richardson JS: Neurochemical aspects of depression: the past and the future? International Journal of Neuroscience 27:19–47, 1985. 415, 419

Jessen G. 420

Jessup BA, Neufeld RWJ, Merskey H: Biofeedback therapy for headache and other pain: an evaluative review. Pain 7:225–270, 1979. 251

Jimerson DC. 255, 389, 390, 430

John K. 275, 348, 352, 354–358, 360, 361, 363, 364

Johnson C, Larson R: Bulimia: an analysis of moods and behavior. Psychosomatic Medicine 44:342–350, 1982. 713

Johnson DAW: The use of benzodiazepines in depression. British Journal of Clinical Pharmacology 19:315–355, 1985. 702

Johnson J. 577

Johnson JH. 466

Johnson M. 505

Johnson O, Crockett D: Changes in perceptual asymmetries with clinical improvement of depression and schizophrenia. Journal of Abnormal Psychology 91:45–54, 1982. 572

Johnson R. 574

Johnson R, Donchin E: Sequential expectancies and decision making in a changing environment: an electrophysiological approach. Psychophysiology 19:183–200, 1982. 574

Johnstone EC, Cunningham O, Owens DG, Frith CD, McPherson K, Dowie C, Riley G, Gold A: Neurotic illness and its response to anxiolytic and antidepressant treatment. Psychological Medicine 10:321–329, 1980. 700

Jonas JM. 151, 255

Jones AP. 157

Jones D. 411

Jones DA. 395

Jones K. 390, 392

Jones M. 49, 51, 476, 480

Jones MS. 310

Joschke K. 660

Josiassen RC. 575

Judd FK. 393

Judd FK, Norman TR, Burrows GD, McIntyre IM: The dexamethasone suppression test in panic disorder. Pharmacopsychiatry 20:99–101, 1987. 387

Judd LL, Risch SC, Parker DC, Janowsky DS, Segal DS, Huey LY: Blunted prolactin response: a neuroendocrine abnormality manifested by depressed patients. Archives of General Psychiatry 39:1413–1416, 1982. 407

Judiesch KJ. 595

Jue SG. 703

Jung KG. 666, 667

Kachi T. 244

Kafka MS, Nurnberger JI, Siever L, Targum S, Uhde TW, Gershon ES: Alpha-2 adrenergic receptor function in patients with unipolar and bipolar affective disorder. Journal of Affective Disorders 10:163–169, 1986. 393

Kagan J, Reznick JS, Snidman N, et al: Origins of panic disorder, in Neurobiology of Anxiety. Edited by Ballenger JC. New York, Alan R Liss, 1988. 354, 355, 357

Kahn RJ. 703

Kahn RJ, McNair DM, Frankenthaler LM: Tricyclic treatment of generalized anxiety disorder. Journal of Affective Disorders 13:145–151, 1987. 702

Kahn RJ, McNair DM, Lipman RS, Covi L, Rickels K, Downing R, Fisher S, Frankenthaler LM: Imipramine and chlordiazepoxide in depressive and anxiety disorders, II: efficacy in anxious outpatients. Archives of General Psychiatry 43:79–85, 1986. 676, 702

Kaiser S. 660

Kalant H. 290

Kales A. 327

Kales JD. 327

Kalin NH. 423

Kalivas PW, Duffy P, Latimer LG: Neurochemical and behavioral effects of corticotropin-releasing factor in the ventral tegmental area of the rat. Journal of Pharmacology and Experimental Therapeutics 242:757–763, 1987. 420

Kalton GW. 247

Kammeier ML, Hoffman H, Loper RG. Personality characteristics of alcoholics as college freshmen and at time of treatment. Quarterly Journal of Studies on Alcohol, 34:390–399, 1973. 283, 284

Kandel DB, Davies M: Epidemiology of depressive mood in adolescents. Archives of General Psychiatry 39:1205–1212, 1982. 362

Kandel DB, Davies M: Adult sequelae of adolescent depressive symptoms. Archives of General Psychiatry 43:255–265, 1986. 362

Kandell RE: The stability of psychiatric diagnosis. British Journal of Psychiatry 124:352–356, 1974. 501

Kane JM. 387, 573

Kanfer FH: Self-regulation: research issues and speculations, in Behavior Modification in Clinical Psychology. Edited by Neuringer C, Michael JL. New York, Appleton-Century-Crofts, 1970. 642

Kania J. 189

Kanner L: Child Psychiatry, 2nd Edition. Springfield, IL, Charles C Thomas, 1948. 315

Kantor JS. 573

Kaplan C. 713

Kaplan JE. 151

Kaplan M. 414

Kaplan MH, Feinstein AR: The importance of classifying initial co-morbidity in evaluating the outcome of diabetes mellitus. Journal of Chronic Diseases 27:387–404, 1974. 6, 7, 331

Kaplan RD. 190, 201, 325

Kaplan RF. 289

Karlsson I. 427, 428, 430

Karno M. 6, 44, 45, 61, 63, 93, 95, 97, 109, 115, 116, 118, 120, 137, 190, 204, 206, 221, 246, 305, 307, 308, 311, 332, 333, 364, 439, 455, 649, 650, 661

Karno M, Hough RL, Burnham MA, Escobar JI, Timbers DM, Santana F, Boyd JH: Lifetime prevalences of specified psychiatric disorders among Mexican-Americans and non-Hispanic whites in Los Angeles. Archives of General Psychiatry 44:695–701, 1987. 317, 322

Kashani JH: Depression in the preschool child. Journal of the Child in Contemporary Society 15:11–17, 1982. 365

Kashani JH, Beck NC, Hoeper EW, Fallahi C, Corcoran CM, McAllister JA, Rosenberg TK, Reid JC: Psychiatric disorders in a community sample of adolescents. American Journal of Psychiatry 144:584–589, 1987. 360, 361

Kashani JH, Carlson GA, Beck NC, Hoeper EW, Corcoran CM, McAllister JA, Fallahi C, Rosenberg TK, Reid JC: Depression, depressive symptoms, and depressed mood among a community sample of adolescents. American Journal of Psychiatry 144:931–934, 1987. 275, 279, 317, 322, 360, 361

Kashani JH, McGee RO, Clarkson SE, Anderson JC, Walton LA, Williams S, Silva PA, Robins AJ, Cytryn L, McKnew DH: Depression in a sample of 9-year-old children: prevalence and associated characteristics. Archives of General Psychiatry 40:1217–1223, 1983. 279

Kasvikis YG, Tsakiris F, Marks IM, Basoglu M, Noshirvani HF: Past history of anorexia nervosa in women with obsessive compulsive disorder. International Journal of Eating Disorders 5:1069–1075, 1986. 310

Kathol RG. 389

Katon W: Depression: Somatic symptoms and medical disorders in primary care. Comprehensive Psychiatry 23:274–287, 1982. 242, 248

Katon W: Panic disorder and somatizaton: review of 55 cases. American Journal of Medicine 77:101–106, 1984. 476

Katon W, Kleinman A, Rosen G: Depression and somatization: a review, Part I. American Journal of Medicine 72:127–135, 1982. 243

Katon W, Vitaliano PP, Russo J, Jones M, Anderson K: Panic disorder:

spectrum of severity and somatization. Journal of Nervous and Mental Disease 175:12–19, 1987. 49, 51, 476, 480

Katschnig H: Measuring life stress: a comparison of the checklist and panel technique, in Life Events and Psychiatric Disorders: Controversial Issues. Edited by Katschnig H. Cambridge, England, Cambridge University Press, 1986. 467, 468, 471

Katz GM, Itil TM: Video methodology for research in psychopathology and psychopharmacology. Archives of General Psychiatry 31:204–210, 1974. 264

Katz JL. 255

Katz JL, Kuperberg A, Pollack CP, Walsh BT, Zumoff B, Weiner H: Is there a relationship between eating disorder and affective disorder? New evidence from sleep recordings. American Journal of Psychiatry 141:753–758, 1984. 255

Katz MM. 256, 260, 264, 265, 505

Katz M, Cole JO, Barton WE: The role of methodology of classification in psychiatry and psychopathology (No HSM 72-9015). Washington, DC, Department of Health, Education and Welfare, 1968. 22

Katz MM, Secunda SK, Hirschfeld RMA, Koslow SH: NIMH Clinical Research Branch Collaborative Program on the Psychobiology of Depression. Archives of General Psychiatry 36:765–771, 1979. 296, 297, 684

Katz RJ. 490

Katz RJ: Animal model of depression: pharmacological sensitivity of a hedonic deficit. Pharmacology, Biochemistry and Behavior 16:965–968, 1982. 424

Katz RJ, Roth K: Tail pinch induced stress-arousal facilitates brain stimulation reward. Physiology and Behavior 22:193–194, 1979. 424

Katz RJ, Roth KA, Carroll BJ: Acute and chronic stress effects on open field activity in the rat: implications for a model of depression. Neuroscience and Biobehavioral Reviews 5:247–251, 1981. 424

Kaufman I: Mother-infant separation in monkeys: an experimental model, in Separation and Depression: Clinical and Research Aspects. Edited by Scott JP, Senay E. Washington, DC, American Association for the Advancement of Science, 1973. 521

Kaufman IC, Rosenblum LA: The reaction to separation in infant monkeys: anaclitic and conservation withdrawal. Psychosomatic Medicine 29:648–675, 1967. 521

Kaye WH. 254, 255

Kaye WH, Gwirtsman HE, George DT, Ebert MH, Jimerson DC, Tomai TP, Chrousos GP, Gold PW: Elevated cerebrospinal fluid levels of immunoreactive corticotropin-releasing hormone in anorexia nervosa: relation to state of nutrition, adrenal function, and intensity of depression. Journal of Clinical Endocrinology and Metabolism 64:203–208, 1987. 430

Kayne NT. 516, 517

Kayser A. 673

Kazdin AE. 277, 359, 360

Kazdin AE: Research Design in Clinical Psychology. New York, Harper & Row, 1980. 623, 629

Kazdin AE, French NH, Unis AS, Esveldt-Dawson K, Sherick RB: Hopelessness, depression, and suicidal intent among psychiatrically disturbed inpatient children. Journal of Consulting and Clinical Psychology 51:504–510, 1983. 528

Keefe P. 479

Keegan D. 290

Keeler MH, Taylor CI, Miller WC: Are all recently detoxified alcoholics depressed? American Journal of Psychiatry 136: 586–588, 1979. 287

Keener JJ. 284, 285, 288, 290

Keith RM. 245

Kelleher R. 422

Keller MB. 298, 300, 346, 347, 354, 378, 666, 684

Keller MB, Beardslee WR, Dorer DJ, Lavori PW, Samuelson H, Klerman GL: Impact of severity and chronicity of parental affective illness on adaptive functioning and psychopathology in children. Archives of General Psychiatry 43:930–937, 1986. 354, 355, 356, 357

Keller MB, Herzog DB, Lavori PW, Bridges A, Ott I, Klerman GL: One-year course of bulimia and affective disorder. Presented at the annual meeting of the American Psychiatric Association, Washington, DC, May 1986. 255

Keller MB, Klerman GL, Lavori PW, Coryell W, Endicott J, Taylor J: Long-term outcome of episodes of major depression: clinical and public health significance. Journal of the American Medical Association 252:788–792, 1984. 236, 296, 301

Keller MB, Lavori PW, Coryell W, Andreasen NC, Endicott J, Clayton PJ, Klerman GL, Hirschfeld RMA: Differential outcome of pure manic, mixed/cycling, and pure depressive episodes in patients with bipolar illness. Journal of the American Medical Association 255:3138–3142, 1986. 301

Keller MB, Lavori PW, Endicott J, Coryell W, Klerman GL: "Double depression": two-year follow-up. American Journal of Psychiatry 140:689–694, 1983. 322, 325, 494

Keller MB, Lavori PW, Friedman B, Nielsen E, Endicott J, MacDonald-Scott P, Andreasen NC: The longitudinal interval follow-up evaluation: a comprehensive method for assessing outcome in prospective longitudinal studies. Archives of General Psychiatry 44:540–548, 1987. 297, 556

Keller MB, Lavori PW, Lewis CE, Klerman GL: Predictors of relapse in major depressive disorder. Journal of the American Medical Association 250:3299–3304, 1983. 236, 296, 301

Keller MB, Shapiro RW: "Double depression": super-imposition of acute depressive episodes on chronic depressive disorders. American Journal of Psychiatry 139:438–442, 1982a. 318, 322

Keller MB, Shapiro RW: Longitudinal Interval Follow-up Evaluation (LIFE), version II. Boston, Massachusetts General Hospital, 1982b. 556

Kelley HH: Attribution theory in social psychology, in Nebraska Symposium on Motivation, vol 15. Edited by Levine D. Lincoln, NE, University of Nebraska Press, 1967. 516

Kellner CH. 395, 396, 430, 433

Kellner R: Neurosis in general practice. British Journal of Clinical Practice 19:681–682, 1965. 247

Kellner R: Functional somatic symptoms and hypochondriasis: a survey of empirical studies. Archives of General Psychiatry 42:821–833, 1985. 240, 246

Kellner R: Somatizaton and Hypochondriasis. New York, Praeger, 1986. 239, 240, 242, 243, 245, 246, 247, 249

Kellner R: Anxiety and somatic complaints, in Handbook of Anxiety II. Edited by Noyes R, Roth M. Amsterdam, the Netherlands, Elsevier Science Publishers, 1988a. 240, 243, 245

Kellner R: Treatment of functional somatic symptoms and undifferentiated somatoform disorders, in Treatment Manual of Mental Disorders. Edited by Karasu T. Washington, DC, American Psychiatric Association, 1988b. 250, 251

Kellner R, Abbott PJ, Winslow WW, Pathak D: Fears, beliefs and attitudes in

DSM-III hypochondriasis. Journal of Nervous and Mental Disease 175:20–25, 1987. 246

Kellner R, Pathak D, Romanik R, Winslow WW: Life events and hypochondriacal concerns. Psychiatric Medicine 1:133–141, 1983. 244, 246, 247

Kellner R, Sheffield BF: A self-rating scale of distress. Psychological Medicine 3:88–100, 1973. 247

Kellner R, Simpson GM, Winslow WW: The relationship of depressive neurosis to anxiety and somatic symptoms. Psychosomatics 13:358–362, 1972. 245

Kellner R, Slocumb JC, Wiggins RG, Abbott PJ, Winslow WW, Pathak D: Hostility, somatic symptoms and hypochondriacal fears and beliefs. Journal of Nervous and Mental Disease 173:554–561, 1985. 243

Kemper K. 254

Kendall PC. 641

Kendall PC, Hollon SD, Beck AT, Hammen CL, Ingram RE: Issues and recommendations regarding the use of the Beck Depression Inventory. Cognitive Therapy and Research 11:289–300, 1987. 615, 617

Kendell RE. 79, 90, 653

Kendell RE: The stability of psychiatric diagnoses. British Journal of Psychiatry 124:352–356, 1974. 164, 599, 620, 696

Kendell RE: The Role of Diagnosis in Psychiatry. Oxford, Blackwell Scientific Publications, 1975. 76, 90

Kendell RE: The classification of depressions: a review of contemporary confusion. British Journal of Psychiatry 125:15–28, 1976. 605

Kendell RE: The choice of diagnostic criteria for biological research. Archives of General Psychiatry 39:1334–1339, 1982. 445, 448

Kendell RE, Discipio WJ: Obsessional symptoms and obsessional personality traits in patients with depressive illnesses. Psychological Medicine 1:65–72, 1970. 309

Kendler KS. 100

Kendler KS: A twin study of mortality in schizophrenia and neurosis. Archives of General Psychiatry 43:643, 1986. 180

Kendler K: Schizophrenia and other psychotic disorders, in An Annotated Bibliography of DSM-III. Edited by Skodol AE, Spitzer RL. Washington, DC, American Psychiatric Press, 1987. 84

Kendler KS, Eaves LJ: Models for the joint effect of genotype and environment on liability to psychiatric illness. American Journal of Psychiatry 143:279–289, 1986. 120

Kendler KS, Hays P: Paranoid psychosis (delusional disorder) and schizophrenia. Archives of General Psychiatry 38:547–551, 1981. 30

Kendler KS, Heath A, Martin NG, Eaves LJ: Symptoms of anxiety and depression in a volunteer twin population: the etiological role of genetic and environmental factors. Archives of General Psychiatry 43:213–221, 1986. 344, 370, 580

Kendler KS, Heath AC, Martin NG, Eaves LJ: Symptoms of anxiety and symptoms of depression: same genes, different environments? Archives of General Psychiatry 44:451–457, 1987. 370, 478, 487, 490, 497

Kennedy HG: Fatigue and fatigability. British Journal of Psychiatry 153:1–5, 1988. 151

Kennedy J. 288

Kennedy RE, Craighead WE: Differential effects of various types of reinforcement and punishment on learning, expectations and recall in depression and anxiety. Paper presented at the Annual Meeting of the Association for the Advancement of Behavior Therapy. Chicago, Illinois, 1979. 505, 617

Kennedy S. 256

Kenny M. 386, 387

Kern R. 331, 466

Kernberg OF: Borderline Conditions and Pathological Narcissism. Northvale, NJ, Jason Aronson, 1975. 35, 546, 554

Kerr TA. 54, 506, 508, 509, 599, 619

Kessel WIN: Psychiatric morbidity in a London general practice. British Journal of Prev Soc Medicine 14:16–22, 1960. 247

Kessler LG. 115, 116

Kessler LG, Cleary PD, Burke JD: Psychiatric disorders in primary care. Archives of General Psychiatry 42:583–587, 1985. 588, 593

Kessler RC, McRae JA: Trends in stress and psychological distress. American Sociology Review 41:443–452, 1981. 168

Kessler RM. 577

Kety SS. 30, 415, 425, 431

Kety SS, Rosenthal D, Wender P, Schulsinger F: The types and prevalence of mental illness in the biological and adoptive families of adopted schizophrenics, in The Transmission of Schizophrenia. Edited by Rosenthal D, Kety SS. Oxford, England, Pergamon, 1968, pp 345–362. 29

Keys DJ. 228

Khan A. 414

Khan A, Ciraulo DA, Nelson WH, Becker JT, Nies A, Jaffe JH: Dexamethasone suppression test in recently detoxified alcoholics: clinical implications. Journal of Clinical Psychopharmacology 4:94–97, 1984. 290

Khan A, Lee E, Dager S, Hyde T, Raisys V, Avery D, Dunner D: Platelet MAO-B activity in anxiety and depression. Biological Psychiatry 21:847–849, 1986. 394

Khantzian EJ, Treece C: DSM-III psychiatric diagnosis of narcotic addicts: recent findings. Archives of General Psychiatry 42:1067–1071, 1985. 189, 200

Khouri P, Akiskal H: The bipolar spectrum reconsidered, in Contemporary Directions in Psychopathology. Edited by Millon T, Klerman G. New York, Guilford, 1986. 52

Kidd KK. 272, 336, 346, 348, 350, 352, 580, 649, 650

Kidd RF. 516

Kielholz P. 655

Kielholz P: Alcohol and depression. British Journal of Addiction 65:187–193, 1969. 295

Kilts CD. 418, 424–428, 430

Kilts CD, Bissett G, Krishnan KRR, Smith MA, Chappell P, Nemeroff CB: The preclinical and clinical neurobiology of corticotropin-releasing factor (CRF), in Hormones and Depression. Edited by Halbreich U, Rose RM. New York, Raven, 1987, pp 297–312. 430

Kim M. 386

Kimber NM. 393

King AC. 577

King D. 47, 322, 599, 603

King R, Margraf J, Ehlers A: Panic disorder-overlap with symptoms of somatization disorder, in Panic and Phobias: Empirical Evidence of Theoretical Models and Long Term Effects of Behavioral Treatments. Edited by Hand I, Wittchen HU. New York, Springer-Verlag, 1986. 227

Kingston R. 623

Kirk R: Experimental Design: Procedures for the Behavioral Sciences. Belmont, CA, Brooks/Cole, 1982. 627, 628, 629

Kirmayer LJ: Culture, affect and somatization, part I. Transcultural Psychiatric Research Review 21:159–188, 1984. 239, 246

Kirmayer L: Somatization and the social construction of illness experience, in Illness Behavior: A Multidisciplinary Model. New York, Plenum, 1986, pp 111–133. 246

Kiss JZ. 418

Kjellman BF. 394

Kleber HD. 294, 296, 302, 323

Klein DF. 272, 318, 323, 327, 415, 432, 604, 659, 673–677

Klein DF: Delineation of two drug-responsive anxiety syndromes. Psychopharmacologia 5:397–408, 1964. 675, 700

Klein DF: Importance of psychiatric diagnosis in prediction of clinical drug effects. Archives of General Psychiatry 16:118–126, 1967. 675

Klein DF: Drug therapy as a means of syndromal identification and nosological revision, in Psychopathology and Psychopharmacology. Edited by Cole JO, Freedman AM, Friedhoff AJ. Baltimore, Johns Hopkins University Press, 1973. 598

Klein DF: Endogenomorphic depression, a conceptual and terminological revision. Archives of General Psychiatry 31:447–454, 1974. 603

Klein DF: Anxiety reconceptualized: early experience with imipramine and anxiety. Comprehensive Psychiatry 21:411–427, 1980. 281, 367, 500

Klein D: Anxiety reconceptualized, in Anxiety: New Directions and Changing Concepts. Edited by Klein D, Rabkin J. New York, Raven, 1981, pp 235–262. 43, 44, 675

Klein DF, Rabkin JG, Gorman JM: Etiological and pathophysiological inferences from the pharmacological treatment of anxiety, in Anxiety and the Anxiety Disorders. Edited by Tuma AH, Maser JD. Hillsdale, NJ, Lawrence Erlbaum Associates, 1985. 570

Klein D, Zitrin C, Woerner M, Ross D: Treatment of phobias. Archives of General Psychiatry 40:139–145, 1983. 43, 675

Klein DN, Dickstein S, Taylor EB, Harding K: Identifying chronic affective disorders in outpatients: validation of the General Behavior Inventory. Journal of Consulting and Clinical Psychology 57:106–111, 1989. 323

Klein DN, Taylor EB, Harding K, Dickstein S: Double depression and episodic major depression: demographic, clinical, familial, personality, and socioenvironmental characteristics and short-term outcome. American Journal of Psychiatry 145:1226–1231, 1988. 322

Klein L. 588, 592, 593

Kleinman AM. 15, 243

Kleinman A: Social Origins of Distress and Disease. New Haven, CT, Yale University Press, 1986. 473, 474, 487

Kleitman N: Sleep and Wakefulness, 2nd Edition. Chicago, University of Chicago Press, 1963. 709

Klerman GL. 54, 161, 168, 236, 249, 255, 296, 301, 322, 323, 325, 328, 354–357, 475, 483, 494, 499, 505, 508, 509, 554, 622, 624, 629, 700, 719

Klerman G: Anxiety and depression, in Handbook of Studies on Depression. Edited by Burrows G. New York, Excerpta Medica, 1977. 504

Klerman GL: Affective disorders, in The Harvard Guide to Modern Psychiatry. Edited by Nicholi AM. Cambridge, MA, The Belknap Press of the Harvard University Press, 1978a, pp 253–281. 160

Klerman GL: The evolution of a scientific nosology, in Schizophrenia: Science and Practice. Edited by Shershow JC. Cambridge, MA, Harvard University Press, 1978b. 61

Klerman GL: Other specific affective disorders, in Comprehensive Textbook of Psychiatry, Vol. 3, 3rd Edition. Edited by Kaplan HI, Freedman AM, Sadock BJ. Baltimore, Williams & Wilkins, 1980. 328

Klerman GL: Overview of the Cross-National Collaborative Panic Study. Archives of General Psychiatry 45:407–412, 1988. 592

Klerman GL, Lavori PW, Rice J, Reich T, Endicott J, Andreasen NC, Keller MB, Hirschfeld RMA: Birth cohort trends in rates of major depressive disorder among relatives of patients with affective disorders. Archives of General Psychiatry 42:689–693, 1985. 666

Klerman GL, Weissman MM, Rounsaville BJ, Chevron ES: Interpersonal Psychotherapy of Depression. New York, Basic Books, 1984. 603

Klett CJ. 23

Kling M. 388

Klinger E, Barta S, Maxeimer M: Motivational correlates of thought content frequency and commitment. Journal of Personality and Social Psychology 39:1222–1237, 1980. 712

Klosko JS. 226, 227

Kneip J. 421

Knesevich MA. 689

Knight AF. 422

Knight DL. 415

Knight RP: The psychodynamics of chronic alcoholism. The Journal of Nervous and Mental Disease 86:538–543, 1937. 283

Knott VJ, Lapierre YD: Computerized EEG correlates of depression and antidepressant treatment. Progress in Neuro-Psychopharmacology and Biological Psychiatry 11:213–221, 1987. 573

Koch R. 125

Kocsis JH. 390

Kocsis JH, Frances AJ: A critical discussion of DSM-III dysthymic disorder. American Journal of Psychiatry 144:1534–1542, 1987. 317

Kocsis JH, Frances AJ, Mann JJ, Sweeney J, Voss C: Imipramine for the treatment of chronic depression. Psychopharmacology Bulletin 21:698–700, 1985. 318

Kocsis JH, Frances AJ, Voss C, Mann JJ, Mason BJ, Sweeney J: Imipramine for treatment of chronic depression. Archives of General Psychiatry 45:253–257, 1988. 318, 325

Kocsis JH, Voss C, Mann JJ, Frances A: Chronic depression: demographic and clinical characteristics. Psychopharmacology Bulletin 22:192–195, 1986. 326

Koegel P, Burnam A, Farr RK: The prevalence of specific psychiatric disorders among homeless individuals in the inner city of Los Angeles. Archives of General Psychiatry 45:1085–1092, 1988. 322

Koenigsberg HW, Kaplan RD, Gilmore MM, Cooper AM: The relationship between syndrome and personality disorder in DSM-III: experience with 2,462 patients. American Journal of Psychiatry 142:207–212, 1985. 190, 201, 325

Koening LJ. 518

Kofoed L, Kania J, Walsh T, Atkinson RM: Outpatient treatment of patients with substance abuse and coexisting psychiatric disorders. American Journal of Psychiatry 143:867–872, 1986. 189

Kohout J. 503

Kolb B, Taylor L: Affective behavior in patients with localized cortical excisions: role of lesion site and side. Science 214:89–91, 1981. 565

Kolden G. 513, 518, 530, 541, 543, 640

Kraepelin E: (1899): Psychiatrie. En Lehrbuch für Studierende und Ärzte (6th German edn.). Barth, Leipzig. Translated (1902) as Clinical Psychiatry by AR Diefendorf. The MacMillan Company, New York. 151

Kraepelin E: Manic-Depressive Insanity and Paranoia. Translated by Barclay RM. Edited by Robertson GM. Edinburgh, E & S Livingstone, 1921. 598, 605

Kraepelin E: Comparative psychiatry, in Themes and Variations in European Psychiatry. Edited by Hirsch SR, Shepherd M. Charlottesville, VA, University Press of Virginia, 1974. 31

Krahenguhl V. 362

Krahn DD, Gosnell BA, Grace M, Levine AS: CRF antagonist partially reverses CRF- and stress-induced effects on feeding. Brain Research Bulletin 17:285–289, 1986. 421, 423

Kramer M. 115, 159, 165, 168, 171, 321, 588, 589, 661, 705

Kramer PA. 289

Kramer-Fox M. 395

Krantz S, Hammen C: Assessment of cognitive bias in depression. Journal of Abnormal Psychology 88:611–619, 1979. 641

Kranzler HR. Preliminary studies on the effects of buspirone on craving in alcoholics. Presented at the annual meeting of the American College of Neuropsychopharmacology, 1987. 291

Kranzler HR, Liebowitz N: Depression and anxiety in substance abuse: clinical implications. Medical Clinics of North America 72:867–885, 1988. 288

Krasnoff L. 180, 466

Kravitz HM. 281

Kravitz M. 472

Krejci MJ. 508

Krieger D. 429, 432

Kringlen EE: Obsessional neurotics: a long-term follow-up. British Journal of Psychiatry 111:709–722, 1965. 308, 311, 314

Kripke DF: Phase advance theories for affective illnesses, in Circadian Rhythms in Psychiatry: Basic and Clinical Studies. Edited by Goodwin F, Wehr T. Pacific Grove, CA, Boxwood Press, 1983. 709

Krishnan KRR. 415, 430

Kronfol Z. 387, 403, 427, 613

Kronfol Z, Hamsher K de S, Digre K, Waziri R: Depression and hemisphere functions: changes associated with unilateral ECT. British Journal of Psychiatry 132:560–567, 1978. 567, 570

Krummel SJ. 389

Kubal L. 504

Kuhn TS: The Structure of Scientific Revolutions. Chicago, University of Chicago Press, 1962. 14, 23

Kuhn TS: The Structure of Scientific Revolutions, 2nd Edition. International Encyclopedia of Unified Science, Vol 2, No 2. Chicago, University of Chicago Press, 1970. 14, 15, 23, 25

Kuiper K. 509

Kuiper NA. 643

Kuiper NA, MacDonald MR: Schematic processing in depression: the self-based consensus bias. Cognitive Therapy and Research 7:469–484, 1983. 643

Kukopulos A, Reginaldi R, Floris G, Serra G, Tondo L: Course of the manic-depressive cycle and changes caused by treatment. Pharmakopsychiatrie Neuro-psykopharmakologie 13:156–167, 1980. 605

Kung LS. 431

Kuperberg A. 255

Kupfer DJ. 233, 235, 237
Kupfer DJ, Ehlers CL: Two roads to rapid eye movement latency. Archives of General Psychiatry 46:945–948, 1989. 409
Kupfer DJ, Freedman DX: Treatment for depression: "standard" clinical practice as an unexamined topic. Archives of General Psychiatry 43:509–511, 1986. 237
Kurlander HM. 505, 617
Kurthen I. 388
Kushner M. 570
Kvetnansky R. 424
Lacey BC. 244
Lacey JI: Individual differences in somatic response patterns. Journal of Comparative and Physiological Psychology 43:338, 1950. 244
Lacey JI, Bateman DE, Van Lehn R: Autonomic response specificity: an experimental study. Psychosomatic Medicine 15:8, 1953. 244
Lacey JI, Lacey BC: Verification and extension of the principle of autonomic response-stereotypy. American Journal of Psychology 71:50, 1958. 244
Lader M: The Psychophysiology of Mental Illness. London, Routledge & Kegan Paul, 1975. 599
Lader MH, Wing L: Physiological measures in agitated and retarded patients. Journal of Psychiatric Research 7:89–100, 1969. 700
Laffer PS. 255
Lahti RA, Barsuhn C: The effect of various doses of minor tranquilizers on plasma corticosteroids in stressed and nonstressed rats. Research Communications in Chemical Pathology and Pharmacology 11:595–603, 1975. 422
Laird N, Olivier DC: Covariance analysis of censored survival data using log-linear analysis techniques. Journal of the American Statistical Association 76:231–240, 1981. 169
Lake CR. 600
Lake MD. 254
Lake R. 276, 571
Lalakea ML. 308, 571, 574
Lambert MJ, Hatch DR, Kingston R, Edwards BC: Zung, Beck and Hamilton rating scales as measures of treatment outcome: a meta-analytic comparison. Journal of Consulting and Clinical Psychology 54:54–59, 1986. 623
Lamberts S: Neuroendocrine aspects of the dexamethasone suppression test in psychiatry. Life Sciences 39:91–95, 1986. 386
Lambo TA. 154
Lamborn KR. 673
Lambourn J. 700
Lamiell J: Toward an idiothetic psychology of personality. American Psychologist 36:276–289, 1981. 708, 710
Lampertico M. 255
Landau S. 574
Lander ES, Botstein D: Mapping complex genetic traits in humans: new methods using a complete RFLP linkage map. Cold Spring Harbor Symposia on Quantitative Biology 51:49–62, 1986. 683
Landerman R. 159
Lane LA. 404–406
Lang PJ. 635
Lang PJ: A bio-informational theory of emotional imagery. Psychophysiology 16:495–512, 1979. 636
Lang PJ: Cognition in emotion: concept and action, in Emotion, Cognition

and Behavior. Edited by Izard C, Kagan J, Zajonc R. New York, Cambridge University Press, 1983. 636, 646

Lang PJ: The cognitive psychophysiology of emotion: fear and anxiety, in Anxiety and the Anxiety Disorders. Edited by Tuma AH, Maser JD. Hillsdale, NJ, Lawrence Erlbaum Associates, 1985. 54, 509, 527, 636

Langer DH. 276, 571

Langer SZ. 414

Langner TS. 177, 245

Langner TS: A twenty-two item screening score of psychiatric symptom indicating impairment. Journal of Health and Human Behavior 3:269–272, 1962. 173

Langston K. 577

Lanke J. 144, 147, 168

Lantz S. 254

Lapierre YD. 573

Laraia MT. 387

Larsen S. 251

Larson DW. 630

Larson R. 712–716

Larson R: Adolescents' daily experience with family and friends: contrasting opportunity systems. Journal of Marriage and the Family 45:739–750, 1983. 715

Larson R, Csikszentmihalyi M: The experience sampling method, in New Directions for Naturalistic Methods in the Behavioral Sciences. Edited by Reis H. San Francisco, Jossey-Bass, 1984. 708

Larssen SE. 251

Larsson H. 140

Lasègue D: De l'anorexie hystérique. Archives Générales de Medicine, 1873. Reprinted in Evolution of Psychosomatic Concepts. Anorexia Nervosa: A Paradigm. Edited by Kaufman RM, Heiman M. International Universities Press, 1964, pp 141–155. 253, 254

Lasky JJ. 23

Last CG, Francis G, Hersen M, Kazdin AE, Strauss CC: Separation anxiety and school phobia: a comparison using DSM-III criteria. American Journal of Psychiatry 144:653–657, 1987. 277, 359, 360, 361

Last CG, Hersen M, Kazdin AE, Finkelstein R, Strauss CC: Comparison of DSM-III separation anxiety and overanxious disorders: demographic characteristics and patterns of comorbidity. Journal of the American Academy of Child and Adolescent Psychiatry 26:527–531, 1987. 277

Latimer LG. 420

Latimer PL. 229

Latimer PR: Irritable bowel syndrome. Psychosomatics 24:205–218, 1983. 244, 249

Laude R. 225

Laux D. 673

Lavori PW. 236, 255, 297, 298, 301, 322, 325, 354–357, 494, 556, 666

Lavori PW, Keller MB: Improving the aggregate performance of psychiatric diagnostic methods when not all subjects receive the standard test. Statistics in Medicine 7:727–737, 1988. 684

Laws ER Jr. 394

Lawson SG. 261

Layden MA. 517

Lazarus RS. 637, 640

Lazarus RS: Psychological Stress and the Coping Process. New York, McGraw-Hill, 1966. 519

Lazarus RS: Emotions and adaptation: conceptual and empirical relations, in Nebraska Symposium on Motivation. Edited by Arnold WJ. Lincoln, NE, University of Nebraska Press, 1968. 519

Lazarus RS: Psychological stress and coping in adaptation and illness. International Journal on Psychiatry in Medicine 5:321–333, 1974. 637

Lazarus RS, Averill JR: Emotion and cognition: with special reference to anxiety, in Anxiety: Current Trends in Theory and Research. Edited by Spielberger CD. New York, Academic, 1972. 519

Leaf PJ. 116, 165, 168, 171, 317, 321, 323, 327, 589

Leckman JF. 275, 310, 350, 363, 377, 499, 563, 580

Leckman J, Merikangas K, Pauls D, Prusoff B, Weissman M: Anxiety disorders and depression: contradictions between family study data and DSM-III conventions. American Journal of Psychiatry 140:880–882, 1983. 44, 45, 94, 109, 346, 499, 505

Leckman JF, Weissman MM, Merikangas KR, Pauls DL, Prusoff BA: Panic disorder and major depression: increased risk of major depression, alcoholism, panic and phobic disorders in families of depressed probands with panic disorder. Archives of General Psychiatry 40:1055–1060, 1983. 45, 206, 364, 377, 478, 487, 499, 605, 619

Leckman JF, Weissman MM, Merikangas KR, Pauls DL, Prusoff BA: Methodologic differences in major depression and panic disorder studies. Archives of General Psychiatry 41:722–723, 1984. 346, 347, 364

Lecrubier Y. 599

Lee E. 394

Lee G. 420

Lee NF, Rush AJ, Mitchell JE: Depression and bulimia. Journal of Affective Disorders 9:231–238, 1985. 255

Leff JP. 487

Leff JP: Psychiatrists versus patients concept of unpleasant emotions. British Journal of Psychiatry 133:306–313, 1978. 696

LeGoc Y. 599

Lehman AF. 387

Lehmann HE. 655

Leight KA, Ellis HC: Emotional mood states, strategies and state-dependency in memory. Journal of Verbal Learning and Verbal Behavior 20:251–266, 1981. 643

Leighton AH. 137, 154, 155, 157, 159, 161, 162, 165–172, 174, 333

Leighton AH: My Name Is Legion: The Stirling County Study of Psychiatric Disorder and Sociocultural Environment. New York, Basic Books, 1959. 154

Leighton AH, Lambo TA, Hughes CC, Leighton DC, Murphy JM, Macklin DB: Psychiatric Disorder Among the Yoruba: A Report from the Cornell-Aro Mental Health Research Project in the Western Region, Nigeria. Ithaca, NY, Cornell University Press, 1963. 154

Leighton DC. 154

Leighton DC, Harding JS, Macklin DB, Macmillan AM, Leighton AH: The Character of Danger: The Stirling County Study. New York, Basic Books, 1963a. 154, 155, 165

Leighton DC, Harding JS, Macklin DB, Hughes CC, Leighton AH: Psychiatric findings of the Stirling County Study. American Journal of Psychiatry 119:1021–1026, 1963b. 171

Leitch IM. 700

Lemmi H. 47, 318, 325, 327, 599, 603, 604

Le Moal M. 420, 421, 423

Lenane MC. 315

Lengvari I. 418

Lentz RD. 327

Lenz HJ, Raedler A, Greten H, Brown MR: CRF initiates biological actions within the brain that are observed in response to stress. American Journal of Physiology 252:34–39, 1987. 420

Leonard HL. 315

Leonhard K: The classification of Endogenous Psychoses. New York, John Wiley, 1979. 505

Lesse S: The relationship of anxiety to depression. American Journal of Psychotherapy 36:332–348, 1982. 414, 433

Lesser IM. 387, 404–406, 586, 592, 594

Lesser IM, Ford CV, Friedmann CTH: Alexithymia in somatizing patients. General Hospital Psychiatry 1:256–261, 1979. 246

Lesser IM, Poland RE, Holcomb C, Rose DE: Electroencephalographic study of nighttime panic attacks. Journal of Nervous and Mental Disease 173:744–746, 1985. 575

Lesser IM, Rubin RT, Finder E, Forster B, Poland RE: Situational depression and the dexamethasone suppression test. Psychoneuroendocrinology 8:441–445, 1983. 488

Lesser IM, Rubin RT, Pecknold JC, Rifkin A, Swinson RP, Lydiard RB, Burrows GD, Noyes R Jr, DuPont RL Jr: Secondary depression in panic disorder and agoraphobia. Archives of General Psychiatry 45:437–443, 1988. 594, 607

Lesser M. 387

Levav I. 180, 181

Levav I, Krasnoff L, Dohrenwend BS: Israeli PERI life event scale: ratings of events by community sample. Israel Journal of Medical Sciences 17:176–183, 1981. 180

Levin A. 672, 676–678

Levine AS. 420, 421, 423

Levine AS, Rogers B, Kneip J, Grace M, Morley JE: Effect of centrally administered corticotropin releasing factor (CRF) on multiple feeding paradigms. Neuropharmacology 22:337–339, 1983. 421

Levine PH. 392

Levine S. 503, 521

Levitt K.523, 622

Levy JC. 287

Levy J: Individual differences in cerebral hemisphere asymmetry, theoretical issues and experimental considerations, in Cerebral Hemisphere Asymmetry: Method, Theory and Application. Edited by Hellige J. New York, Praeger, 1983. 564, 572

Lewinsohn PM. 639, 640

Lewinsohn PM: A behavioral approach to depression, in The Psychology of Depression: Contemporary Theory and Research. Edited by Friedman RJ, Katz MM. Washington, DC, VH Winston, 1974a. 508

Lewinsohn PM: Clinical and theoretical aspects of depression, in Innovative Treatment Methods of Psychopathology. Edited by Calhoun KS, Adams HE, Mitchell KM. New York, John Wiley, 1974b. 639

Lewinsohn PM: Activity schedules in treatment of depression, in Counseling Methods. Edited by Krumboltz JD, Thoresen CE. New York, Holt, Rinehart

& Winston, 1976. 640

Lewinsohn PM, Steinmetz JL, Larson DW, Franklin J: Depression-related cognitions: antecedent or consequence? Journal of Abnormal Psychology 90:213–219, 1981. 630

Lewinsohn PM, Talkington J: Studies on the measurement of unpleasant events and relations with depression. Applied Psychological Measurement 3:83–101, 1979. 639, 640

Lewis A: Problems of obsessional illness. Proceedings of the Royal Society of Medicine 36:325–336, 1936. 307, 309, 314

Lewis AJ: Melancholia: a clinical survey of depressive states. Journal of Mental Science 80:277–278, 1934. 499

Lewis AJ: States of depression and their clinical and aetiological differentiation. British Medical Journal 21:183–186, 1938. 499

Lewis BI: Hyperventilation syndrome: a clinical and physiological evaluation. Cal Med 3:121, 1959. 249

Lewis CE. 236, 296, 301

Ley RG, Bryden MP: A dissociation of right and left hemispheric effects for recognizing emotional tone and verbal content. Brain and Cognition 1:3–9, 1982. 564

Lieberman JA, Brenner R, Lesser M, Coccaro E, Borenstein M, Kane JM: Dexamethasone suppression test in patients with panic disorder. American Journal of Psychiatry 117:25, 1983. 387

Liebowitz JH. 36

Liebowitz MR. 673, 674, 677

Liebowitz M, Fyer A, Gorman J: Lactate provocation of panic attacks, I: clinical and behavioral findings. Archives of General Psychiatry 41:764–770, 1984. 391

Liebowitz MR, Fyer AJ, Gorman JM, Campeas R, Levin A, Davies SO, Klein DF: Alprazolam in the treatment of panic disorders. Journal of Clinical Psychopharmacology 6:13–20, 1986a. 676

Liebowitz MR, Fyer A, Gorman J, Campeas R, Levin A: Phenelzine in social phobia. Journal of Clinical Psychiatry 43:613–614, 1986b. 677

Liebowitz MR, Fyer AJ, Gorman JM, Dillon D, Davies S, Stein JM, Cohen BS, Klein DF: Specificity of lactate infusions in social phobia versus panic disorders. American Journal of Psychiatry 142:947–950, 1987. 392

Liebowitz MR. Fyer AJ, McGrath P, Klein DF: Clonidine treatment of panic disorder. Psychopharmacology Bulletin 17:122–123, 1981. 415, 432

Liebowitz M, Gorman J, Fyer A: Lactate provocation of panic attacks, II: biochemical and physiological findings. Archives of General Psychiatry 42:709–719, 1985. 391

Liebowitz MR, Gorman JM, Fyer AJ, Campeas R, Levin A, Sandberg D, Hollander E, Papp L, Goetz D: Pharmacotherapy of social phobia: a placebo-controlled comparison of phenelzine and atenolol. Journal of Clinical Psychiatry 49:252–257, 1988. 672, 678

Liebowitz MR, Gorman JM, Fyer AJ, Klein DF: Social phobia: review of a neglected anxiety disorder. Archives of General Psychiatry 40:139–145, 1983. 677

Liebowitz MR, Quitkin FM, Stewart JW, McGrath PJ, Harrison WM, Markowitz JS, Rabkin JG, Tricamo E, Goetz DM, Klein DF: Antidepressant specificity in atypical depression. Archives of General Psychiatry 45:129–137, 1988. 673

Liebowitz MR, Quitkin FM, Stewart JW, McGrath PJ, Harrison W, Rabkin J, Tricamo E, Markowitz JS, Klein DF: Phenelzine vs imipramine in atypical depression: a preliminary report. Archives of General Psychiatry 41:669–677, 1984. 604, 673

Liebowitz N. 288

Liese BS. 284, 285

Liljeberg P. 288, 290

Lin TY, Standley CC: The Scope of Epidemiology in Psychiatry. Geneva, World Health Organization, 1962. 33

Lindall A. 425

Lindenthal JJ. 483, 629

Lindy JD. 503

Ling N. 420, 426

Link BG. 180, 466

Link BG, Dohrenwend BP: Formulation of hypotheses about the ratio of untreated to treated cases in the true prevalence studies of functional psychiatric disorders in adults in the United States, in Mental Illness in the United States: Epidemiological Estimates. Edited by Dohrenwend BP, Dohrenwend BS, Gould MS, Link B, Neugegauer R, Wursch-Hitzig, R. New York, Praeger. 1980a. 182

Link B, Dohrenwend BP: Formulation of hypotheses about the true prevalence of demoralization in the United States, in Mental Illness in the United States: Epidemiological Estimates. Edited by Dohrenwend BP, Dohrenwend BS, Gould MS, Link B, Neugegauer R, Wursch-Hitzig R. New York, Praeger, 1980b. 178, 477

Linnoila M. 488

Linton EA. 418

Liotti G. 525

Lipinski DP. 716

Lipman RS. 54, 158, 234, 240, 256, 261, 508, 509, 624, 674, 676, 702

Lipman RS: Differentiating anxiety and depression in anxiety disorders: use of rating scales. Psychopharmacology Bulletin 18:69–77, 1982. 621, 700

Lipman RS, Rickels K, Covi L, Derogatis LR, Uhlenhuth EH: Factors of symptom distress: doctor ratings of anxious neurotic outpatients. Archives of General Psychiatry 21:328–338, 1969. 158

Liposits Z, Lengvari I, Vigh S, Schally AV, Fierko B: Immunohistological detection of degenerating CRF-immunoreactive nerve fibers in the median eminence after lesion of paraventricular nucleus of the rat: a light and electron microscopic study. Peptides 4:941–953, 1983. 418

Lipowski ZJ: Somatization: A borderland between medicine and psychiatry. Canadian Medical Association Journal 135:609–614, 1986. 239

Lipper S. 407

Lipsey JR. 327

Livesey J. 417

Livingston R, Nugent H, Rader L, Smith RC: Family histories of depressed and severely anxious children. American Journal of Psychiatry 142:1497–1499, 1985. 359

Ljunggren JG. 394

Lo WH: A follow-up study of obsessional neurotics in Hong Kong Chinese. British Journal of Psychiatry 113:823–832, 1967. 306, 311

Locke BZ. 115, 159, 321, 588, 649, 650, 664, 666, 705

Loewenstein RJ, Hamilton JA, Alagna S, Reid N, deVries MW: Experiential sampling in the study of multiple personality disorder. American Journal of Psychiatry 144:19–24, 1987. 712

Lohr N. 387, 403, 427, 613

Loke J. 391, 392

Lolas F, de la Para G: Cerebral psychophysiology of depression preliminary results. Invest Clin 20:33–47, 1979. 574

Loosen PT. 427, 428, 430

Loosen PT, Garbutt JC, Prange AJ: Evaluation of the diagnostic utility of the TRH-induced TSH response in psychiatric disorders. Pharmacopsychiatry 20:90–95, 1987. 394

Loosen PT, Prange AJ, Wilson IC: TRH (Protirelin) in depressed alcoholic men. Archives of General Psychiatry 36:540–547, 1979. 290

Lopatka C. 622

Loper RG. 283, 284

Lopez JF. 389

Loriaux DL. 255, 430, 431, 433

Loriaux L. 417

Lorr M. 554

Lorr M, McNair DM, Klett CJ, Laskey JJ. Evidence of ten psychotic syndromes. Journal of Consulting Psychology 26:185–189, 1962. 23

Lorr M, Sohn T, Katz M: Toward a definition of depression. Archives of General Psychiatry 17:183–186, 1967. 505

Losito BG. 425

Loudon JB. 555

Lovland B. 251

Lowenstein LM. 283, 284

Lowenthal DT. 247

Lowry PJ. 418

Lubin B. 613, 614, 615, 630

Luborsky L. 292

Lucki I. 388

Ludlow C. 276, 571

Lum LC: The syndrome of habitual chronic hyperventilation, in Modern Trends in Psychosomatic Medicine, Vol. 3. Edited by Hill O. Boston, Butterworths, 1976, p 196. 249

Lundberg D. 425

Lunde I. 30

Lushene RE. 213, 554, 613, 644, 716, 719

Lustman PJ. 249

Lydiard RB. 387, 594, 607

Lyketsos GC. 120

Lyons JS. 11, 305

Maas JW. 415, 432

MacDonald MR. 643

MacDonald-Scott P. 297, 556

MacFadyen J. 254

Mackay AVP. 431

Macklin DB. 154, 155, 165, 171

MacLeod C. 509, 527, 531, 533

MacLeod C, Mathews A, Tata P: Attentional bias in emotional disorders. Journal of Abnormal Psychology 95:15–20, 1986. 509, 527, 531

Macmillan AM. 154, 155, 165

Macmillan AM: The Health Opinion Survey: technique for estimating prevalence of psychoneurotic and related types of disorder in communities. Psychological Reports 3:325–329, 1957. 157, 177

MacMillen SR. 661

MacPhillamy DJ, Lewinsohn PM: The Pleasant Events Schedule: studies on reliability, validity, and scale intercorrelation. Journal of Consulting and Clinical Psychology 50:363–380, 1982. 639, 640

Maddock RJ. 392, 712

Maderdrut JL. 424

Maggini C. 604, 606

Maggioni M. 255

Maguire KP. 388, 406

Mahoney MJ: The self-management of covert behavior: a case study. Behavior Therapy 2:575–578, 1971. 638

Maier SF, Seligman MEP: Learned helplessness: theory and evidence. Journal of Experimental Psychology: General 105:3–46, 1976. 528

Maier W. 45

Maier W, Buller R, Hallmayer J: Comorbidity of panic disorder and major depression: results from a family study, in Panic and Phobias: Treatments and Variables Affecting Course and Outcome. Edited by Hand I, Wittchen H-U. Berlin, Springer-Verlag, 1988, pp 180–185. 339, 340, 346, 347

Maisami M. 272

Maislin G. 388

Makara GB. 418

Malinowski B: Coral Gardens and Their Magic: Soil Tilling and Agricultural Rites, Vol 1. Bloomington, IN, Indiana University Press, 1935. 709

Mallya G. 606

Malmo RB, Shagass C: Physiologic study of symptom mechanisms in psychiatric patients under stress. Psychosomatic Medicine 11:25–29, 1949. 244

Mandler G: Helplessness: theory and research in anxiety, in Anxiety: Current Trends in Theory and Research, Vol 3. Edited by Spielberger CD. New York, Academic, 1972. 508, 509, 519, 525, 527

Manier DH. 432

Mann JJ. 318, 325, 326

Mann L. 571, 572

Mann SA. 487

Mannisto P. 408

Mannuzza S, Fyer AJ, Klein DF, Endicott J: Schedule for Affective Disorders and Schizophrenia–Lifetime Version (modified for the study of anxiety disorders): rational and conceptual development. Journal of Psychiatric Research 20:317–325, 1986. 659

Manton KG. 159

Maples CW. 528

Mapother E: Discussion on manic-depressive psychosis. British Medical Journal 2:872–879, 1926. 475, 499

March S. 254

Marder SR. 716

Maremmani I. 599

Margolin R. 577

Margraf J. 227, 392, 712

Margraf J, Ehlers A, Roth WT: Biological models of panic disorder and agoraphobia: a review. Behavior Research and Therapy 24:553–567, 1986. 712

Margraf J, Taylor B, Ehlers A, Roth WT, Agras WS: Panic attacks in the natural environment. Journal of Nervous and Mental Disease 175:558–566, 1987. 713

Market JR. 414

Markowitz JS. 466, 604

Marks IM. 310

Marks I: Fear and Phobias. London, Heinemann, 1969. 624, 677

Marks IM: Review of behavioral psychotherapy, I: obsessive compulsive disorders. American Journal of Psychiatry 138:584–592, 1981. 309

Marks IM: Obsessive compulsive disorder, in Fears, Phobias, and Rituals: Panic Anxiety and Their Disorders. New York, Oxford University Press, 1987, pp 423–456. 309

Marks IM, Hodgson R, Rachman S: Treatment of chronic OCD 2 years after in vivo exposure. British Journal of Psychiatry 127:349–364, 1975. 308

Marks IM, Matthews AM: Brief standard self-rating for phobic patients. Behaviour Research and Therapy 17:263–267, 1979. 213, 716, 719

Marks T. 518, 629

Marlatt GA: Relapse prevention: theoretical rationale and overview of the model, in Relapse Prevention. Edited by Marlatt GA, Gordon JR. New York, Guilford, 1985. 292

Marriott P. 390

Marrosu F, Mereu G, Fratta W, Carcangiu P, Camarri F, Gessa GL: Different epileptogenic activities of murine and ovine corticotropin-releasing factor. Brain Research 408:394–398, 1987. 420

Marsella AJ, Sartorius N, Jablensky A, Fenton FR: Cross-cultural studies of depressive disorders: an overview, in Culture and Depression. Edited by Kleinman A, Good G. Berkeley, CA, University of California Press, 1985. 474

Martin D. 404, 407

Martin JB, Reichlin S: Clinical Neuroendocrinology, 2nd Edition. Philadelphia, FA Davis, 1987, p 160. 417

Martin JL. 180

Martin NG. 344, 345, 370, 478, 487, 490, 497, 580

Martin NG, Jardine R, Andrews G, Heath AC: Anxiety disorders and neuroticism: are there genetic factors specific to panic? Acta Psychiatrica Scandinavica 77:698–700, 1988. 371

Martin RL. 84, 317, 321, 337, 338, 378, 447, 453, 455–457

Martin RL, Cloninger CR, Guze SB, Clayton PJ: Mortality in a follow-up of 500 psychiatric outpatients. Archives of General Psychiatry 42:47–54, 1985. 10, 180, 439, 440, 449, 457

Martinez R. 500, 660

Mason BJ. 318, 325

Massimini F, Csikszentmihalyi M, Carli M: The monitoring of optimal experience: a tool for psychiatric rehabilitation. Journal of Nervous and Mental Disease 175:545–550, 1987. 712, 713

Masuda A. 420, 426

Matar A. 302

Mathe A. 429, 432

Mathew RJ, Meyer JS, Francis DJ, Semchuk KM, Mortel K, Claghorn JL: Cerebral blood flow in depression. American Journal of Psychiatry 137:1449–1450, 1980. 576

Mathews A. 509, 527, 531, 631, 632, 716, 719

Mathews A, Eysenck M: Clinical anxiety and cognition, in Theoretical Foundations of Behavior Therapy. Edited by Eysenck H, Martin I. New York, Plenum, 1987. 532

Mathews A, MacLeod C: Discrimination of threat cues without awareness in anxiety states. Journal of Abnormal Psychology 95:131–138, 1986. 509, 527, 531, 533

Mathura CB. 661

Matousek M. 574, 580

Matthews AM. 213

Mattsson NB. 158

Mattsson NB, Williams HV, Rickels K, Lipman RS, Uhlenhuth EH: Dimensions of symptom distress in anxious neurotic outpatients. Psychopharmacology Bulletin 5:19–32, 1969. 158

Matussek P, Wiegand M: Partnership problems as causes of endogenous and neurotic depressions. Acta Psychiatrica Scandinavica 71:95–104, 1985. 476

Matuzas, W. 586

Mavissakalian MR, Barlow DH: Assessment of obsessive-compulsive disorders, in Behavioral Assessment of Adult Disorders. Edited by Barlow DH. New York, Guilford, 1981. 523

Mavissakalian M, Michelson L: Two-years follow-up of exposure and imipramine treatment of agoraphobia. American Journal of Psychiatry 143:1106–1112, 1986. 368

Mavreas VG, Beis A, Mouyias A, Rigoni F, Lyketsos GC: Prevalence of psychiatric disorders in Athens: a community study. Social Psychiatry 21:172–181, 1986. 120

Max D. 508

Maxeimer M. 712

Mayfield DG: Alcohol and affect: experimental studies, in Alcoholism and Affective Disorders. Edited by Goodwin DW, Erickson CK. New York, Spectrum Publications, 1979. 288, 290

Mayfield DG, Coleman LL: Alcohol use and affective disorder. Diseases of the Nervous System 29:467–474, 1968. 288

Mayman M. 585

Mayol A. 516, 518, 629

Mayou R: The nature of bodily symptoms. British Journal of Psychiatry 129:55–60, 1976. 239, 246, 248

Mazure C, Nelson JC, Price LH: Reliability and validity of the symptoms of major depressive illness. Archives of General Psychiatry 43:451–456, 1986. 660

Mazziotta JC. 577

McAllister JA. 275, 279, 317, 322, 360, 361

McAllister TW, Hays LR: TRH test, DST, and response to desipramine in primary degenerative dementia. Biological Psychology 22:189–193, 1987. 386

McArthur LA: The how and what of why: some determinants and consequences of causal attribution. Journal of Personality and Social Psychology 22:171–193, 1972. 516

McCabe S. 621

McCain GA. 251

McCann BS. 230

McCarthy G, Donchin E: A metric for thought: a comparison of P300 latency and reaction time. Science 211:77–80, 1981. 574

McCauley PA, Di Nardo PA, Barlow DH: Differentiating anxiety and depression using a modified scoring system for the Hamilton scales. Paper presented at the Association for Advancement of Behavior Therapy, Boston, November 1987. 219

McCauley PA, Di Nardo PA, Barlow DH: A cluster analysis application in anxiety disorders. Poster presented at the Association for Advancement of Behavior Therapy, New York, November 1988. 230

McChesney CM. 478, 580, 590, 594

McClanahan KL. 392

McCord J. 283

McCord W, McCord J: Origins of Alcoholism. Stanford, Stanford University Press, 1960. 283

McCue, RE. 386

McEvoy L. 6, 44, 45, 61, 63, 93, 95, 97, 109, 118, 120, 137, 190, 204, 206, 221, 305, 307, 308, 311, 315, 321, 332, 333, 364, 439, 455, 590, 649, 650, 661

McFarland RE. 503

McGee RO. 279

McGlashan TH. 307

McGrath PH, Stewart JW, Harrison WH, Wager S, Quitkin FM: Phenelzine treatment of melancholia. Journal of Clinical Psychiatry 47:420–422, 1986. 675

McGrath PJ. 260, 415, 432, 604, 673, 674

McGuiness B. 480, 490

McGuire MT, Polsky RH: Behavioral changes in hospitalized acute schizophrenics: an ethological perspective. Journal of Nervous and Mental Disease 167:651–657, 1979. 709

McInnes A. 574

McIntyre IM. 387, 393

McIntyre IM, Norman T, Marriott P, Burrows GD: The pineal hormone melantonin in panic disorder. Journal of Affective Disorders 12:203–206, 1987. 390

McKeon J. 235

McKeon P, Murray R: Familial aspects of obsessive-compulsive neurosis. British Journal of Psychiatry 151:528–534, 1987. 306

McKernon J. 288

McKinley JC. 256, 283

McKinney WT Jr. 600, 601

McKnew DH. 279

McLaughlin DE. 247

McLellan AT, Luborsky L, Woody GE, O'Brien CP, Droler K: Predicting response to alcohol and drug abuse treatments: role of psychiatric severity. Archives of General Psychiatry 40:620–625, 1983. 292

McLeod DR, Hoehn-Saric R, Stefan RL: Somatic symptoms of anxiety: comparison of self-report and physiological measures. Biological Psychiatry 21:301–310, 1986. 227

McNair DM. 23, 676, 702

McNair DM, Kahn RJ: Imipramine compared with a benzodiazepine for agoraphobia, in Anxiety: New Research and Changing Concepts. Edited by Klein DF, Rabkin J. New York, Raven, 1981, pp 69–79. 703

McNair DM, Lorr M, Droppleman LF: Profile of Mood States. San Diego, Educational and Industrial Testing Service, 1971. 554

McNally RJ. 223

McPherson FM. 90

McPherson FM, Antram MC, Bagshaw VE, Carmichael SK: A test of the hierarchical model of personal illness. British Journal of Psychiatry 131:56–58, 1977. 79, 90

McPherson K. 700

McRae JA. 168

Meadow R. 245

Meehl P: Specific etiology and other forms of strong influence: some quantitative meanings. The Journal of Medicine and Philosophy 2:33–53, 1977. 492, 496

Meissner WW: Theories of personality and psychopathology: classical psychoanalysis, in Comprehensive Textbook of Psychiatry, Vol I, 4th Edition. Edited by Kaplan HI, Sadock BJ. Baltimore, Williams & Wilkins, 1985, pp 337–418. 546

Melancon SM. 712

Melby JC. 386

Melby JM. 255

Melges FT, Bowlby J: Types of hopelessness in psychopathological process. Archives of General Psychiatry 20:690–699, 1969. 509, 511, 519

Meller, WH. 389

Mellinger GD. 477, 590

Mellman TA, Uhde TW: Obsessive compulsive symptoms in panic disorder. American Journal of Psychiatry 144:1573–1576, 1987.

Mello NK. 283, 284, 313

Meltzer HY. 408

Melville ML. 415

Mendels J. 254, 427

Mendels J, Weinstein N, Cochrane C: The relationship between depression and anxiety. Archives of General Psychiatry 27:649–653, 1972. 51, 54, 499, 505, 616, 623, 626, 631

Mendelsohn S. 178

Mendelson JH, Mello NK: Experimental analysis of drinking behavior in chronic alcoholics. Annals of the New York Academy of Sciences 133:828–845, 1966. 283, 284

Mendelson M. 213, 226, 613, 644

Mendelson WB. 276, 571, 575

Menkes DB. 419, 432

Menninger K: The Vital Balance: The Life Process in Mental Health and Mental Illness. New York, Viking, 1963. 20, 32

Menninger K, Mayman M, Pruyser P: The Vital Balance. Middlesex, England, Penguin Books, 1967. 585.

Merchant A. 661

Merchenthaler I. 424

Merchenthaler I: Corticotropin releasing factor (CRF)-like immunoreactivity in the rat central nervous system: extrahypothalamic distribution. Peptides 5:53–69, 1984. 418

Merchenthaler I, Vigh S, Petrusz P, Schally AV: The paraventriculo-infundibular corticotropin releasing factor (CRF)-pathway as revealed by immunocytochemistry in long-term hypophysectomized or adrenalectomized rats. Regulatory Peptides 5:295–305, 1983. 418

Mercier P. 703

Mereu G. 420

Merikangas KR. 44, 45, 94, 109, 189, 200, 206, 275, 346, 347, 348, 352, 354–358, 360, 361, 363, 364, 377, 478, 487, 499, 508, 605, 619

Merikangas KR, Weissman MM: Epidemiology of anxiety disorders in adulthood, in Psychiatry, Vol 3. Edited by Cavenar JO Jr. Philadelphia, JB Lippincott, 1986. 152

Merluzzi TV, Rudy TE, Krejci MJ: Social skill and anxiety: information processing perspectives, in Information Processing Approaches to Clinical Psychology. Edited by Ingram RE. New York, Academic, 1986. 508

Merskey H. 251, 255, 389, 390, 430

Merskey H: Conversion disorders, in Treatments of Psychiatric Disorders: A Task Force Report of the American Psychiatric Association. Edited by American Psychiatric Association. Washington, DC, American Psychiatric Press, 1989, pp 2152–2158. 248

Mertens CJ. 154, 157, 159

Messick S. 80

Mesulam M. 310, 312

Mesulam MM: A cortical network for directed attention and unilateral neglect. Annals Neurology 10:309–325, 1981. 582

Metalsky GI. 510–513, 515, 517, 518, 527, 528, 541, 543

Metalsky GI, Abramson LY: Attributional styles: toward a framework for conceptualization and assessment, in Cognitive-Behavioral Interventions: Assessment Methods. Edited by Kendall PC, Hollon SD. New York, Academic, 1981. 516

Metalsky GI, Abramson LY, Seligman MEP, Semmel A, Peterson C: Attributional styles and life events in the classroom: vulnerability and invulnerability to depressive mood reactions. Journal of Personality and Social Psychology 43:612–617, 1982. 517

Metalsky GI, Halberstadt LJ, Abramson LY: Vulnerability to depressive mood reactions: toward a more powerful test of the diathesis-stress and causal mediation components of the reformulated theory of depression. Journal of Personality and Social Psychology 52:386–393, 1987. 517

Metropolitan Life Insurance Tables. New York, Metropolitan Life Insurance Co., 1964. 267

Meyer BG. 213

Meyer JS. 576

Meyer RE. 235, 284, 285, 286, 288, 290, 300, 302, 661

Meyer RE: How to understand the relationship between psychopathology and addictive disorders: another example of the chicken and the egg, in Psychopathology and Addictive Disorders. Edited by Meyer RE. New York, Guilford, 1986. 284, 291

Meyer-Gross W, Slater E, Roth M: Clinical Psychiatry. Baltimore, Williams & Wilkins, 1954. 24

Meyers JK. 483, 629

Mezzich A. 52

Mezzich JE. 52, 53, 230

Mezzich J: Multiaxial systems in psychiatry, in Comprehensive Textbook of Psychiatry, Vol 1, 3rd Edition. Edited by Freeman AM, Sadock BJ. Baltimore, Williams & Wilkins, 1980. 26

Mezzich JE: International use and impact of DSM-III, in An Annotated Bibliography of DSM-III. Edited by Skodol AE, Spitzer RL. Washington, DC, American Psychiatric Press, 1987. 190

Mezzich JE, Dow JT, Coffman GA: Developing an efficient clinical information system for a comprehensive psychiatric institute, I: principles, design and organization. Behavior Research Methods and Instrumentation 13:459–463, 1981. 192

Mezzich JE, Dow JT, Ganguli R, Munetz MR, Zettler-Segal M: Computerized initial and discharge evaluations, in Clinical Care and Information Systems in Psychiatry. Edited by Mezzich JE. Washington, DC, American Psychiatric Press, 1986. 192

Mezzich JE, Dow JT, Rich CL, Costello AJ, Himmelhoch JM: Developing an efficient clinical information system for a comprehensive psychiatric institute, II: the initial evaluation form. Behavior Research Methods and Instrumentation 13:464–478, 1981. 191
Michael J. 189, 200
Michael ST. 171, 245
Michelson L. 368
Michelson W (ed): Public policy in temporal perspective. The Hague, Mouton, 1978. 710
Midanik L: Alcohol problems and depressive symptoms in a national survey, in Psychosocial Constructs of Alcoholism and Substance Abuse. Edited by Stimmel B. New York, Haworth Press, 1983. 287, 291
Miles HWM, Barrabee EL, Finesinger JE: Evaluation of psychotherapy, with a follow-up study of 62 cases of anxiety neurosis. Psychosomatic Medicine 13:83, 1951. 242
Millar WM. 173
Miller H. 643
Miller LM. 252
Miller MD. 273
Miller P. 302
Miller RD. 260, 603
Miller SM. 499, 500, 506–509, 511, 518, 519, 528–530
Miller WC. 287
Miller WR: Psychological deficit in depression. Psychological Bulletin 82:238–260, 1975. 508
Miller WR, Seligman MEP: Learned helplessness, depression, and the perception of reinforcement. Behaviour Research and Therapy 14:7–17, 1976. 528
Miller WR, Seligman MEP, Kurlander HM: Learned helplessness, depression, and anxiety. Journal of Nervous and Mental Disease 161:347–357, 1975. 505, 617
Mineka S. 503
Mineka S: Depression and helplessness in primates, in Child Nurturance Series, Vol 3: Studies of Development in Nonhuman Primates. Edited by Fitzgerald H, Mullins A, Gage P. New York, Plenum, 1982. 503
Mineka S, Suomi S: Social separation in monkeys. Psychological Bulletin 85:1376–1400, 1978. 503
Mineka S, Suomi S, Delizio R: Multiple separations in adolescent monkeys: an opponent-process interpretation. Journal of Experimental Psychology: General 110:56–85, 1981. 504, 522
Minichiello WE. 314
Minkoff K, Bergman E, Beck AT, Beck R: Hopelessness, depression and attempted suicide. American Journal of Psychiatry 130:455–459, 1973. 528
Minors DS, Waterhouse JM: Circadian Rhythms and the Human. Bristol, J Wright & Sons Ltd, Stonebridge Press, 1981. 710
Mirin SM. 189, 200
Mirkin P. 661
Mirsky AF. 579
Mirsky A, Duncan C: Etiology and expression of schizophrenia: neurobiological and psychological factors. Annual Review of Psychology 37:291–319, 1986. 52
Mischel W: Personality and Assessment. New York, John Wiley, 1968. 710
Mitchell JE. 255

Mobley PL. 415, 432

Mochizuki T. 420

Mock J. 213, 226, 613, 644

Moga MM, Gray TS: Evidence for corticotropin-releasing factor, neurotensin, and somatostatin in the neural pathway from the central nucleus of the amygdala to the parabrachial nucleus. Journal of Comparative Neurology 241:275-284, 1985. 418

Mogg K, Mathews A, Weinman J: Memory bias in clinical anxiety. Journal of Abnormal Psychology 96:94–98, 1987. 632

Mohs R. 429, 432

Moldofsky H. 258

Moller MB. 396

Monakhov K, Perris C, Botskarev VK, von Knorring L, Nikiforov AI: Functional interhemispheric differences in relation to various psychopathological components of the depressive syndromes: a pilot international study. Neuropsychobiology 5:143–155, 1979. 573

Monroe SM. 477, 475, 481, 490, 491, 493, 494

Monroe SM: Assessment of life events: retrospective versus concurrent strategies. Archives of General Psychiatry 39:606–610, 1982a. 465

Monroe SM: Life events and disorder: event-symptom associations and the course of disorder. Journal of Abnormal Psychology 91:14–24, 1982b. 466

Monroe SM: Life events assessment: current practices, emerging trends. Clinical Psychology Review 2:435–453, 1982c. 465

Monroe SM: Major and minor life events as predictors of psychological distress: further issues and findings. Journal of Behavioral Medicine 6:189–205, 1983. 491

Monroe SM: Stress and social support: assessment issues, in Handbook of Research Methods in Cardiovascular Behavioral Medicine. Edited by Schneiderman P, Kaufman P, Weiss SM. New York, Plenum, 1989. 470

Monroe SM, Peterman AM: Life stress and psychopathology, in Research on Stressful Life Events: Theoretical and Methodological Issues. Edited by Cohen L. New York, Sage, 1988. 467, 468, 478, 479, 492, 493

Monroe SM, Steiner SC: Social support and psychopathology: interrelations with preexisting disorder, stress, and personality. Journal of Abnormal Psychology 95:29–39, 1986. 470, 492

Monroe SM, Thase ME, Hersen M, Bellack AS, Himmelhoch JM: Life events and the endogenous-nonendogenous distinction in the treatment course of depression. Comprehensive Psychiatry 26:175–186, 1985. 476

Monroe SM, Wade SL: Life events and anxiety disorders, in Handbook of Anxiety Disorders. Edited by Last CL, Hersen M. New York, Guilford, 1988. 478, 479

Monson RA. 250, 251, 252

Monson RR. 161, 167, 168, 169, 170, 171

Monson RR: Analysis of relative survival and proportional mortality. Computers and Biomedical Research 7:325–332, 1974. 169

Montgomery MA, Clayton PJ, Friedhof AJ: Psychiatric disorders in Tourette syndrome patients and first degree relatives, in Gilles de la Tourette Syndrome. Edited by Friedhof AJ, Chase TN. New York, Raven, 1982, pp 335–339. 310

Montgomery SA, Asberg M: A new depression scale designed to be sensitive to change. British Journal of Psychiatry 134:382–389, 1979. 256

Montgomery TA. 661

Moore TV: The essential psychoses and their fundamental syndromes. Catholic University Studies in Psychiatry and Psychology 3:1–2, 1933. 72, 80

Moos RM. 632

Moraitis S. 247

Morey LC: A comparative validation of the Foulds and Bedford hierarchy of psychiatric symptomatology. British Journal of Psychiatry 146:424–428, 1985. 79, 90

Morey LC: The Foulds hierarchy of personal illness: a review of recent research. Comprehensive Psychiatry 28:159–168, 1987. 78, 90

Morey LC, Skinner HA, Blashfield RK: A typology of alcohol abuse: correlates and implications. Journal of Abnormal Psychology 93:408–417, 1984. 80

Morgan J. 422

Morihisa J. 577

Morley JE. 421

Morley JE, Levine AS: Corticotropin releasing factor, grooming and ingestive behavior. Life Sciences 31:1459–1464, 1982. 420, 421

Moron P. 576

Morrell W. 254

Morris JN: The Uses of Epidemiology, 2nd Edition. Baltimore, Williams & Wilkins, 1964. 114

Morris RJ. 158, 159

Morse W. 422

Mortel K. 576

Moscovitch M, Strauss E, Olds J: Handedness and dichotic listening performance in patients with unipolar endogenous depression who received ECT. American Journal of Psychiatry 138:988–990, 1981. 572

Moser E. 576

Moss HB. 341, 342, 502

Mossberg D, Liljeberg P, Borg S: Clinical conditions in alcoholics during long-term abstinence: a descriptive longitudinal treatment study. Alcohol 2:551–553, 1985. 288, 290

Mould DE: Differentiation between depression and anxiety: a new scale. Journal of Consulting and Clinical Psychology 43:592, 1975.

Mountjoy CQ. 6, 48, 49, 54, 499, 707

Mountjoy CQ, Roth M: Studies in the relationship between depressive disorders and anxiety states, part 1: rating scales. Journal of Affective Disorders 4:127–147, 1982a. 414, 626

Mountjoy CQ, Roth M: Studies in the relationship between depressive disorders and anxiety states, part 2: clinical items. Journal of Affective Disorders 4:149–161, 1982b. 48, 54, 414

Mountjoy CQ, Roth M, Garside RF, Leitch IM: A clinical trial of phenelzine in anxiety, depressive and phobic neurosis. British Journal of Psychiatry 13:486–492, 1977. 700

Mouri T. 430

Mouyias A. 120

Mueller EA. 308

Mueller-Spahn F. 576

Muenz L. 570

Mukherjee B. 422

Mullaney JA: The relationship between anxiety and depression: a review of some principal component analytic studies. Journal of Affective Disorders 7:139–148, 1984. 54, 477

Mullaney JA, Trippett CJ: Alcohol dependence and phobias: clinical description and relevance. British Journal of Psychiatry 135:565–573, 1979. 290

Muller EE. 255

Muller JC, Pryor WW, Gibbons JE, Orgain ES: Depressions and anxiety during Rauwolfia therapy. Journal of the American Medical Association 159:836–840, 1955. 431

Muller OA. 430

Munetz MR. 192

Munjack DJ. 415

Munjack DJ, Moss HB: Affective disorder and alcoholism in families of agoraphobics. Archives of General Psychiatry 38:869–871, 1981. 341, 342

Munoz R. 8, 10, 24, 91, 114, 205, 254, 294, 337, 439, 449, 455, 457, 502, 694

Munro A: Some familial and social factors in depressive illness. British Journal of Psychiatry 112:429–441, 1966. 294

Munroe RH, Munroe RL: Effects of environmental experience on spatial ability in an East African society. Journal of Social Psychology 83:15–22, 1971a. 709

Munroe RH, Munroe RL: Household density and infant care in an East African society. Journal of Social Psychology 83:9–13, 1971b. 709

Munroe RL. 709

Murphy DL. 276, 308, 407, 571, 574, 643

Murphy GE. 332, 602

Murphy JM. 154, 159

Murphy JM: Psychiatric labeling in cross-cultural perspective. Science 191:1019–1028, 1976. 154

Murphy JM: War stress and civilian Vietnamese: a study of psychological effects. Acta Psychiatrica Scandinavica 56:92–108, 1977. 157, 158

Murphy JM: Continuities in community-based psychiatric epidemiology. Archives of General Psychiatry 37:1215–1223, 1980. 154, 155

Murphy JM: Psychiatric Instrument Development for Primary Care Research (NIMH Contract No. 80M014280101D). Rockville, MD, Division of Biometry and Epidemiology, 1981. 156

Murphy JM: Diagnosis, screening and "demoralization": epidemiologic implications. Psychiatric Developments 2:101–133, 1986a. 155

Murphy JM: The Stirling County Study, in Community Surveys of Psychiatric Disorders. Edited by Weissman MM, Myers JK, Ross C, in Monographs in Psychosocial Epidemiology. New Brunswick, NJ, Rutgers University Press, 1986b, pp 135–155. 155

Murphy JM: Trends in depression and anxiety: men and women. Acta Psychiatrica Scandinavica 73:113–127, 1986c. 168

Murphy JM: Depression screening instruments: history and issues, in Screening for Depression in Primary Care. Edited by Attkisson C, Zich J. New York, Routledge, Chapman & Hall, 1988. 156

Murphy JM, Berwick DM, Weinstein MC, Borus JF, Budman SH, Klerman GL: Performance of screening and diagnostic tests: application of receiver operating characteristic (ROC) analysis. Archives of General Psychiatry 44:550–555, 1987. 161

Murphy JM, Monson RR, Olivier DC, Sobol AM, Leighton AH: Affective disorders and mortality: a general population study. Archives of General Psychiatry 44:473–480, 1987. 169, 170, 171

Murphy JM, Monson RR, Olivier DC, Sobol AM, Pratt LA, Leighton AH: Mortality risk and psychiatric disorders: results of a general physician survey. Social Psychiatry and Psychiatric Epidemiology 24:134–142, 1989. 171, 172, 174

Murphy JM, Neff RK, Sobol AM, Rice JX Jr, Olivier DC: Computer diagnosis of depression and anxiety: the Stirling County Study. Psychological Medicine 15:99–112, 1985. 160

Murphy JM, Olivier DC, Sobol AM, Monson RR, Leighton AH: Diagnosis and outcome: depression and anxiety in a general population. Psychological Medicine 16:117–126, 1986. 167, 168

Murphy JM, Sobol AM, Neff RK, Olivier DC, Leighton AH: Stability of prevalence: depression and anxiety disorders. Archives of General Psychiatry 41:990–997, 1984. 137, 162, 165, 166, 167, 172, 333

Murphy JM, Sobol AM, Olivier DC, Monson RR, Leighton AH, Pratt LA: Prodromes of depression and anxiety: the Stirling County Study. British Journal of Psychiatry 155:490–495, 1989. 161

Murphy MC. 279

Murray RM. 306, 344, 345

Murray RM, Gurling HMD, Bernadt M, Ewusi-Mensah I, Saunders JD, Clifford CA: Do personality and psychiatric disorders predispose to alcoholism? in Pharmacological Treatments for Alcoholism. Edited by Edwards G, Littleton J. New York, Methuen, 1984. 287, 289

Myers JK. 115, 286, 287, 290, 294, 311, 317, 321, 414, 588, 705

Myers JK, Weissman MM, Tischler GL, Holzer CE, Leaf PJ, Orvaschel H, Anthony JC, Boyd JH, Burke JD, Kramer M, Stoltzman R: Six month prevalence of psychiatric disorders in three communities. Archives of General Psychiatry 41:959–967, 1984. 165, 168, 171, 589

Myren J, Lovland B, Larssen SE, Larsen S: Psychopharmacologic drugs in the treatment of the irritable bowel syndrome. Annales de Gastroenterologie et Hepatologie 20:117–123, 1984. 251

Naraghi M. 655

Narang RL. 505

Nash EH. 250

Nasrallah A. 294, 296, 301, 302, 305

Nathan PE, O'Brien JS, Lowenstein LM: Operant studies of chronic alcoholism: interaction of alcohol and alcoholics, in Biological Aspects of Alcohol. Edited by Roach PMK, McIsaac WM, Creaven PJ. Austin, TX, University of Texas Press, 1971. 283, 284

National Institute of Mental Health: NIMH Diagnostic Interview Schedule: Version III. Rockville, MD, National Institute of Mental Health, 1981. 321

National Institute of Mental Health, U.S. Department of Health and Human Services, Public Health Service, Alcohol, Drug Abuse, and Mental Health Administration: D/ART Program: Depression/Awareness, Recognition, Treatment. Washington, DC. National Institute of Mental Health, 1987. 251

Nee LE, Polinsky RJ, Ebert MH: Tourette's syndrome: clinical and family study, in Gilles de la Tourette Syndrome. Edited by Friedhof AJ, Chase TN. New York, Raven, 1982, pp 291–295. 310

Neff RK. 137, 160, 162, 165, 166, 167, 172, 333

Nelson JC. 327, 660

Nelson RO: Assessment and therapeutic functions of self-monitoring, in Progress in Behavior Modification, Vol 5. Edited by Hersen M, Eisler RM, Miller P. New York, Academic, 1977. 709, 716

Nelson RO, Lipinski DP, Boykin RA: The effect of self-recorders' training and the obtrusiveness of the self-recording device on the accuracy and reactivity of self-monitoring. Behavior Therapy 9:200–208, 1978. 716

Nelson WH. 290

Nemeroff CB. 404, 418, 424–428, 430–432

Nemeroff CB, Bissette G, Akil H, Fink M: Cerebrospinal fluid neuropeptides in depressed patients treated with ECT: corticotropin-releasing factor, β-endorphin, and somatostatin. British Journal of Psychiatry (in press). 433

Nemeroff CB, Knight DL, Krishnan KRR, Slotkin TA, Bissette G, Melville ML, Blazer DG: Marked reduction in the number of platelet ³H-imipramine binding sites in geriatric depression. Archives of General Psychiatry 45:919–923, 1988. 415

Nemeroff CB, Owens MJ, Bissette G, Andorn AC, Stanley M: Reduced corticotropin-releasing factor (CRF) binding sites in the frontal cortex of suicides. Archives of General Psychiatry 45:577–579, 1988. 428

Nemeroff CB, Widerlov E, Bissette G, Walleus H, Karlsson I, Eklund K, Kilts CD, Loosen PT, Vale W: Elevated concentrations of CSF corticotropin-releasing factor-like immunoreactivity in depressed patients. Science 226:1342–1344, 1984. 427, 428, 430

Nemiah JC: Hypochondriasis (hypochondriacal neurosis), in Comprehensive Textbook of Psychiatry, Vol. 2. Edited by Freedman AM, Kaplan HI, Sadock BJ. Baltimore, Williams & Wilkins, 1980, pp 1538–1543. 239

Nemiah JC, Sifneos PE: Psychosomatic illness: a problem in communication. Psychotherapy and Psychosomatics 18:154–160, 1970. 246

Nemzer E. 254

Nesse RM. 43, 53, 387, 586, 590

Nestadt G. 6, 44, 45, 61, 63, 93, 95, 97, 109, 118, 120, 137, 190, 204, 206, 221, 305, 307, 308, 311, 332, 333, 364, 439, 455, 649, 650, 661

Neufeld RWJ. 251

Neville B. 511

Newberry P. 288

Newman H. 158, 159

Neziroglu FA. 315

Nicassio P. 528

Nicholls MG. 417

Nichols MA. 247

Nicolson N. 710

Nielsen E. 297, 556

Nieman L. 255

Nies A. 290, 673

Nies A: Differential response patterns to MAO inhibitors and tricyclics. Journal of Clinical Psychiatry 45:70–77, 1984. 673

Nikiforov AI. 573

Nishikawa T, Scatton B: Neuroanatomical site of the inhibitory influence of anxiolytic drugs on central serotonergic transmission. Brain Research 371:123–132, 1986. 415

Nixon JM. 487

Noam GG. 548, 549, 550

Norman TR. 387, 390

Norman TR, Judd FK, Gregory M, James RH, Kimber NM, McIntyre IM, Burrows GD: Platelet serotonin uptake in panic disorder. Journal of Affective Disorders 11:69–72, 1986. 393

Norman WT: On estimating psychological relationships: social desirability and self report. Psychological Bulletin 67:273–293, 1967. 716

Norton GR, Harrison B, Hauch J, Rhodes L: Characteristics of people with infrequent panic attacks. Journal of Abnormal Psychology 94:216–221, 1985. 223

Norvell N, Brophy C, Finch AJ: The relationship of anxiety to childhood depression. Journal of Personality Assessment 49:150–153, 1985. 274

Noshirvani HF. 310

Noyes AP: Modern Clinical Psychiatry. Philadelphia, WB Saunders, 1949. 314

Noyes R Jr. 217, 335, 337, 338, 340, 341, 342, 344, 364, 386, 387, 472, 586, 592, 594, 607, 619

Noyes R Jr: Is panic disorder a disease for the medical model? Psychosomatics 28:582–586, 1987. 248

Noyes R Jr, Anderson DJ, Clancy J, Crowe RR, Slymen DJ, Ghoneim MM, Hinrichs JV: Diazepam and propranolol in panic disorder and agoraphobia. Archives of General Psychiatry 41:287–292, 1984. 703

Noyes R Jr, Clancy J, Crowe R, Hoenk PR, Slymen DJ: The familial prevalence of anxiety neurosis. Archives of General Psychiatry 35:1057–1059, 1978. 335, 337, 338, 344

Noyes R Jr, Clancy J, Hoenk PR, Slymen D: The prognosis of anxiety neurosis. Archives of General Psychiatry 37:173–178, 1978. 334

Noyes R Jr, Clarkson C, Crowe RR: A family study of generalized anxiety disorder. American Journal of Psychiatry 144:1019–1024, 1987. 343, 344

Noyes R Jr, Clarkson C, Crowe RR, Yates WR, McChesney CM: A family study of generalized anxiety disorder. American Journal of Psychiatry 144:1019–1024, 1987. 590, 594

Noyes R Jr, Crowe RR, Harris EL, Hamra BJ, McChesney CM, Chaudhry DR: Relationship between panic disorder and agoraphobia: a family study. Archives of General Psychiatry 43:227–232, 1986. 478, 580

Nugent H. 359

Nunnally JC. 505

Nurnberger JI. 254, 393, 394

Nutt DJ, Fraser S: Platelet binding studies in panic disorder. Journal of Affective Disorders 12:7–11, 1987. 394

Nystrom C, Matousek M, Hallstrom T: Relationships between EEG and clinical characteristics in major depressive disorder. Acta Psychiatrica Scandinavica 73:390–394, 1986. 574, 580

Oberg RGE. 581

O'Brien CP. 292

O'Brien GT. 207, 208, 209, 228, 590, 591, 635

O'Brien JS. 283, 284

Obrist WD. 570

O'Connor J. 255

O'Connor L. 404, 427

Oei TI, Zwart FM: The assessment of life events: self-administered questionnaire versus interview. Journal of Affective Disorders 10:185–190, 1986. 467, 468

O'Hara MW. 699, 701

Öhman A, Dimberg U, Öst LG: Animal and social phobias: biological constraints on learned fear responses, in Theoretical Issues in Behavior Therapy. Edited by Resis S, Bootzin RR. Orlando, FL, Academic, 1985. 636

Öjesjö L. 144, 168

Öjesjö L: Long-term outcome in alcohol abuse and alcoholism among males in the Lundby general population, Sweden. British Journal of Addiction 76:391–400, 1981. 300

Öjesjö L, Hagnell O, Lanke J: Incidence of alcoholism among men in the Lundby community cohort, Sweden, 1957-1972. Probabilistic baseline calculations. Journal of Studies on Alcohol 11:1190–1198, 1982. 147

Okada F. 432

Okada M. 613, 635

O'Keefe D. 251

Oldfield EH. 417, 430, 431, 433

Olds J. 572

Olivier DC. 137, 160, 161, 162, 165, 166, 167, 168, 169, 170, 171, 172, 333

Olivier DC, Neff RK: LOGLIN 1.0 User's Guide. Boston, Harvard University School of Public Health, 1974.

Olmstead MP. 261

O'Neill P. 285, 290

Opler MK. 171, 245

Oreland L. 491

Orgain ES. 431

Orley J, Wing JK: Psychiatric disorders in two African villages. Archives of General Psychiatry 36:513–520, 1979. 120

Ormel J. 42

Ornsteen M. 388

Ortman J. 30

Orvaschel H. 165, 168, 171, 317, 321, 589, 707

Orvaschel H: Parental depression and child psychopathology, in Childhood Psychopathology and Depression. Edited by Guze SB, Earls FJ, Barrett JE. New York, Raven, 1983, pp 53–66. 354, 355

Orvaschel H: Psychiatric interviews suitable for use in research with children and adolescents. Psychopharmacology Bulletin 21:737–745, 1985. 356

Orvaschel H, Walsh-Allis G, Ye W: Psychopathology in children of parents of recurrent depression. Journal of Abnormal Psychiatry 16:17–28, 1988. 354, 357

Oscar-Berman M, Zola-Morgan SM: Comparative neuropsychology and Korsakoff's syndrome, I: spatial and visual reversal learning. Neuropsychologia 18:499–512, 1980a. 581

Oscar-Berman M, Zola-Morgan SM: Comparative neuropsychology and Korsakoff's syndrome, II: two-choice visual discrimination learning. Neuropsychologia 18:513–525, 1980b. 581, 582

Oscar-Berman M, Zola-Morgan SM, Oberg RGE, Bonner RT: Comparative neuropsychology and Korsakoff's syndrome, III: delayed response, delayed alternation and DRL performance. Neuropsychologia 20:187–202, 1982. 581

Osgood CE, Suci GJ, Tannenbaum PH: The Measurement of Meaning. Urbana, IL, University of Illinois Press, 1957. 646

Osgood TB. 386, 387

Öst LG. 635

Oswald I, Brezinova V, Dunleavy DLF: On the slowness of action of tricyclic antidepressant drugs. British Journal of Psychiatry 120:673–677, 1972. 431

Othmer E. 284, 285

Othmer S. 296, 302

Ott I. 255

Otto W. 571, 575

Ottoson JO. 250

Overall JE. 414

Overall JE: The Brief Psychiatric Rating Scale psychopharmacology research: psychological measurements in psychopharmacology. Modern Problems in Pharmacopsychiatry 7:67–78, 1974. 719

Overall JE, Hollister LE, Johnson M, Pennington V: Nosology of depression and differential response to drugs. The Journal of the American Medical Association 195:946–948, 1966. 505

Overall JE, Zisook S: Diagnosis and the phenomenology of depressive disorders. Journal of Consulting and Clinical Psychology 48:626–634, 1980. 505

Owens DG. 700

Owens MJ. 256, 428

Owens MJ, Bissette G, Lundberg D, Nemeroff CB: Acute effects of antidepressant and anxiolytic drugs on CRF-LI in microdissected rat brain regions. Proceedings of the 26th annual meeting of the American College of Neuropsychopharmacology, 1987. 425

Padian NS. 327

Paez P. 273

Pahwa S. 151

Palkovits M. 418

Palmer CD, Harrison GA: Intercorrelation between sleep and activity patterns in Otmoor villages. Human Biology 55:749–762, 1983. 710

Palmer HD, Jones MS: Anorexia nervosa as a manifestation of compulsion neurosis. Archives of Neurological Psychiatry 41:856–858, 1939. 310

Palmer R. 415

Panerai AE. 255

Papp L. 672, 678

Pardes H. 653

Parker DC. 407

Parker RR. 673

Parkes C: Separation anxiety: an aspect of the search for a lost object, in British Journal of Psychiatry, Special Publication #3, Studies of Anxiety. Edited by Lader M, 1969. 536

Parkes C: The first year of bereavement: a longitudinal study of the reaction of London widows to the death of their husbands. Psychiatry 33:444–467, 1971. 536

Parkes CM: Bereavement: Studies of Grief in Adult Life, 2nd Edition. London, Tavistock, 1986. 602

Parrella D. 713

Parrish RT. 590

Pathak D. 243, 244, 246, 247

Patrie LE. 288

Patterson MB. 453

Paul SM. 429, 430, 432, 488

Paulauskas SL. 276, 279, 280, 281, 322, 360, 362

Pauls DC. 346, 347

Pauls DL. 44, 45, 94, 109, 206, 335, 337, 338, 340, 344, 364, 377, 478, 487, 499, 505, 580, 605, 607, 619

Pauls DL, Towbin KE, Leckman JF, Zahner GEP, Cohen DJ: Gilles de la Tourette's syndrome and obsessive-compulsive disorder: evidence supporting a genetic relationship. Archives of General Psychiatry 43:1180–1182, 1986. 310, 563

Paulus PB. 528

Paykel ES. 489, 622, 673

Paykel ES: Depressive typologies and response to amitriptyline. British Journal of Psychiatry 120:147–156, 1972. 505

Paykel ES: Life events and psychiatric disorder, in Stressful Life Events: Their Nature and Effects. Edited by Dohrenwend BS, Dohrenwend BP. New York, John Wiley, 1974, pp 135–149. 480, 483

Paykel ES: Depression and appetite. Journal of Psychosomatic Research 21:401–407, 1977. 257, 260

Paykel ES: Life events and early environment, in Handbook of Affective Disorders. Edited by Paykel ES. New York, Guilford, 1982. 465, 466, 475, 476, 479, 481, 488

Paykel ES: The clinical interview for depression. Development, reliability, and validity. Journal of Affective Disorders 9:85–96, 1985. 261

Paykel ES, McGuiness B, Gomez J: An Anglo-American comparison of the scaling of life events. British Journal of Medical Psychology 49:237–243, 1976. 480

Paykel ES, Meyers JK, Dienelt MN, Klerman GL, Lindenthal JJ, Pepper MP: Life events and depressions: a controlled study. Archives of General Psychiatry 21:753–760, 1969. 483, 629

Paykel ES, Parker RR, Penrose RJJ, Rassaby ER: Depressive classification and prediction of response to phenelzine. British Journal of Psychiatry 134:572–581, 1979. 673

Paykel ES, Prusoff BA, Klerman GL, DiMascio A: Self-report and clinical interview ratings in depression. Journal of Nervous and Mental Disease 156:166–182, 1973. 719

Paykel ES, Rowan PR, Parker RR, Bhat A: Response to phenelzine and amitriptyline in subtypes of outpatient depression. Archives of General Psychiatry 39:1041–1049, 1982. 673

Paykel ES, Rowan PR, Rao BM, Bhat A: Atypical depression: nosology and response to antidepressants, in Treatment of Depression: Old Controversies and New Approaches. Edited by Clayton R, Barrett J. New York, Raven, 1983. 673

Pearson ES: The analysis of variance in cases of non-normal variation. Biometrika 23:114–133, 1931. 628

Pecknold JC. 586, 592, 594, 607

Pecknold JC, McClure DJ, Appeltauer L: Does tryptophan potentiate clomipramine in the treatment of agoraphobic and social phobic patients. British Journal of Psychiatry 140:484–490, 1982. 703

Peeke HVS. 502

Pendleton L. 453

Penick EC, Powell BJ, Othmer E, Bingham SF, Rice AS, Liese BS: Subtyping alcoholics by coexisting psychiatric syndromes: course, family history, outcome, in Longitudinal Research in Alcoholism. Edited by Goodwin DW, Van Dusen KT, Mednick SA. Boston, Kluwer-Nijhoff, 1984. 284, 285

Pennebaker JW: The Psychology of Physical Symptoms. New York, Springer-Verlag, 1982. 246

Pennebaker JW: Traumatic experience and psychosomatic disease: exploring the roles of behavioural inhibition, obsession, and confiding. Canadian Journal of Psychology 26:82–95, 1985. 246

Pennebaker JW, Burnam MA, Schaeffer MA, Harper DC: Lack of control as a determinant of perceived physical symptoms. Journal of Personality and Social Psychology 35:167–174, 1977. 247

Pennington V. 505

Penrose RJJ. 673

Pepper MP. 483, 629

Perez FM Jr. 417

Perlmutter J. 396, 577, 586

Perris C. 573

Perris H, von Knorring L, Oreland L, Perris C: Life events and biological vulnerability: a study of life events and platelet MAO activity in depressed patients. Psychiatric Research 12:111–120, 1984. 491

Perry JC: Depression in borderline personality disorder: lifetime prevalence at interview and longitudinal course of symptoms. American Journal of Psychiatry 142:15–21, 1985. 326

Perry JC: A prospective study of life stress, defenses, psychotic symptoms, and depression in borderline and antisocial personality disorders and bipolar type II affective disorder. Journal of Personality Disorders 2:49–59, 1988. 558

Perry JC, Cooper SH: A preliminary report on defenses and conflicts associated with borderline personality disorder. Journal of the American Psychoanalytic Association 34:863–893, 1986a. 548, 549, 551

Perry JC, Cooper SH: What do cross-sectional measures of defenses predict? in Empirical Studies of the Ego Mechanisms of Defense. Edited by Vaillant GE. Washington, DC, American Psychiatric Press, 1986b. 548, 549, 550, 551

Perry JC, Cooper SH: Empirical Studies of Psychological Defense Mechanisms, in Psychiatry. Edited by Michels R, Cavenar JO. Philadelphia, JB Lippincott, 1987. 547, 551

Perry JC, Cooper SH: An empirical study of defense mechanisms, I: clinical interview and life vignette ratings. Archives of General Psychiatry 46:444–452, 1989. 548, 549, 551, 555

Perry JC, Lavori PW, Pagano CJ, O'Connell ME, Hoke L: The relationship between stressful life events and recurrence of depression in borderline and antisocial personality disorders and bipolar type II affective disorder, manuscript submitted for publication.

Persson R. 432

Perugi G. 599

Perus C. 491

Pervin LA: Personality: current controversies, issues and directions. Annual Review of Psychology 36:83–114, 1985. 708

Peselow ED, Baxter N, Fieve RR, Barouche F: The dexamethasone suppression test as a monitor of clinical recovery. American Journal of Psychiatry 144:130–135, 1987. 388

Peterman AM. 467, 468, 478, 479, 492, 493

Peterson C. 517

Peterson C, Seligman MEP: Causal explanations as a risk factor for depression: theory and evidence. Psychological Review 91:347–374, 1984. 581

Peterson GA, Ballenger JC, Cox DP, Hucek A, Lydiard RB, Laraia MT, Trockman C: The dexamethasone suppression test in agoraphobia. Journal of Clinical Psychopharmacology 5:100–102, 1985. 387

Peterson RA. 223

Petraglia F, Sutton S, Vale W, Plotsky P: Corticotropin-releasing factor decreases plasma luteinizing hormone levels in female rats by inhibiting gonadotropin-releasing hormone release into hypophysial-portal circulation. Endocrinology 120:1083–1088, 1987. 422

Petrie A: Individuality in Pain and Suffering. Chicago, University of Chicago Press, 1967. 244

Petrie K, Chamberlain K: Hopelessness and social desirability as moderator variables in predicting suicidal behavior. Journal of Consulting and Clinical Psychology 51:485–487, 1983. 528

Petrusz P. 418

Petrusz P, Merchenthaler I, Maderdrut JL, Heitz PU: Central and peripheral distribution of corticotropin-releasing factor. Fed Proc 44:229–235, 1985. 424

Petsche H. 574

Petzel TP. 645

Pfeffer JM: Hyperventilation and the hyperventilation syndrome. Postgraduate Medical Journal 60 (Suppl 2):12–15, 1984. 249

Pfefferbaum A, Wenegrat BG, Ford JM, Roth WT, Kopell BS: Clinical application of the P3 component of event-related potentials, II: dementia, depression and schizophrenia. Electroencephalography and Clinical Neurophysiology 59:104–124, 1984. 574

Pfister H. 660, 662, 664

Pfohl B. 386, 388, 392, 468

Pfohl B, Coryell W, Zimmerman M: DSM-III personality disorders: diagnostic overlap and internal consistency of individual DSM-III criteria. Comprehensive Psychiatry 27:21–34, 1986. 331

Phelps M. 577

Phil M. 419, 432

Phillips S. 572

Phol R. 387

Pickar D. 429, 430, 432, 488, 577

Pickens R. 656, 664

Picton TW. 574

Pinsker H. 502

Piran N, Kennedy S, Garfinkel PE, Owens M: Affective disturbance in eating disorders. Journal of Nervous and Mental Disease 173:395–400, 1985. 256

Pitman RK, Green RC, Jenike MA, Mesulam M: Clinical comparison of Tourette's disorder and obsessive-compulsive disorder. American Journal of Psychiatry 144:1166–1171, 1987. 310, 312

Pitts FN: Biochemical factors in anxiety neurosis. New England Journal of Medicine 277:1329–1336, 1971. 707

Pliner LF. 249

Plotsky P. 422

Plotsky PM, Vale W: Hemorrhage-induced secretion of corticotropin-releasing factor-like immunoreactivity into the rat hypophyseal portal circulation and its inhibition by glucocorticoids. Endocrinology 114:164–169, 1984. 417

Plutchik R: Measurement implications of a psychoevolutionary theory of emotions, in Assessment and Modification of Emotional Behavior. Edited by Blankstein KR, Pliner P, Polivy J. New York, Plenum, 1980. 645

Pockberger H, Petsche H, Rappelsberger P, Zidek B, Zapotoczky HG: Ongoing EEG in depression: a topographic spectral analytical pilot study. Electroencephalography and Clinical Neurophysiology 61:349–358, 1985. 574

Pohl R. 411

Poland RE. 387, 488, 575

Poland RE, Rubin RT, Lane LA, Martin DJ, Rose DE, Lesser IM: A modified dexamethasone suppression test for endogenous depression. Psychiatry Research 15:293–299, 1985. 404

Poland RE, Rubin RT, Lesser IM, Lane LA, Hart PJ: Neuroendocrine aspects of primary endogenous depression, II: serum dexamethasone concentrations and hypothalamic-pituitary-adrenal cortical activity as determinants of the dexamethasone suppression test response. Archives of General Psychiatry 44:790–795, 1987. 405, 406

Polinsky RJ. 310

Polivy J. 261

Pollack CP. 255

Pollak JM: Obsessive-compulsive personality: a review. Psychological Bulletin 86:225–241, 1979. 313

Pollitt J: Natural history of obsessional states. British Medical Journal 1:194–198, 1957. 306, 315

Pollock M. 322

Polsky RH. 709

Popa GT, Fielding U: A portal circulation from the pituitary to the hypothalamic region. Journal of Anatomy 65:88, 1930. 416

Pope HG. 255

Popkin MK, Callies AL, Lentz RD, Colon EA, Sutherland DE: Prevalence of major depression, simple phobia, and other psychiatric disorders in patients with longstanding type I diabetes mellitus. Archives of General Psychiatry 45:64–68, 1988. 327

Popper C. 200

Porjesz B. 290

Porjesz B, Begleiter H: Human brain electrophysiology and alcoholism, in Alcohol and the Brain. Edited by Tarter RE, Van Thiel DH. New York, Plenum, 1985. 290

Portwood MF: Chronic fatigue syndrome: a diagnosis for consideration. Nurse Practitioner 2:11–12, 15–18, 23, 1988. 151

Post RM. 388, 393, 395, 415, 430, 433, 523, 570, 575, 577, 602, 603, 607, 703

Postpischil F. 311

Poterzio F. 255

Pottash ALC. 407

Pottenger M. 294, 296, 323

Pottenger M, McKernon J, Patrie LE, Weissman MM, Ruben HL, Newberry P: The frequency and persistence of depressive symptoms in the alcohol abuser. Journal of Nervous and Mental Disease 166:562–570, 1978. 288

Potter L. 414

Powell BJ. 284, 285

Powers SI. 548, 549, 550

Poznanski EO, Krahenguhl V, Zrull JP: Childhood depression: a longitudinal perspective. Journal of the American Academy of Child Psychiatry 15:491–501, 1976. 362

Prabucki K. 354–357

Prange AJ. 290, 394

Pratt LA. 161, 171, 172, 174

Presly AS. 90

Price DT. 273

Price LH. 390, 660

Price LH, Charney DS, Rubin L, Heninger GR: Alpha-2 adrenergic receptor function in depression. Archives of General Psychiatry 43:849–858, 1986. 389

Price RA, Kidd KK, Weissman MM: Early onset (under age 30 years) and panic disorder as markers for etiologic homogeneity in major depression. Archives of General Psychiatry 44:434–440, 1987. 272, 649, 650

Price TR. 327

Pringuey D. 597

Pritchard WS: Psychophysiology of P300. Psychological Bulletin 89:506–540, 1981.

Proctor JD. 528

Prudo R, Harris T, Brown GW: Psychiatric disorder in a rural and an urban population, 3: social integration and the morphology of affective disorder. Psychological Medicine 14:327–345, 1984. 470, 474, 486, 488, 493, 494

Prusoff BA. 44, 45, 94, 109, 206, 275, 318, 322, 327, 336, 346, 347, 348, 352,

354–358, 360, 361, 363, 364, 377, 478, 487, 499, 505, 580, 605, 619, 719

Prusoff BA, Klerman GL: Differentiating depressed from anxious neurotic outpatients. Archives of General Psychiatry 30:302–308, 1974. 54, 475, 499, 505, 508, 509, 624, 700

Prusoff BA, Klerman GL, Paykel ES: Concordance between clinical assessments and patients' self-report in depression. Archives of General Psychiatry 26:546–552, 1972. 622

Pruyn JP. 237

Pruyser P. 585

Pry G. 642

Pryor WW. 431

Przybeck TR. 286

Puig-Antich J. 260, 273

Puig-Antich J: Affective disorders in childhood: a review and perspectives. Psychiatric Clinics of North America 3:403–424, 1980. 353

Puig-Antich J: Affective disorders in children and adolescents: diagnostic validity and psychobiology, in Psychopharmacology: A Third Generation of Progress. Edited by Meltzer H. New York, Raven, 1987, pp 843–861. 360, 361

Puig-Antich J, Rabinovich H: Relationship between affective and anxiety disorders in childhood, in Anxiety Disorders of Childhood. Edited by Gittelman R. New York, Guilford, 1986. 273

Pulver AE, Carpenter WT Jr: Lifetime psychotic symptoms assessed with the DIS. Schizophrenia Bulletin 9:377–382, 1983. 179

Purtell JJ. 248

Purtillo D. 151

Puthezhath N. 53, 712

Puzantian VR. 341, 346, 378, 478, 602, 606, 709, 719

Pyke R. 414

Pyszczynski T, Greenberg J: Self-regulatory perseveration and the depressive self-focusing style: a self-awareness theory of reactive depression. Psychological Bulletin 102:122–138, 1987. 509, 527

Qualls CB. 404

Quinlan DM. 327, 554

Quitkin FM. 572, 604, 673, 675

Quitkin FM, Liebowitz MR, Klein DF: Comparison of monoamine oxidase inhibitors and tricyclic antidepressants in the treatment of depression, in Treatment of Depression: Old Controversies and New Approaches. Edited by Clayton P, Barrett J. New York, Raven, 1983. 673

Quitkin FM, Rabkin JG, Stewart JW, McGrath PJ, Harrison W, Davies M, Goetz R, Puig-Antich J: Sleep of atypical depressives. Journal of Affective Disorders 8:61–67, 1985. 260

Quitkin FM, Stewart JW, McGrath PJ, Liebowitz MR, Harrison WM, Tricamo E, Klein DF, Rabkin JG, Markowitz J, Wager SG: Phenelzine vs. imipramine in probable atypical depression: defining syndrome boundaries of selective MAOI responders. American Journal of Psychiatry 145:3, 1988. 673, 674

Rabinovich H. 273

Rabkin JG. 260, 570, 604, 673, 674

Racagni G, Smeraldi E: Anxious Depression: Assessment and Treatment. New York, Raven, 1987. 597

Rachman S. 308

Rachman S: The conditioning theory of fear acquisition: a critical examination. Behaviour Research Therapy 15:375–387, 1977. 635

Rachman SJ, Hodgson RJ: Obsessions and Compulsions. Englewood Cliffs, NJ, Prentice-Hall, 1980. 503

Rachman S, Levitt K: Panics and their consequences. Behaviour Research Therapy 23:585–600, 1985. 523

Rachman SJ, Levitt K, Lopatka C: Panic: the links between cognitions and bodily symptoms, I. Behaviour Research Therapy 25:411–423, 1987. 622

Raczynski JM. 227, 244

Rader L. 359

Rae DS. 6, 44, 45, 61, 63, 93, 95, 97, 109, 115, 116, 118, 120, 137, 190, 204, 206, 221, 305, 307, 308, 311, 332, 333, 364, 439, 455, 649, 650, 664, 666

Rahe RH. 465, 466

Raichle ME. 396, 577, 589

Rainey JM. 387

Rainey M, Ettedugi E, Pfohl B, Balon R, Weinberg P, Yelonek S, Berchou R: The beta receptor: isoproterenol anxiety states. Psychopathology 17:40–51, 1984. 392

Raisman R. 414

Raisys V. 394

Rao BM. 673

Rao K. 327

Rapee RM. 223

Rapee RM, Sanderson WC, Barlow DH: Social phobia features across the DSM-III-R anxiety disorders. Journal of Psychopathology Behavior Assessment, in press. 228

Rapoport JL. 315, 571

Rapoport J, Elkins R, Langer DH, Sceery W, Buchsbaum MS, Gillin JC, Murphy DL, Zahn TP, Lake R, Ludlow C, Mendelson W: Childhood obsessive compulsive disorder. American Journal of Psychiatry 138:1545–1554, 1981. 276, 571

Rapoport RN. 154

Rappelsberger P. 574

Raskin A. 256

Raskin A, Schulterbrandt J, Reatig N, McKeon J: Replication of factors of psychopathology in interview, word behavior and self-report ratings of hospitalized depressives. Journal of Nervous and Mental Disease 148:87–98, 1969. 235

Raskin M, Peeke HVS, Dickman W, Pinsker H: Panic and generalized anxiety disorders: developmental antecedents and precipitants. Archives of General Psychiatry 39:687–689, 1982. 502

Rasmussen SA, Tsuang MT: Clinical characteristics in family history in DSM-III obsessive compulsive disorder. American Journal of Psychiatry 143:317–322, 1986a. 310, 312

Rasmussen SA, Tsuang MT: Epidemiology and clinical features of obsessive compulsive disorder, in Obsessive Compulsive Disorders: A Theory of Management. Edited by Jenike MA, Baer L, Minichiello WE. Littleton, MA, PSG Publishing, 1986b, pp 23–44. 307, 312, 314

Rassaby ER. 673

Ratcliff KS. 93, 159, 592, 656, 661

Ravaris CL. 673

Ravaris L, Robinson DS, Ives O, Nies A, Bartett D: Phenelzine and amitriptyline in the treatment of depression. Archives of General Psychiatry 37:1075–1080, 1980. 673

Ravel JL. 154, 157

Watson D. Orlando, FL, Academic, 1989, pp 55–79. 648

Rehm LP: Self-management and cognitive processes in depression, in Cognitive Processes in Depression. Edited by Alloy LB. New York, Guilford (in press). 648

Rehm LP, Fuchs CZ, Roth DM, Kornblith SJ, Romano JM: A comparison of self-control and assertion skills treatments of depression. Behavior Therapy 10:429–442, 1979. 642

Rehm LP, O'Hara MW: Item characteristics of the Hamilton Rating Scale for Depression. Journal of Psychiatric Research 19:31–41, 1985. 699, 701

Reich J: The epidemiology of anxiety. Journal of Nervous and Mental Disease 174:129–136, 1986. 590, 623, 624

Reich LH, Davis RK, Himmelhoch JM: Excessive alcohol use in manic-depressive illness. American Journal of Psychiatry 131:83–85, 1974. 288

Reich T. 285, 296, 302, 308, 453, 666, 684

Reich W. 666, 713

Reichler RJ. 354–358

Reichlin S. 417

Reid DE. 248

Reid JC. 275, 279, 317, 322, 360, 361

Reid N. 712

Reidenberg MM, Lowenthal DT: Adverse non-drug reactions. New England Journal of Medicine 279:678–679, 1968. 247

Reiman EM, Raichle ME, Butler FK, Herscovitch P, Robins E: A focal brain abnormality in panic disorder, a severe form of anxiety. Nature 310:683–685, 1984. 577

Reiman EM, Raichle ME, Robins E, Butler FK, Herscovitch P, Fox P, Perlmutter J: The application of positron emission tomography to the study of panic disorder. American Journal of Psychiatry 143:469–477, 1986. 396, 577, 586

Reisberg B. 386

Reiss S, Peterson RA, Gursky DM, McNally RJ: Anxiety sensitivity, anxiety frequency and the prediction of fearfulness. Behaviour Research and Therapy 24:1–8, 1986. 223

Reivich M. 570

Reker D. 574

Remington M. 472

Rennie TAC. 171, 245

Renshaw DC: Suicide and depression in children. Journal of School Health 44:487–489, 1974. 272

Resnick JS. 354, 355, 357

Resnick SM. 570

Rey AC. 570

Reynolds GP. 430

Reynolds TD: Fluctuations in schizophrenic behavior. Medical Annals of the District of Columbia 34:520-549, 1965. 709, 710

Rhodes L. 223

Rholes WS. 512

Rholes WS, Riskind JH, Neville B: The relationship of cognitions and hopelessness to depression and anxiety. Social Cognition 3:36–50, 1985. 511

Rice AS. 284, 285

Rice J. 160, 666, 684

Rice JP, Endicott J, Knesevich MA, Rochberg N: The estimation of diagnostic sensitivity using stability data: an application to major depressive disorder. Journal of Psychiatric Research 21:337–345, 1987. 689

Rich CL. 191

Richards C. 276, 279, 280, 281

Richardson JS. 415, 419

Rickels K. 54, 158, 159, 240, 256, 388, 414, 506, 508, 509, 619, 624, 627, 674, 676, 702

Rickels K, Feighner JP, Smith WT: Alprazolam, amitriptyline, doxepin and placebo in the treatment of depression. Archives of General Psychiatry 42:134–141, 1985. 699, 703

Rider E. 548, 549, 550

Rifkin A. 586, 592, 594, 607

Riggi SJ. 431

Rigoni F. 120

Riley G. 700

Rimoldi HJA: Behavior Inventory. Chicago, University of Chicago Press, 1950. 157

Risch SC. 407, 420

Risch SC, Janowsky DS, Gillin JC: Muscarinic supersensitivity of anterior pituitary ACTH and beta-endorphin release in major depressive illness. Peptides 789–792, 1983. 411

Riskind JH. 218, 225, 496, 509, 511, 528, 529, 631

Riskind JH: Attributional patterns in anxiety: a model of appraisal, semantic space, and associative pathways, manuscript under editorial review. 500

Riskind JH, Beck AT, Berchick RJ, Brown G, Steer RA: Reliability of DSM-III diagnoses for major depression and generalized anxiety disorder using the Structured Clinical Interview for DSM-III. Archives of General Psychiatry 44:817–820, 1987. 700

Riskind JH, Beck AT, Brown GB, Steer RA: Taking the measure of anxiety and depression: validity of reconstructed Hamilton scales. Journal of Nervous and Mental Disease 175:474–479, 1987. 219

Riskind JH, Rholes WS, Brannon WS, Burdick CA: Attributions and expectations: a confluence of vulnerabilities in mild depression in a college student population. Journal of Personality and Social Psychology 53:349–354, 1987. 512

Ritchie J. 418, 424–426, 431

Rittmaster R. 255

Rivier C. 416, 417, 420

Rivier C, Rivier J, Vale W: Inhibition of adrenocorticotropic hormone secretion in the rat by immunoneutralization of corticotropin-releasing factor. Science 218:377–378, 1982. 417, 423

Rivier C, Rivier J, Vale W: Stress-induced inhibition of reproductive functions: role of endogenous corticotropin-releasing factor. Science 20:607–609, 1986. 422

Rivier JE. 416–422, 425

Rivinus T. 254

Rivinus TM, Biederman J, Herzog DB, Kemper K, Harper GP, Harmatz JS, Houseworth S: Anorexia nervosa and affective disorders: a controlled family history study. American Journal of Psychiatry 141:1414–1418, 1984. 254

Robbins DR. 277, 280

Roberts AH: Housebound wives: a follow-up study of a phobic anxiety state. British Journal of Psychiatry 110:191–194, 1964. 479

Roberts N. 273, 274

Robertson AG, Jackman H, Meltzer HY. Prolactin response to morphine in depression. Psychiatry Research 11:353–364, 1984. 408

Robertson J, Bowlby J: Responses of young children to separation from their mothers. Courrier Centre Inter Enfance 2:131–142, 1952. 503

Robertson MM. 310

Robertson MM, Trimble MR: Major tranquilizers used as antidepressants. Journal of Affective Disorders 4:173–193, 1982. 700

Robins AJ. 279

Robins E. 8, 22, 24, 42, 91, 92, 114, 181, 205, 232, 248, 254, 256, 273, 286, 294, 297, 306–308, 318, 321, 337, 339, 396, 405, 427, 439, 449, 455, 457, 483, 502, 577, 589, 593, 673, 682, 694

Robins E, Guze SB: Establishment of diagnostic validity in psychiatric illness: its application to schizophrenia. American Journal of Psychiatry 126:983–987, 1970. 8, 52, 113, 163, 598

Robins E, Guze SB: Classification of affective disorders: the primary-secondary, the endogenous-reactive, and the neurotic-psychotic concepts, in Recent Advances in the Psychobiology of the Depressive Illnesses (DHEW Publication 70-9053). Edited by Williams TA, Katz MM, Shield JA Jr. Washington, DC, U.S. Government Printing Office, 1972, pp 283–293. 294

Robins LN. 115, 159, 315, 321, 588, 590, 661, 705

Robins L: Psychiatric epidemiology. Archives of General Psychiatry 35:697–702, 1978. 24

Robins LN, Bates WM, O'Neill P: Adult drinking patterns of former problem children, in Society, Culture, and Drinking Patterns. Edited by Pittman DJ, Snyder CR. New York, John Wiley, 1962. 285, 290

Robins LN, Helzer JE, Croughan J, Ratcliff KS: National Institute of Mental Health Diagnostic Interview Schedule: its history, characteristics, and validity. Archives of General Psychiatry 38:381–389, 1981. 93, 159, 592, 656, 661

Robins LN, Helzer JE, Przybeck TR: Epidemiological perspective on alcoholism: ECA data. Presented at the annual meeting of the American Psychopathological Association, 1986. 286

Robins LN, Helzer JE, Ratcliff KS, Seyfried W: Validity of the Diagnostic Interview Schedule, Version II: DSM-III diagnoses. Psychological Medicine 12:855–870, 1982. 656, 661

Robins LN, Helzer JE, Weissman MM, Orvaschel H, Gruenberg E, Burke JD Jr, Regier DA: Lifetime prevalence of specific psychiatric disorders in three sites. Archives of General Psychiatry 41:949–958, 1984. 165, 313, 317, 321, 589, 707

Robins LN, Wing J, Wittchen H-U, Helzer JE, Babor TF, Burke JD, Farmer A, Jablensky A, Pickens R, Regier DA, Sartorius N, Towle LH: The Composite International Diagnostic Interview: an epidemiologic instrument suitable for use in conjunction with different diagnostic systems and in different cultures. Archives of General Psychiatry 45:1069–1077, 1988. 656, 664

Robinson DS. 322, 673

Robinson DS, Kayser A, Corcella J, Laux D, Yingling K, Howard D: Panic attacks in outpatients with depression: response to antidepressant treatment. Psychopharmacology Bulletin 21:562–566, 1985. 673

Robinson DS, Nies A, Ravaris CL, Lamborn KR: The monoamine oxidase inhibitor, phenelzine, in the treatment of depressive-anxiety states. Archives of General Psychiatry 29:407–413, 1973. 673

Robinson J: How Americans Use Time: A Social-Psychological Analysis of Everyday Behavior. New York, Praeger, 1977. 710, 715

Robinson RG, Lipsey JR, Rao K, Price TR: Two year longitudinal study of poststroke mood disorders: comparison of acute-onset with delayed-onset depression. American Journal of Psychiatry 143:1238–1244, 1986. 327

Robson AM. 456

Rochberg N. 689

Rock JP, Oldfield EH, Schulte HM, Gold PW, Kornblith PL, Loriaux L, Chrousos GP: Corticotropin releasing factor administered into the ventricular CSF stimulates the pituitary-adrenal axis. Brain Research 323:365–368, 1984. 417

Roelofs SM: Hyperventilation, anxiety, craving for alcohol: a subacute alcohol withdrawal syndrome. Alcohol 2:501–505, 1985. 291

Roemer RA. 575

Roffwarg H. 255, 427

Rogan WJ, Gladen B: Estimating prevalence from the results of a screening test. American Journal of Epidemiology 107:71–76, 1978. 692

Rogers B. 421

Rollnick S. 300

Romanik R. 244, 246, 247

Romano JM. 642

Romanoski AJ. 661

Romer D. 517

Room R: Measurement and distribution of drinking patterns and problems in general populations, in Alcohol-Related Disabilities (WHO Offset Publication No 32). Edited by Edwards G, Gross MM, Keller M, Moser J, Room R. Geneva, World Health Organization, 1977, pp 61–87. 302, 303

Roose SP. 255, 256

Rorer LG: The great response-style myth. Psychological Bulletin 63:129–156, 1965. 716

Rorsman B. 144, 168

Rorsman B, Hagnell O, Lanke J, Öjesjö L: Incidence of anxiety in the Lundby study: changes over time during a quarter of a century. Neuropsychobiology 18:13–20, 1987. 144

Rose DE. 404, 575

Rose RM. 465

Rosen G. 243

Rosen G: Social stress and mental disease from the eighteenth century to the present: some origins of social psychiatry. The Milbank Memorial Fund Quarterly 1:5–32, 1958. 464

Rosen I: The clinical significance of obsessions in schizophrenia. Journal of Mental Science 103:773–785, 1957. 306, 307

Rosenbaum JF. 676

Rosenberg CM: Personality and obsessional neurosis. British Journal of Psychiatry 113:471–477, 1967. 312, 314

Rosenberg CM: Complications of obsessional neurosis. British Journal of Psychiatry 114:477–478, 1968. 306, 307

Rosenberg L. 503

Rosenberg S: The relationship of certain personality factors to prognosis in psychotherapy. Journal of Clinical Psychology 10:341–345, 1954. 250

Rosenberg TK. 275, 279, 317, 322, 360, 361

Rosenblum LA. 521

Rosenfeld H. 158, 159

Rosenhan DL: On being sane in insane places. Science 179:250–258, 1973. 20

Rosenthal D. 29, 30

Rosenthal D: Genetics of Psychopathology. New York, McGraw-Hill, 1971. 336

Rosenthal M. 420

Rosenthal RH. 318, 325, 327

Rosenthal TL. 53, 317, 322, 325, 341, 346, 378, 602, 606, 709, 719

Ross DC. 43, 675

Ross E. 395

Rossi J. 713

Rosvold HE, Mirsky AF, Sarason I, Bransome ED, Beck LH: A continuous performance test of brain damage. Journal of Consulting Psychology 20:343–350, 1956. 579

Roth DM. 642

Roth D, Rehm LP, Rozensky RA: Self-reward, self-punishment and depression. Psychological Reports 47:3–7, 1980. 642

Roth KA. 424

Roth M. 24, 48, 54, 71, 414, 599, 626, 700

Roth M: The phobic anxiety-depersonalization syndrome. Proceedings of The Royal Society of Medicine 52:587–595, 1959. 536

Roth M: The phobic anxiety-depersonalization syndrome and some general etiological problems in psychiatry. Journal of Neuropsychiatry 1:293, 1960. 536

Roth M, Gurney C, Garside R, Kerr T: Studies in the classification of affective disorders: the relationship between anxiety states and depressive illness–I. British Journal of Psychiatry 121:147–161, 1972. 54, 331, 506, 508, 509, 599, 619

Roth M, Mountjoy CQ: The distinction between anxiety states and depressive disorders, in Handbook of Affective Disorders. Edited by Paykel ES. New York, Guilford, 1982. 6, 48, 49, 54, 499, 707

Roth RH. 425

Roth RS. 581

Roth S, Kubal L: Effects of noncontingent reinforcement on tasks of differing importance: facilitation and learned helplessness. Journal of Personality and Social Psychology 32:680–691, 1975. 504

Roth WT. 392, 574, 712, 713

Rothenberg A: Eating disorder as a modern obsessive-compulsive syndrome. Psychiatry 49:45–53, 1986. 311

Rothschild AJ. 386

Roubicek J. 573

Rounsaville BJ. 603

Rounsaville BJ, Dolinisky ZS, Babor TF, and Meyer RE: Psychopathology as a predictor of treatment outcome in alcoholics. Archives of General Psychiatry 44:505–513, 1987. 235, 285, 286, 288, 300, 302

Rounsaville BJ, Kosten TR, Weissman MM, Kleber HD: Prognostic significance of psychopathology in treated opiate addicts. Archives of General Psychiatry 43:739–745, 1986. 302

Rounsaville BJ, Sholomkas D, Prusoff BA: Chronic mood disorders in depressed outpatients. Journal of Affective Disorders 2:73–88, 1980. 318, 322

Rowan PR. 673

Rowan PR, Paykel ES, Parker RR: Phenelzine and amitriptyline: effects on symptoms of neurotic depression. British Journal of Psychiatry 140:475–483, 1982. 673

Roy A. 430, 433

Roy A, Pickar D, Linnoila M, Doran AR, Paul SM: Cerebrospinal fluid monoamine and monoamine metabolite levels and the dexamethasone suppression test: relationship to life events. Archives of General Psychiatry 43:356-

360, 1986. 488

Roy A, Pickar D, Paul S, Doran A, Chrousos GP, Gold PW: CSF corticotropin-releasing hormone in depressed patients and normal control subjects. American Journal of Psychiatry 144:641–645, 1987. 429, 430, 432

Roy-Byrne PP. 255, 393, 415, 523, 575, 602, 607

Roy-Byrne PP, Bierer LM, Uhde TW: The dexamethasone suppression test in panic disorder: comparison with normal controls. Biological Psychiatry 20:1234–1237, 1985. 387

Roy-Byrne PP, Uhde TW, Post RM: Effects of one night's sleep deprivation on mood and behavior in patients with panic disorder: comparison with depressed patients and normal controls. Archives of General Psychiatry 43:895–899, 1986. 388, 395, 603

Roy-Byrne P, Uhde TW, Post RM, Gallucci W, Chrousos GP, Gold PW: The corticotropin-releasing hormone stimulation test in patients with panic disorder. American Journal of Psychiatry 143:896–899, 1986. 388

Rozensky RA. 642

Rozensky RA, Rehm LP, Pry G, Roth D: Depression and self-reinforcement behavior in hospital patients. Journal of Behavior Therapy and Experimental Psychiatry 8:35–38, 1977. 642

Ruben HL. 288, 294, 296, 323

Rubin L. 389

Rubin RT. 404–406, 488, 594, 607

Rubin RT, Poland RE, Lesser IM, Winston RA, Blodgett AN: Neuroendocrine aspects of primary endogenous depression. Archives of General Psychiatry 44:328–336, 1987. 387

Rubio-Stipec M. 317, 321, 660

Rudin E: Ein Beitrag zur Frage der Zwang Krankheit insbesondere ihrer hereditaren Beizel ungen. Arch Psychiat Nervenkr 191:14–54, 1953. 306

Rudy TE. 508

Rush AJ. 255, 256, 513, 543, 581, 641

Russell J: A circumplex model of affect. Journal of Personality and Social Psychology 39:1161–1178, 1980. 54, 55, 506, 645, 646

Russo J. 49, 51, 476, 480

Rutt C. 296, 302

Rutter M: Meyerian psychobiology, personality development, and the role of life experiences. American Journal of Psychiatry 143:1077–1087, 1986. 491, 492, 493

Rutter M, Tizard J, Whitmore K: Education, Health and Behavior. New York, Krieber, 1981. 272

Saavedra JM: Changes in dopamine, noradrenaline and adrenaline in specific septal and preoptic nuclei after acute immobilization stress. Neuroendocrinology 35:396–401, 1982. 424

Saavedra JM, Kvetnansky R, Kopin IJ: Adrenaline, noradrenaline and dopamine levels in specific brain stem areas of acutely immobilized rats. Brain Research 160:271–280, 1979. 424

Sabanes F. 387

Sachar EJ, Hellman L, Roffwarg H: Disrupted 24 hour patterns of cortisol secretion in psychotic depression. Archives of General Psychiatry 28:19–24, 1973. 427

Sackheim HA, Greenburg MS, Weinman AL, Gur RC, Hungerbuhler JP, Geschwind N: Hemispheric asymmetry in the expression of positive and negative emotions: neurological evidence. Archives of Neurology 39:210–218, 1982. 565

Sadik C. 255, 256

Sainsbury P, Gibson JG: Symptoms of anxiety and tension and the accompanying physiological changes in the muscular system. Journal of Neurology, Neurosurgery and Psychiatry 17:216–224, 1954. 244

Sakai T: Clinico-genetic study on obsessive-compulsive neurosis. Bulletin of the Osaka Medical School Supplement 12:323–331, 1967. 306

Salamero M. 387

Sali L. 255

Salkin B. 254, 311

Samuelson H. 354–357

Sandberg D. 672, 678

Sanders-Bush E, Bushing JA, Snyder SH: Long-term effects of p-chloroamphetamine and related drugs on central serotonergic mechanisms. Journal of Pharmacology and Experimental Therapeutics 192:33–41, 1975. 409

Sanderson WC. 228

Sanderson WC, Barlow DH: Domains of worry within the proposed DSM-III-revised generalized anxiety disorder categories: reliability and description. Paper presented at the annual meeting of the Association for Advancement of Behavior Therapy. Chicago, October 1986. 224

Sanderson WC, Rapee RM, Barlow DH: The influence of an illusion of control on panic attacks induced via inhalation of 5% CO_2 enriched air. Archives of General Psychiatry 46:157–162, 1989. 223

Sanderson WC, Rapee RM, Barlow DH: Differences in panic symptoms experienced by the DSM-III-revised anxiety disorder categories, submitted for publication.

Sansone RA. 254

Santana F. 317, 322

Sarason I. 579

Sarason IG: Cognitive processes, anxiety, and the treatment of anxiety disorders, in Anxiety and the Anxiety Disorders. Edited by Tuma AH, Maser JD. Hillsdale, NJ, Lawrence Erlbaum Associates, 1985. 508, 509, 527

Sarason IG, Johnson JH, Siegel JM: Assessing the impact of life changes: development of the Life Experience Survey. Journal of Consulting and Clinical Psychology 46:932–946, 1978. 466

Sargant W: Drugs in the treatment of depression. British Medical Journal 1:225–227, 1961. 603

Sartorius N. 79, 90, 372, 474, 484, 487, 651, 652, 653, 655, 656, 664

Sartorius N, Davidian H, Ernberg G, Fenton FR, Fujii I, Gaspar M, Gulbinat W, Jablensky A, Kielholz P, Lehmann HE, Naraghi M, Shimizu M, Shinfuku N, Takahasi R: Depressive disorders in different cultures: report on the WHO collaborative study on standardized assessment of depressive disorders. Geneva, World Health Organization, 1983. 655

Sashidarian SP. 120

Saunders JD. 287, 289

Savard RJ, Rey AC, Post RM: Halstead-Reitan category test in bipolar and unipolar affective disorders: relationship to age and phase of illness. Journal of Nervous and Mental Disease 168:297–304, 1980.

Sawchenko PE. 418, 425, 570

Saykin AJ. 570

Scatton B. 415

Sceery W. 276

Schaefer MR, Sobieraj K, Hollyfield RL: Severity of alcohol dependence and its relationship to additional psychiatric symptoms in male alcoholic inpatients. American Journal of Drug and Alcohol Abuse 13:435–447, 1987.

Schaeffer MA. 247

Schaffer CB. 256, 260, 264, 265

Schally AV. 418

Schapira K. 599

Schatzberg AF. 386

Schatzberg AF, Cole JO: Benzodiazepines in depressive disorders. Archives of General Psychiatry 35:1359–1365, 1987a. 702

Schatzberg AF, Cole JO: Benzodiazepines in the treatment of depressive, borderline personality and schizophrenic disorders. British Journal of Clinical Pharmacology 11:175–225, 1987b. 702

Scheftner WA. 346, 347, 378

Scheier MF. 509, 715

Schilder P: The organic background of obsessions and compulsions. American Journal of Psychiatry 94:1397–1416, 1938. 310

Schildkraut JJ: The catecholamine hypothesis of depression: a review of supporting evidence. American Journal of Psychiatry 122:509–522, 1965. 415, 431

Schildkraut JJ, Kety SS: Biogenic amines and emotion. Science 156:21–30, 1967. 415, 431

Schildkraut JJ, Klein DF: The classification and treatment of depressive disorder, in Manual of Psychiatric Therapeutics. Edited by Shader RI. Boston, Little, Brown, 1975. 318, 327

Schlemmer RF. 260

Schlesser MA, Winokur G, Sherman BM: Genetic subtypes of unipolar primary depressive illness distinguished by hypothalamic-pituitary-adrenal axis activity. Lancet 1:739–741, 1979. 385, 563

Schneider K: Klinische Psychopathologie, 5th Edition. Translated by Hamilton MW. New York, Grune & Stratton, 1959. 88

Schneider LS, Munjack D, Severson JA, Palmer R: Platelet [3H]-imipramine binding in generalized anxiety disorder, panic disorder, and agoraphobia with panic attacks. Biological Psychiatry 22:59–66, 1987. 415

Schonberger LB. 151

Schooley R. 151

Schopflocher D. 571, 575

Schreiber JL. 254

Schrier SS. 254

Schubert DSP. 453

Schuckit MA: Alcoholism and affective disorders: diagnostic confusion, in Alcoholism and Affective Disorders. Edited by Goodwin DW, Erickson CK. New York, Spectrum Publications, 1979. 288

Schuckit M: Alcoholic patients with secondary depression. American Journal of Psychiatry 140:711–714, 1983a. 295

Schuckit MA: Alcoholism and other psychiatric disorders. Hospital and Community Psychiatry 34:1022–1026, 1983b. 189, 200, 285

Schuckit M: The clinical implications of primary diagnostic groups among alcoholics. Archives of General Psychiatry 42:1043–1049, 1985. 284, 285, 286, 290

Schuckit MA, Winokur G: A short-term follow-up of women alcoholics. Diseases of the Nervous System 33:672–678, 1972. 288

Schulberg HC. 178, 489, 661

Schulsinger F. 29, 30

Schulte HM. 417, 430, 433

Schulte HM, Chrousos GP, Gold PW, Booth JD, Oldfield EH, Cutler GB Jr, Loriaux DL: Continuous administration of synthetic ovine corticotropin-releasing factor in man: physiological and pathophysiological implications. Journal of Clinical Investigation 75:1781, 1985. 431

Schulterbrandt J. 235

Schulterbrandt J, Raskin A, Reatig N: Further application of factors of psychopathology in the interview, ward behavior, and self-reported ratings of hospitalized depressed patients. Psychological Reports 34:23–32, 1974. 256

Schwartz CE. 314

Schwartz DM, Thompson MG: Do anorectics get well? current research and future needs. American Journal of Psychiatry 138:319–323, 1981. 173

Schwartz GE, Davidson RJ, Goleman DJ: Patterning of cognitive and somatic processes in the self-regulation of anxiety: effects of medication versus exercise. Psychosomatic Medicine 40:321–328, 1978. 213

Schwartz JM. 577

Scott R. 120, 659

Scott-Strauss A. 318, 322, 325

Sechter D. 414

Secord PF. 712

Secunda SK. 296, 297, 684

Seeligson M. 420

Segal DS. 407

Segal Z: Appraisal of the self-schema construct in cognitive models of depression. Psychological Bulletin 103:147–162, 1988. 632

Segal Z, Shaw BF: Cognitive assessment, in Handbook of Cognitive-Behavioral Therapies. Edited by Dobson KS. New York, Guilford, 1988. 622, 631

Seggie J, Uhlir J, Brown GM: Adrenal stress responses following septal lesions in the rat. Neuroendocrinology 16:225–236, 1974. 424

Seligman MEP. 505, 509, 516, 517, 527, 528, 581, 617, 640

Seligman ME: Phobias and preparedness. Behavior Therapy 2:307–320, 1971. 636

Seligman MEP: Depression and learned helplessness, in The Psychology of Depression: Contemporary Theory and Research. Edited by Friedman RJ, Katz MM. New York, Winston-Wiley, 1974. 640

Seligman MEP: Helplessness: On Depression, Development, and Death. San Francisco, WH Freeman, 1975. 504, 508, 509, 510, 511, 521, 527, 528, 640

Seligman MEP, Abramson LY, Semmel A, von Baeyer C: Depressive attributional style. Journal of Abnormal Psychology 88:242–247, 1979. 641

Selin CE. 577

Sellers D. 295

Sellers EM, Kalant H: Alcohol intoxication and withdrawal. New England Journal of Medicine 294:757–762, 1976. 290

Selye H: A syndrome produced by diverse nocuous agents. Nature 138:32, 1936. 416, 420, 465

Selye H: The Stress of Life. New York, McGraw-Hill, 1956. 34

Semchuk KM. 576

Semler G. 660, 661, 662, 664

Semler G, Wittchen H-U, Joschke K, Zaudig M, von Geiso T, Kaiser S, von Cranach M, Pfister H: Test-retest Reliability of a Standardized Psychiatric Interview (DIS/CIDI). European Archives of Psychiatry and Neurological Sciences 236:214–222, 1987. 660

Semmel A. 517, 641

Semrad E, Grinspoon L, Fienberg SE: Development of an Ego Profile Scale.

Archives of General Psychiatry 28:70–77, 1973. 547

Serra G. 605

Sesman M. 317, 321, 660

Severson JA. 415

Seyfried W. 656, 661

Shadick R. 226

Shagass C. 244

Shagass C: Differentiation between anxiety and depression by the photically activated electroencephalogram. American Journal of Psychiatry 112:41–66, 1955. 700

Shagass C, Roemer RA, Straumanis JJ, Josiassen RC: Distinctive somatosensory evoked potential features in obsessive-compulsive disorder. Biological Psychiatry 19:1507–1524, 1984. 575

Shapiro MF, Lehman AF: The diagnosis of depression in different clinical settings: an analysis of the literature on the dexamethasone suppression test. Journal of Nervous and Mental Disease 171:714–720, 1983. 387

Shapiro RW. 318, 322, 556

Shapiro S. 588, 592, 593, 661

Shapiro S, Skinner EA, Kessler LG, VonKorff M, German PS, Tischler GL, Leaf PJ, Benham L, Cottler L, Regier DA: Utilization of health and mental health services: three epidemiologic catchment area sites. Archives of General Psychiatry 41:971–978, 1984. 116

Sharbrough FW. 394

Sharpe L. 572, 653

Shaw BF. 513, 543, 581, 622, 631

Shaw BF, Dobson KS: Cognitive assessment of depression, in Cognitive Assessment. Edited by Merluzzi T, Glass C, Genest M. New York, Guilford, 1979. 622

Shaw BF, Vallis TM, McCabe S: The assessment of the severity and symptom patterns in depression, in Handbook of Depression: Treatment, Assessment and Research. Edited by Beckham E, Leber W. Homewood, IL, Dorsey Press, 1985. 621

Shaw P. 677

Shear M, Devereux R, Kramer-Fox M: Low prevalence of MVP in patients with panic disorder. American Journal of Psychiatry 141:302–303, 1984. 395

Shearer SL. 581

Sheehan DV. 390, 392

Sheehan DV: The Anxiety Disease. New York, Charles Scribner's Sons, 1986. 607

Sheehan DV, Ballenger J, Jacobsen G: Treatment of endogenous anxiety with phobic, hysterical and hypochondriacal symptoms. Archives of General Psychiatry 35:51–59, 1980. 703

Sheehan DV, Claycomb B, Surman OS, Baer L, Coleman J, Gelles L: Panic attacks and dexamethasone suppression test. American Journal of Psychiatry 140:1063, 1983. 387

Sheehan D, Sheehan K: The classification of phobic disorders. International Journal of Psychiatry in Medicine 12:243–266, 1983. 53

Sheehan K. 53

Sheffield BF. 247

Sheier I. 613

Sheikh J. 392, 712

Shepard RA: Behavioral effects of GABA agonists in relation to anxiety and benzodiazepine action. Life Science 40:2429–2436, 1987. 415

Shepherd M, Cooper B, Brown AC, Kalton GW: Psychiatric Illness in General Practice. London, Oxford University Press, 1966. 247

Sherick RB. 528

Sherman BM. 385, 563

Sherman JE. 423

Sherrod A. 225

Shibasaki T. 420, 426

Shimizu M. 655

Shinfuku N. 655

Shipko S: Alesithymia and somatization. Psychotherapy and Psychosomatics 37:193–201, 1982. 246

Shizume K. 420, 426, 430

Sholomskas D. 318, 322, 354–358, 360, 361

Shrout PE. 178, 180, 181, 317, 321, 466, 660

Shrout PE, Dohrenwend BP, Levav I. Development of a discriminant rule for screening cases of diverse diagnostic types. Journal of Consulting and Clinical Psychology 54:314–319, 1986. 180, 181

Shulman BH. 525

Siassi I. 157

Sicotte N. 575

Siegel JM. 466

Siegel SJ, Alloy LB: Interpersonal perceptions and consequences of depressive-significant other interactions: a naturalistic study of college roommates (in press). 505

Sierles FS, Chen JJ, McFarland RE, Taylor MA: Post-traumatic stress disorder and concurrent psychiatric illness: a preliminary report. American Journal of Psychiatry 140:1177–1179, 1983. 503

Siever LJ. 308, 393, 394, 703

Siever LJ, Murphy DL, Slater S, de la Vega E, Lipper S. Plasma prolactin changes following fenfluramine in depressed patients compared to controls: an evaluation of central serotonergic responsivity in depression. Life Science 34:1029–1039, 1984. 407

Siever LJ, Uhde TW, Jimerson DC: Differential inhibitory noradrenergic responses to clonidine in 25 depressed patients and 25 normal control subjects. American Journal of Psychiatry 141:733–741, 1984. 389, 390

Sifneos PE. 246

Siggins GR. 419

Sigman M: Children with Emotional Disorders and Developmental Disabilities. Orlando, FL, Grune & Stratton, 1985. 190, 200

Sigvardsson S. 285, 440, 447, 453, 461, 626

Sigvardsson S, Bohman M, Cloninger CR: Structure and stability of childhood personality: prediction of later social adjustment. Journal of Child Psychology and Psychiatry and Allied Disciplines 28:929–946, 1987. 461

Sigvardsson S, Bohman M, von Knorring AL, Cloninger CR: Symptom patterns and causes of somatization in men, I: differentiation of two discrete disorders. Genetic Epidemiology 3:153–169, 1986. 245, 447, 448, 453

Silva PA. 279

Silver FL. 570

Simison D. 247

Simmonds M: Ueber Hypophysisschwund mit todlichem Ausgang. Deutsche Medizinische Wochenschrift 1:322–323, 1914. 254

Simon HA. 712

Simon HA: Sciences of the Artificial. Boston, MIT Press, 1969. 712

Simon R. 653

Simpson GG: Principles of Animal Taxonomy. San Francisco, Freeman, 1961. 64

Simpson GM. 245

Simson PG, Weiss JM, Ambrose MJ, Webster A: Infusion of a monoamine oxidase inhibitor into the locus coeruleus can prevent stress-induced behavioral depression. Biological Psychiatry 21:724–734, 1986. 419, 425

Simson PG, Weiss JM, Hoffman LJ, Ambrose MJ: Reversal of behavioral depression by infusion of an alpha-2 adrenergic agonist into the locus coeruleus. Neuropharmacology 25:385–389, 1986. 419, 425

Sinaiko E. 386

Singer JL: Navigating the Stream of Consciousness: Research in Daydreaming and Related Inner Experience. New York, Plenum, 1975. 717

Singer JL: Experimental studies of daydreaming and the stream of thought, in The Stream of Consciousness. Edited by Pope KS, Singer JL. New York, Plenum, 1978. 717

Sipprelle CN. 638

Sirinathsinghji DJS: Modulation of lordosis behaviour in the female rat by corticotropin releasing factor, β-endorphin and gonadotropin releasing hormone in the mesencephalic central gray. Brain Research 336:45–55, 1985. 421

Sirinathsinghji DJS: Inhibitory influence of corticotropin releasing factor on components of sexual behaviour in the male rat. Brain Research 407:185–190, 1987. 421

Sirinathsinghji DJS, Rees LH, Rivier J, Vale W: Corticotropin-releasing factor is a potent inhibitor of sexual receptivity in the female rat. Nature 305:230–235, 1983. 421, 422

Siris SG. 716

Sitaram N. 395

Sitaram N, Dube S, Jones D, Pohl R, Gershon S. Acetylcholine and alpha$_1$-adrenergic sensitivity in the separation of depression and anxiety. Psychopathology 17:24–39, 1984. 411

Sitaram N, Gillin JC. Development and use of pharmacological probes of the CNS in man: evidence of cholinergic abnormality in primary affective illness. Biological Psychology 15:925–955, 1980. 411

Sjodin I. 250

Sjodin I, Svedlund J, Ottosson JO, Doterall G: Controlled study of psychotherapy in chronic peptic ulcer disease. Psychosomatics 27:187, 1986. 250

Skinner EA. 116, 588, 592, 593

Skinner HA. 80

Skinner HA: Dimensions and clusters: a hybrid approach to classification. Applied Psychological Measurement 3:327–341, 1979. 71

Skinner HA: Construct validation approach to psychiatric classification, in Contemporary Directions in Psychopathology. Edited by Millon T, Klerman GL. New York, Guilford, 1986. 71

Skinner HA, Jackson DN: A model of psychopathology based on an integration of MMPI actuarial systems. Journal of Consulting and Clinical Psychology 46:231–238, 1978. 283

Skodol AE. 180, 190

Skolnick BE. 570

Slater E. 24

Slater E, Slater P: A heuristic theory of neurosis. Journal of Neurological Psychiatry 7:49–55, 1944. 472

Slater JF. 323

Slater P. 472

Slater S. 407

Slocumb JC. 243

Slotkin TA. 415

Slymen DJ. 217, 334, 335, 337, 338, 344, 364, 472, 619, 703

Slymen DS. 340, 607

Smail P. 291

Smail P, Stockwell T, Canter S, Hodgson R: Alcohol dependence and phobic anxiety states, I: a prevalence study. British Journal of Psychiatry 144:53–57, 1984. 291

Smart ED, Beaumont VJP, George WCG: Some personality characteristics of patients with anorexia nervosa. British Journal of Psychiatry 128:57–60, 1976. 311

Smeltzer DJ. 254

Smeraldi E. 597

Smith A. 468, 471

Smith GR, Miller LM, Monson RA, Ray DC: Consultation-liaison intervention in somatization disorder. Hospital and Community Psychiatry 37:1207–1210, 1986. 252

Smith GR, Monson RA, Ray DC: Patients with multiple unexplained symptoms. Archives of Internal Medicine 146:69–72, 1986. 250, 251

Smith MA. 418, 424–426, 430, 431

Smith MD. 456

Smith RC. 359

Smith WT. 699, 703

Smouse PE. 261

Snidman N. 354, 355, 357

Snyder DR. 415, 431

Snyder SH. 409

Sobol AM. 137, 160, 161, 162, 165, 166, 167, 168, 169, 170, 171, 172, 174, 333

Sobue I. 244

Sohn T. 505

Soldatos CR. 327

Sollogub AC. 189, 200

Solyum L. 676, 703

Soubrie P. 415

Spellman M. 260

Spielberger CD: The measurement of state and trait anxiety: conceptual and methodological issues, in Emotions: Their Parameters and Measurement. Edited by Levi L. NewYork, Raven, 1975. 614

Spielberger CD, Gorsuch RL, Lushene RE: Manual for the State-Trait Anxiety Inventory. Palo Alto, CA, Consulting Psychologists Press, 1970. 213, 554, 613, 644, 716, 719

Spier SA, Tesar GE, Rosenbaum JF, Woods SW: Treatment of panic disorder and agoraphobia with clonazepam. Journal of Clinical Psychiatry 47:238–242, 1986. 676

Spiess J. 416, 417, 420

Spiro HR, Siassi I, Crocetti GM: What gets surveyed in a psychiatric survey? Journal of Nervous and Mental Disease 154:105–114, 1972. 157

Spitz RA: Anaclitic depression. Psychoanalytic Study of the Child 2:313–347, 1946. 503

Spitzer RL. 22, 24, 32, 42, 101, 115, 181, 256, 297, 299, 488, 613, 621, 667, 681

Spitzer RL: Nosology, in An Annotated Bibliography of DSM-III. Edited by Skodol AE, Spitzer RL. Washington, DC, American Psychiatric Press, 1987. 96

Spitzer RL, Andreasen NC, Endicott J: Schizophrenia and other psychotic disorders in DSM-III. Schizophrenia Bulletin 4:489–509, 1978. 84

Spitzer RL, Endicott J: Schedule for Affective Disorders and Schizophrenia: Life-Time Version (SADS-L), 3rd Edition. New York, New York State Psychiatric Institute, 1977. 593, 684

Spitzer RL, Endicott J: Schedule for Affective Disorders and Schizophrenia (SADS). New York, Biometrics Research Division, New York State Psychiatric Institute, 1978. 93, 657

Spitzer RL, Endicott J, Robins E: Research Diagnostic Criteria: rationale and reliability. Archives of General Psychiatry 35:773–782, 1978a. 22, 24, 42, 92, 114, 181, 205, 232, 256, 273, 286, 297, 339, 405, 427, 483, 502, 593, 673, 682, 694

Spitzer RL, Endicott J, Robins E: Research Diagnostic Criteria (RDC) for a Selected Group of Functional Disorders, Third Edition. New York, Biometric Research, 1978b. 318, 694

Spitzer RL, Endicott J, Robins E: Research Diagnostic Criteria (RDC) for a Selected Group of Functional Disorders, Updated 2/4/85. New York Department of Assessment and Training, New York State Psychiatric Institute, 1985. 92

Spitzer RL, Fleiss J: A re-analysis of the reliability of psychiatric diagnosis. British Journal of Psychiatry 125:341–347, 1974. 208

Spitzer RL, Williams JBW: Classification of mental disorders, in Comprehensive Textbook of Psychiatry, Vol 4. Edited by Kaplan HI, Sadek BJ. Baltimore, Williams & Wilkins, 1980. 26

Spitzer R, Williams J: Classification of mental disorders, in Comprehensive Textbook of Psychiatry, Vol 1, 4th Edition. Edited by Kaplan H, Sadock B. Baltimore, Williams & Wilkins, 1985a. 42

Spitzer RL, Williams J: Instruction Manual for the Structured Clinical Interview for DSM-III (SCID). New York, New York State Psychiatric Institute, 1985b. 43, 44, 46, 621

Spitzer R, Williams J: Proposed revisions in the DSM-III classification of anxiety disorders based on research and clinical experience, in Anxiety and the Anxiety Disorders. Edited by Tuma AH, Maser JD. Hillsdale, NJ, Lawrence Erlbaum Associates, 1985c. 45, 207

Spitzer RL, Williams JBW: Structured Clinical Interview for DSM-III–Patient Version (SCID-P) (3/1/85). New York, Biometrics Research Department, New York State Psychiatric Institute, 1985d. 323

Spitzer R, Williams JBW: Revising DSM-III: the process and major issues, in Diagnosis and Classification in Psychiatry: A Critical Appraisal of DSM-III. Edited by Tischler GL. New York, Cambridge University Press, 1987. 95

Spitzer RL, Williams JBW, First MB, Kendler K: A proposal for DSM-IV: solving the "organic/nonorganic" problem (editorial). Journal of Neuropsychiatry and Clinical Neuroscience 1:126–127, 1989. 100

Spitzer RL, Williams JBW, Gibbon M: Structured Clinical Interview for DSM-III-R–Personality Disorders (SCID-II) (10/15/86). New York, Biometrics Research Department, New York State Psychiatric Institute, 1986. 323

Spitzer RL, Williams JBW, Gibbon M: Structured Clinical Interview for DSM-III-R–Patient Version (4/1/87). New York, New York State Psychiatric Institute, 1987. 657, 658, 681

Spitzer RL, Williams JBW, Skodol A: DSM-III: the major achievements and an overview. American Journal of Psychiatry 137:151–164, 1980. 190

Spitznagel E. 661

Squires KC. 574

Squires KC, Wickens CD, Squires NK, Donchin E: The effect of stimulus sequence on the waveform of the cortical event-related potential. Science 193:1142–1146, 1976. 574

Squires NK. 574

Srole L, Fisher AK: The Midtown Manhattan Longitudinal Study vs. "The Mental Paradise Lost" Doctrine: a controversy joined. Archives of General Psychiatry 37:209–221, 1980. 22, 168

Srole L, Langner TS, Michael ST, Opler MK, Rennie TAC: Mental Health in the Metropolis: The Midtown Manhattan Study. New York, McGraw-Hill, 1962. 171, 245

Stabenau JR. 661

Stalla GK. 430

Standley CC. 33

Stangl D. 468

Stanley M. 428

Star SA: The screening of psychoneurotics: comparison of psychiatric diagnoses and test scores at all induction stations, in Measurement and Prediction. Edited by Stouffer SA, Guttman L, Suchman EA, Lazarsfeld P, Star SA, Clausen JA. Princeton, NJ, Princeton University Press, 1950a, pp 548–567. 156, 177

Star SA: The screening of psychoneurotics in the army: technical development of tests, in Measurement and Prediction. Edited by Stouffer SA, Guttman L, Suchman EA, Lazarsfeld P, Star SA, Clausen JA. Princeton, NJ, Princeton University Press, 1950b, pp 486–547. 156

Staton RD. 570

Stavrakaki C, Vargo B: The relationship of anxiety and depression: a review of the literature. British Journal of Psychiatry 149:7–16, 1986. 271, 274, 414, 493, 626, 709

Stavrakaki C, Vargo B, Boodoosingh L, Roberts N: The relationship between anxiety and depression in children: rating scales and clinical variables. Canadian Journal of Psychiatry 32:433–439, 1987. 273, 274

St. Clair DM. 574

Steckel W: The Interpretation of Dreams. New York, Liveright, 1943. 239

Steer RA. 218, 219, 496, 509, 528, 529, 631, 700

Stefan RL. 227

Stein L, Belluzzi JD, Wise CD: Benzodiazepines: behavioral and neurochemical mechanisms. American Journal of Psychiatry 134:665–669, 1977. 415

Stein M. 387, 575

Steiner M. 403, 427, 613

Steiner S. 470, 492

Steinhausen HC, Glanville K: Follow-up studies of anorexia nervosa: a review of research findings. Psychological Medicine 13:239–249, 1983. 311

Steinmetz JL. 630

Steketee GS. 11, 229

Stenbäck A: Hypochondria in duodenal ulcer. Advances in Psychosomatic Medicine 1:307–312, 1960. 246

Stengel E: A study on some clinical aspects of the relationships between obsessional neurosis and psychotic reaction types. Journal of Mental Science 91:166–187, 1945. 307

Stenslie CE. 572, 581

and characterization of immunoreactive corticotropin-releasing factor in human tissues. Journal of Clinical Endocrinology and Metabolism 59:861–867, 1984. 430

Sugarman AA. 427

Sullivan FM. 422

Sullivan JL. 260, 603

Sulser F, Janowsky AJ, Okada F, Manier DH, Mobley PL: Regulation of recognition and action function of the norepinephrine (NE) receptor-coupled adenylate cyclase system in brain: implications for the therapy of depression. Neuropharmacology 22:425–431, 1983. 432

Sulser F, Vetulani J, Mobley PL: Mode of action of antidepressant drugs. Biochemical Pharmacology 27:257–261, 1978. 415, 432

Sumida RM. 577

Suomi S. 503, 504, 522

Suomi SJ, Mineka S, Harlow HF: Social separation in monkeys from several motivational perspectives, in Motivation. Edited by Teitelbaum P, Satinoff E. New York, Plenum, 1984. 503

Surman OS. 387, 392

Surman O, Williams J, Sheehan D, Strome T, Jones K, Coleman J: Immunological response to stress in agoraphobia and panic attacks. Biological Psychiatry 21:768–774, 1986. 390

Surtees P. 120

Surtees PE, Kendell RE: The hierarchy model of psychiatric symptomatology: an investigation based on Present State Examination ratings. British Journal of Psychiatry 135:438–443, 1979. 79, 90

Sussman PS. 571, 575

Sutherland DE. 327

Sutker TP. 285

Sutton RE. 420

Sutton RE, Koob GF, LeMoal M, Rivier J, Vale W: Corticotropin releasing factor produces behavioural activation in rats. Nature 297:331–333, 1982. 420, 421

Sutton S. 422, 572

Svedlund J. 250

Svedlund J, Ottosson J, Sjodin I, Dotevall G: Controlled study of psychotherapy in irritable bowel syndrome. Lancet 2:589–592, 1983. 250

Svensson TH: Peripheral, autonomic regulation of locus coeruleus noradrenergic neurons in brain: putative implications for psychiatry and psychopharmacology. Psychopharmacology 92:1–7, 1987. 419, 425

Svensson TH, Persson R, Wallin L, Walinder J: Anxiolytic action of clonidine. Nordisk Psyk Tidskr 32:439–441, 1978. 432

Swann AC. 575

Swanson LW, Sawchenko PE, Rivier J, Vale WW: Organization of ovine corticotropin-releasing factor immunoreactive cells and fibers in the rat brain: an immunohistochemical study. Neuroendocrinology 36:165–186, 1983. 418, 425

Swartz MS, Blazer DG, Woodbury MA, George LK, Landerman R: Somatization disorder in a US Southern community: use of a new procedure for analysis of medical classification. Psychological Medicine 16:595–609, 1986. 159

Swedo SE, Leonard HL, Rapoport JL, Lenane MC, Goldberger EL, Cheslow DL: A double-blind comparison of clomipramine and desipramine in the treatment of trichotillomania (hair pulling). New England Journal of Medi-

Journal of Psychiatry 141:196–201, 1984. 570

Taylor MA, Abrams R: Cognitive impairment patterns in schizophrenia and affective disorder. Journal of Neurology, Neurosurgery and Psychiatry 50:895–899, 1987. 567, 570

Taylor MA, Redfield J, Abrams R: Neuropsychological dysfunction in schizophrenia and affective disorder. Biological Psychiatry 16:467–478, 1981. 567

Taylor S, Crocker J: Schematic bases of social information processing, in The Ontario Symposium on Personality and Social Psychology, Vol 1. Edited by Higgens E, Hermann P, Zanna M. Hillsdale, NJ, Lawrence Erlbaum Associates, 1980. 530

Tazi A, Dantzer R, LeMoal M, Rivier J, Vale W, Koob GF: Corticotropin-releasing factor antagonist blocks stress-induced fighting in rats. Regulatory Peptides 18:37–42, 1987. 421, 423

Tazi A, Swerdlow NR, LeMoal M, Rivier J, Vale W, Koob GF: Behavioral activation by CRF: evidence for the involvement of the ventral forebrain. Life Science 41:41–49, 1987. 420

Tearnan BH, Telch MJ, Keefe P: Etiology and onset of agoraphobia: a critical review. Comprehensive Psychiatry 125:51–62, 1984. 479

Teasdale JD. 509, 516, 517, 527, 528, 640, 643

Teasdale JD: Affect and accessibility. Philosophical Transactions of the Royal Society of London B302:403–412, 1983a. 642

Teasdale JD: Negative thinking in depression: cause, effect, or reciprocal relationship? Advances in Behavior Research Therapy 5:27–49, 1983b. 642

Teasdale JD, Fogarty SJ: Differential effects of induced mood on retrieval of pleasant and unpleasant events from episodic memory. Journal of Abnormal Psychology 88:248–257, 1979. 643

Teder W. 664, 666

Teders SJ. 251

Teitlebaum M. 588, 592, 593

Teja JS, Narang RL, Aggarwal AK: Depression across cultures. British Journal of Psychiatry 119:253–260, 1971. 505

Telch MJ. 479

Tellegen A. 55, 645

Tellegen A: Structures of mood and personality and their relevance to assessing anxiety, with an emphasis on self-report, in Anxiety and the Anxiety Disorders. Edited by Tuma AH, Maser JD. Hillsdale, NJ, Lawrence Erlbaum Associates, 1985. 48, 54, 55, 506, 508, 580, 581, 599, 645, 646

Tennant C. 120, 659

Tennant C, Bebbington P: The social causation of depression: a critique of the work of Brown and his colleagues. Psychological Medicine 8:565–575, 1978. 468

Tennant C, Bebbington P, Hurry J: The role of life events in depressive illness: is there a substantial causal relation? Psychological Medicine 11:379–389, 1981a. 468

Tennant C, Bebbington P, Hurry J: The short-term outcome of neurotic disorder in the community: the relation of remission to clinical factors and to 'neutralizing' life events. British Journal of Psychiatry 139:213–220, 1981b. 487

Tennant C, Hurry J, Bebbington P: The relation of childhood separation experiences to adult depressive and anxiety states. British Journal of Psychiatry 141:475–482, 1982. 478

Tennant C, Smith A, Bebbington P, Hurry J: The contextual threat of life events: the concept and its reliability. Psychological Medicine 9:525–528,

1979. 468, 471

Tennen H, Herzberger S: Depression, self-esteem, and the absence of self-protective attributional biases. Journal of Personality and Social Psychology 52:72–80, 1987. 516

Termansen PG. 571, 575

Tesar GE. 676

Thase ME. 476

Thatcher-Britton K. 420

Theander S: Research on outcome and prognosis of anorexia nervosa and some results from a Swedish long term study. International Journal of Eating Disorders 2:167–174, 1983. 254, 255

Theunissen J. 712

Thiebot MH, Hamon M, Soubrie P: Attenuation of induced-anxiety in rats by chlordiazepoxide: role of raphe dorsalis benzodiazepine binding sites and serotonergic neurons. Neuroscience 7:2287–2294, 1982. 415

Thierry A, Javoy F, Glowinski J, Kety S: Effects of stress on the metabolism of norepinephrine, dopamine, and serotonin in the central nervous system of the rat. I. Modification of norepinephrine turnover. Journal of Pharmacology and Experimental Therapeutics 163:163–171, 1968. 425

Thomas E, Dewald L: Experimental neuroses: neuropsychological analysis, in Psychopathology: Experimental Models. Edited by Maser JD, Seligman MEP. San Francisco, WH Freeman, 1977. 504

Thomas JW. 415

Thomas KB: The consultation and the therapeutic illusion. British Medical Journal 1:1327–1328, 1978. 251

Thompson MG. 173

Thompson WD. 294, 296, 323, 580

Thyer BA, Himle J, Curtis GC, Cameron OG, Nesse RM: A comparison of panic disorder and agoraphobia with panic attacks. Comprehensive Psychiatry 26:208–214, 1985. 43, 53, 586

Thyer BA, Parrish RT, Curtis GC, Nesse RM, Cameron OG: Ages of onset of DSM-III anxiety disorders. Comprehensive Psychiatry 26:113–122, 1985. 590

Tiller JWG, Biddle N, Maguire KP, Davies BM: The dexamethasone suppression test and plasma dexamethasone in generalized anxiety disorder. Biological Psychiatry 23:261–270, 1988. 388, 406

Timbers DM. 317, 322

Tiongco D. 386, 387

Tischler GL. 116, 165, 171, 589

Tizard J. 272

Tomai TP. 430

Tomori N. 430

Tondo L. 605

Toolan JM. Depression in children and adolescents. American Journal of Orthopsychiatry 32:404–415, 1962. 272, 280

Torellas A, Guaza C, Borrell J: Effects of acute and prolonged administration of chlordiazepoxide upon the pituitary-adrenal activity and brain catecholamines in sound stressed and unstressed rats. Neuroscience 5:2289–2295, 1980. 422

Torgersen S: Genetic factors in anxiety disorders. Archives of General Psychiatry 40:1085–1089, 1983. 372, 375

Torgersen S: Developmental differentiation of anxiety and affective neurosis. Acta Psychiatrica Scandinavica 71:304–310, 1985a. 481, 490, 496

Torgersen S: Hereditary differentiation of anxiety and affective neuroses. British Journal of Psychiatry 146:530–534, 1985b. 344, 372, 481, 482, 607

Torgersen S: Genetic factors in moderately severe and mild affective disorders. Archives of General Psychiatry 43:222–226, 1986. 372, 580

Torgerson WS: Theory and Methods of Scaling. New York, John Wiley, 1958. 626

Tosato G. 151

Towbin KE. 310, 563

Towle LH. 656

Tozawa F. 430

Treece C. 189, 200

Tremblay MA. 154

Tricamo E. 604, 673, 674

Trimble MR. 310, 700

Trippett CJ. 290

Trockman C. 387

Troughton EP. 242, 285

Tsakiris F. 310

Tsuang MT. 307, 310, 312, 314

Tsuang MT, Woolson RF: Mortality in patients with schizophrenia, mania, depression and surgical conditions. British Journal of Psychiatry 130:162–166, 1977. 173

Tuason V. 53

Tucker DM. 581

Tucker DM, Antes JR, Stenslie CE, Barnhardt TM: Anxiety and lateral cerebral function. Journal of Abnormal Psychology 87:380–383, 1978. 572, 581

Tucker DM, Stenslie CE, Roth RS, Shearer SL: Right frontal lobe activation and right hemisphere performance: decrement during a depressed mood. Archives of General Psychiatry 38:169–174, 1981. 581

Tucker DM, Williamson PA: Asymmetric neural control systems in human self-regulation. Psychological Review 91:185–215, 1984. 565

Tunving K. 147

Tuomisto J, Mannisto P. Neurotransmitter regulation of anterior pituitary hormones. Pharmacological Reviews 37:249–332, 1985. 408

Turk DC. 244

Turner RM. 229

Turner RW. 588, 592, 593

Turner SM. 396

Turner SM, Beidel DC, Dancu CY, Keys DJ: Psychopathology of social phobia and comparison to avoidant personality disorder. Journal of Abnormal Psychology 95:389–394, 1986. 228

Turner SM, McCann BS, Beidel DC, Mezzich JE: DSM-III classification of the anxiety disorders: a psychometric study. Journal of Abnormal Psychology 95:168–172, 1986. 230

Turner S, Williams S, Beidel D, Mezzich J: Panic disorder and agoraphobia with panic attacks: covariation along the dimensions of panic and agoraphobic fear. Journal of Abnormal Psychology 95:384–388, 1986. 53

Tye NC, Iversen SD, Green AR: The effects of benzodiazepines and serotonergic manipulations on punished responding. Neuropharmacology 18:689–695, 1979. 415

Tyler SK, Tucker DM: Anxiety and perceptual structure: individual differences in neuropsychological function. Journal of Abnormal Psychology 91:210–220, 1982. 581

Tyrer PJ. 593

Tyrer P: The Role of Bodily Feelings in Anxiety. London, Oxford University Press, 1976. 244

Tyrer P: Classification of anxiety. British Journal of Psychiatry 144:78–83, 1984. 703

Tyrer P: Neurosis divisible? Lancet 1:685–688, 1985. 472, 493, 605

Tyrer P: Classification of anxiety disorders: a critique of DSM-III. Journal of Affective Disorders 11:99–104, 1986a. 43, 45, 332, 594

Tyrer P: New rows of neuroses: are they an illusion? Integrative Psychiatry 4:25–31, 1986b. 472, 473, 497

Tyrer P, Gardner M, Lambourn J, Whitford M: Clinical and pharmacokinetic factors affecting response to phenelzine. British Journal of Psychiatry 136:359–365, 1980. 700

Tyrer P, Remington M, Alexander J: The outcome of neurotic disorders after out-patient and day hospital care. British Journal of Psychiatry 151:57–62, 1987. 472

Uddenberg CE. 140

Uhde TW. 313, 387, 388, 389, 390, 393, 394, 395, 603

Uhde TW, Berrettini WH, Roy-Byrne PP, Boulenger J-P, Post RM: Platelet [³H]imipramine binding in patients with panic disorder. Biological Psychiatry 22:52–58, 1987. 393, 415

Uhde TW, Kellner CH: Cerebral ventricular size in panic disorder. Journal of Affective Disorders 12:175–178, 1987. 395, 396

Uhde TW, Roy-Byrne P, Gillin JC, Mendelson WB, Boulenger JP, Vittone BJ, Post RM: The sleep of patients with panic disorder: a preliminary report. Psychiatry Research 12:251–259, 1984. 575

Uhde TW, Roy-Byrne PP, Vittone BJ, Boulenger J-P, Post RM: Phenomenology and neurobiology of panic disorder, in Anxiety and the Anxiety Disorders. Edited by Tuma AH, Maser JD. Hillsdale, NJ, Lawrence Erlbaum Associates, 1985. 523, 602, 607

Uhde TH, Siever LJ, Post RM: Clonidine: Acute challenge and clinical trial paradigms for the investigation and treatment of anxiety disorders, affective illness and pain syndromes, in Neurobiology of Mood Disorders. Edited by Post RM, Ballenger PC. Baltimore, Williams & Wilkins, 1984, pp 554–571. 703

Uhlenhuth EH. 158, 240, 256, 586, 674

Uhlenhuth EH, Balter MB, Mellinger GD, Cisin IH, Clinthorne J: Symptom checklist syndromes in the general population. Archives of General Psychiatry 40:1167–1173, 1983. 477, 590

Uhlir J. 424

Ulett PC, Gildea EF: Survey of surgical procedures in psychoneurotic women. Journal of the American Medical Association 143:960–963, 1950. 248

Unden F, Ljunggren JG, Kjellman BF, Beck-Friis J, Wetterberg L: Unaltered 24 h serum PRL levels and PRL response to TRH in contrast to decreased 24 h serum TSH levels and TSH response to TRH in major depressive disorder. Acta Psychiatrica Scandinavica 75:131–138, 1987. 394

Unis AS. 528

Uytdenhoef P, Portelange P, Jacquy J, Charles G, Linkowski P, Mendlewicz J: Regional cerebral blood flow and lateralized hemispheric dysfunction in depression. British Journal of Psychiatry 143:128–132, 1983.

Vaccarino FJ. 420

Vaglum P. 201

Vaglum S, Vaglum P: Borderline and other mental disorders in alcohol female psychiatric patients: a case control study. Psychopathology 18:50–60, 1985. 201

Vaillant GE: Natural history of male psychological health: the relation of choice of ego mechanisms of defense to adult adjustment. Archives of General Psychiatry 33:535–545, 1976. 547, 549, 550, 552

Vaillant GE: Adaptation to Life. Boston, Little, Brown, 1977. 546, 547

Vaillant G: The Natural History of Alcoholism. Cambridge, Harvard University Press, 1983. 283

Vaillant GE, Drake RE: Maturity of ego defenses in relation to DSM-III Axis II personality disorder. Archives of General Psychiatry 42:597–601, 1985. 549, 550, 552

Vale WW. 417, 418, 419, 420–423, 425, 427–430, 432

Vale W, Spiess J, Rivier C, Rivier J: Characterization of a 41-residue ovine hypothalamic peptide that stimulates secretion of corticotropin and β-endorphin. Science 213:1394–1397, 1981. 416, 417

Valentino RJ, Foote SL: Corticotropin-releasing factor disrupts sensory responses of brain noradrenergic neurons. Neuroendocrinology 45:28–36, 1987. 419

Valentino RJ, Foote SL, Aston-Jones G: Corticotropin-releasing factor activates noradrenergic neurons of the locus coeruleus. Brain Research 270:363–367, 1983. 419, 420, 425, 426, 431

Vallacher RR. 716

Vallis TM. 621

Van Den Burgt JA. 423

Van der Brink. 42

Van Doren T. 308

van Kammen DP. 716

Van Lehn R. 244

Van Meter K: Block-modeling and cross-classification techniques for estimating population parameters from network data. Paper presented at the Workshop on the Methodology of Applied Drug Research, European Community Health Directorate, Luxemburg, January 1986. 713

Van Meter K, de Vries MW, Kaplan C: Cross-classification analysis of psychiatric syndromes. BMS (Paris) 15 (July), 1987. 713

Van Valkenburg C. 24, 599, 603

Van Valkenburg C, Akiskal HS, Puzantian V, Rosenthal T: Anxious depressions: clinical, family history, and naturalistic outcome: comparisons with panic and major depressive disorders. Journal of Affective Disorders 6:67–82, 1984. 53, 341, 346, 378, 478, 602, 606, 709, 719

Varela M. 420, 421

Vargo B. 271, 273, 274, 414, 493, 626, 709

Vasquez CV. 500, 505, 509, 530

Vaughan M: The relationship between obsessional personality, obsessions in depression and symptoms of depression. British Journal of Psychiatry 129:36–39, 1976. 309

Vermilyea BB. 43, 44, 45, 46, 49, 51, 55, 62, 63, 64, 67, 69, 70, 71, 76, 190, 200, 207, 209, 213, 221, 223, 227, 472, 619

Vermilyea JA. 43, 44, 45, 46, 49, 51, 55, 62, 63, 64, 67, 69, 70, 71, 76, 190, 200, 207, 209, 213, 221, 223, 225, 472, 619

Vetulani J. 415, 432

Videbech T: The psychopathology of anancastic endogenous depression. Acta Psychiatrica Scandinavica 52:336–373, 1975. 309, 311

Viesselman J. 296, 302

Waterhouse JM. 710

Waternaux C. 237

Watkins JT, Rush AJ: Cognitive response test. Cognitive Therapy and Research 7:425–436, 1983. 641

Watkins WD. 392

Watson D, Clark L: Negative affectivity: the disposition to experience aversive emotional states. Psychological Bulletin 96:465–490, 1984. 508, 621

Watson D, Clark L, Tellegen A: Cross-cultural convergence in the structure of mood: a Japanese replication and a comparison with U.S. findings. Journal of Personality and Social Psychology 47:127–144, 1984. 55

Watson D, Tellegen A: Toward a consensual structure of mood. Psychological Bulletin 98:219–235, 1985. 645

Waziri R. 567, 570

Webb V. 423

Weber H. 417

Webster A. 419, 425, 496

Weckowitz TE. 646

Wegner DM, Vallacher RR: The Self in Social Psychology. Oxford, Oxford University Press, 1980. 716

Wegner JT, Struve FA, Kantor JS, Kane JM: Relationship between the B-Mitten EEG pattern and tardive dyskinesia. Archives of General Psychiatry 36:599–603, 1979. 573

Wehr TA, Goodwin FK: Can antidepressants cause mania and worsen the course of affective illness? American Journal of Psychiatry 144:1403–1411, 1987. 605

Weinberg P. 392

Weinberger DR. 570, 577

Weiner B. 515

Weiner B: An attributional theory of achievement motivation and emotion. Psychological Review 92:548–573, 1985. 509, 515

Weiner H. 255

Weiner HM: Psychobiology and Human Disease. New York, Elsevier 1977. 496

Weiner MF. 255

Weingartner H, Miller H, Murphy DL: Mood-state-dependent retrieval of verbal associations. Journal of Abnormal Psychology 86:276–284, 1977. 643

Weinman AL. 565

Weinman J. 632

Weinshilboum RM. 394

Weinstein MC. 161

Weinstein N. 51, 54, 499, 505, 616, 623, 626, 631

Weiss JM. 419, 425

Weiss JM, Goodman PA, Ambrose MJ, Webster A, Hoffman LJ: Neurochemical basis of behavioral depression, in Advances in Behavioral Medicine, Vol 1. Edited by Katkin ES, Manuck SB. Greenwich, CT, JAI Press, 1984. 496

Weiss JM, Goodman PA, Losito BG, Corrigan S, Charry JM, Bailey WH: Behavioral depression produced by an uncontrollable stressor: relationship to norepinephrine, dopamine, and serotonin levels in various regions of rat brain. Brain Research Review 3:167–205, 1981. 425

Weiss RD, Mirin SM, Michael J, Sollogub AC: Psychopathology in chronic cocaine abusers. American Journal of Drug and Alcohol Abuse 12:17–29, 1986. 189, 200

Weissenburger A, Rush AJ, Giles DE, Stunkard AJ: Weight change in depression. Psychiatry Research 17:275–283, 1986. 256

Weissman A, Beck AT: Development and validation of the Dysfunctional Attitude Scale (DAS). Paper presented at the meeting of the Association of the Advancement of Behavior Therapy, Chicago, November 1978. 641

Weissman MM. 44, 45, 94, 109, 152, 165, 171, 206, 272, 288, 302, 313, 317, 321, 327, 346, 347, 364, 377, 487, 499, 505, 528, 589, 603, 605, 619, 623, 649, 650, 707

Weissman M: The epidemiology of anxiety disorders: rates, risks, and familial patterns, in Anxiety and the Anxiety Disorders. Edited by Tuma AH, Maser JD. Lawrence Erlbaum Associates, Hillside, NJ, 1985. 670

Weissman MM, Gammon GD, John K, Merikangas KR, Warner V, Prusoff BA, Sholomskas D: Children of depressed parents. Archives of General Psychiatry 44:847–853, 1987. 275, 354, 355, 356, 357, 358, 360

Weissman MM, Gershon ES, Kidd KK, Prusoff BA, Leckman JF, Dibble E, Hamovit J, Thompson WD, Pauls DL, Guroff JJ: Psychiatric disorders in the relatives of probands with affective disorders. Archives of General Psychiatry 41:13–21, 1984. 580

Weissman MM, Kidd KK, Prusoff BA: Variability in rates of affective disorders in relatives of depressed and normal probands. Archives of General Psychiatry 39:1397–1403, 1982. 336, 346

Weissman MM, Klerman GL: The chronic depressive in the community: underrecognized and poorly treated. Comprehensive Psychiatry 18:523–531, 1977a. 323, 328

Weissman MM, Klerman GL: Sex differences and the epidemiology of depression. Archives of General Psychiatry 34:98–111, 1977b. 168

Weissman MM, Leaf PJ, Bruce ML: The epidemiology of dysthymia in the community. Presented in Symposium 101, Diagnosis and Treatment of Chronic Depression, annual meeting of the American Psychiatric Association, Chicago, May 1987. 317, 321

Weissman MM, Leaf PJ, Bruce ML, Florio L: The epidemiology of dysthymia in five communities: rates, risks, comorbidity, and treatment. American Journal of Psychiatry 145:815–819, 1988. 317, 321, 323, 327

Weissman M, Leckman J, Merikangas K, Gammon G, Prusoff B: Depression and anxiety disorders in parents and children: results from the Yale Family Study. Archives of General Psychiatry 41:845–852, 1984. 45, 275, 363, 377, 499

Weissman MM, Leckman JF, Merikangas KR, Prusoff BA, Gammon GD: Depression and anxiety disorders in parents and children: results from the Yale family study. 38:139–152, 1983.

Weissman MM, Merikangas KR: The epidemiology of anxiety and panic disorders: an update. Journal of Clinical Psychiatry 47 (Suppl):11–17, 1986. 189, 200

Weissman MM, Merikangas KR, John K, Wickramaratne P, Prusoff BA, Kidd KK: Family-genetic studies of psychiatric disorders: developing technologies. Archives of General Psychiatry 43:1104–1116, 1986. 348, 352

Weissman MM, Myers JK: Affective disorders in a US urban community. Archives of General Psychiatry 35:1304–1311, 1978. 317, 321

Weissman MM, Myers JK: Clinical depression in alcoholism. American Journal of Psychiatry 137:372–373, 1980. 294

Weissman MM, Myers JK, Harding PS: Psychiatric disorders in a U.S. urban community. American Journal of Psychiatry 135:459–462, 1978. 311

Weissman MM, Myers JK, Harding PS: Prevalence and psychiatric heterogeneity of alcoholism in a United States urban community. Journal of Studies on Alcohol 41:672–781, 1980. 286, 287, 290

Weissman MM, Paykel ES: The Depressed Woman: A Study of Social Relationships. Chicago, University of Chicago Press, 1974. 489

Weissman MM, Pottenger M, Kleber H, Ruben HL, Williams D, Thompson WD: Symptom patterns in primary and secondary depression: a comparison of primary depressives with depressed opiate addicts, alcoholics and schizophrenics. Archives of General Psychiatry 34:854–862, 1977. 294, 296, 323

Weissman MM, Wickramaratne P, Merikangas KR, Leckman JF, Prusoff BA, Caruso KA, Kidd KK, Gammon GD: Onset of major depression in early adulthood: increased familial loading and specificity. Archives of General Psychiatry 41:1136–1143, 1984. 350

Weissman MM, Wickramaratne P, Warner V, John K, Prusoff BA, Merikangas KR, Gammon GD: Assessing psychiatric disorders in children: discrepancies between mothers' and childrens' reports. Archives of General Psychiatry 44:747–753, 1987. 364

Wells RT. 247

Wells V. 287

Welner A, Reich T, Robins E, Fishman R, Van Doren T: Obsessive compulsive neurosis: record, follow-up, and family studies, I: inpatient record study. Comprehensive Psychiatry 17:527–539, 1976. 308

Welner Z, Reich W, Herjanic B, Jung KG, Amado H: Reliability, validity, and parent-child agreement studies of the Diagnostic Interview for Children and Adolescents (DICA). Journal of the American Academy of Child and Adolescent Psychiatry 26:649–653, 1987. 666–667

Wender P. 29

Wender PH, Kety SS, Rosenthal D, Schulsinger F, Ortman J, Lunde I: Psychiatric disorders in the biological and adoptive families of adopted individuals with affective disorders. Archives of General Psychiatry 43:923–929, 1986. 30

Wenegrat BG. 574

West ED, Dally PJ: Effects of Iproniazid in depressive syndromes. British Medical Journal. June: 1491–1494, 1959. 603

Wetterberg L. 394

Wetzel R. 453

Wetzel R, Cloninger CR, Hong B, Reich T: Personality as a subclinical expression of affective disorders. Comprehensive Psychiatry 21:197–205, 1980. 453

Wexler BE, Heninger GR: Alterations in cerebral laterality during acute psychotic illness. Archives of General Psychiatry 36:278–284, 1979. 572

Whalley LJ. 574

Wheeler EO, White PD, Reed EW, Cohen ME: Neurocirculatory asthenia (anxiety neurosis, effort syndrome, neurasthenia). Journal of the American Medical Association 142:878–888, 1950. 585, 586

Wheeler EO, Williamson CR, Cohen ME: Heart scare, heart surveys, and iatrogenic heart disease. Journal of the American Medical Association 167:1096, 1958. 242

White G. 140

White PD. 585

White R: Motivation reconsidered: the concept of competence. Psychological Review 66:297–333, 1959. 527

Whiteford HA, Evans L: Agoraphobia and the dexamethasone suppression test. Australian and New Zealand Journal of Psychiatry 18:374, 1984. 387

Whitford M. 700

Wilson H. 570

Wilson IC. 290

Wilson LG. 337, 338, 386, 387, 414, 472, 502, 505, 619, 676

Wine J: Test anxiety and direction of attention. Psychological Bulletin 76:92–104, 1971. 638

Wing JK. 120, 656, 659, 664

Wing JK: A technique for studying psychiatric morbidity in in-patient and out-patient series and in general population samples. Psychological Medicine 6:665–671, 1976. 484

Wing J, Babor T, Brugha T, Burke J, Cooper JE, Giel R, Jablensky A, Regier D, Sartorius N: SCAN: Schedules for Clinical Assessment in Neuropsychiatry. Archives of General Psychiatry (in press). 653, 655

Wing JK, Bebbington P: Epidemiology of depression, in Handbook of Depression: Treatment, Assessment and Research. Edited by Beckham E, Leber W. Homewood, IL, Dorsey Press, 1985. 624

Wing JK, Cooper JE, Sartorius N: Description and Classification of Psychiatric Syndromes. Cambridge, Cambridge University Press, 1974a. 79, 90, 484

Wing JK, Cooper JE, Sartorius N: The measurement and classification of psychiatric symptoms: an introduction manual for the Present State Examination and CATEGO Programme. London, Cambridge University Press, 1974b. 372, 474, 487, 651, 652, 655

Wing JK, Nixon JM, Mann SA, Leff JP: Reliability of the PSE (ninth edition) used in a population study. Psychological Medicine 7:505–516, 1977. 487

Wing L. 700

Winokur A, March S, Mendels J: Primary affective disorders in relatives of patients with anorexia nervosa. American Journal of Psychiatry 137:695–698, 1980. 254

Winokur G. 8, 10, 24, 91, 114, 205, 254, 288, 294, 295, 296, 301, 305, 337, 346, 347, 378, 385, 388, 389, 390, 439, 449, 455, 457, 563, 694

Winokur G: Alcoholism and depression. Substance and Alcohol Actions/Misuse 4:111–119, 1983. 302

Winokur G, Behar D, VanValkenburg C: Is a familial definition of depression both feasible and valid? Journal of Nervous and Mental Disease 166:764, 1978. 24

Winokur G, Black DW: Psychiatric and medical diagnoses as risk factors for mortality in psychiatric patients: a case-control study. American Journal of Psychiatry 144:208–211, 1987. 294

Winokur G, Black DW, Nasrallah A: Depressions secondary to other psychiatric disorders and medical illnesses. American Journal of Psychiatry 145:233–237, 1988. 294, 296, 302

Winokur G, Zimmerman M, Cadoret R: Cause the bible tells me so. Archives of General Psychiatry 45:683–684, 1988. 9

Winslow WW. 243, 245, 246, 247

Winston M. 300

Winston RA. 387

Wise CD. 415

Wittchen H-U. 656, 660, 664

Wittchen H-U: Epidemiology of panic attacks and panic disorders, in Panic and Phobias. Edited by Hand I, Wittchen H-U. Berlin, Springer-Verlag, 1986. 707

Wittchen H-U: Natural course and spontaneous remissions of untreated anxiety disorders: results of the Munich follow-up study, in Panic and Phobias: Treatments and Variables Affecting Course and Outcome. Edited by Hand I, Wittchen H-U. Berlin, Springer-Verlag, 1988, pp 5–17. 332, 333

Wittchen H-U, Burke JD, Semler G, Pfister H, von Cranach M, Zaudig M: Recall and dating of psychiatric symptoms: test-retest reliability of time-related symptom questions in a standardized psychiatric interview (CIDI/DIS). Archives of General Psychiatry 46:437–443, 1989. 660, 662, 664

Wittchen H-U, Semlar G: Reliability of the German DIS, Version 2. Final Report. Unpublished report (NIMH Internal Document). 661

Wittchen H-U, Semlar G, von Zerssen D: Comparing ICD diagnoses with DSM-III and RDC using the Diagnostic Interview Schedule (Version II). Archives of General Psychiatry 42:677–684, 1985. 661

Wittchen H-U, Teder W: Reliability of life-event assessments: test-retest reliability and fall-off effects of the Munich interview for life-events and conditions (MEL), submitted for publication. 664, 666

Woerner MG. 43, 675

Wohlfahrt S. 140

Wolf AW, Schubert DSP, Patterson MB, Grande TP, Brocco KJ, Pendleton L: Associations among major psychiatric diagnoses. Journal of Consulting and Clinical Psychology 56:292–294, 1988. 453

Wolfman MG. 572

Wolfstetter-Kausch H. 323

Wolpe J: Psychotherapy by Reciprocal Inhibition. Stanford, CA, Stanford University Press, 1958. 634

Wolpe J: The positive diagnosis of neurotic depression as an etiological category. Comprehensive Psychiatry 27:449–460, 1986. 605

Wolpe J, Lang PJ: A Fear Survey Schedule for use in behavior therapy. Behaviour Research and Therapy 2:27–30, 1964. 635

Wong PTP, Weiner B: When people ask "why" questions, and the heuristics of attributional search. Journal of Personality and Social Psychology 40:650–663, 1981. 515

Wood D, Othmer S, Reich T, Viesselman J, Rutt C: Primary and secondary affective disorder, I: past social history and current episodes in 92 depressed inpatients. Comprehensive Psychiatry 18:201–210, 1977. 296, 302

Woodbury MA. 159

Woodbury MA, Manton KG: A new procedure for analysis of medical classification. Methods of Information in Medicine 21:210–220, 1982. 159

Woodruff RA Jr. 8, 10, 24, 91, 114, 205, 254, 286, 294, 295, 296, 337, 439, 449, 455, 457, 602, 694

Woodruff RA Jr, Guze SB, Clayton PJ: Anxiety neurosis among psychiatric outpatients. Comprehensive Psychiatry 13:165–170, 1972. 291

Woodruff RA, Guze SB, Clayton PJ: Alcoholics who see a psychiatrist compared with those who do not. Quarterly Journal of Studies on Alcohol 34:1162–1171, 1973. 287

Woodruff RA, Guze SB, Clayton PJ, Carr D: Alcoholism and depression, in Alcoholism and Affective Disorders. Edited by Goodwin DN, Erickson CK. New York, Spectrum Publications, 1979. 289

Woodruff RA, Murphy GE, Herjanic N: The natural history of affective disorders, 1: symptoms of 72 patients at the time of index hospital admission. Journal of Psychiatric Research 5:255–263, 1967. 332

Woods, SW. 389, 390, 391, 392, 676

Woods SW, Charney DS, Loke J, Goodman WK, Redmond DE, Heninger GR: Ventilatory and anxiogenic response to carbon dioxide in healthy subjects and patients with panic anxiety before and after alprazolam treatment. Archives of General Psychiatry 43:900–909, 1986. 392

Woody GE. 292

Woolson RF. 173

Workman K. 300

Workman-Daniels KL. 302

World Health Organization: International Classification of Diseases, 8th Revision. Geneva, World Health Organization, 1969. 42

World Health Organization: International Classification of Diseases, 9th Revision. Geneva, World Health Organization, 1977. 17, 372, 653

World Health Organization: International Classification of Diseases: Clinical Modification, 9th Revision. Ann Arbor, MI, Edwards Brothers, 1978. 4

World Health Organization: 1987 Draft of ICD-10 Chapter V: Mental, Behavioral and Developmental Disorders (Clinical Descriptions and Diagnostic Guidelines). Geneva, World Health Organization, 1987. 140, 204

Wortman CB, Brehm JW: Responses to uncontrollable outcomes: an integration of reactance theory and the learned helplessness model, in Advances in Experimental Social Psychology, Vol 8. Edited by Berkowitz L. New York, Academic, 1975. 504, 521, 527

Wortman CB, Dintzer L: Is an attributional analysis of the learned helplessness phenomenon viable? A critique of the Abramson-Seligman-Teasdale reformulation. Journal of Abnormal Psychology 87:75–90, 1978. 516

Wu J. 577, 575

Yager J. 255

Yanaihara C. 420

Yanaihara N. 420

Yarmey D: The Psychology of Eyewitness Testimony. New York, Free Press, 1979. 710

Yates E. 273

Yates WR. 590, 594

Yayura-Tobias JA, Neziroglu FA: Related Disorders in Obsessive-compulsive Disorders: Pathogenesis, Diagnosis, Treatment. New York, Marcel Dekker, 1983, pp 105–122. 315

Ye W. 354, 355, 357

Yeh C-M. 406

Yelonek S. 392

Yeragani VK. 387

Yerevanian B. 47, 599, 603

Yerkes RM, Dodson JD: The relation of strength of stimulus to rapidity of habit formation. Journal of Comparative Neurology and Psychiatry 18:458–482, 1908. 570

Yeudall LT. 571, 574, 575

Yeudall LT, Schopflocher D, Sussman PS, Barabash W, Warnake LB, Gill D, Otto W, Howarth B, Termansen PG: Panic attack syndrome with and without agoraphobia: neuropsychological and evoked potential correlates, in Laterality and Psychopathology. Edited by Flor-Henry P, Gruzelier J. Amsterdam, Elsevier Science Publishers, 1983. 571, 575

Yingling K. 673

Yorgelun-Todd D. 255

Young EA. 387, 403, 427, 613

Young JZ: The Life of Vertebrates, 2nd Edition. New York, Oxford University Press, 1962. 413

Young WF Jr, Laws ER Jr, Sharbrough FW, Weinshilboum RM: Human monoamine oxidase. Archives of General Psychiatry 43:604–609, 1986. 394

Yozawitz A, Bruder G, Sutton S, Sharpe L, Gurland B, Fleiss J, Costa L:

Dichotic perception: evidence for right hemisphere dysfunction in affective psychosis. British Journal of Psychiatry 135:224–237, 1979. 572

Zahn TP. 276, 571, 572

Zahner GEP. 310, 563

Zahner GEP: Chronic stress pathways to psychological morbidity: social correlates of anxiety and depression in urban locales. Ph.D. dissertation, Yale University, New Haven, 1983. 154

Zanarini MC, Gunderson JG, Frankenburg FR: Axis I phenomenology of borderline personality disorder. Comprehensive Psychiatry 30:149–156, 1989. 326

Zapotoczky HG. 574

Zaudig M. 660, 662, 664

Zec RF. 570

Zegans L. 151

Zerifian E. 411

Zetin M. 575

Zettler-Segal M. 192

Zevon M, Tellegen A: The structure of mood change: an idiographic/nomothetic analysis. Journal of Personality and Social Psychology 43:111–122, 1982. 55

Zidek B. 574

Zimmerman M. 9, 331

Zimmerman M: Methodological issues in the assessment of life events: a review of issues and research. Clinical Psychology Review 3:339–370, 1983. 467, 468

Zimmerman M, Coryell W: Reliability of follow-up assessments of depressed inpatients. Archives of General Psychiatry 43:468–470, 1985. 489

Zimmerman M, Coryell W, Pfohl B: The validity of the dexamethasone suppression test as a marker for endogenous depression. Archives of General Psychiatry 43:347–355, 1986. 385, 386

Zimmerman MM, Coryell W, Pfohl B: Prognostic validity of the dexamethasone suppression test: results of a six-month prospective follow-up. American Journal of Psychiatry 144:212–214, 1987. 388

Zimmerman M, Pfohl B, Stangl D: Life events assessment of depressed patients: a comparison of self-report and interview formats. Journal of Human Stress 11:13–19, 1986. 468

Zisook S. 505

Zitrin CM. 43, 675

Zitrin CM, Klein DF, Woerner MG, Ross DC: Treatment of phobias, I: comparison of imipramine hydrochloride and placebo. Archives of General Psychiatry 40:125–138, 1983. 675

Zola-Morgan SM. 581, 582

Zrull JP. 362

Zuckerman DM, Prusoff BA, Weissman MM, Padian NS: Personality as a predictor of psychotherapy and pharmacotherapy outcome for depressed patients. Journal of Consulting and Clinical Psychology 48:730–735, 1980. 327

Zuckerman M, Lubin B: The Multiple Affect Adjective Checklist. San Diego, CA, Educational and Industrial Testing Service, 1965. 613, 614, 615, 630

Zumoff B. 255

Zung WW: A self-rating depression scale. Archives of General Psychiatry 12:63–70, 1965. 23, 613, 719

Zwart FM. 467, 468

Subject Index

Acetylcholine, 407, 417
Acoustic startle. *See* Startle response
Acquired immune deficiency syndrome
    (AIDS), 312, 382–384, 513, 541, 692
Addison's disease, 397
Adenylate cyclase, 432
Adinazolam, 425
Adjustment disorder with anxious mood,
    590, 594
Adjustment disorders with "mixed-
    emotional" features, 602
Admixtures. *See* Co-variation, anxiety/
    depression
Adolescents, 287, 322, 361
Adrenal cortex, 34, 416
Adrenal medulla, 416
Adrenocorticotropic hormone (ACTH),
    389, 397, 404, 409, 410, 416, 430
Affect
    positive, 55, 506, 565, 599
    negative, 55, 506, 508, 564
Affective disorder. *See* Depression; Mood
    disorder
"Affective equivalents," 604
Age neurosis, 142
Age of onset, 271–272, 341, 350, 365
Agoraphobia, 43, 94, 96, 98, 125–126, 342,
    367, 479, 502, 505, 523, 536, 586, 587
    and defense mechanisms, 558
    without history of panic, 106, 591
Agoraphobia comorbidities, 106
    depression, 218
    generalized anxiety, 128
    panic, 6, 128, 229, 383, 535
    simple phobia, 213
    social phobia, 213, 228
Alarm reaction, 416, 420
Alcohol abuse/dependence, 89, 193, 589
    antecedent psychopathology, 284, 295
    "biaxial" concept, 300
    "functional" view, 283

mania, 288
methodological issues, 287
prognosis, 286
relapse, 292
risk factors, 284
treatment, 291
Type 1, 461
Type 2, 285
withdrawal, 289, 290, 295, 386, 390
Alcohol dependence syndrome (ADS),
    300
Alcoholism, 142, 147, 171, 284, 449, 461,
    563, 713
Alcoholism comorbidities
    adjustment, 193
    agoraphobia, 291
    antisocial personality disorder (ASP),
    285, 286
    anxiety, 5, 120, 286, 291, 302, 360
    bipolar, 2, 288, 300
    depression, major, 119, 193, 200, 287,
    288, 299–301, 360, 451
    dramatic personality cluster, 197
    dysphoria, 6, 285, 286, 288
    generalized anxiety disorder, 291
    impulse control, 200
    irritability, 283, 286
    mental retardation, 172
    mood disorder, 5
    panic, 190, 291
    personality disorder, 172, 197, 302
    schizoaffective disorder, 300
    substance abuse disorder, other, 193,
    200
Alexithymia, 246
Algorithm, 160–163
Alpha-1-adrenergic receptor system, 389
Alpha-2-adrenergic receptor system, 389,
    390, 394, 432
Alprazolam, 399, 425, 586, 601, 602, 675,
    699, 703